T0401944

SpringerWienNewYork

Paul Kosma • Sven Müller-Loennies
Editors

Anticarbohydrate Antibodies

From Molecular Basis to Clinical Application

SpringerWienNewYork

Editors
Prof. Paul Kosma
Department of Chemistry
University of Natural Resources
and Life Sciences
Muthgasse 18
1190 Vienna
Austria
paul.kosma@boku.ac.at

PD Dr. Sven Müller-Loennies
Research Center Borstel
Leibniz-Center for Medicine and Biosciences
Parkallee 22
23845 Borstel
Germany
sml@fz-borstel.de

SpringerWienNewYork is a part of Springer Science+Business Media
springer.at

Typesetting: SPi, Pondicherry, India

Printed on acid-free and chlorine-free bleached paper
SPIN: 80063492

With 113 Figures

Library of Congress Control Number: 2011941770

ISBN 978-3-7091-0869-7 e-ISBN 978-3-7091-0870-3
DOI 10.1007/978-3-7091-0870-3
SpringerWienNewYork

Preface

Despite major scientific efforts over more than half a century infectious diseases and cancer remain important threats to human health. The increasing resistance against chemotherapeutics currently in medical use presents a new challenge to develop additional strategies for treatment of these diseases.

The unique carbohydrate signatures at the cell surface of infectious pathogens, bacteria, viruses, fungi and parasites, or aberrant cancer cells and their exposed location at the cell surface render carbohydrates ideal targets for vaccination and the development of therapeutic or diagnostic antibodies.

Recent advances in the identification, structural analysis and chemical synthesis of protective epitopes and an improved understanding of carbohydrate – protein interactions have paved the way for numerous efforts currently under way to exploit anticarbohydrate antibodies for the treatment of human infectious and non-infectious diseases such as cancer. Moreover, anticarbohydrate antibodies play an important role in xenotransplantation and may be used as diagnostic tools in inherited diseases. For the development of advanced diagnostics as well as therapies an in-depth understanding of the antigenic and immunogenic properties of carbohydrates is a prerequisite.

The book **Anticarbohydrate Antibodies – from molecular basis to clinical application** – provides an account of the current methodological approaches for the identification of carbohydrate epitopes in saccharides, glycopeptides and glycolipids, and their presentation and recognition by antibodies at atomic resolution.

Contributions written by experts in the field outline how anticarbohydrate antibodies may be used for the diagnosis of, e.g., inherited and infectious diseases and how novel vaccination strategies may be derived from this knowledge, including the reverse engineering of protective antibodies and the development of mimetic peptides. Thus, major carbohydrate epitopes from biomedically important pathogens such as *Bacillus anthracis, Vibrio cholerae, Shigella flexneri, Neisseria meningitidis,* group B *Streptococcus, Escherichia coli, Chlamydiae, Candida albicans,* and human immunodeficiency virus have been thoroughly defined. These studies have been aided by x-ray diffraction data, nuclear magnetic resonance spectroscopy, oligosaccharide synthesis and isolation of native glycan fragments, respectively, providing an insight into the immunological recognition of carbohydrates in general and a basis for rational-vaccine design including the options for fully synthetic vaccines in the future for a number of diseases.

A substantial part of the volume addresses antibody-dependent features of xenotransplantation, tumor biology and the prospects of carbohydrate-based tumor therapies, including strategies to enhance the inherently weak carbohydrate-protein binding interactions by peptide mimetics. In addition, increasing evidence of the importance of the peptide portion towards glycopeptide recognition and antigenicity has been demonstrated.

The controversial discussion on the impact of cross-reactive IgE antibodies directed against insect and plant *N*-glycans and their contribution to allergic responses has been summarized and extended with recent data on allergenic *O*-glycan and α-Gal epitopes.

The valuable application of well-defined epitopes and antibody specificity is reflected in chapters focused on diagnostic applications using modern glycoarray technology for detection and evaluation of tumor-associated antibodies as well as on specific diagnosis of mucolipidosis.

The book concludes with insightful coverage of relevant techniques to generate valid binding and structural data by surface plasmon resonance and NMR spectroscopy, supported by the increasing power of modern modeling approaches.

Long neglected due to the tremendous success of antibiotics and due to the particular immunological properties of carbohydrates, being T-cell independent antigens and often only weakly bound by antibodies, characteristics which have prevented their introduction into the clinics apart from a few successful examples so far, the recent launch of a large number of clinical trials and examples summarized in this book show that carbohydrates and anticarbohydrate antibodies are on the way to play a major role in future medicine.

Paul Kosma
Sven Müller-Loennies

Contents

Contributors

Mark Agostino Medicinal Chemistry and Drug Action, Monash Institute of Pharmaceutical Sciences, Monash University, Parkville, VIC 3052, Australia

Toshio Ariga Institute of Molecular Medicine and Genetics and Institute of Neuroscience, Medical College of Georgia, Georgia Health Science University, 11 20 15th Street, Augusta, USA

Ryan J. Blackler Department of Biochemistry and Microbiology, University of Victoria, Victoria, BC, Canada V8P 3P6

Ola Blixt Department of Cellular and Molecular Medicine, Copenhagen Center for Glycomics, University of Copenhagen, Blegdamsvej 3, DK-2200 Copenhagen, Denmark

Irene Boos Department of Cellular and Molecular Medicine, Copenhagen Center for Glycomics, University of Copenhagen, Blegdamsvej 3, DK-2200 Copenhagen, Denmark

Helmut Brade Research Center Borstel, Leibniz-Center for Medicine and Biosciences, Parkallee 22, D-23845 Borstel, Germany

Lore Brade Research Center Borstel, Leibniz-Center for Medicine and Biosciences, Parkallee 22, D-23845 Borstel, Germany

Thomas Braulke Department of Biochemistry, Children's Hospital, University Medical Center Hamburg-Eppendorf, Martinistr. 52; Bldg. N27, 20246 Hamburg, Germany

David R. Bundle Department of Chemistry, University of Alberta, Edmonton, AB, Canada, T6G 2G2

Javier F. Cañada Chemical and Physical Biology, CIB-CSIC, Ramiro de Maeztu 9, 28040 Madrid, Spain

Pierre Chassagne Institut Pasteur, Unité de Chimie des Biomolécules, 25-28 rue du Dr Roux, 75724 Paris Cedex 15, France; Université Paris Descartes 12 rue de l'Ecole de Médecine, 75006 Paris, France

Casey Costello Department of Chemistry, University of Alberta, Edmonton, AB, Canada, T6G 2G2

Muriel Delepierre Insitut Pasteur, Unité de Chimie des Biomolécules, 25–28 rue du Dr Roux, 75724 Paris Cedex 15, France; CNRS URA 2185, Institut Pasteur, 75015 Paris, France

Stephen V. Evans Department of Biochemistry and Microbiology, University of Victoria, Victoria, BC, Canada V8P 3P6

William Farrugia Centre for Immunology, Burnet Institute Melbourne, VIC 3004, Australia

Wolfgang Hemmer Floridsdorf Allergy Centre, Franz Jonas Platz 8/6, 1210 Vienna, Austria

James P. Hewitson Institute of Immunology and Infection Research, University of Edinburgh, West Mains Road, Edinburgh, EH9 3JT, UK

Tim Horlacher Department of Biomolecular Systems, Max-Planck Institute for Colloids and Interfaces, D-14476 Potsdam, Germany; Freie Universität Berlin, Arnimallee 22, 14195 Potsdam, Germany

Harold J. Jennings Institute for Biological Sciences, National Research Council of Canada, 100 Sussex Drive, Ottawa, ON, Canada K1A 0R6

Jesús Jiménez-Barbero Chemical and Physical Biology, CIB-CSIC, Ramiro de Maeztu 9, 28040 Madrid, Spain

Ann Marie Kieber-Emmons Department of Pathology, Winthrop P. Rockefeller Cancer Institute, University of Arkansas for Medical Sciences Little Rock, Little Rock, AR, USA

Thomas Kieber-Emmons Department of Pathology, Winthrop P. Rockefeller Cancer Institute, University of Arkansas for Medical Sciences Little Rock, Little Rock, AR, USA

Paul Kosma Department of Chemistry, University of Natural Resources and Life Sciences, A-1190 Vienna, Austria

Renate Kunert University of Natural Resources and Life Sciences, Muthgasse 18, 1190 Vienna, Austria

Horst Kunz Johannes Gutenberg-Universität Mainz, Institut für Organische Chemie, Duesbergweg 10–14, D-55128 Mainz, Germany

Tomasz Lipinski Department of Chemistry, University of Alberta, Edmonton, AB, Canada, T6G 2G2; Institute of Immunology and Experimental Therapy, Polish Academy of Sciences, ul. Rudolfa Weigla 12, 53–114 Wroclaw, Poland

Roger MacKenzie Institute for Biological Sciences, National Research Council Canada, 100 Sussex Drive, Ottawa, ON K1A OR6, Canada

Ulla Mandel Department of Cellular and Molecular Medicine, Copenhagen Center for Glycomics, University of Copenhagen, Blegdamsvej 3, DK-2200 Copenhagen, Denmark

Rick M. Maizels Institute of Immunology and Infection Research, University of Edinburgh, West Mains Road, Edinburgh, EH9 3JT, UK

Filipa Marcelo Chemical and Physical Biology, CIB-CSIC, Ramiro de Maeztu 9, 28040 Madrid, Spain

Behjatolah Monzavi-Karbassi Department of Pathology, Winthrop P. Rockefeller Cancer Institute, University of Arkansas for Medical Sciences Little Rock, Little Rock, AR, USA

Sven Müller-Loennies Research Center Borstel, Leibniz-Center for Medicine and Biosciences, Parkallee 22, D-23845 Borstel, Germany

Laurence A. Mulard Institut Pasteur, Unité de Chimie des Biomolécules, 25–28 rue du Dr Roux, 75724 Paris Cedex 15, France; Université Paris Descartes 12 rue de l'Ecole de Médecine, 75006 Paris, France

Ramachandran Murali Department of Biomedical Sciences, Cedars Sinai Medical Center, Los Angeles, CA, USA

Corwin Nycholat Department of Chemistry, University of Alberta, Edmonton, AB, Canada, T6G 2G2; The Scripps Research Institute, 10550 North Torrey Pines Road, MEM-L71, La Jolla, CA 92037 USA

Matthias A. Oberli Department of Biomolecular Systems, Max-Planck Institute for Colloids and Interfaces, D-14476 Potsdam, Germany; Freie Universität Berlin, Arnimallee 22, 14195 Berlin, Germany

Akashi Otaki Department of Biomedical Sciences, Cedars Sinai Medical Center, Los Angeles, CA, USA

Anastas Pashov Department of Pathology, Winthrop P. Rockefeller Cancer Institute, University of Arkansas for Medical Sciences Little Rock, Little Rock, AR, USA

Armelle Phalipon Institut Pasteur, Unité de Pathogénie Microbienne Moléculaire, 25–28 rue du Dr Roux, 75724 Paris Cedex 15, France; INSERM U786, Institut Pasteur, 75015 Paris, France

Sandra Pohl Department of Biochemistry, Children's Hospital, University Medical Center Hamburg-Eppendorf, Martinistr. 52; Bldg. N27, 20246 Hamburg, Germany

Paul A. Ramsland Centre for Immunology, Burnet Institute Melbourne, VIC 3004, Australia; Department of Surgery Austin Health, University of Melbourne, Heidelberg, VIC 3084, Australia; Department of Immunology, Monash University, Alfred Medical Research and Education Precinct, Melbourne, VIC 3004, Australia

Robert Rennie The Department of Laboratory Medicine & Pathology, University of Alberta Hospitals, Edmonton, AB, Canada, T6G 2G2

Somdutta Saha Department of Pathology, Winthrop P. Rockefeller Cancer Institute, University of Arkansas for Medical Sciences Little Rock, Little Rock, AR, USA

Mauro S. Sandrin Department of Surgery Austin Health, University of Melbourne, Heidelberg, VIC 3084, Australia

Andrew M. Scott Tumour Targeting Program, Ludwig Institute for Cancer Research Melbourne, VIC 3084, Australia

Peter H. Seeberger Department of Biomolecular Systems, Max-Planck Institute for Colloids and Interfaces, D-14476 Potsdam, Germany; Freie Universität Berlin, Arnimallee 22, 14195 Berlin, Germany

François-Xavier Theillet Insitut Pasteur, Unité de Chimie des Biomolécules, 25–28 rue du Dr Roux, 75724 Paris Cedex 15, France; CNRS URA 2185, Institut Pasteur, 75015 Paris, France; Leibniz-Institut für Molekulare Pharmakologie (FMP), Robert-Roessle-Strasse 10, 13125 Berlin, Germany

Seigo Usuki Institute of Molecular Medicine and Genetics and Institute of Neuroscience, Medical College of Georgia, Georgia Health Science University, 11 20 15th Street, Augusta, USA

Daniel B. Werz Institut für Organische und Biomolekulare Chemie der Georg-August-Universität Göttingen, Tammannstr. 2, D-37077 Göttingen, Germany

Ulrika Westerlind Gesellschaft zur Förderung der Analytischen Wissenschaften e.V, ISAS – Leibniz Institute for Analytical Sciences, Otto-Hahn-Str. 6b, D-44227 Dortmund, Germany

Robert J. Woods Complex Carbohydrate Research Center, University of Georgia, 315 Riverbend Road, Athens, GA 30602, USA; School of Chemistry, National University of Ireland at Galway, Galway, Ireland

Austin B. Yongye Complex Carbohydrate Research Center, University of Georgia, 315 Riverbend Road, Athens, GA 30602, USA; Torrey Pines Institute for Molecular Studies, 11350 SW Village Parkway, Port St. Lucie, FL 34987, USA

Robert K. Yu Institute of Molecular Medicine and Genetics and Institute of Neuroscience, Medical College of Georgia, Georgia Health Science University, 11 20 15th Street, Augusta, USA

Elizabeth Yuriev Medicinal Chemistry and Drug Action, Monash Institute of Pharmaceutical Sciences, Monash University, Parkville, VIC 3052, Australia

1 Multidisciplinary Approaches to Study O-Antigen: Antibody Recognition in Support of the Development of Synthetic Carbohydrate-Based Enteric Vaccines

François-Xavier Theillet, Pierre Chassagne, Muriel Delepierre, Armelle Phalipon, and Laurence A. Mulard

1.1 Introduction

Enteric infections, including bacterium-induced diarrhoeal diseases, represent a major health burden worldwide. In developed countries, infectious diarrhoea contributes primarily to morbidity. It remains the second leading cause of death in children below 5 years of age living in the developing world (Cheng et al. 2005; You et al. 2010). It is anticipated that improved living conditions will contribute to diminish the transmission of enteric pathogens and lower the incidence of enteric diseases. In the meantime, the introduction of vaccines could play an active part in

F.-X. Theillet
Insitut Pasteur, Unité de Chimie des Biomolécules, 25-28 rue du Dr Roux, 75724 Paris Cedex 15, France

CNRS URA 2185, Institut Pasteur, 75015 Paris, France

Leibniz-Institut für Molekulare Pharmakologie (FMP), Robert-Roessle-Strasse 10, 13125 Berlin, Germany

P. Chassagne • L.A. Mulard (✉)
Institut Pasteur, Unité de Chimie des Biomolécules, 25-28 rue du Dr Roux, 75724 Paris Cedex 15, France

Université Paris Descartes 12 rue de l'Ecole de Médecine, 75006 Paris, France
e-mail: laurence.mulard@pasteur.fr

M. Delepierre
Insitut Pasteur, Unité de Chimie des Biomolécules, 25-28 rue du Dr Roux, 75724 Paris Cedex 15, France

CNRS URA 2185, Institut Pasteur, 75015 Paris, France

A. Phalipon
Institut Pasteur, Unité de Pathogénie Microbienne Moléculaire, 25-28 rue du Dr Roux, 75724 Paris Cedex 15, France

INSERM U786, Institut Pasteur, 75015 Paris, France

P. Kosma and S. Müller-Loennies (eds.), *Anticarbohydrate Antibodies*,
DOI 10.1007/978-3-7091-0870-3_1, © Springer-Verlag/Wien 2012

reducing the vulnerability of the target populations to the predominant enteric pathogens. Along this line, *Shigella*, ETEC, cholera, and typhoid fever were identified by WHO since the early 1990s as the highest bacterial disease priorities for the development of new or improved enteric vaccines. Substantial progress was made (Levine 2006). In this context, polysaccharide-based parenteral vaccines have been investigated with some success. The licensure of the purified capsular Vi polysaccharide against typhoid fever was an important achievement, especially since recent evidence of herd protection conferred by the vaccine has highlighted the benefit of large-scale use in endemic countries (Khan et al. 2010). Moreover, encouraging investigational studies on a Vi polysaccharide–protein conjugate vaccine, which could be introduced into the infant immunization schedule, were reported (Canh et al. 2004; Cui et al. 2010).

Gram-negative bacteria lacking a capsular polysaccharide (CP) are the most frequent causes of the above mentioned enteric infections. Lipopolysaccharide (LPS), the most abundant component of their cell wall, is a major factor of virulence (Reeves 1995). This three component molecule (Fig. 1.1) comprises (1) the lipid A, anchored in the outer leaflet of the membrane, (2) the core, a short oligosaccharide (OS) showing limited structural diversity among members of a given species, and (3) the O-antigen (O-Ag), a polysaccharide built of repeating units (RUs), the diversity of which provides major determinants for classification into serogroups and serotypes (Raetz and Whitfield 2002). Evidence suggests that LPS, and in particular the O-Ag, is a dominant target of the host's protective immunity, and as such a strategic element in enterobacterial vaccine development (Nagy and Pal 2008). However, in contrast to CP antigens, the lipid A-mediated LPS toxicity precludes immunization with purified LPS. Masking toxicity by means of liposomal preparations has been attempted (Dijkstra et al. 1987). Thus far, protein conjugates of detoxified LPS (dLPS), issued from lipid A removal by mild acid hydrolysis, have emerged as a promising concept. It was hypothesized that O-Ag specific serum IgG antibodies (Abs) could confer protective immunity to diseases caused by homologous enterobacterial pathogens by inactivating the inoculum (Robbins et al. 1992, 1995). A number of such dLPS-based conjugates have evolved towards successful pre-clinical and clinical trials (Nagy and Pal 2008).

In the past decades however, the use of glycoconjugate immunogens derived from enterobacterial O-Ag fragments, as pioneered by Svenson and Lindberg (Svenson et al. 1979; Svenson and Lindberg 1981), has been the subject of intensive investigations. In line with the ground-breaking demonstration that disaccharides of synthetic origin could act as surrogates of the native *Streptococcus pneumoniae* type 3 CP (Goebel 1939), it was postulated that protein conjugates of well-defined synthetic OSs shorter than the native O-Ag might serve as potent immunogens able to elicit high titers of anti-O-Ag IgG Abs. In theory, OSs corresponding to the pertinent epitopes, anticipated to reach a maximum of 6–7 residues based on early work of Kabat and others (Kabat 1960; Mage and Kabat 1963), could be as immunogenic as the parent O-Ag following covalent linkage to an appropriate carrier. As successfully exemplified with QuimiHib® (Verez-Bencomo et al. 2004), the strategy may provide an answer to induce long-term immunity to

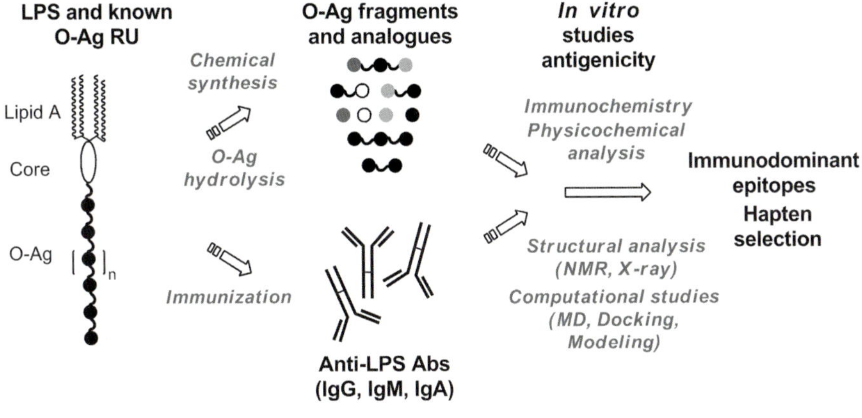

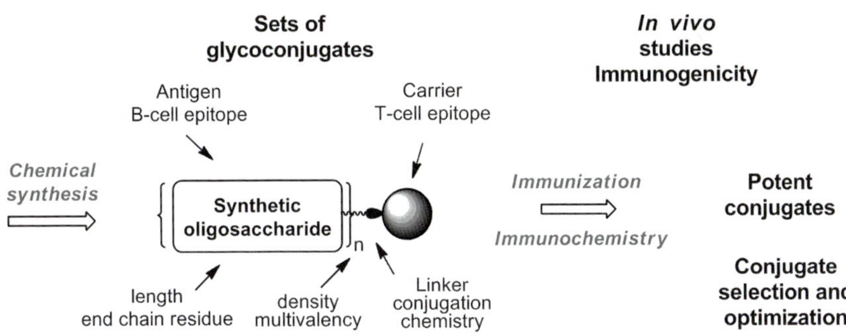

Fig. 1.1 LPS structure and general strategy towards synthetic OS-based vaccines. *Top*: Characterization of immunodominant epitopes. *Bottom*: Selection of promising glycoconjugate immunogens (RU, repeating units, *NMR* nuclear magnetic resonance, *X-ray* X-ray crystallography, *MD* molecular dynamics)

enterobacterial infections in a wide spectrum of individuals, including in the pediatric population at risk.

The synthetic OS-based conjugate approach offers several advantages over that involving dLPS. On one hand, product homogeneity ensures hapten integrity and facilitates reproducibility and analytical issues. On the other hand, risks and limitations associated to bacterial cell cultures, LPS extraction and absolute requirement for detoxification are avoided. Nevertheless, several parameters are thought to be critical for a successful approach (Fig. 1.1). Major ones include (1) the carrier, which brings in the required T-helper arm, (2) the composition and length of the OS hapten, and (3) the density of the hapten i.e. the molar OS:protein ratio, and mode of attachment of the former onto the carrier. Although those factors were shown to be interdependent to some extent, the choice of the OS hapten often serves as starting point. Detailed information on the Ab:LPS mode of recognition may aid in the identification of the appropriate carbohydrate components, which can then be turned into effective, protective immunogens. With recent technological advances in glycochemistry, major contributions towards new developments in the field of carbohydrate-based vaccines were thus often combined with molecular studies towards a deeper understanding of O-Ag:Ab recognition. The rational is that immunization with a hapten mimicking the natural target of protection, i.e. recognized by a set of protective Abs, could elicit sera with similar recognition and protection abilities.

This chapter will report on promising multidisciplinary approaches aimed at developing synthetic OS-based vaccines against diseases caused by selected enterobacterial pathogens including *Vibrio cholerae* O1, *Shigella dysenteriae* type 1 (SD1), and *Shigella flexneri* (SF). Whenever appropriate, most recent achievements in the field of dLPS conjugates and peptide mimics will also be highlighted.

1.2 *Vibrio cholerae*

1.2.1 LPSs as the Targets of Protection

V. cholerae is the causative agent of cholera, a highly contagious diarrhoeal disease, often occurring as devastating outbreaks (Sack et al. 2004). O-Ag composition allowed the classification of vibrios into some 200 serogroups (Chatterjee and Chaudhuri 2003), two of which – serogroup O1 and the emergent serogroup O139 – account for the vast majority of epidemic cholera. Recovery from disease confers serogroup-specific immunity against subsequent infections, and the presence of anti-*V. cholerae* LPS Abs is generally considered to be a marker for immunity to cholera (Provenzano et al. 2006). Two whole-cell vaccines are in use today, although their efficacy varies among recipients. In the search for an improved vaccine that would induce long-term immunity for those at risk, better defined immunogens could emerge from the use of glycoconjugates encompassing multiple copies of dLPS (Boutonnier et al. 2001; Paulovicova et al. 2006; Grandjean et al. 2009) or synthetic O-Ag fragments thereof (Chernyak et al. 2002; Kovac 2006; Wade et al. 2006).

V. cholerae O139 bears both a CP and a LPS. Interestingly, the O-Ag moiety of the LPS is made of a single RU, which is identical to that of the CP (Chatterjee and Chaudhuri 2003). Both dLPS and CP conjugates were shown to induce vibriocide IgG Abs in mice (Kossaczka et al. 2000; Boutonnier et al. 2001). Nevertheless, in the absence of any comprehensive molecular data on the protective epitopes – the smallest structural elements that fill a protective Ab binding site –, the most promising vaccine strategy against *V. cholerae* O139 infection remains to be identified.

In contrast, extensive studies have been performed on the more established *V. cholerae* serotype O1. As a general trend, pathogenic strains of *V. cholerae* O1 belong to two related serotypes, Ogawa and Inaba, which are equally prevalent in the field. The corresponding O-Ags both consist of 12–18 α-(1→2)-linked 4-amino-4,6-dideoxy-D-mannopyranose (D-perosamine), in which the amino group is acylated with 3-deoxy-L-*glycero*-tetronic acid (Fig. 1.2). Their structures differ by their terminal residue. The presence of an end-chain residue bearing a 2-*O*-methyl group

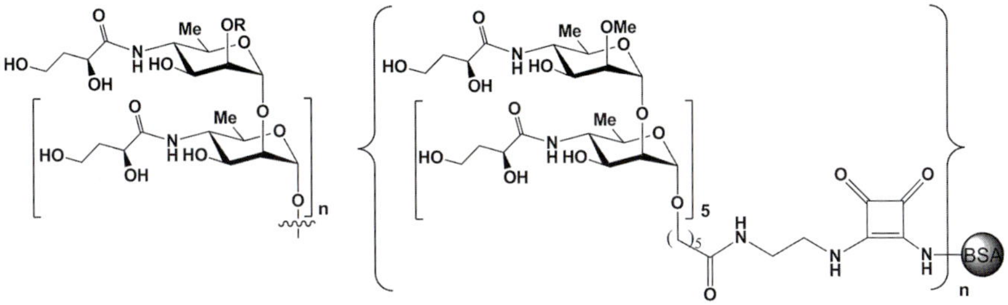

Fig. 1.2 *Left*: Structure of the O-Ags of *V. cholerae* serotypes Inaba (R = H) and Ogawa (R = Me). *Right*: Structure of an Ogawa hexasaccharide–bovine serum albumin (BSA) conjugate (Chernyak et al. 2002)

is characteristic of the Ogawa O-Ag, whereas a *N*-(3-deoxy-L-*glycero*-tetronyl)-D-perosamine is present at the nonreducing terminus of the Inaba O-Ag (Hisatsune et al. 1993; Chatterjee and Chaudhuri 2003). The two O-Ags were shown to have similar conformational behaviour (Gonzalez et al. 1999). Field experiments have demonstrated that a killed whole-cell Inaba vaccine protected against both serotypes. On the contrary, Ogawa vaccines protected against cholera caused by the homologous serotype only (Provenzano et al. 2006). Interestingly, sera resulting from immunization with either Ogawa or Inaba synthetic OS-conjugates could cross-react with both serotypes (Meeks et al. 2004; Saksena et al. 2005). However, Inaba synthetic OS-conjugates were less prone to induce a potent anti-LPS vibriocidal Ab response than their Ogawa counterparts (Meeks et al. 2004; Wade et al. 2006), although related dLPS conjugates were found efficient (Gupta et al. 1992; Grandjean et al. 2009). Put together, these data show the need to elicit a good immune response against the Inaba serotype, which probably calls for a better understanding of the different recognitions of Ogawa and Inaba O-Ags by protective Abs.

1.2.2 Immune Recognition of Ogawa and Inaba LPSs

1.2.2.1 On the Antigenic Determinants

Rabbit and mouse antisera allowed to distinguish three antigenic determinants (A, B, and C) present in Ogawa or Inaba LPSs. One of these determinants, i.e. motif A, is expressed substantially by both serotypes. In addition, Ogawa LPS displays the C epitope, but to a lesser extent than Inaba LPS, whereas the latter lacks the B epitope (Chatterjee and Chaudhuri 2006). Murine mAbs representative of the three classes of *V. cholerae* O1 dLPS-epitope specificity have been isolated (Gustafsson and Holme 1985; Sciortino et al. 1985; Adams et al. 1988; Ito and Yokota 1988; Bougoudogo et al. 1995; Iredell et al. 1998). This allowed localization of the A, B, and C epitopes, and in some cases, identification of their molecular structure, respectively.

Immunochemical Investigation Towards Ogawa and Inaba Common Antigenic Motifs

On the whole, immunoelectrophoresis and agglutination tests demonstrated that motif A occurs as multiple copies in the O-Ag (Gustafsson and Holme 1985; Iredell et al. 1998), which is consistent with epitopes defined by one or more intrachain residues.

Motif C is present as a single determinant recognized by mAb I-24-2, an IgG3 of low vibriocidal potency. Its exact localization was found ambiguous, despite two independent studies relying on LPS:I-24-2 ELISA inhibition, which led to convergent hypotheses. On one hand, the data issued from synthetic O-Ag fragments and core analogues indicated a partial specificity for the core (Wang et al. 1998; Villeneuve et al. 1999). On the other hand, experiments carried out with purified core and various dLPS fragments strongly suggested recognition of a motif sitting at the junction between the O-Ag component and the core moiety (Wang et al. 1998; Villeneuve et al. 1999). Despite the lack of any irrefutable validation, the latter hypothesis also agrees with additional data from the former study indicating moderate inhibition of LPS:mAb recognition by Inaba O-Ag monosaccharide. To resolve this ambiguity, the crystal structure of IgG1 F22-30, a mAb of related specificity (Grandjean et al. 2009), was solved at a 2.5 Å resolution (pdb code: 2UYL) (Ahmed et al. 2008). Attempted docking of various monosaccharides in the paratope predicted a preferred anchoring of the perosamine residue and its tetronic acid side chain in the putative binding pocket, displayed in what otherwise appeared as a rather shallow surface. Nevertheless, in the absence of any bound ligand in the crystal structure, information about the LPS:mAb recognition mode remains elusive (Ahmed et al. 2008).

Ogawa O-Ag Specificity Derived from Structural Analysis and Immunochemistry

Motif B was identified as the end-chain residue of the Ogawa O-Ag by fluorescence titration of two closely related murine vibriocidal mAbs (IgG1 S-20-4 and IgG1 A-20-6) with synthetic segments of *V. cholerae* O1 O-Ags, ranging from mono- to hexasaccharides. Interestingly, 90% of the maximal contribution to mAb binding resided in the single 2-*O*-methylated terminal monosaccharide, known to discriminate between the Ogawa and Inaba O-Ags. The hydrogen bonding network involved in O-Ag:mAb recognition was revealed using deoxy and deoxyfluoro analogues of the evoked residue (Wang et al. 1998; Liao et al. 2002). In particular, the contribution of the C-3 and C-2′ hydroxyl groups was set to light, while the crucial role played by the methoxy group was confirmed (Wang et al. 1998). Observations made in the course of the above mentioned study were subsequently supported by crystallographic data on the complex formed between Fab S-20-4 and the nonreducing end mono- and disaccharides of Ogawa O-Ag (Villeneuve et al. 2000, pdb codes: 1F4W, 1F4X, 1F4Y). A cavity defined by the CDRs L3, H1 and H3, ligates the terminal residue through six hydrogen bonds, and accommodates the Ogawa-specific 2-*O*-methyl group, in a somewhat flexible hydrophobic pocket (Fig. 1.3). The downstream residue is involved in only one hydrogen bond with the mAb paratope. Although the total buried surface at the Ab-disaccharide interface is

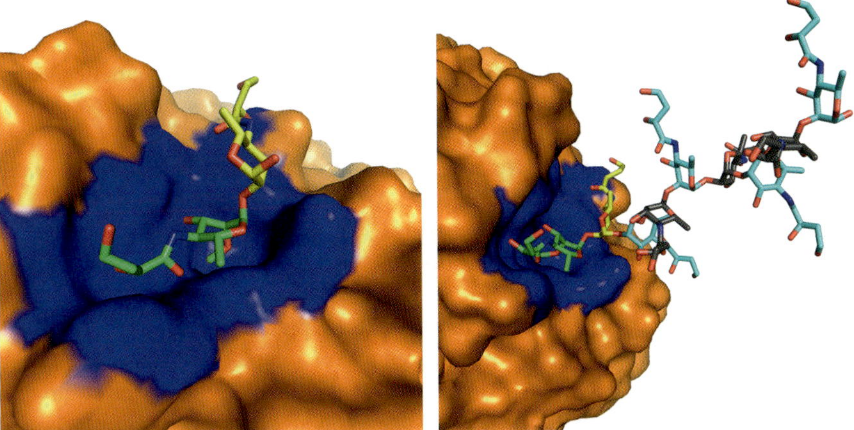

Fig. 1.3 Structure of Fab S-20-4 in complex with fragments of *V. cholerae* Ogawa O-Ag. *Left*: View of the interaction between S-20-4 and the synthetic non-reducing end disaccharide in the crystal structure of the complex (pdb code: 1F4Y). Contacting or buried Ab atoms are in deep blue. The terminal *O*-methylated residue and the inner O-Ag residue are represented with green and yellow carbons, respectively. *Right*: Model of the interaction between S-20-4 and an extended Ogawa-specific O-Ag segment, according to Alzari and collaborators (Villeneuve et al. 2000). For the sake of visibility, inner residues of the extension are alternatively represented with cyan and black carbons. The dihedral angles of the glycosidic linkages are set to the value adopted in the crystal

only 550 Å^2, the corresponding Ab binding constant equals to $1.2 \times 10^6\ M^{-1}$. Since ligand elongation does not increase affinity further, this showed that the O-Ag end-chain residue is a major antigenic determinant for the Ogawa serotype, obviously taking part in the B motif. The following model of the mAb S-20-4:Ogawa O-Ag complex was proposed: the polysaccharide in a linear extended conformation, matching the absence of O-Ag folding set to light by circular dichroism (Bystricky et al. 1998), was attached to the mAb paratope by its endchain disaccharide and protruded without any further contacts (Villeneuve et al. 2000).

1.2.2.2 On the Search for Potent Synthetic OS-Based Immunogens

Considering the potential antigenic and/or immunogenic cross-reactivity between Ogawa and Inaba serotypes, the design of a glycoconjugate vaccine against *V. cholerae* O1 infection can be challenged according to at least two strategies, focusing either on serotype-specific epitopes or on shared epitopes. With the information gained from the LPS:mAb recognition studies described above, both avenues of inquiry were pursued.

Vibrio cholerae O1 Serotype Ogawa

Knowledge of the minimal OS length required to induce a vibriocidal response is a major step forward in the development of a synthetic carbohydrate-based cholera vaccine. As demonstrated for at least three vibriocidal mAbs, two IgGs and an IgA, the Ogawa-specific antigenic determinant encompasses the O-Ag nonreducing terminus, and is fully exposed within the outermost disaccharide. Potent Ogawa glycoimmunogens were expected to be in reach, possibly by use of haptens as short as a disaccharide. Along this line, numerous protein conjugates of synthetic Ogawa O-Ag fragments ranging from mono- to hexasaccharides were synthesized (Kovac 2006) and evaluated for their immunogenicity in mice. Mono- to pentasaccharide conjugates were mostly ineffective at inducing vibriocidal sera, although they were immunogenic and even induced protective Abs in a few animals (Saksena et al. 2005). The hexasaccharide conjugates (Fig. 1.2), in contrast, were identified as potent immunogens able to induce vibriocidal Abs, whose potency was correlated to protection (Chernyak et al. 2002).

The discrepancy in the reported data cannot be explained by relying exclusively on the present knowledge of the fine specificity of interactions controlling mAb recognition of antigenic motif B. However, the use of different hapten-to-protein linkers seems to contribute towards an explanation since the mode of attachment was subsequently shown to influence the induction of vibriocidal Abs (Saksena et al. 2006). Additional complexity arose from the observation that, independently of the hapten length, several Ogawa OS conjugate-induced sera cross-reacted with Inaba LPS (Saksena et al. 2005). In spite of the fact that glycoconjugates derived from the end chain monosaccharide of the Ogawa O-Ag were likely to boost the immune response against Ogawa bacteria (Wade et al. 2006), these results question the immunodominance of the 2-*O*-methylated acylated perosamine in synthetic OS-based immunogens. Overall, available data for this system suggest the unreliability of isolated structural and/or antigenicity data on predicting protective efficacy, as measured by the vibriocidal activity of the immune sera.

Vibrio cholerae O1 Serotype Inaba

In the absence of any conclusive data on the nature of an immunodominant Inaba protective epitope, that is an epitope recognized by vibriocidal Abs, it was hypothesized that similarly with Abs specific for the Ogawa B epitope, Abs to the terminal residues of Inaba O-Ag would be protective. Accordingly, BSA-conjugates of Inaba di-, tetra- and hexasaccharides were synthesized (Kovac 2006), and shown to be immunogenic in mice (Meeks et al. 2004). However, in contrast to the Ogawa hexasaccharide immunogens (Chernyak et al. 2002), all Inaba synthetic OS conjugates failed to induce Abs, which were vibriocidal *in vitro* or protective in the infant mouse assay (Meeks et al. 2004). Changing BSA for rEPA confirmed the initial data (Wade et al. 2006). It was suggested that the induced Abs did not bind with enough affinity or specificity to Inaba LPS when expressed on the bacterial cell surface. Alternatively, these results also raised concerns on the protective nature of Inaba O-Ag terminal segments or on the conjugate delivery (Meeks et al. 2004; Wade et al. 2006), and promoted subsequent analyses on the mAb gene family usage in relation to protective capacity (Wade and Wade 2008).

Interestingly, original studies with hydrazine-treated Inaba LPS conjugates had demonstrated some potential, since the conjugates were shown to induce vibriocidal Abs against both Ogawa and Inaba serotypes in mice (Gupta et al. 1992), and even in human (Gupta et al. 1998). The latter study, however, called for further improvements since the vibriocidal activity was mostly correlated to the induction of IgM Abs. Along this line, chemically defined glycoconjugate immunogens prepared from acid-detoxified Inaba LPS were reinvestigated by taking advantage of the presence of a unique D-glucosamine core residue suitable for site-specific conjugation (Grandjean et al. 2009). The preserved integrity of the Ogawa/Inaba common motif C, which supposedly engages residues from both the core and the O-Ag (see above), was ascertained prior to any immunization. In support of the presumed role of this shared epitope as the target of functional Abs, the conjugate-elicited sera had similar vibriocidal activity for the homologous (Inaba) and heterologous (Ogawa) serotypes (Grandjean et al. 2009). Nevertheless, as with hydrazine-treated Inaba LPS conjugates, a deficiency in the switch from a T-independent to a T-dependent immune response was outlined. Considered as a whole, these unpredictable outcomes raise concerns on the intrinsic properties of the Inaba glycoimmunogens, and underscore the challenge faced in the development of an efficient bivalent *V. cholerae* O1 vaccine.

1.2.2.3 On the Quality of the Anti-LPS Ab Response

As a whole, the above results suggest that selected antigenicity data, possibly supported by X-ray analysis, may provide important knowledge of the minimal structural elements required for the design of efficient *V. cholerae* O1 glycoconjugate immunogens. In this perspective, delineating the exact molecular features of antigenic motifs C and A, as well as the protective capacity of Abs directed against the latter, may contribute to a better understanding of the available immunogenicity data and improve vaccine design. However, in the Ogawa context, data also underline that although informative and contributive to vaccine design, fine knowledge of the structural characteristics of LPS:Ab recognition may not be predictive of the immunogenic potency of the ensuing glycoconjugates. As stated in the introduction to this chapter, besides the carbohydrate hapten component and carrier, numerous factors govern the quality of the induced immune response and as such, require optimization. Investigations on additional parameters, such as the necessary presence of strong immunomodulators (Paulovicova et al. 2010), the importance of hapten density for triggering the activation of appropriate B-cell receptors (Paulovicova et al. 2006), or the input of the prime-boost strategy (Wade et al. 2006), would be useful.

1.3 *Shigella* the Causing Agent of Bacillary Dysentery

1.3.1 On the *Shigella* O-Ag Targets

1.3.1.1 Need for a Pediatric Vaccine Against Prevalent Serotypes

Shigellosis, also known as bacillary dysentery, stands as one of the big five diarrhoeal diseases. It represents a significant public health burden, which causes high morbidity and mortality, particularly in the 1 to 5-years old population living in low development index countries (Kotloff et al. 1999; Kosek et al. 2003). This mucosal infection, which occurs only in humans, is recognized as a major cause of malnutrition and impairs childhood development, in endemic areas (Petri et al. 2008; Moore et al. 2010). The infection originates through contacts with *Shigella*, a Gram-negative enteroinvasive bacterium. The species *Shigella* is divided into four groups, namely, *S. flexneri* (SF), *S. sonnei*, *S. dysenteriae* (SD) and *S. boydii*, which are subdivided into some 50 serotypes and subserotypes according to the structure of their O-Ag RU (Simmons and Romanowska 1987; Liu et al. 2008). Several serotypes trigger infection, and the prevalence of antibiotic-resistant strains is markedly on the rise (Kosek et al. 2010). Of utmost concern, SD1 sets off devastating epidemics, whereas *S. sonnei* and SF – most of the 15 known serotypes – account for endemic infections. While SF is prevalent in developing countries, *S. sonnei* causes occasional outbreaks in developed countries and tends to gain importance in emerging countries. Despite the persisting need for a vaccine and the breadth of candidate vaccines that have undergone and/or reached clinical trials, no convincing viable vaccine is available so far (Levine et al. 2007; Kweon 2008; Kaminski and Oaks 2009). Promising results have emerged, but important issues indicative of the difficulty in selecting an optimal strategy remain unanswered (Phalipon et al. 2008).

1.3.1.2 dLPS Conjugates as Advanced Investigational *Shigella* Vaccines

The strong indication that *Shigella* O-Ags are major targets of the host's humoral protective immune response against bacillary dysentery (Cohen et al. 1991) has been exploited advantageously (Levine et al. 2007; Kweon 2008; Kaminski and Oaks 2009). Prime investigations on dLPS conjugates capable of inducing anti-LPS IgG-mediated protection (Robbins et al. 1992) focused on the most prevalent serotypes, namely SD1, SF serotype 2a (SF2a), and *S. sonnei*. Candidate vaccines against SF2a and *S. sonnei* were shown to have excellent safety records and to be immunogenic in adults. Subsequently, immunogenicity in 1 to 4-year-old children, the age group at greatest risk for shigellosis, was also demonstrated (Passwell et al. 2003). Of particular merit is the finding that a *S. sonnei* conjugate provided protection in young adult volunteers (Cohen et al. 1997) and more importantly, in the 3 to 4 years old (Passwell et al. 2010). A further support to the concept resides in the evidence that anti-LPS Abs from individuals immunized with a *Shigella* conjugate vaccine have anti-invasive activity (Chowers et al. 2007). Interestingly, in line with the alternative discussed below, the most recent tendency is towards the search for neoglycoprotein type immunogens stemming from dLPS haptens encompassing 1 to 4 O-Ag RUs only (Robbins et al. 2009; Kubler-Kielb et al. 2010).

1.3.1.3 Towards Better Standardized *Shigella* Glycoconjugate Vaccines

In the search for well-defined *Shigella* conjugate vaccines, a molecular oriented approach involving synthetic O-Ag fragments was initiated in the 1980s. The most advanced studies paved the way to novel promising candidate vaccines against SD1 (Pozsgay et al. 2003) and SF2a infections (Mulard and Phalipon 2008). Extensive analysis of serotype-specific O-Ag:Ab recognition permitted the identification of immunodominant epitopes exposed on the O-Ags, prior to any immunogenicity study.

1.3.2 SD1: Knowledge and Hopes from Synthetic O-Ag Fragments

1.3.2.1 Molecular Modeling in Support to Immunochemistry to Uncover a SD1 Immunodominant Epitope

Investigation of the molecular recognition of SD1 O-Ag by murine mIgM 3707 E9 involved intact O-Ag, a linear polymer with a tetrasaccharide biological RU ($A^1B^1C^1D^1$, Fig. 1.4) (Dmitriev et al. 1976; Liu et al. 2008) and 26 synthetic mono- to octasaccharide fragments or analogues thereof (Pavliak et al. 1993). Affinity measurements using ligand-induced protein fluorescence change showed that mIgM 3707 E9 recognizes intrachain epitopes and that α-D-galactopyranose (C^1) is the only residue that exhibits detectable Ab binding by itself. Upon further analysis, it was found that the mAb displays fine specificity for the α-L-Rha*p*-(1→2)-α-D-Gal*p* sequence (B^1C^1), showing submillimolar affinity (Miller et al. 1998). Deoxy- and deoxyfluoro analogues of the latter further demonstrated that mIgM 3707 E9 recognition was mediated by hydrophobic interactions with the B^1 moiety in complement to strong hydrogen bonds involving all three C^1 hydroxyl groups (Coxon et al. 1997; Miller et al. 1998). Moreover, it was shown that extension of this immunodominant disaccharide by flanking residues did not influence binding significantly and that any concomitant decrease in affinity could be restored upon further elongation (Pavliak et al. 1993).

A similar pattern of recognition was reported for IgG 5338 H4 (Miller et al. 1996), produced by immunizing mice with a dLPS-tetanus toxoid conjugate. In contrast, none of the SD1 di- and trisaccharides significantly inhibited the binding of IgMs 5286 F2 and 5297 Cl, although both Abs showed fine specificity for the entire O-Ag RUs overlapping at the $B^1C^1D^1$ segment where D^1 is a *N*-acetyl-α-D-glucosamine residue (Miller et al. 1996). Moreover, inhibition studies that engaged additional mouse and rat mIgMs generated against LPS expressed in *E. coli* K-12/SD1 hybrids brought to light three closely related patterns of specificity. SD1 LPS: Ab recognition was inhibited by partially overlapping di- or trisaccharide segments of the RU, all of which comprised an α-D-galactopyranosyl and/or an α-L-rhamnopyranosyl residue (C^1 or B^1) (Falt and Lindberg 1994).

Fig. 1.4 Structure of the RU of the SD1 O-Ag: $A^1B^1C^1D^1$ (Dmitriev et al. 1976)

Investigations on the conformational properties of selected O-Ag sequences by use of NMR spectroscopy (Pozsgay et al. 1998; Coxon et al. 2000) and extensive molecular modeling computations (Nyholm et al. 2001) pointed to a peculiar behaviour of the α-D-Gal*p*-(1→3)-α-D-Glc*p*NAc (C^1-D^1) linkage, which adopts two favoured conformations. For pentasaccharide $A^1B^1C^1D^1A^{1\prime}$ and larger O-Ag fragments, a hairpin conformation predominates (Nyholm et al. 2001). Modeling of the $[A^1B^1C^1D^1]_4$ hexadecasaccharide in its "all hairpin" fixed conformation put forward a helix-type arrangement, whereby the D-galactopyranosyl residues protrude radially with some exposure of the adjacent L-rhamnose (B^1) and *N*-acetyl-D-glucosamine residues. The ensuing docking of the pentasaccharide hairpin conformer in the homology modeled mIgM 3703 E9 binding site was in full agreement with the binding data previously obtained for the modified B^1C^1 disaccharides (Miller et al. 1998). This set of immunochemical and modeling data strengthened the former NMR-based observations suggesting that pentasaccharide $A^1B^1C^1D^1A^{1\prime}$ is the shortest fragment that shows the conformational features of the natural O-Ag (Pozsgay et al. 1993). It was hypothesized that the preferred conformation adopted within this O-Ag segment is involved in Ab recognition and possibly also in inducing a strong anti-O-Ag Ab response (Nyholm et al. 2001).

1.3.2.2 Synthetic OS-Protein Conjugates are more Potent Immunogens than Their dLPS-Protein Counterparts

A major initiative towards the use of synthetic SD1 O-Ag fragments as optimized haptens in the design of original glycovaccines against the homologous infection emerged at the edge of the above summarized study on SD1 O-Ag:Ab recognition. The first outstanding report on the immunogenicity of synthetic SD1 carbohydrate–protein conjugates involved haptens ranging from 1 to 4 frame-shifted RUs, whose nonreducing end residue was B^1 (Pozsgay et al. 1999) (Fig. 1.5). The reasoning for hapten selection favoured the synthetic accessibility of the OS targets. Indeed, while a convergent strategy was designed to reach oligomers equipped with a spacer at their reducing end, the best outcome for building block condensation was anticipated to take place for the construction of the A^1-B^1 glycosidic linkage (Pozsgay et al. 2003). In support of the hypothesis stemming from the modeling data (see above), the tetrasaccharide–HSA conjugates did not evoke statistically significant levels of anti-LPS IgG Abs. In contrast, all conjugates of the di-, tri- and tetramers – 2, 3, and 4 RUs, respectively – elicited a better anti-LPS IgG Ab response than that achieved by a lattice type dLPS-HSA (Pozsgay et al. 1999). Moreover, the use of synthetic haptens demonstrated that OS length and OS density are two correlated variables that govern the immunogenicity of the conjugates. A subsequent study was performed in an attempt to define the role of the nonreducing end residues in dictating the immunogenicity of neoglycoproteins made up of short OSs (Pozsgay et al. 2007). Analysis of the anti-LPS IgG titers induced by conjugates, which comprised synthetic hexa- to tridecasaccharides differing by their nonreducing terminus and/or length, provided convincing evidence that the impact of the terminus could prevail over that of the length in this range of SD1 OS length, and therefore underscored a new variable prone to control neoglycoprotein immunogenicity.

Fig. 1.5 Potent synthetic OS-based conjugates against SD1 infection. *Bottom*: First generation showing a hexadecasaccharide hapten linked to human serum albumin (HSA) (Pozsgay et al. 1999). *Top*: Second generation showing a heptasaccharide hapten linked to BSA (Pozsgay et al. 2007)

In agreement with the Ab binding experiments (Pavliak et al. 1993; Falt and Lindberg 1994; Miller et al. 1996) and molecular modeling studies (Nyholm et al. 2001), conjugates with galactose-terminated haptens, among which a heptasaccharide (Fig. 1.5), were identified as potent immunogens (Pozsgay et al. 2007). The potency of haptens with a nonreducing D^1 terminus was also substantiated.

Interestingly, competitive inhibition of the hyperimmune anti-SD1 serum binding to homologous LPS by the same hexa- to tridecasaccharides suggested the absence of correlation between binding inhibition potency, structural characteristics, and immunogenicity for this range of SD1 OSs (Pozsgay et al. 2007). Without questioning the relevance of the former *in vitro* antigenicity data or modeling investigations, these new results outline the extreme complexity of understanding and possibly governing the parameters involved in immunogenicity and its *in vivo* context.

1.3.3 *S. flexneri*: A Fabulous System Thanks to O-Ag Large Antigenic Diversity but High Chemical Similarity

1.3.3.1 α-D-Glucosylation and *O*-Acetylation as Sources of Serotype and Serogroup Specificity

Interest in the structure and biology of SF O-Ags was already manifest in the 1960s (Simmons 1971) and has since remained very active. Over the years, numerous studies contributed to solve the antigenic determinants responsible for SF type and group factors and thus, to provide the molecular basis of serological specificity and

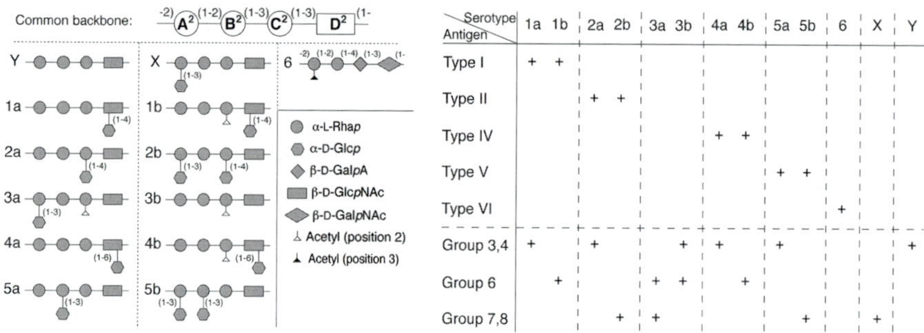

Antigen \ Serotype	1a	1b	2a	2b	3a	3b	4a	4b	5a	5b	6	X	Y
Type I	+	+											
Type II			+	+									
Type IV							+	+					
Type V									+	+			
Type VI											+		
Group 3,4	+		+			+	+		+				+
Group 6		+			+	+		+					
Group 7,8				+	+					+		+	

Fig. 1.6 Basic structures of the SF O-Ags accounting for distinct serotypes and subserotypes (Simmons and Romanowska 1987; Levine et al. 2007). The non stoichiometric *O*-acetylation patterns are not indicated

cross-reactivity (Simmons and Romanowska 1987). It is generally acknowledged that all SFs – except SF6 – O-Ags consist of a common backbone made of multiple 2-α-L-Rha*p*-(1→2)-α-L-Rha*p*-(1→3)-α-L-Rha*p*-(1→3)-β-D-Glc*p*NAc-1→ tetrasaccharide repeats ($A^2B^2C^2D^2$, Fig. 1.6), whose α-D-glucosylation (E^2) and/or *O*-acetylation at selected positions govern classification into serotypes and subtypes (Simmons and Romanowska 1987; Allison and Verma 2000).

As could be anticipated from their chemical structure, some O-Ags share basic type and/or group motifs, a feature which is indicative of serological cross-reactivity. Indeed, early studies demonstrated that polyclonal rabbit sera collected for diagnostic purposes could react with a large variety of SF LPSs (Ewing and Carpenter 1966; Carlin and Lindberg 1983). A subsequent report on MASF B, a mIgM isolated by immunizing BALB/c mice with SFY, the only SF strain that lacks O-Ag substitutions (Fig. 1.6), and shown to recognize all SF strains in addition to SD1, provided strong evidence of the presence of a group determinant common to all SF O-Ags. This peculiar epitope was thought to be as small as a disaccharide since MASF B bound to an α-L-Rha*p*-(1→2)-α-L-Rha*p*-BSA conjugate as well as to BSA conjugates encompassing larger OS haptens (Carlin and Lindberg 1987a). On a more general basis, group- or type-specific mAbs, whether of seric (IgM, IgG) or mucosal origin (sIgA), could be produced provided that an appropriate immunization and selection protocol was set up (Fukazawa et al. 1969; Carlin and Lindberg 1983, 1986c, 1987b; Carlin et al. 1986b; Hartman et al. 1996). Protective mAbs specific for the immunizing strain were also isolated (Phalipon et al. 1995, 2006).

1.3.3.2 Potential for Inducing Cross-Protective Abs: Insights Gained from Molecular Dynamics Simulations

The above observations are consistent with the fact that early reports on SF cross-protection, induced in patients having recovered from natural infection or volunteers immunized with one particular SF serotype, are scarce (Karnell et al. 1995; van de Verg et al. 1996). The topic remains understudied (Formal et al. 1966), although the absence of cross-reactivity between species has been documented (Mel et al. 1965; Formal et al. 1966, 1991; Rasolofo-Razanamparany et al. 2001). An interesting outcome of a recent clinical trial was the cross-protection against non-vaccine SF types found to be stimulated in 1 to 4 year-old children receiving a SF2a dLPS-rEPA conjugate (Passwell et al. 2010). Although the modest number of events impaired any statistical significance, this first hint on the ability of dLPS conjugates at inducing SF cross-protective sera in young children is a step forward to a conjugate vaccine, which would provide multiple serotype coverage in the targeted population by use of few LPSs. In a previous study, it was postulated that immunizing with type 2a, 3a and 6 SF O-Ags could protect against almost every SF serotypes (Noriega et al. 1999).

A recent report on the preferred conformations adopted by 12 SF O-Ags, as predicted by NMR-supported molecular dynamics simulations, revealed the fundamentals of the influence of stoichiometric backbone substitutions on O-Ag conformation and consequently, Ab recognition (Theillet et al. 2011b). It was found that except for SF1a and SF1b, a given serotype defining O-Ag backbone alteration, α-D-glucosylation and/or *O*-acetylation, does not induce new backbone conformations but only restrains the preexisting ones i.e. those reached for the glycosidic linkages in the SFY O-Ag. Hence, Abs against epitopes made of backbone residues arranged in shared favoured conformations, thus binding most SF O-Ag, are likely to exist. The identification of MASF B (Carlin and Lindberg 1987a) substantiated these predictions. Detailed calculations supported the original assumption that certain structural domains of the SF O-Ags would remain the same and accessible irrespective of the presence of substituents on the linear polysaccharide (Carlin and Lindberg 1983). The study further demonstrated that α-D-glucosylation or *O*-acetylation do not affect the backbone conformational behaviour beyond the nonreducing glycosidic linkage adjacent to the site of substitution and do not influence the impact of any other occurring backbone modification (Theillet et al. 2011b). Data also showed that individual O-Ag substitutions induce branching pattern-specific conformations, which occur steadily along the polysaccharide chain and to a lesser extent in the terminal RU. This observation called attention to the immunodominant contributions of the serotype-specific epitopes, which necessarily comprise more than three backbone residues. Alternatively, the data provided strong indications that broader cross-reactive Abs may be induced, although to a lesser extent, against epitopes located in unsubstituted backbone segments, which adopt favoured conformations shared amongst several SF O-Ags. Obviously, the study provides a conformation-based rational for the cross-protection occasionally observed following natural infection or immunization with experimental vaccines and encourages further efforts towards a carbohydrate-based broad coverage SF vaccine (Theillet et al. 2011b).

Although conformational analysis may come in support, recourse to chemically defined OSs representing restricted O-Ag segments is mandatory to map the fine specificity of Ab-binding to the natural polymer. Similarly with *V. cholerae* O1 and SD1, major contributions to current knowledge on SF O-Ag:Ab recognition involved large panels of synthetic serotype-specific OSs and analogues thereof, combined to a diversity of state-of-the-art techniques. The latter has evolved over the past three decades to include solved crystal structures of selected OS:Ab complexes.

1.3.3.3 Multidisciplinary Approaches to Identify SF5a Immunodominant Epitopes: On the α-D-Glc*p*-(1→3)-α-L-Rha*p* Branching Pattern

Investigation on the Seric Immune Response

The α-D-Glc*p*-(1→3)-α-L-Rha*p* branching pattern is the most frequently encountered antigenic factor in SF O-Ags (Figs. 1.6 and 1.7). When rhamnose A^2 is involved (E^2A^2), the O-Ags carry the group 7,8 factor as in SFX, SF2b, SF3a, and SF5b. Alternatively, if glucosylation occurs at residue B^2 (E^2B^2) as in SF5a and SF5b, the type V factor is expressed (Backinowsky et al. 1985; Simmons and Romanowska 1987). A study aimed at generating mAbs toward the antigenic determinants of SF variants X, Y, and 5b (Carlin et al. 1986a) showed that all SF5b-induced mAbs bound SF5b and SF5a O-Ags to the same extent, thereby exhibiting typical group V binding characteristics. Additional data also suggested that α-D-(1→3)-glucosylation at rhamnose A^2 did not interfere with binding (Carlin and Lindberg 1987b). Along the same lines, immunization with SFX strains generated Abs which reacted with SF3a O-Ag as well as with SFX O-Ag. While emphasizing the supremacy of the group 7,8 antigenic marker in this immunization context, the fact that some mAbs – but not all – could also bind SF2b and SF5b O-Ags indicated a broad range of fine specificity in the induced sera (Carlin et al. 1986a).

In another study (Clement et al. 2003), epitope mapping of IgG C20, a protective mAb generated against SF5a bacteria, used 20 synthetic mono- to pentasaccharides representative of frame-shifted SFY and/or SF5a O-Ag fragments. Inhibition ELISA against SF5a LPS showed that the E^2B^2 moiety was essential for recognition and that contributions from both the C^2 and $D^{2\prime}$ residues adjacent to the branched $A^2(E^2)B^2$ trisaccharide were required for binding in the submillimolar range. The binding of IgG C20 was highest for $D^{2\prime}A^2(E^2)B^2C^2$ (Fig. 1.7), which suggested recognition of an intra-chain epitope. NMR and molecular modeling indicating that among the four possible type-specific pentasaccharides, $D^{2\prime}A^2(E^2)B^2C^2$ was the sequence which best adopted the O-Ag conformation, strengthened the conclusions derived from the binding data.

Investigation on the Mucosal Immune Response: The Input of Secretory IgAs

Keeping in mind that a serotype-specific mucosal Ab response is induced by *Shigella* (Islam et al. 1995; Rasolofo-Razanamparany et al. 2001), the study described above was extended to two protective secretory IgAs, namely IgA C5 and IgA I3 (Clement et al. 2006). Using the same set of synthetic SF5a OSs, inhibition ELISA against the cognate LPS indicated a pattern of recognition closely resembling that of IgG C20. Once more, $D^{2\prime}A^2(E^2)B^2C^2$ was the sequence best recognized by the two mAbs. In both cases however, the measured IC_{50} for

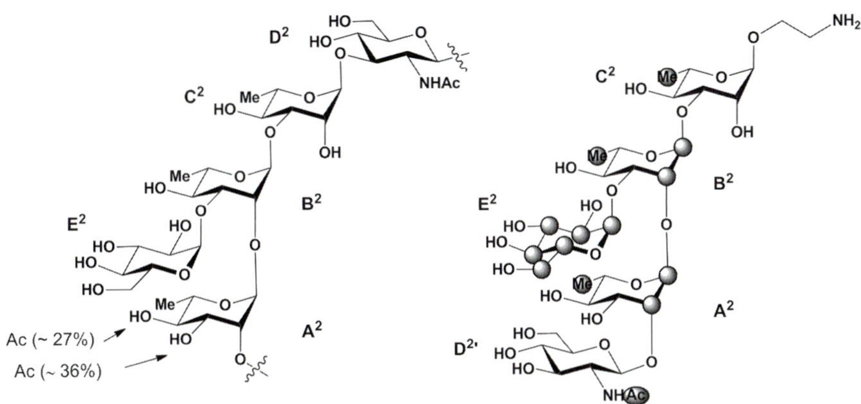

Fig. 1.7 *Left*: Structure of the RU of SF5a O-Ag ($A^2(E^2)B^2C^2D^2$), also showing the recently revealed *O*-acetylation pattern (Perepelov et al. 2010). *Right*: Frame-shifted pentasaccharide hapten – $D^{2\prime}A^2(E^2)B^2C^2$ – with highlights on alkyl protons interacting with IgA C5 and IgA I3, based on measured STD-NMR intensities (Clement et al. 2006). For the sake of visibility, alkyl proton contributions are reported on their bound carbons

$D^{2\prime}A^2(E)\,^2B^2C^2$ was close to 25 mM, strongly suggesting that the sIgAs recognized the O-Ag with a much lower affinity than IgG C20 ($IC_{50} \approx 40\ \mu M$) (Clement et al. 2003). In this range of affinity, trNOE- and STD-NMR experiments were used as the techniques of choice in addressing the fine specificity of O-Ag:Ab recognition, while avoiding the need for modified synthetic OSs. Whereas the former provided evidence that the bound conformation of $D^{2\prime}A^2(E^2)B^2C^2$ did not differ from that adopted when free in solution, the latter indicated that binding of $D^{2\prime}A^2(E^2)B^2C^2$ to the IgAs was mostly driven by glucose E^2 and that rhamnose B^2 played a major role. Moreover, all rhamnose methyl groups were shown to be in close contact with the Ab paratope, which denoted hydrophobic-mediated interactions (Fig. 1.7). In conformity with NMR data, the docking of the $B^{2\prime}C^{2\prime}D^{2\prime}A^2(E^2)B^2C^2D^2A^{2\prime\prime}$ nonasaccharide and a four RU O-Ag segment in the homology-modeled Fab I3 led to putative pictures of the O-Ag:Ab complex whereby the glucose E^2 served as an anchor (Clement et al. 2006). They also put forward the key contribution of chain elongation in governing the O-Ag binding mode. This independent observation fully corroborates the more recent assumption that SF mAbs selected for serotype specificity bind fragments large enough to exclude cross-reactivity, i.e. comprising more than three backbone residues (Theillet et al. 2011b).

Is Short OS Antigenicity Predictive of Their Immunogenicity?

In the absence of larger serotype-specific O-Ag fragments, these data converged to surmise that $D^{2\prime}A^2(E^2)B^2C^2$ (Fig. 1.7) is likely to induce SF5a O-Ag-specific Abs in the context of a conjugate vaccine. Selected conjugates were thus synthesized and their immunogenicity was evaluated in mice. The low IgG Ab titer against the SF5a O-Ag (A. Phalipon and L. Mulard, unpublished data) was suggestive of chain elongation playing a key role in this system as already hypothesized from the low binding affinity and the modeling data. These results also strengthen the idea that the identification of said "immunodominant protective epitopes" is only one step on the way to an OS-based vaccine, but that antigenicity data obtained for short O-Ag fragments may not necessarily warrant potent immunogenicity of the cognate conjugates.

1.3.3.4 Multidisciplinary Approaches Towards Potent SFY O-Ag Mimics

Combined Immunochemical, Physicochemical, Conformational and Structural Analysis to Identify SFY Immunodominant Epitopes

SFY displays the simplest of the SF O-Ags (Figs. 1.6 and 1.8). The polysaccharide expresses the group 3,4 antigen, which happens to be found on several other O-Ags (Carlin and Lindberg 1987a; Simmons and Romanowska 1987). Hence, OS haptens directing the immune response towards the corresponding epitope could pave the way to a broad serotype-coverage vaccine. Immunization of mice or rats with whole heat-killed SFY bacteria generated numerous mAbs, whose propensity to bind various O-Ag structural domains was probed by use of defined OSs and synthetic OS–BSA conjugates in addition to a variety of SF LPSs. Attempts to elucidate the exact nature of the epitope associated to group 3,4 were somewhat unsuccessful since the isolated anti-SFY mAbs showed diverse patterns of SF LPS specificity (Carlin et al. 1986a; Carlin and Lindberg 1987a). Mapping the combining site of five of those mAbs – the MASF Y1 to Y4 IgGs and the MASF Y5 IgM – with chemically defined OSs ranging from di- to dodecasaccharides, by use of the ELISA and Farr inhibition assays, suggested their classification into roughly two families, recognizing endchain or intrachain epitopes, respectively (Carlin et al. 1987b). In brief, MASF Y3 and Y4 bound a rather small combining site that adjusts to the O-Ag terminus. Further inspection by use of modified OSs demonstrated that the two Abs recognize different epitopes. On the other hand, the bindings of MASF Y1, Y2 and Y5 to SFY O-Ag were best inhibited by the $[C^2D^2A^2B^2]_3$ dodecasaccharide,

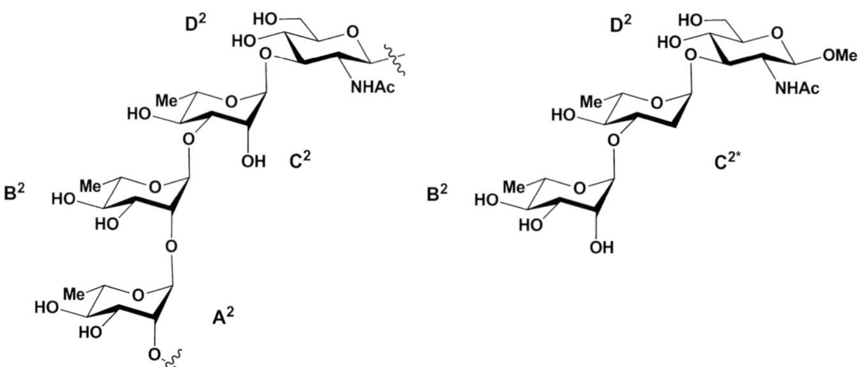

Fig. 1.8 *Left*: Structure of the RU of the SFY O-Ag ($A^2B^2C^2D^2$). *Right*: Structure of the $B^2C^{2*}D^2$ trisaccharide deoxygenated at position 2 of residue C^2 (Vyas et al. 2002)

although the minimal OS size necessary for inhibition varied from one Ab to another. Groove type combining site Abs recognizing intrachain antigenic determinants were hypothesized. In agreement with the observed differences in epitope size, LPS cross-reactivities were at variance. In particular, MASF Y2, which accommodates epitopes larger than an octasaccharide had a specificity restricted to SFY. Overall, in addition to emphasizing the contributions of well-characterized OSs in probing the fine specificity of O-Ag:Ab complementarity, these findings revealed the complexity of the SFY O-Ag antigenic repertoire (Carlin et al. 1987b). They also substantiated the more recent understanding that Abs recognizing large epitopes were more likely to discriminate between different serotypes (Theillet et al. 2011b).

Additional knowledge of the molecular recognition of the SFY O-Ag by homologous Abs was inferred from the mapping of the combining site of IgM GC-4 and IgG SYA/J6 by use of synthetic SFY OSs and analogues thereof. The affinity for the Abs was measured by EIA (Bundle 1989; Hanna and Bundle 1993). Both Abs showed similar trends with $B^2C^2D^2$ being the essential recognition element (Hanna and Bundle 1993). New insights from the crystallographic analysis of the SYA/J6 Fab domain, and its complexes with pentasaccharide $A^2B^2C^2D^2A^{2\prime}$ and trisaccharide $B^2C^{2*}D^2$ missing the 2_{C2}-OH (Fig. 1.8) were consistent with previous reports. In combination with titration microcalorimetry experiments involving SYA/J6 in interaction with the above mentioned pentasaccharide, $A^2B^2C^2D^2$, and a set of $B^2C^2D^2$ trisaccharides modified at specific sites, they revealed relatively weak hydrogen bonds to individual hydroxyls with the exception of the 4_{D2}-OH, as well as significant contributions from the acetamide, and more generally from van der Waals and nonpolar interactions (Vyas et al. 2002). In agreement with former studies (Hanna and Bundle 1993), deoxygenation at position 2_{C2} of the trisaccharide improved binding as a consequence of a better burying fit of the ligand and more favourable hydrophobic interactions than those involving the non deoxygenated pentasaccharide. Indeed, in contrast to $B_2C_2{*}D_2$, NMR and modeling studies of the O-Ag fragments in the free form (Bock et al. 1982; Kreis et al. 1997) suggested that $A^2B^2C^2D^2A^{2\prime}$ binding to SYA/J6 entailed changes in the pentasaccharide conformation, which essentially took place at the C^2-D^2 and D^2-$A^{2\prime}$ linkages. As a direct consequence, residue C^2 is completely buried into a deep pocket, and the partially solvent-exposed residue D^2 was evidenced as being crucial for recognition. Rhamnoses A^2 and $A^{2\prime}$ are the most exposed residues. They also contribute to binding through contacts at the edges of the combining site, albeit to a lesser extent. Overall, interaction with the $A^2B^2C^2D^2A^{2\prime}$ pentasaccharide ($K_a = 2.5 \times 10^5\ M^{-1}$) takes place in a large groove, approximately 25 Å long, 10 Å deep, and 12 Å wide. The groove runs parallel to the V_H–V_L interface and encompasses a deep pocket in the bottom. A plausible model of the bound O-Ag was built by elongating the pentasaccharide in both directions, using the crystal conformations for the glycosidic linkages that match the preferred conformation of the free SFY O-Ag (Kreis et al. 1997; Theillet et al. 2011b). As revealed from the portrayed $[A^2B^2C^2D^2]_3$ dodecamer:Ab complex, this model provided further indications that SYA/J6 is likely to recognize intrachain segments fitted into the combining site *via* the $A^2B^2C^2D^2A^{2\prime}$ epitope (Fig. 1.9) (Vyas et al. 2002).

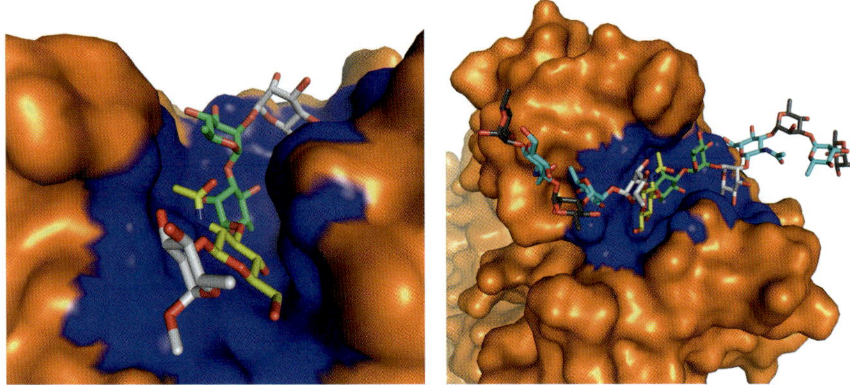

Fig. 1.9 Structure of Fab SYA/J6 in complex with fragments of the SFY O-Ag. *Right*: View of the interaction between SYA/J6 and pentasaccharide $A^2B^2C^2D^2A^{2\prime}$ in the crystal structure of the complex (pdb code: 1M7I). Contacting or buried atoms of the Ab are in deep blue. Residues B^2 and C^2 are represented with green carbons, residue D^2 with yellow carbons and residues A^2 and $A^{2\prime}$ with white carbons. *Left*: Model of the interaction of SYA/J6 with an O-Ag segment extended at both sides of the pentasaccharide (Vyas et al. 2002). For the sake of visibility, residues of the extension are alternatively represented with cyan and black carbons. This extension was built with dihedral angles set to the values adopted by the corresponding glycosidic linkages in the crystal

On the Search for Functional Mimics of SFY O-Ag

The knowledge gained on the SFY O-Ag:SYA/J6 system was subsequently exploited in the design of potent high affinity ligands. Two strategies were investigated. On one hand, intramolecular tethering paired with functional group replacement was employed in the design of analogues of $B^2C^2D^2$, which was shown to induce anti-LPS IgG Abs in mice when used as its BSA conjugate (Bundle et al. 2005). By pre-organizing the trisaccharide into its SYA/J6-bound conformation through the introduction of a β-alanyl linker between C-1_{B2} and the acetamide in D^2 (Fig. 1.10), a nice 15-fold increase in binding was observed (McGavin et al. 2005). However, contrary to expectations from crystallographic and thermodynamic data (Vyas et al. 2002), combining monochlorination or monodeoxygenation at 2_{C2} with tethering (Fig. 1.10) did not yield any substantial affinity enhancement. This result indicated the absence of strong additive free energy gains and suggested the need for a more detailed computational model (McGavin and Bundle 2005).

An alternative strategy focused on the identification of peptide mimotopes to replace OS haptens. Along this line, octapeptide MDWNMHAA was identified upon screening of phage-displayed libraries with SYA/J6. Interestingly, comparison of the peptide crystal structure in complex with the Fab fragment of SYA/J6 to that of $A^2B^2C^2D^2A^{2\prime}$ suggested that mimicry was functional rather than structural (Vyas et al. 2003; Borrelli et al. 2008). Unfortunately, the peptide was poorly immunogenic (Borrelli et al. 2008). In line with the above strategy dealing with constrained OSs, it was hypothesized that predisposition of Ab-bound epitopes in the free peptide would lead to a more rapid cross-reactive anti-PS response. Accordingly, taking advantage of the available structural and molecular modeling

Fig. 1.10 Structures of selected SFY O-Ag analogues. *Right*: Set of tethered $B^2C^2D^2$ trisaccharide analogues (McGavin et al. 2005). *Left*: Chimeric glycopeptide comprising the rhamnose trisaccharide $A^2B^2C^2$ α-linked to a MDW tripeptide aglycone (Hossany et al. 2009)

data, a chimeric glycopeptide whereby the NMHAA portion was replaced by the α-linked $A^2B^2C^2$, was designed to ensure appropriate fit of rhamnose C^2 in the deep pocket within the SYA/J6 combining site and prevent major entropic loss upon binding. However, competitive inhibition ELISA studies demonstrated that the chimeric glycopeptide did not inhibit SYA/J6 binding to SFY LPS (Hossany et al. 2009).

Altogether, the outcome of these various attempts provided additional evidences to the tremendous complexity of the network of parameters governing O-Ag functional mimicry. Despite notable progress emerging from structural and computational knowledge, there is still a long way to go in the search for a potent surrogate of SFY LPS.

1.3.3.5 Towards Potent SF2a Glycovaccines: The α-D-Glc*p*-(1→4)-α-L-Rha*p* Branching Pattern

Combined Immunochemical and Physicochemical Analysis to Identify SF2a Immunodominant Epitopes

SF2a remains the most prevalent SF serotype worldwide. Its O-Ag has the characteristic α-D-Glc*p*-(1→4)-α-L-Rha*p* (E^2C^2) branching pattern common with the SF2b O-Ag, resulting in a basic pentasaccharide RU ($A^2B^2(E^2)C^2D^2$, Fig. 1.11) (Simmons and Romanowska 1987). In a study dedicated to SF2a mAbs, upon i.p. immunization of mice with heat-killed SF2a bacteria, 15 hydridomas were obtained. None of the clones recognized the SF2b O-Ag and nine reacted exclusively with the

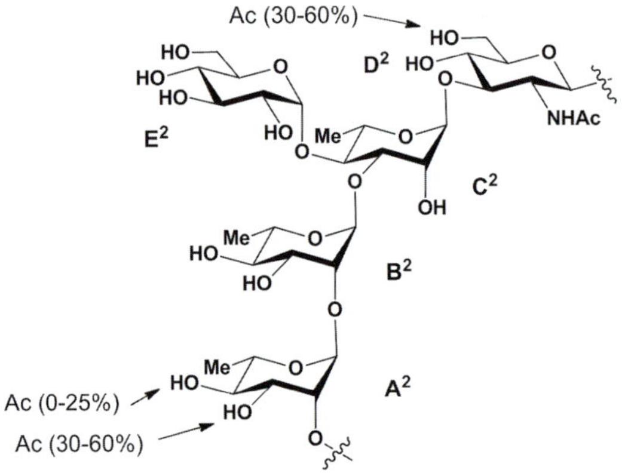

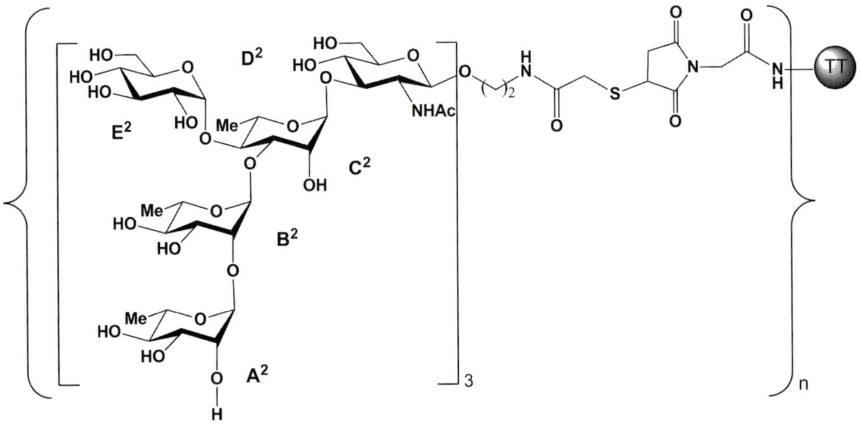

Fig. 1.11 *Top*: Structure of the basic RU of the SF2a O-Ag ($A^2B^2(E^2)C^2D^2$), also showing the recently disclosed *O*-acetylation pattern (Kubler-Kielb et al. 2007; Perepelov et al. 2009). *Bottom*: Structure of the first synthetic OS-based SF2a vaccine candidate (Phalipon et al. 2009)

SF2a O-Ag. This observation suggested a highly discrete specificity of recognition, which was confirmed following mice immunization with SF2b heat-killed bacteria (Carlin and Lindberg 1983). An independent analysis of the binding specificity of four mAbs generated following mucosal immunization of mice with SF2a virulent bacteria supported those findings. All Abs cross-reacted with LPS expressing the group 3,4 antigen, but none of them recognized the SF2ba LPS. Although the Abs showed a variety of antigenic specificities, this suggested that the response to the 3,4 group antigen was the most prevalent one (Hartman et al. 1996).

In a more recent study, appropriate combinations of the various strategies exemplified above were successfully adapted to characterize the recognition pattern of five mAbs representing all IgG subtypes. All five mAbs were shown to protect passively against SF2a in a murine model of pulmonary infection, mimicking the disease-induced inflammation (Phalipon et al. 2006). Analogously to the above described systems, mapping of the mIgG combining sites took advantage of a panel of 22 synthetic OSs representing frame-shifted di- to pentasaccharides and selected larger fragments occurring in the O-Ag (Phalipon et al. 2006, 2009; Mulard and Phalipon 2008). The finding that $E^2C^2D^2$ was the sole trisaccharide recognized at a submillimolar concentration and that larger OSs lacking the $E^2C^2D^2$ sequence did not show any binding whereas $E^2C^2D^2A^{2\prime}$ did, revealed the crucial contributions to Ab recognition of both the α-(1→4)-glucosyl residue (E^2) and the neighbouring *N*-acetylglucosamine (D^2). Monoclonal IgG F22-4, which was the only mAb showing measurable affinity for $E^2C^2D^2$, $E^2C^2D^2A^{2\prime}$, and $E^2C^2D^2A^{2\prime}B^{2\prime}$, exemplified a first category of Abs. Being at variance with the other four IgGs, this Ab V_H germline gene resembles that of SYA/J6, which is specific for SFY O-Ag (cf. Sect. 1.3.3.4) (Phalipon et al. 2006). Similar binding of F22-4 to the three ligands suggested a minor – if any – contribution of residues $A^{2\prime}$ and $B^{2\prime}$ to recognition. In contrast, addition of rhamnose B^2 improved the binding free energy ΔG by −2 kcal·mol^{-1}, on average. The key role of residue B^2 in Ab recognition was more general, since $B^2(E^2)C^2D^2$ was also recognized by IgG D15-7 and IgG E4-1. However, the minimal sequences necessary for recognition by IgG A2-1 and IgG C1-7 was the $B^2(E^2)C^2D^2$ tetrasaccharide flanked by residue $A^2/A^{2\prime}$ at either end (Phalipon et al. 2006). Analysis of the length-dependent OS:Ab recognition using larger OSs highlighted a favourable input of an endchain $D^{2\prime\prime}A^2$ moiety to all Ab bindings except F22-4 (Table 1.1), thus constricting Ab classification into two major families. Overall, the $B^2(E^2)C^2D^2$ fragment was seen as an immunodominant "protective" determinant, where OS elongation correlated with an increase in mAb binding. The major improvement in IC_{50}, observed when going from a one RU ligand to its dimer, was turned into a moderate or even absent positive contribution when the latter was elongated into the corresponding trimer (Table 1.1) (Phalipon et al. 2009). It is suggested that for all Abs, optimal O-Ag antigenic mimicry was reached within this range of OS length. Additional support to this assumption emerged from the appreciation that the recognition of O-Ag fragments by human sera from patients naturally infected with SF2a was either similar or increasing with the number of RUs in this range of OS length. This finding also demonstrated that O-Ag epitopes recognized by human sera are, to some extent, present in haptens corresponding to a small number of RUs (Phalipon et al. 2009).

Table 1.1 Recognition of the synthetic deca- and pentadecasaccharides ($[A^2B^2(E^2)C^2D^2]_2$ and $[A^2B^2(E^2)C^2D^2]_3$, respectively) by SF2a-specific protective mIgGs and comparison to available data for selected SF2a O-Ag fragments[a,b]

	IgG F22-4	IgG D15-7	IgG A2-1	IgG E4-1	IgG C1-7
$A^2B^2(E^2)C^2D^2$	21 ± 9	490 ± 100	378 ± 24	287 ± 66	734 ± 200
$B^2(E^2)C^2D^2A^{2\prime}B^{2\prime}(E^{2\prime})C^{2\prime}$	0.22 ± 0.02	60.8 ± 23	15 ± 5	12 ± 4	242 ± 124
$[D^2A^2B^2(E^2)C^2]_2$	5 ± 1.4	12 ± 3.6	3 ± 1.8	4 ± 1.7	19 ± 4
$[A^2B^2(E^2)C^2D^2]_2$	0.7 ± 0.6	38 ± 6	2.7 ± 0.3	17 ± 3	52 ± 21
$[A^2B^2(E^2)C^2D^2]_3$	0.32 ± 0.07	13 ± 2	14 ± 4	7 ± 4	21 ± 9

[a]Measurement of IC_{50} (μM) by inhibition ELISA. SD is indicated

[b]Extracted from those published (Phalipon et al. 2006, 2009), with corrections

On the Importance of OS Length for Ab Recognition: Input from Structural and Conformational Analysis

Crystallographic data were obtained for the complexes of Fab F22-4 bound to a SF2a synthetic deca- (pdb code: 3BZ4) and pentadecasaccharide (pdb code: 3C6S), corresponding to two and three biological RUs, respectively (Vulliez-Le Normand et al. 2008). Out of the 11 residues visible in the electron density map of the $[A^2B^2(E^2)C^2D^2]_3$ complex, ten corresponded to two consecutive RUs as in the decasaccharide. The binding modes of $[A^2B^2(E^2)C^2D^2]_2$ and $[A^2B^2(E^2)C^2D^2]_3$ to F22-4 were almost identical, showing a nonasaccharide epitope – $A^2B^2(E^2)$ $C^2D^2A^{2\prime}B^{2\prime}(E^{2\prime})C^{2\prime}$ – encompassing six residues in direct interaction with the Ab. The buried accessible area at the Ab-decasaccharide interface of 1,125 $Å^2$ does not totally contribute to the $9.6 \times 10^6\ M^{-1}$ affinity (Theillet et al. 2011a). Ligands are accommodated in a groove shaped binding site approximately 20 Å long, 8 Å deep, and 15 Å wide, which is defined by CDR-L1, H1 and H2 on its sides, and CDR-L3 and H3 on its floor. In agreement with the key role of $E^2C^2D^2$ in F22-4 recognition, narrowing of the groove at the center of the binding site generates a small cavity and a deep pocket, which are ideally suited to ligate the *N*-acetylglucosamine D^2 and the branched glucose E^2, respectively (Fig. 1.12). Consistent with the need for at least two consecutive RUs to reach optimal Ab recognition, both the branched glucose $E^{2\prime}$ and rhamnose C^2 make intermediate contacts. Residues A^2, $A^{2\prime}$ and $B^{2\prime}$ also contribute, albeit to a lesser extent. Interestingly, the bound conformation of the $B^2C^2D^2$ segment in the SF2a ligands is similar to that of the same trisaccharide in

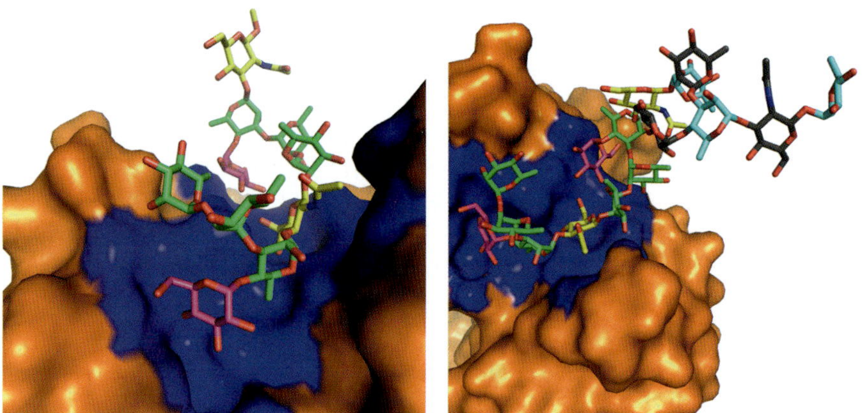

Fig. 1.12 Structure of Fab F22-4 in complex with fragments of the SF2a O-Ag. *Right*: View of the interaction between F22-4 and decasaccharide $[A^2B^2(E^2)C^2D^2]_2$ in the crystal structure of the complex (pdb code: 3BZ4). Contacting or buried atoms of the Ab are in deep blue. Residues A^2, B^2, and C^2 are represented with green carbons, residues D^2 with yellow carbons and residues E^2 with magenta carbons. *Left*: Model of the interaction of F22-4 with an O-Ag segment extended at the nonreducing side of the decasaccharide (Vulliez-Le Normand et al. 2008). This extension was built with dihedral angles set to the values adopted by the corresponding glycosidic linkages in the crystal. For the sake of visibility, residues of the extension are alternatively represented with cyan and black carbons

the SYA/J6:$A^2B^2C^2D^2A^{2\prime}$ complex (Vyas et al. 2002). Similar backbone dihedral angles characterize the two RUs in the F22-4:OS complexes. However, the E^2C^2 and $E^{2\prime}C^{2\prime}$ dihedral angles differ widely from each other, with the former linkage adopting a high energy non-exoanomeric (*anti*, *anti*) conformation (Vulliez-Le Normand et al. 2008). This conformation was also seen in the free form albeit to a much lesser extent than the normal exoanomeric conformation (Theillet et al. 2011b). A more recent investigation on F22-4 in complex with tri- to hexasaccharides, using STD-NMR combined with MD simulations in explicit solvent, indicated that interaction was mediated by constant tight binding of $E^2C^2D^2$ to the mAb *via* persistent hydrogen bonds forcing the trisaccharide segment in the conformation seen in the co-crystal, whereas residues A^2, B^2, $A^{2\prime}$, $B^{2\prime}$ and $D^{2\prime\prime}$ show a higher degree of flexibility and do not strongly interact with the Ab (Theillet et al. 2011a). Corroborating with information generated by antigenicity and crystallographic data, STD-NMR analysis of F22-4 ligand recognition also provided strong indications that in contrast to SYA/J6, F22-4 is likely to recognize both intrachain and endchain epitopes on the SF2a O-Ag, with a preference for the upstream O-Ag terminus (Theillet et al. 2011a).

On a more general basis, NMR investigation of the conformational behaviour of synthetic SF2a O-Ag fragments in solution suggested a similar environment for 11 of the 13 internal residues within the $[A^2B^2(E^2)C^2D^2]_3$ pentadecasaccharide and the corresponding constituents in the de-*O*-acetylated SF2a O-Ag (Theillet et al. 2011b). Besides providing a possible explanation for the slight increase in Ab recognition of the pentadecasaccharide over the decasaccharide segment, this observation ascertained that conformational O-Ag mimicry by synthetic OSs was feasible, provided that the OSs comprised at least three RUs.

Knowledge Gained from Immunological Studies: En Route Towards a Clinical Trial for the First SF2a Synthetic OS-Based Vaccine Candidate

To better understand the relationship between antigenicity and immunogenicity, haptens of potential interest to the design of synthetic SF2a OS-based immunogens emerged from the available antigenicity data. The reasoning favored the hapten composition rather than the synthetic access. Ranging from the $E^2C^2D^2$ trisaccharide to the $[A^2B^2(E^2)C^2D^2]_3$ pentadecasaccharide, the selected haptens differed in terms of OS length and endchain residue (Phalipon et al. 2006). All the corresponding conjugates, except one, were immunogenic in mice even though they were administered in the absence of an adjuvant. Interestingly, only the conjugates that contained haptens corresponding to two or three O-Ag RUs, respectively, induced a significant anti-LPS IgG Ab response (Phalipon et al. 2006). Similar to SD1, Ab titers increased with the number of RUs per hapten and correlated to hapten density for a given OS length (Phalipon et al. 2009). The three RU hapten also showed promising immunogenicity when presented as B,T-bi-epitope liposomal constructs. The latter were proposed as alternatives to the conventional neoglycoprotein immunogens (Said Hassane et al. 2009). Independently of the nature of the immunogen, the induced sera demonstrated protective capacity, underlining the potency of the pentadecasaccharide hapten (Phalipon et al. 2009). Moreover, analysis of the recognition profile of the sera induced in mice by a pentadecasaccharide-tetanus toxoid conjugate (Fig. 1.11) provided outstanding evidence that the conjugate mimicked LPS presentation at the bacterial surface and that the immune response was highly specific for the SF2a O-Ag (Phalipon et al. 2009).

On one hand, NMR and crystallographic data suggested that the synthetic $[A^2B^2(E^2)C^2D^2]_3$ pentadecasaccharide is both a structural and conformational mimic of the natural O-Ag. On the other hand, physicochemical, immunochemical and *in vivo* data converged towards the identification of $[A^2B^2(E^2)C^2D^2]_3$ as an antigenic and potent immunogenic mimic of that same O-Ag moiety, when associated to an appropriate carrier containing the required T-helper arm. However, immunity to carbohydrate antigens is species-specific, and in the absence of any relevant animal model of shigellosis, promising data in mice are not necessarily predictive of efficiency in humans. In this context, all data converge to the conclusion that probing the efficacy in human of a selected SF2a synthetic pentadecasaccharide-based conjugate was mandatory.

Encouraging data emerged in the course of a phase III clinical trial. Although an insufficient number of episodes prevented any conclusive statement on efficacy, SF2a dLPS–protein conjugates were found to be safe and immunogenic in humans, including in 1 to 4 year old children (Passwell et al. 2010). Moreover, measurable protection against homologous infection was demonstrated in children above 3 years of age that received a *S. sonnei* dLPS–protein conjugate vaccine. Efficacy was age-dependent, suggesting the need for improvement (Passwell et al. 2010).

Future Prospects: The SF2a O-Ag is *O*-Acetylated

O-Acetylation is another important issue in the field of glycoconjugate vaccines, whether in regards to tailoring synthetic OS-based conjugates of optimal immunogenicity or ensuring consistency of the final vaccine formulations (Szu et al. 1991). SF2a O-Ag *O*-acetylation had been noted (Simmons and Romanowska 1987), but the *O*-acetylation in a non stoichiometric fashion at two positions of the RU was only recently disclosed (Kubler-Kielb et al. 2007). Thereafter, the non stoichiometric *O*-acetylation of the SF1a, SF1b and SF5a O-Ags was documented (Perepelov et al. 2009, 2010). Similarities in the *O*-acetylation pattern at rhamnose A^2 of these four SF O-Ags were obvious (Kubler-Kielb et al. 2007; Perepelov et al. 2009, 2010), suggesting a potential site for Ab cross-reactivity. Interestingly, the same reasoning was proposed to explain the cross-protection towards SF6, observed in the field following young children immunization with a SF2a dLPS-protein investigational vaccine (Passwell et al. 2010). Moreover, concomitant removal of the LPS *O*-acetyl groups and ester bound fatty acids resulted in the partial loss of antigenicity (Kubler-Kielb et al. 2007), suggesting the need for a better understanding of the contribution of *O*-acetylation on antigenicity, immunogenicity, and cross-protection. In an attempt to investigate further, a set of three decasaccharides made of two consecutive biological RUs, either mono- or di-*O*-acetylated at the required positions (Fig. 1.11), were synthesized (Mulard and Gauthier 2010) to complement the already available synthetic $[A^2B^2(E^2)C^2D^2]_2$ decasaccharide (Belot et al. 2005).

1.3.3.6 On the Road Towards a SF Glycovaccine in the Context of Multivalency

As already stated, the number and highly variable geographical distribution of SF serotypes causing shigellosis may hamper the development of a broadly efficient vaccine (Levine et al. 2007). Based on type and group antigenic determinants (Fig. 1.6), SF3a, which also predominates in several countries, is an attractive serotype to include in a broad serotype coverage vaccine comprised of a limited number of serotypes. In this context, it was included as a major component of several cocktail vaccine candidates (Levine et al. 2007). In particular, a bivalent attenuated construct combining SF3a and SF2a provided a high level of cross-protection among other SF serotypes (Noriega et al. 1999). In line with the above mentioned studies, investigations on the immunodominant epitopes on SF3a O-Ag was initiated recently (Boutet and Mulard 2008; Boutet et al. 2009).

Another serotype of interest is SF6, the only serotype whose O-Ag is not built from the $A^2B^2C^2D^2$ tetrasaccharide backbone (Fig. 1.6). Like SF3a, the development of a vaccine against SF6 has been tackled along two lines, including as a monovalent dLPS-based immunogen. The later study exemplifies a recent tendency towards the search for neoglycoprotein type immunogens stemming from low molecular weight dLPS haptens, also known as core–OS haptens, as initiated for *S. sonnei* (Robbins et al. 2009; Kubler-Kielb et al. 2010), and subsequently adapted to SD1, SF2a and SF6 (Robbins et al. 2009; Kubler-Kielb et al. 2010). Similarly with the other *Shigella* strains, the potential of this strategy was demonstrated for SF6. In line with previous observations, the immunogenicity of the SF6 core–OS conjugates did not necessarily match their antigenicity, but was obviously dependent on the number of O-Ag RUs within the core–OS haptens. A BSA-conjugate made of haptens comprising an average of seven O-Ag RUs induced anti-LPS Ab levels similar to that generated by the conventional dLPS conjugate in mice (Robbins et al. 2009; Kubler-Kielb et al. 2010).

This novel strategy combines the expertise gained on lattice-type dLPS-based conjugates with the more recent understanding that glycoconjugate immunogens, made of short synthetic haptens of defined lengths bound at single site to the protein carrier, may contribute significantly in enhancing the anti-LPS Ab response (Pozsgay et al. 1999). As such, this attractive alternative to existing methodologies may find wide applications especially when synthetic haptens are not easily accessible due to O-Ag chemical complexity. In the context of further developments, the characterization at the molecular level of the epitopes recognized by this new generation of dLPS conjugate vaccines may help additional tailoring of the constructs towards improved immunogenicity. The above detailed successful interdisciplinary approaches may be extended towards this aim.

1.3.4 Conclusion and Perspectives: OS-Based Enteric Vaccines: Dream or Reality?

Polysaccharide vaccines have found widespread use in preventing infections caused by capsulated bacteria either in the form of purified polysaccharides or conjugates thereof. Its proven track record has encouraged broader developments to include conjugate vaccine candidates based on dLPSs instead of capsular polysaccharides. Some dLPS-based conjugates have been shown to be safe and immunogenic in healthy volunteers including young children. With regards to enteric infections, the protective efficacy of a *S. sonnei* vaccine candidate has been demonstrated.

Complying with the quality control and safety standards requested by the Health Authorities is a complex challenge, especially if using dLPS antigens of natural source. However, as illustrated in this chapter, recent advances in glycochemistry have paved the way to promising well-characterized conjugates derived from synthetic OS haptens, acting as functional mimics of the natural polysaccharide antigen. Towards this aim, numerous structural, theroretical, physicochemical and/or immunochemical investigations on the recognition of synthetic OS by protective mAbs have revealed key immunodominant components of several O-Ags of interest. As a whole, available data suggest that the identification of such epitopes, by use of complementary multidisciplinary approaches, streamlines the efficient design of experimental conjugate vaccines encompassing synthetic LPS components. They also underline that the numerous factors that govern the quality of the induced immune response prevented simple translation of antigenicity data into optimal immunogenicity. However, they also demonstrate that part of these limitations may be overcome by taking into account the information derived from structural, conformational and physicochemical analysis.

In contrast to a recent report on *S. pneumoniae* 14, which suggests that a synthetic frame-shifted RU of the CP may be a serious candidate for a conjugate vaccine against homologous infections (Safari et al. 2008), the general trend highlighted in this chapter confirms former findings with *Salmonella* (Lindberg et al. 1983). Thus, conjugates of synthetic OSs composed of at least two RUs – more advantageously three and six RUs in the case of hetero- and homopolysaccharides, respectively – were identified as efficient immunogens in mice.

The data in this chapter show that converting synthetic O-Ag fragments into immunogens able to achieve a potent Ab-mediated, broadly protective, immunity and a long-lasting memory response in all target populations remains a significant challenge. As for other novel vaccine strategies, the present developments urge for a proof-of-concept in humans.

Particularly for *Shigella*, the considerable diversity amongst the pathogenic species and the possible emergence of new serotypes (Ye et al. 2010) introduce a new layer of complexity to the concern. A dominant issue deals with the capacity to design easy-to-manufacture standardized conjugates, which combine the strongest possible immunogenicity and the highest crossprotective ability with the mandatory accessibility to the poorest populations.

Acknowledgments We wish to thank all the former and present collaborators who participated in our own *V. cholerae* and *Shigella* LPS-based vaccine programs. We warmly thank Prof. Philippe J. Sansonetti for his unfailing support and Dr. Marie-Aline Bloch for her trust in the SF2a project. L.M. is extremely grateful to Dr. Cornelis P.J. Glaudemans, Dr. Paul Kovac, Dr. John B. Robbins and Dr. Rachel Schneerson for their valuable role in instigating her interest for the field of synthetic OS-based vaccines.

Besides support from the Institut Pasteur, our work has been funded by the following agencies and fundations: NIH (to L.M.), Ministère Français de la Recherche, DGA, FRM, CANAM, KOSEF, ANR, Ms Frank Howard fellowship, Roux fellowship, Vasant & Kusum Joshi fellowship.

References

Adams LB, Henk MC, Siebeling RJ (1988) Detection of *Vibrio-cholerae* with monoclonal-antibodies specific for serovar-O1 lipopolysaccharide. J Clin Microbiol 26:1801–1809

Ahmed F, Andre-Leroux G, Haouz A, Boutonnier A, Delepierre M, Qadri F, Nato F, Fournier JM, Alzari PM (2008) Crystal structure of a monoclonal antibody directed against an antigenic determinant common to Ogawa and Inaba serotypes of *Vibrio cholerae* O1. Proteins 70:284–288

Allison GE, Verma NK (2000) Serotype-converting bacteriophages and O-antigen modification in *Shigella flexneri*. Trends Microbiol 8:17–23

Backinowsky LV, Gomtsyan AR, Byramova NE, Kochetkov NK, Yankina NF (1985) Synthesis of oligosaccharide fragments of *Shigella-flexneri* O-specific polysaccharide. 4. The synthesis of the trisaccharide Glc-α-1-3Rha-α-1-3Rha-α-OMe, and tetrasaccharides Rha-α-1-2(Glc-α-1-3) Rha-α-1-3Rha-α-OMe and GlcNAc-β-1-2Rha-α-1-2(Glc-α-1-3)Rha-α-OMe. Localization of the O-factor-V. Bioorg Khim 11:1562–1571

Belot F, Guerreiro C, Baleux F, Mulard LA (2005) Synthesis of two linear PADRE conjugates bearing a deca- or pentadecasaccharide B epitope as potential synthetic vaccines against *Shigella flexneri* serotype 2a infection. Chem Eur J 11:1625–1635

Bock K, Josephson S, Bundle DR (1982) Lipopolysaccharide solution conformation – antigen shape inferred from high-resolution H-1 and C-13 nuclear magnetic-resonance spectroscopy and hard-sphere calculations. J Chem Soc Perkin Trans 2:59–70

Borrelli S, Hossany RB, Pinto BM (2008) Immunological evidence for functional rather than structural mimicry by a *Shigella flexneri* Y polysaccharide-mimetic peptide. Clin Vaccine Immunol 15:1106–1114

Bougoudogo F, Vely F, Nato F, Boutonnier A, Gounon P, Mazie JC, Fournier JM (1995) Protective activities of serum immunoglobulin G on the mucosal surface to *Vibrio cholerae* O1. Bull Inst Pasteur 93:273–283

Boutet J, Mulard LA (2008) Synthesis of 2 tetra- and 4 pentasaccharide fragments of *Shigella flexneri* serotypes 3a and/or X O-antigens from a common tetrasaccharide intermediate. Eur J Org Chem 5526–5542

Boutet J, Guerreiro C, Mulard LA (2009) Efficient synthesis of six tri- to hexasaccharide fragments of *Shigella flexneri* serotypes 3a and/or X O-antigen, including a study on acceptors containing *N*-trichloroacetylglucosamine versus N-acetylglucosamine. J Org Chem 74:2651–2670

Boutonnier A, Villeneuve S, Nato F, Dassy B, Fournier JM (2001) Preparation, immunogenicity, and protective efficacy, in a murine model, of a conjugate vaccine composed of the polysaccharide moiety of the lipopolysaccharide of *Vibrio cholerae* O139 bound to tetanus toxoid. Infect Immun 69:3488–3493

Bundle DR (1989) Antibody combining sites and oligosaccharide determinants studied by competitive-binding, sequencing and X-ray crystallography. Pure Appl Chem 61:1171–1180

Bundle DR, Rich JR, Jacques S, Yu HN, Nitz M, Ling CC (2005) Thiooligosaccharide conjugate vaccines evoke antibodies specific for native antigens. Angew Chem Int Ed Engl 44:7725–7729

Bystricky S, Szu SC, Zhang J, Kovac P (1998) Conformational differences among mono- and oligosaccharide fragments of O-specific polysaccharides of *Vibrio cholerae* O1 revealed by circular dichroism. Carbohydr Res 314:135–139

Canh DG, Lin FY, Thiem VD, Trach DD, Trong ND, Mao ND, Hunt S, Schneerson R, Robbins JB, Chu C, Shiloach J, Bryla DA, Bonnet MC, Schulz D, Szu SC (2004) Effect of dosage on immunogenicity of a Vi conjugate vaccine injected twice into 2- to 5-year-old Vietnamese children. Infect Immun 72:6586–6588

Carlin NI, Lindberg AA (1983) Monoclonal antibodies specific for O-antigenic polysaccharides of *Shigella flexneri*: clones binding to II, II:3,4, and 7,8 epitopes. J Clin Microbiol 18:1183–1189

Carlin NI, Gidney MA, Lindberg AA, Bundle DR (1986a) Characterization of *Shigella flexneri*-specific murine monoclonal antibodies by chemically defined glycoconjugates. J Immunol 137:2361–2366

Carlin NI, Wehler T, Lindberg AA (1986b) *Shigella flexneri* O-antigen epitopes: chemical and immunochemical analyses reveal that epitopes of type III and group 6 antigens are identical. Infect Immun 53:110–115

Carlin NI, Lindberg AA (1986c) Monoclonal antibodies specific for *Shigella flexneri* lipopolysaccharides: clones binding to type I and type III:6,7,8 antigens, group 6 antigen, and a core epitope. Infect Immun 53:103–109

Carlin NI, Lindberg AA (1987a) Monoclonal antibodies specific for *Shigella flexneri* lipopolysaccharides: clones binding to type IV, V, and VI antigens, group 3,4 antigen, and an epitope common to all *Shigella flexneri* and *Shigella dysenteriae* type 1 strains. Infect Immun 55:1412–1420

Carlin NI, Bundle DR, Lindberg AA (1987b) Characterization of five *Shigella flexneri* variant Y-specific monoclonal antibodies using defined saccharides and glycoconjugate antigens. J Immunol 138:4419–4427

Chatterjee SN, Chaudhuri K (2003) Lipopolysaccharides of *Vibrio cholerae*. I. Physical and chemical characterization. Biochim Biophys Acta 1639:65–79

Chatterjee SN, Chaudhuri K (2006) Lipopolysaccharides of *Vibrio cholerae*: III. Biological functions. Biochim Biophys Acta 1762:1–16

Cheng AC, McDonald JR, Thielman NM (2005) Infectious diarrhea in developed and developing countries. J Clin Gastroenterol 39:757–773

Chernyak A, Kondo S, Wade TK, Meeks MD, Alzari PM, Fournier JM, Taylor RK, Kovac P, Wade WF (2002) Induction of protective immunity by synthetic *Vibrio cholerae* hexasaccharide derived from *V. cholerae* O1 Ogawa lipopolysaccharide bound to a protein carrier. J Infect Dis 185:950–962

Chowers Y, Kirschner J, Keller N, Barshack I, Bar-Meir S, Ashkenazi S, Schneerson R, Robbins J, Passwell JH (2007) O-specific polysaccharide conjugate vaccine-induced antibodies prevent invasion of *Shigella* into Caco-2 cells and may be curative. Proc Natl Acad Sci USA 104:2396–2401

Clement MJ, Imberty A, Phalipon A, Perez S, Simenel C, Mulard LA, Delepierre M (2003) Conformational studies of the O-specific polysaccharide of *Shigella flexneri* 5a and of four related synthetic pentasaccharide fragments using NMR and molecular modeling. J Biol Chem 278:47928–47936

Clement MJ, Fortune A, Phalipon A, Marcel-Peyre V, Simenel C, Imberty A, Delepierre M, Mulard LA (2006) Toward a better understanding of the basis of the molecular mimicry of polysaccharide antigens by peptides: the example of *Shigella flexneri* 5a. J Biol Chem 281:2317–2332

Cohen D, Green MS, Block C, Slepon R, Ofek I (1991) Prospective study of the association between serum antibodies to lipopolysaccharide O antigen and the attack rate of shigellosis. J Clin Microbiol 29:386–389

Cohen D, Ashkenazi S, Green MS, Gdalevich M, Robin G, Slepon R, Yavzori M, Orr N, Block C, Ashkenazi I, Shemer J, Taylor DN, Hale TL, Sadoff JC, Pavliakova D, Schneerson R, Robbins

JB (1997) Double-blind vaccine-controlled randomised efficacy trial of an investigational *Shigella sonnei* conjugate vaccine in young adults. Lancet 349:155–159

Coxon B, Sari N, Mulard LA, Kovac P, Pozsgay V, Glaudemans CPJ (1997) Investigation by NMR spectroscopy and molecular modeling of the conformations of some modified disaccharide antigens for *Shigella dysenteriae* type 1. J Carbohydr Chem 16:927–946

Coxon B, Sari N, Batta G, Pozsgay V (2000) NMR spectroscopy, molecular dynamics, and conformation of a synthetic octasaccharide fragment of the O-specific polysaccharide of *Shigella dysenteriae* type 1. Carbohydr Res 324:53–65

Cui C, Carbis R, An SJ, Jang H, Czerkinsky C, Szu SC, Clemens JD (2010) Physical and chemical characterization and immunologic properties of *Salmonella enterica* serovar typhi capsular polysaccharide–diphtheria toxoid conjugates. Clin Vaccine Immunol 17:73–79

Dijkstra J, Mellors JW, Ryan JL, Szoka FC (1987) Modulation of the biological activity of bacterial endotoxin by incorporation into liposomes. J Immunol 138:2663–2670

Dmitriev BA, Knirel YA, Kochetkov NK, Hofman IL (1976) Somatic antigens of *Shigella* – structural investigation on O-specific polysaccharide chain of *Shigella-dysenteriae* type-1 lipopolysaccharide. Eur J Biochem 66:559–566

Ewing WH, Carpenter KJ (1966) Recommended designations for the subserotypes of *Shigella flexneri* serotypes. Int J Syst Bacteriol 16:145–149

Falt IC, Lindberg AA (1994) Epitope mapping of six monoclonal antibodies recognizing the *Shigella dysenteriae* type 1 O-antigenic repeating unit expressed in *Escherichia coli* K-12. Microb Pathog 16:27–41

Formal SB, Kent TH, May HC, Palmer A, Falkow S, LaBrec EH (1966) Protection of monkeys against experimental shigellosis with a living attenuated oral polyvalent dysentery vaccine. J Bacteriol 92:17–22

Formal SB, Oaks EV, Olsen RE, Wingfield-Eggleston M, Snoy PJ, Cogan JP (1991) Effect of prior infection with virulent *Shigella flexneri* 2a on the resistance of monkeys to subsequent infection with *Shigella sonnei*. J Infect Dis 164:533–537

Fukazawa Y, Shinoda T, Tsuchiya T (1969) Response and specificity of antibodies for *Shigella flexneri*: demonstration of type-specific factors in immunoglobulin G fraction of antiserum. J Bacteriol 98:1128–1134

Goebel WF (1939) Studies on antibacterial immunity induced by artificial antigens: I. Immunity to experimental pneumococcal infection with an antigen containing cellobiuronic acid. J Exp Med 69:353–364

Gonzalez L, Asensio JL, Ariosa-Alvarez A, Verez-Bencomo V, Jimenez-Barbero J (1999) Solution conformation and dynamics of the trisaccharide fragments of the O-antigen of *Vibrio cholerae* O1, serotypes Inaba and Ogawa. Carbohydr Res 321:88–95

Grandjean C, Boutonnier A, Dassy B, Fournier JM, Mulard LA (2009) Investigation towards bivalent chemically defined glycoconjugate immunogens prepared from acid-detoxified lipopolysaccharide of *Vibrio cholerae* O1, serotype Inaba. Glycoconj J 26:41–55

Gupta RK, Szu SC, Finkelstein RA, Robbins JB (1992) Synthesis, characterization, and some immunological properties of conjugates composed of the detoxified lipopolysaccharide of *Vibrio cholerae* O1 serotype Inaba bound to cholera toxin. Infect Immun 60:3201–3208

Gupta RK, Taylor DN, Bryla DA, Robbins JB, Szu SC (1998) Phase 1 evaluation of *Vibrio cholerae* O1, serotype Inaba, polysaccharide–cholera toxin conjugates in adult volunteers. Infect Immun 66:3095–3099

Gustafsson B, Holme T (1985) Immunological characterization of *Vibrio cholerae* O:1 lipopolysaccharide, O-side chain, and core with monoclonal antibodies. Infect Immun 49:275–280

Hanna HR, Bundle DR (1993) Antibody oligosaccharide interactions – the synthesis of 2-deoxy-alpha-L-rhamnose containing oligosaccharide haptens related to *Shigella-flexneri* variant-Y antigen. Can J Chem 71:125–134

Hartman AB, Van de Verg LL, Mainhart CR, Tall BD, Smith-Gill SJ (1996) Specificity of monoclonal antibodies elicited by mucosal infection of BALB/c mice with virulent *Shigella flexneri* 2a. Clin Diagn Lab Immunol 3:584–589

Hisatsune K, Kondo S, Isshiki Y, Iguchi T, Haishima Y (1993) Occurrence of 2-O-methyl-N-(3-deoxy-L-glycero-tetronyl)-D-perosamine (4-amino-4,6-dideoxy-D-manno-pyranose) in lipopolysaccharide from Ogawa but not from Inaba O forms of O1 *Vibrio cholerae*. Biochem Biophys Res Commun 190:302–307

Hossany BR, Johnston BD, Wen X, Borrelli S, Yuan Y, Johnson MA, Pinto BM (2009) Design, synthesis, and immunochemical characterization of a chimeric glycopeptide corresponding to the *Shigella flexneri* Y O-polysaccharide and its peptide mimic MDWNMHAA. Carbohydr Res 344:1412–1427

Iredell JR, Stroeher UH, Ward HM, Manning PA (1998) Lipopolysaccharide O-antigen expression and the effect of its absence on virulence in rfb mutants of *Vibrio cholerae* O1. FEMS Immunol Med Microbiol 20:45–54

Islam D, Wretlind B, Ryd M, Lindberg AA, Christensson B (1995) Immunoglobulin subclass distribution and dynamics of *Shigella*-specific antibody responses in serum and stool samples in shigellosis. Infect Immun 63:2054–2061

Ito T, Yokota T (1988) Monoclonal-antibodies to *Vibrio-cholerae* O1-serotype Inaba. J Clin Microbiol 26:2367–2370

Kabat EA (1960) The upper limit for the size of the human antidextran combining site. J Immunol 84:82–85

Kaminski RW, Oaks EV (2009) Inactivated and subunit vaccines to prevent shigellosis. Expert Rev Vaccines 8:1693–1704

Karnell A, Li A, Zhao CR, Karlsson K, Minh NB, Lindberg AA (1995) Safety and immunogenicity study of the auxotrophic *Shigella-flexneri* 2a vaccine Sfl1070 with a deleted Arod gene in adult swedish volunteers. Vaccine 13:88–99

Khan MI, Ochiai RL, Clemens JD (2010) Population impact of Vi capsular polysaccharide vaccine. Expert Rev Vaccines 9:485–496

Kosek M, Bern C, Guerrant RL (2003) The global burden of diarrhoeal disease, as estimated from studies published between 1992 and 2000. Bull World Health Organ 81:197–204

Kosek M, Yori PP, Olortegui MP (2010) Shigellosis update: advancing antibiotic resistance, investment empowered vaccine development, and green bananas. Curr Opin Infect Dis 23:475–480

Kossaczka Z, Shiloach J, Johnson V, Taylor DN, Finkelstein RA, Robbins JB, Szu SC (2000) *Vibrio cholerae* O139 conjugate vaccines: synthesis and immunogenicity of *V. cholerae* O139 capsular polysaccharide conjugates with recombinant diphtheria toxin mutant in mice. Infect Immun 68:5037–5043

Kotloff KL, Winickoff JP, Ivanoff B, Clemens JD, Swerdlow DL, Sansonetti PJ, Adak GK, Levine MM (1999) Global burden of *Shigella* infections: implications for vaccine development and implementation of control strategies. Bull World Health Organ 77:651–666

Kovac P (2006) Studies toward a rationally designed conjugate vaccine for cholera using synthetic carbohydrate antigens. In: Bewley C (ed) Protein–carbohydrate interactions in infectious diseases. Royal Society of Chemistry, Cambridge, pp 175–220

Kreis UC, Varma V, Pinto BM (1997) Oligosaccharides corresponding to biological repeating units of *Shigella flexneri* variant Y polysaccharide. 5. Conformational analysis of a heptasaccharide hapten utilizing a combined molecular dynamics and NMR spectroscopic protocol. Theochem J Mol Struct 395:389–409

Kubler-Kielb J, Vinogradov E, Chu C, Schneerson R (2007) O-Acetylation in the O-specific polysaccharide isolated from *Shigella flexneri* serotype 2a. Carbohydr Res 342:643–647

Kubler-Kielb J, Vinogradov E, Mocca C, Pozsgay V, Coxon B, Robbins JB, Schneerson R (2010) Immunochemical studies of *Shigella flexneri* 2a and 6, and *Shigella dysenteriae* type 1 O-specific polysaccharide-core fragments and their protein conjugates as vaccine candidates. Carbohydr Res 345:1600–1608

Kweon MN (2008) Shigellosis: the current status of vaccine development. Curr Opin Infect Dis 21:313–318

Levine MM (2006) Enteric infections and the vaccines to counter them: future directions. Vaccine 24:3865–3873

Levine MM, Kotloff KL, Barry EM, Pasetti MF, Sztein MB (2007) Clinical trials of *Shigella* vaccines: two steps forward and one step back on a long, hard road. Nat Rev Microbiol 5:540–553

Liao X, Poirot E, Chang AH, Zhang X, Zhang J, Nato F, Fournier JM, Kovac P, Glaudemans CP (2002) The binding of synthetic analogs of the upstream, terminal residue of the O-polysaccharides (O-PS) of *Vibrio cholerae* O:1 serotypes Ogawa and Inaba to two murine monoclonal antibodies (MAbs) specific for the Ogawa lipopolysaccharide (LPS). Carbohydr Res 337:2437–2442

Lindberg AA, Wollin R, Bruse G, Ekwall E, Svenson SB (1983) Immunology and immunochemistry of synthetic and semisynthetic *Salmonella* O-antigen-specific glycoconjugates. ACS Symp. Ser 231:83–118

Liu B, Knirel YA, Feng L, Perepelov AV, Senchenkova SN, Wang Q, Reeves PR, Wang L (2008) Structure and genetics of *Shigella* O antigens. FEMS Microbiol Rev 32:627–653

Mage RG, Kabat EA (1963) Immunochemical studies on dextrans. Iii. The specificities of rabbit antidextrans. Further findings on antidextrans with 1,2- and 1,6-specificities. J Immunol 91:633–640

McGavin RS, Bundle DR (2005) Developing high affinity oligosaccharide inhibitors: conformational pre-organization paired with functional group modification. Org Biomol Chem 3:2733–2740

McGavin RS, Gagne RA, Chervenak MC, Bundle DR (2005) The design, synthesis and evaluation of high affinity macrocyclic carbohydrate inhibitors. Org Biomol Chem 3:2723–2732

Meeks MD, Saksena R, Ma X, Wade TK, Taylor RK, Kovac P, Wade WF (2004) Synthetic fragments of *Vibrio cholerae* O1 Inaba O-specific polysaccharide bound to a protein carrier are immunogenic in mice but do not induce protective antibodies. Infect Immun 72:4090–4101

Mel DM, Terzin AL, Vuksic L (1965) Studies on vaccination against bacillary dysentery. 3. Effective oral immunization against *Shigella flexneri* 2a in a field trial. Bull World Health Organ 32:647–655

Miller CE, Karpas A, Schneerson R, Huppi K, Kovac P, Pozsgay V, Glaudemans CPJ (1996) Of four murine, anti-*Shigella dysenteriae* type 1 O-polysaccharide antibodies, three employ V-genes that differ extensively from those of the fourth. Mol Immunol 33:1217–1222

Miller CE, Mulard LA, Padlan EA, Glaudemans CPJ (1998) Binding of modified fragments of the *Shigella dysenteriae* type 1 O-specific polysaccharide to monoclonal IgM 3707 E9 and docking of the immunodeterminant to its modeled Fv. Carbohydr Res 309:219–226

Moore SR, Lima NL, Soares AM, Oria RB, Pinkerton RC, Barrett LJ, Guerrant RL, Lima AAM (2010) Prolonged episodes of acute diarrhea reduce growth and increase risk of persistent diarrhea in children. Gastroenterology 139:1156–1164

Mulard LA, Phalipon A (2008) From epitope characterization to the design of semi-synthetic glycoconjugate vaccines against *Shigella flexneri* 2a infection. ACS Symp. Ser 989:105–136

Mulard LA, Gauthier C (2010) Novel *O*-acetylated decasaccharides. EP10 290 254.1, 12th May 2010

Nagy G, Pal T (2008) Lipopolysaccharide: a tool and target in enterobacterial vaccine development. Biol Chem 389:513–520

Noriega FR, Liao FM, Maneval DR, Ren SX, Formal SB, Levine MM (1999) Strategy for cross-protection among *Shigella flexneri* serotypes. Infect Immun 67:782–788

Nyholm PG, Mulard LA, Miller CE, Lew T, Olin R, Glaudemans CP (2001) Conformation of the O-specific polysaccharide of *Shigella dysenteriae* type 1: molecular modeling shows a helical structure with efficient exposure of the antigenic determinant α-L-Rha*p*-(1 → 2)-α-D-Gal*p*. Glycobiology 11:945–955

Passwell JH, Ashkenazi S, Harlev E, Miron D, Ramon R, Farzam N, Lerner-Geva L, Levi Y, Chu C, Shiloach J, Robbins JB, Schneerson R (2003) Safety and immunogenicity of *Shigella sonnei*-CRM9 and *Shigella flexneri* type 2a-rEPAsucc conjugate vaccines in one- to four-year-old children. Pediatr Infect Dis J 22:701–706

Passwell JH, Ashkenzi S, Banet-Levi Y, Ramon-Saraf R, Farzam N, Lerner-Geva L, Even-Nir H, Yerushalmi B, Chu C, Shiloach J, Robbins JB, Schneerson R (2010) Age-related efficacy of

Shigella O-specific polysaccharide conjugates in 1-4-year-old Israeli children. Vaccine 28:2231–2235

Paulovicova E, Machova E, Hostacka A, Bystricky S (2006) Immunological properties of complex conjugates based on *Vibrio cholerae* O1 Ogawa lipopolysaccharide antigen. Clin Exp Immunol 144:521–527

Paulovicova E, Kovacova E, Bystricky S (2010) *Vibrio cholerae* O1 Ogawa detoxified lipopolysaccharide structures as inducers of cytokines and oxidative species in macrophages. J Med Microbiol 59:158–164

Pavliak V, Nashed EM, Pozsgay V, Kovac P, Karpas A, Chu C, Schneerson R, Robbins JB, Glaudemans CP (1993) Binding of the O-antigen of *Shigella dysenteriae* type 1 and 26 related synthetic fragments to a monoclonal IgM antibody. J Biol Chem 268:25797–25802

Perepelov AV, L'Vov VL, Liu B, Senchenkova SN, Shekht ME, Shashkov AS, Feng L, Aparin PG, Wang L, Knirel YA (2009) A similarity in the *O*-acetylation pattern of the O-antigens of *Shigella flexneri* types 1a, 1b, and 2a. Carbohydr Res 344:687–692

Perepelov AV, Shevelev SD, Liu B, Senchenkova SN, Shashkov AS, Feng L, Knirel YA, Wang L (2010) Structures of the O-antigens of *Escherichia coli* O13, O129, and O135 related to the O-antigens of *Shigella flexneri*. Carbohydr Res 345:1594–1599

Petri WA, Miller M, Binder HJ, Levine MM, Dillingham R, Guerrant RL (2008) Enteric infections, diarrhea, and their impact on function and development. J Clin Invest 118:1277–1290

Phalipon A, Kaufmann M, Michetti P, Cavaillon JM, Huerre M, Sansonetti P, Kraehenbuhl JP (1995) Monoclonal immunoglobulin A antibody directed against serotype-specific epitope of *Shigella flexneri* lipopolysaccharide protects against murine experimental shigellosis. J Exp Med 182:769–778

Phalipon A, Costachel C, Grandjean C, Thuizat A, Guerreiro C, Tanguy M, Nato F, Vulliez-Le Normand B, Belot F, Wright K, Marcel-Peyre V, Sansonetti PJ, Mulard LA (2006) Characterization of functional oligosaccharide mimics of the *Shigella flexneri* serotype 2a O-antigen: implications for the development of a chemically defined glycoconjugate vaccine. J Immunol 176:1686–1694

Phalipon A, Mulard LA, Sansonetti PJ (2008) Vaccination against shigellosis: is it the path that is difficult or is it the difficult that is the path? Microbes Infect 10:1057–1062

Phalipon A, Tanguy M, Grandjean C, Guerreiro C, Belot F, Cohen D, Sansonetti PJ, Mulard LA (2009) A synthetic carbohydrate-protein conjugate vaccine candidate against *Shigella flexneri* 2a Infection. J Immunol 182:2241–2247

Pozsgay V, Coxon B, Yeh H (1993) Synthesis of di- to penta-saccharides related to the O-specific polysaccharide of *Shigella dysenteriae* type 1, and their nuclear magnetic resonance study. Bioorg Med Chem 1:237–257

Pozsgay V, Sari N, Coxon B (1998) Measurement of interglycosidic $^{3}J_{CH}$ coupling constants of selectively ^{13}C labeled oligosaccharides by 2D *J*-resolved ^{1}H NMR spectroscopy. Carbohydr Res 308:229–238

Pozsgay V, Chu C, Pannell L, Wolfe J, Robbins JB, Schneerson R (1999) Protein conjugates of synthetic saccharides elicit higher levels of serum IgG lipopolysaccharide antibodies in mice than do those of the O-specific polysaccharide from *Shigella dysenteriae* type 1. Proc Natl Acad Sci USA 96:5194–5197

Pozsgay V, Coxon B, Glaudemans CPJ, Schneerson R, Robbins JB (2003) Towards an oligosaccharide-based glycoconjugate vaccine against *Shigella dysenteriae* type 1. Synlett:743–767

Pozsgay V, Kubler-Kielb J, Schneerson R, Robbins JB (2007) Effect of the nonreducing end of *Shigella dysenteriae* type 1 O-specific oligosaccharides on their immunogenicity as conjugates in mice. Proc Natl Acad Sci USA 104:14478–14482

Provenzano D, Kovac P, Wade WF (2006) The ABCs (Antibody, B cells, and Carbohydrate epitopes) of cholera immunity: considerations for an improved vaccine. Microbiol Immunol 50:899–927

Raetz CR, Whitfield C (2002) Lipopolysaccharide endotoxins. Annu Rev Biochem 71:635–700

Rasolofo-Razanamparany V, Cassel-Beraud AM, Roux J, Sansonetti PJ, Phalipon A (2001) Predominance of serotype-specific mucosal antibody response in *Shigella flexneri*-infected humans living in an area of endemicity. Infect Immun 69:5230–5234

Reeves P (1995) Role of O-antigen variation in the immune response. Trends Microbiol 3:381–386

Robbins JB, Chu C, Schneerson R (1992) Hypothesis for vaccine development: protective immunity to enteric diseases caused by nontyphoidal *Salmonellae* and *Shigellae* may be conferred by serum IgG antibodies to the O-specific polysaccharide of their lipopolysaccharides. Clin Infect Dis 15:346–361

Robbins JB, Schneerson R, Szu SC (1995) Perspective: hypothesis: serum IgG antibody is sufficient to confer protection against infectious diseases by inactivating the inoculum. J Infect Dis 171:1387–1398

Robbins JB, Kubler-Kielb J, Vinogradov E, Mocca C, Pozsgay V, Shiloach J, Schneerson R (2009) Synthesis, characterization, and immunogenicity in mice of *Shigella sonnei* O-specific oligosaccharide-core-protein conjugates. Proc Natl Acad Sci USA 106:7974–7978

Sack DA, Sack RB, Nair GB, Siddique AK (2004) Cholera. Lancet 363:223–233

Safari D, Dekker HA, Joosten JA, Michalik D, de Souza AC, Adamo R, Lahmann M, Sundgren A, Oscarson S, Kamerling JP, Snippe H (2008) Identification of the smallest structure capable of evoking opsonophagocytic antibodies against *Streptococcus pneumoniae* type 14. Infect Immun 76:4615–4623

Said Hassane F, Phalipon A, Tanguy M, Guerreiro C, Belot F, Frisch B, Mulard LA, Schuber F (2009) Rational design and immunogenicity of liposome-based diepitope constructs: application to synthetic oligosaccharides mimicking the *Shigella flexneri* 2a O-antigen. Vaccine 27:5419–5426

Saksena R, Ma X, Wade TK, Kovac P, Wade WF (2005) Effect of saccharide length on the immunogenicity of neoglycoconjugates from synthetic fragments of the O-SP of *Vibrio cholerae* O1, serotype Ogawa. Carbohydr Res 340:2256–2269

Saksena R, Ma X, Wade TK, Kovac P, Wade WF (2006) Length of the linker and the interval between immunizations influences the efficacy of *Vibrio cholerae* O1, Ogawa hexasaccharide neoglycoconjugates. FEMS Immunol Med Microbiol 47:116–128

Sciortino CV, Yang ZS, Finkelstein RA (1985) Monoclonal-antibodies to outer-membrane antigens of *Vibrio-cholerae*. Infect Immun 49:122–131

Simmons DA (1971) Immunochemistry of *Shigella flexneri* O-antigens: a study of structural and genetic aspects of the biosynthesis of cell-surface antigens. Bacteriol Rev 35:117–148

Simmons DAR, Romanowska E (1987) Structure and biology of *Shigella-flexneri* O-antigens. J Med Microbiol 23:289–302

Svenson SB, Nurminen M, Lindberg AA (1979) Artificial *Salmonella* vaccines: O-antigenic oligosaccharide-protein conjugates induce protection against infection with *Salmonella typhimurium*. Infect Immun 25:863–872

Svenson SB, Lindberg AA (1981) Artificial *Salmonella* vaccine: *Salmonella typhimurium* O-antigen-specific oligosaccharide–protein conjugates elicit protective antibodies in rabbits and mice. Infect Immun 32:490–496

Szu SC, Li XR, Stone AL, Robbins JB (1991) Relation between structure and immunologic properties of the Vi capsular polysaccharide. Infect Immun 59:4555–4561

Theillet FX, Frank M, Vulliez-Le Normand B, Simenel C, Hoos C, Chaffotte A, Bélot F, Guerreiro C, Nato F, Phalipon A, Mulard LA, Delepierre M (2011a) Dynamic aspects of antibody: oligosaccharide complexes characterized by molecular dynamics simulations and STD-NMR. Glycobiology in press

Theillet FX, Simenel C, Guerreiro C, Phalipon A, Mulard LA, Delepierre M (2011b) Effects of backbone substitutions on the conformational behavior of *Shigella flexneri* O-antigens: implications for vaccine strategy. Glycobiology 21:109–121

Van de Verg LL, Bendiuk NO, Kotloff K, Marsh MM, Ruckert JL, Puryear JL, Taylor DN, Hartman AB (1996) Cross-reactivity of *Shigella flexneri* serotype 2a O antigen antibodies following immunization or infection. Vaccine 14:1062–1068

Verez-Bencomo V, Fernandez-Santana V, Hardy E, Toledo ME, Rodriguez MC, Heynngnezz L, Rodriguez A, Baly A, Herrera L, Izquierdo M, Villar A, Valdes Y, Cosme K, Deler ML, Montane M, Garcia E, Ramos A, Aguilar A, Medina E, Torano G, Sosa I, Hernandez I, Martinez R, Muzachio A, Carmenates A, Costa L, Cardoso F, Campa C, Diaz M, Roy R (2004) A synthetic conjugate polysaccharide vaccine against *Haemophilus influenzae* type b. Science 305:522–525

Villeneuve S, Boutonnier A, Mulard LA, Fournier JM (1999) Immunochemical characterization of an Ogawa-Inaba common antigenic determinant of *Vibrio cholerae* O1. Microbiology 145:2477–2484

Villeneuve S, Souchon H, Riottot MM, Mazie JC, Lei P, Glaudemans CPJ, Kovac P, Fournier JM, Alzari PM (2000) Crystal structure of an anti-carbohydrate antibody directed against *Vibrio cholerae* O1 in complex with antigen: molecular basis for serotype specificity. Proc Natl Acad Sci USA 97:8433–8438

Vulliez-Le Normand B, Saul FA, Phalipon A, Belot F, Guerreiro C, Mulard LA, Bentley GA (2008) Structures of synthetic O-antigen fragments from serotype 2a *Shigella flexneri* in complex with a protective monoclonal antibody. Proc Natl Acad Sci USA 105:9976–9981

Vyas NK, Vyas MN, Chervenak MC, Johnson MA, Pinto BM, Bundle DR, Quiocho FA (2002) Molecular recognition of oligosaccharide epitopes by a monoclonal Fab specific for *Shigella flexneri* Y lipopolysaccharide: X-ray structures and thermodynamics. Biochemistry 41: 13575–13586

Vyas NK, Vyas MN, Chervenak MC, Bundle DR, Pinto BM, Quiocho FA (2003) Structural basis of peptide-carbohydrate mimicry in an antibody-combining site. Proc Natl Acad Sci USA 100:15023–15028

Wade TK, Saksena R, Shiloach J, Kovac P, Wade WF (2006) Immunogenicity of synthetic saccharide fragments of *Vibrio cholerae* O1 (Ogawa and Inaba) bound to Exotoxin A. FEMS Immunol Med Microbiol 48:237–251

Wade TK, Wade WF (2008) Variable gene family usage of protective and non-protective anti-*Vibrio cholerae* O1 LPS antibody heavy chains. Microbiol Immunol 52:611–620

Wang J, Villeneuve S, Zhang J, Lei P, Miller CE, Lafaye P, Nato F, Szu SC, Karpas A, Bystricky S, Robbins JB, Kovac P, Fournier JM, Glaudemans CP (1998) On the antigenic determinants of the lipopolysaccharides of *Vibrio cholerae* O:1, serotypes Ogawa and Inaba. J Biol Chem 273:2777–2783

Ye C, Lan R, Xia S, Zhang J, Sun Q, Zhang S, Jing H, Wang L, Li Z, Zhou Z, Zhao A, Cui Z, Cao J, Jin D, Huang L, Wang Y, Luo X, Bai X, Wang P, Xu Q, Xu J (2010) Emergence of a new multidrug-resistant serotype X variant in an epidemic clone of *Shigella flexneri*. J Clin Microbiol 48:419–426

You D, Wardlaw T, Salama P, Jones G (2010) Levels and trends in under-5 mortality, 1990–2008. Lancet 375:100–103

Synthetic Oligosaccharide Bacterial Antigens to Produce Monoclonal Antibodies for Diagnosis and Treatment of Disease Using *Bacillus anthracis* as a Case Study

2

Matthias A. Oberli, Tim Horlacher, Daniel B. Werz, and Peter H. Seeberger

2.1 Introduction

Bacillus anthracis is a Gram-positive, spore-forming soil bacterium that is closely related to *Bacillus cereus* and *Bacillus thuringiensis*. Infections with *Bacillus anthracis* result in a disease called anthrax (Mock and Fouet 2001; Sylvestre et al. 2002). Anthrax is primarily an infection of grazing cattle. Ingested spores germinate within the host to the vegetative form. Vegetative cells multiply, disseminate in the host organism, and kill the host by their virulence factors. Upon contact with air and depending on other environmental factors, the vegetative cells start to sporulate to form the dormant, durable spores again. *B. anthracis* spores are remarkably resistant to physical stress such as extreme temperatures, radiation, harsh chemicals, desiccation, and physical damage. These properties allow them to persist in the soil for decades (Nicholson et al. 2000). Human anthrax infections are very rare and only occur when humans are closely exposed to infected animals, tissue from infected animals or when they are directly exposed to *B. anthracis* spores (Quinn and Turnbull 1998). Depending on the route of infection, anthrax can occur in three forms: cutaneous, gastrointestinal or inhalation anthrax.

More than 95% of all naturally occurring *B. anthracis* infections are cutaneous. This form of anthrax is associated with handling infected animals or products

M.A. Oberli • T. Horlacher • P.H. Seeberger (✉)
Department of Biomolecular Systems, Max-Planck Institute for Colloids and Interfaces, D-14476 Potsdam, Germany

Freie Universität Berlin, Arnimallee 22, 14195 Berlin, Germany
e-mail: peter.seeberger@mpikg.mpg.de

D.B. Werz
Institut für Organische und Biomolekulare Chemie der Georg-August-Universität Göttingen, Tammannstr. 2, D-37077 Göttingen, Germany

P. Kosma and S. Müller-Loennies (eds.), *Anticarbohydrate Antibodies*,
DOI 10.1007/978-3-7091-0870-3_2, © Springer-Verlag/Wien 2012

thereof such as meat, wool, or leather (Lucez 2005). The majority of cutaneous anthrax lesions proceed locally in the area of the exposed tissue. The anthrax lesion begins as a small papule that quickly enlarges and develops a central vesicle, which ruptures, leaving an underlying necrotic ulcer. Historically, case-fatality rates for cutaneous anthrax have been as high as 20% but are now less than 1% with appropriate antimicrobial treatments (Quinn and Turnbull 1998).

Gastrointestinal anthrax typically occurs after eating raw or undercooked contaminated meat. This form is very rare and the case-fatality ratio is unknown, but estimated to range from 25% to 60% (Beatty et al. 2003).

Inhalation anthrax is a systemic infection that is caused by inhalation of *B. anthracis* spores and is associated with very high fatality rates. The highly resistant spores of *B. anthracis* have been a focus of offensive and defensive biological warfare research programs worldwide (Rotz et al. 2002). The high danger of *B. anthracis* spores used as biological weapons was demonstrated by the accidental release of spores from a biological weapons factory in the Soviet Union. This accident killed more than 100 people. The intentional release of anthrax spores through contaminated letters caused the death of five people out of 11 infected with inhalation anthrax and widespread panic among the American population in the autumn of 2001. Following this terrorist attack, *B. anthracis* research programs with the aim to detect, prevent and cure *B. anthracis* were strongly intensified.

Most symptoms of anthrax infections are caused by three *B. anthracis* protein toxins (Moayeri and Leppla 2004). These three toxins work in concert to result in pathogenesis: protective antigen (PA) forms a membrane channel that mediates the entry of two other toxins, the lethal factor (LF) and the edema factor (EF), into host cells. EF, an adenyl cyclase, catalyzes the conversion of ATP to cAMP. LF, a protease, cleaves members of the MEK family and other targets (Moayeri and Leppla 2004). In this way, the toxins interfere with host cell homeostasis and facilitate pathogen survival. The toxins cause the shock-induced death of the host when they are systemically released at the later stages of infection.

The first effective anthrax vaccines using live, attenuated cultures of *B. anthracis* were developed in 1880 by Greenfield (Tigertt 1980) and Pasteur in 1881 (Pasteur 1881). Although effective, the virulence of these heat-attenuated vaccines varied. In 1939, Sterne developed a live, attenuated vaccine from an avirulent, non-encapsulated variant of *B. anthracis* (Sterne 1939). The Sterne-type vaccine replaced the Pasteur heat-attenuated formulation and is still used today as the veterinary vaccine of choice. Due to strong side effects, improved vaccines were developed for human use. While attenuated bacteria are still used in Russia for vaccination, cell free vaccines were developed in the USA and the UK. The only licensed human anthrax vaccine in the United States today is Anthrax Vaccine Adsorbed (AVA), sold as BioThrax (FDA 2005). AVA is a sterile suspension prepared from cell-free filtrates of the non-encapsulated strain *B. anthracis* V770-NP1-R. While effective, considerable adverse effects are observed after AVA vaccination, mild local reactions, including erythema, edema, and indurations, occur in 20% of the recipients and severe local reactions are observed in 1% of those receiving the vaccine. Systemic reactions such as fever, chills, body aches, or nausea occurred in up to 0.2% of AVA immunizations (Brachman et al. 1962). Thus, a safer vaccine is highly desirable.

Like several other bacteria, *B. anthracis* also expresses unique oligosaccharides on the surface. Such strain-specific oligosaccharides create excellent opportunities to generate synthetic anti-bacterial vaccines (Seeberger and Werz 2007). By combination of degradation reactions, extensive NMR spectroscopy and mass spectrometry, two interesting carbohydrate structures of *B. anthracis* were elucidated in recent years. One oligosaccharide antigen, tetrasaccharide **1**, that is probably part of a larger oligosaccharide, was structurally assigned in 2004. This tetrasaccharide is found on the surface of the exosporium glycoprotein BclA of *B. anthracis* spores (Daubenspeck et al. 2004). The BclA tetrasaccharide **1** contains three rhamnose residues and an unusual, non-reducing terminal sugar, 2-*O*-methyl-4-(3-hydroxy-3-methylbutanamido)-4,6-dideoxy-D-glucopyranose, that was named anthrose. This sugar had not been observed previously in other organisms. Tetrasaccharide **1** as well as analogues and truncated sequences thereof have become very attractive targets for the development of a synthetic vaccine and the induction of a highly specific immune response against *Bacillus anthracis*. The second interesting carbohydrate structure, which has been elucidated in 2004, is hexasaccharide **2**. This portion is the repeating unit of the major cell wall polysaccharide from *B. anthracis* vegetative cells (Choudhury et al. 2006). Composition analyses have shown that the structure of this hexasaccharide is different from that of even closely related *B. cereus* strains. Thus, this saccharide may have a function in determining the virulence of *B. anthracis* strains and may become also a component for the development of a multi-subunit vaccine against anthrax (Fig. 2.1).

2.2 The Anthrax Tetrasaccharide

Several groups started synthetic efforts towards the so-called anthrax tetrasaccharide right after its structural characterization. The first complete syntheses were published by Seeberger (Werz and Seeberger 2005) and later Kováč (Saksena et al. 2005, 2006, 2007; Adamo et al. 2005). Other routes leading to the same target structure or the

Fig. 2.1 Anthrax tetrasaccharide **1** released from *B. anthracis* spores and hexasaccharide **2**, a repeating unit of major cell wall polysaccharide from *B. anthracis* vegetative cells shorter trisaccharide portion have been reported by Boons and Crich (Mehta et al. 2006; Crich and Vinogradova 2007). All these protocols start from the chiral pool and utilize readily available carbohydrates such as D-fucose, D-galactose and L-rhamnose as precursors. A completely different route was developed by O'Doherty who used a series of Pd-catalyzed glycosylations as key reactions for the preparation of the oligosaccharide chain (Guo and O'Doherty 2007a,b). A number of enantioselective manipulations are necessary to create the correct stereochemistry starting from 2-acetylfuran. In the following section one synthetic route to the tetrasaccharide is summarized.

2.2.1 Synthesis of Anthrax Tetrasaccharide 1

The synthesis of the unique monosaccharide anthrose is a key step in all syntheses. Seeberger's synthesis of the terminal anthrose started from commercially available D-fucose (**3**) (Scheme 2.1). Acetylation of **3**, followed by immediate protection of the anomeric position with *p*-methoxyphenol (MPOH) and subsequent cleavage of acetate protecting groups furnished **4**. A levulinoyl group proved to be the best choice to protect the C2 hydroxyl group during installation of the β(1→3) glycosidic linkage in anticipation of its selective removal prior to subsequent *O*-2 methylation. Hence, reaction of **4** with 2,2-dimethoxypropane and introduction of the C2-*O*-levulinic ester furnished **5**. Removal of the isopropylidene and tin-mediated, selective benzylation of the C3 hydroxyl group afforded **6**. Inversion of the stereocenter at C4 was achieved by reaction of the hydroxyl group with triflic anhydride to install a triflate that is displaced by sodium azide in an SN2-type fashion to give **7** (Golik et al. 1991). Removal of the anomeric *p*-methoxyphenyl group using wet cerium ammonium nitrate was followed by the formation of the anthrose trichloroacetimidate **8** using conditions reported by Schmidt.

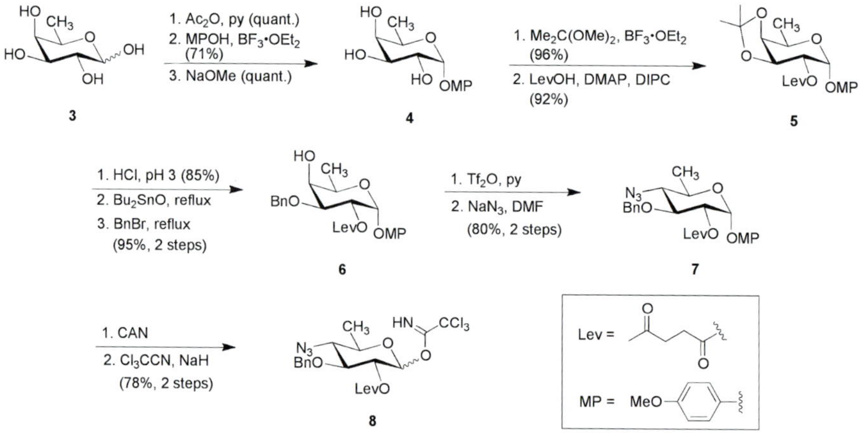

Scheme 2.1 Synthesis of anthrose building block **8** starting from D-fucose **3**

The rhamnose building block **13**, equipped with a robust C2 participating group to ensure α-selectivity and a readily removable temporary protecting group in the C3 position, was synthesized as shown in Scheme 2.2. Placement of an anomeric *p*-methoxyphenol moiety gave **10** (Sarkar et al. 2003). Formation of the *cis*-fused acetal and subsequent benzylation afforded **11**. The transformation of the acetal to the corresponding orthoester and ring-opening resulted in the kinetically preferred axial acetate in **12**. Placement of Fmoc, cleavage of the *p*-methoxyphenyl glycoside and reaction with trichloroacetonitrile in the presence of traces of sodium hydride afforded the trichloroacetimidate building block **13**.

The assembly of the anthrax tetrasaccharide *n*-pentenyl glycoside analogue *via* a (2 + 2) approach commenced with the reaction of building block **14** (Fürstner and Müller 1999) with 4-pentenol (Scheme 2.3a). At a later stage, the *n*-pentenyl moiety can serve as a handle for conjugation to proteins or to glass surfaces for the preparation of microarrays. Removal of acetate, further glycosylation with **13** and subsequent removal of the Fmoc protecting group yielded disaccharide **16**.

The second disaccharide (Scheme 2.3b) was assembled by glycosylation of **12**, an intermediate in the synthesis of building block **13**, with anthrose building block **8**.

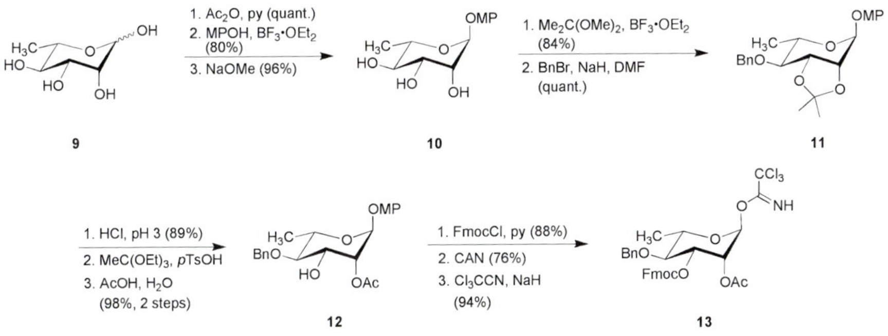

Scheme 2.2 Synthesis of rhamnose building block **13**

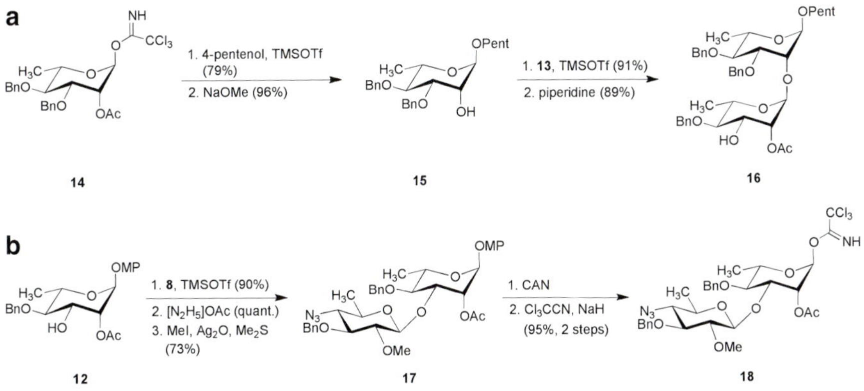

Scheme 2.3 Syntheses of disaccharide building blocks **16** (**a**) and **18** (**b**)

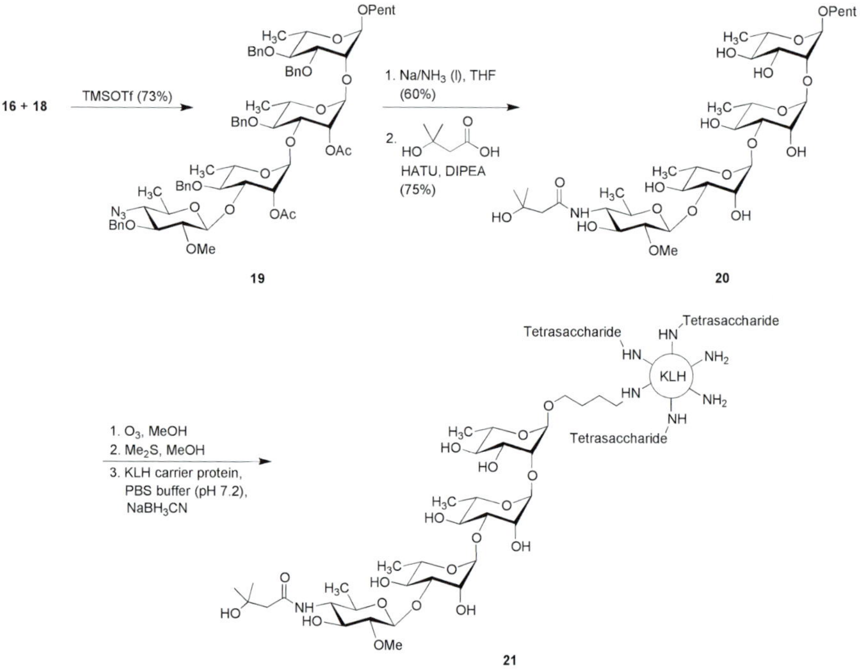

16 + 18 TMSOTf (73%) → 19

1. Na/NH$_3$ (l), THF (60%)
2. 3-hydroxy-3-methylbutyric acid, HATU, DIPEA (75%) → 20

1. O_3, MeOH
2. Me_2S, MeOH
3. KLH carrier protein, PBS buffer (pH 7.2), $NaBH_3CN$ → 21

Scheme 2.4 Completion of the total synthesis and conjugation to a carrier protein

The levulinoyl (Lev) protecting group that ensured β-selectivity was replaced by the final C2 methoxy substituent. Methylation in the presence of acetate was achieved by the action of MeI/Ag_2O in the presence of catalytic amounts of dimethyl sulfide. The commonly used maneuver to convert the methoxyphenyl glycoside into the corresponding trichloroacetimidate furnished disaccharide unit **18**.

To complete the total synthesis, the two disaccharide units **16** and **18** were unified to afford tetrasaccharide **19**. Sodium in liquid ammonia removed all permanent protecting groups and reduced the azide moiety into an amine, thus achieving global deprotection. The formation of the amide with 3-hydroxy-3-methylbutyric acid (Carpino and El-Faham 1995) led to tetrasaccharide **20** including the *n*-pentenyl handle. The double bond in the handle on the reducing terminus was utilized to install a reactive terminal aldehyde moiety *via* ozonolysis. Covalent attachment (Raguputhi et al. 1998; Wang et al. 2000) of tetrasaccharide **20** to keyhole limpet hemocyanine (KLH) carrier protein by reductive amination yielded conjugate **21** that was successfully used as immunogen to produce monoclonal antibodies (mABs) in mice (Tamborrini et al. 2006) (Scheme 2.4).

2.2.2 Immunology

The tetrasaccharide–KLH conjugate was formulated in ImmunEasy^{TM} adjuvant (QIAGEN) and this mixture was injected into mice. Following the second booster immunization, antibodies against tetrasaccharide **1** were detected in the blood of immunized mice as determined by using carbohydrate microarrays bearing the tetrasaccharide **1** structure. Spleen cells of immunized mice were fused with immortalized cell lines to generate hybridoma cell lines. These hybridoma cells were screened for the production of antibodies against tetrasaccharide **1** and cell lines eliciting tetrasaccharide **1** binding IgG antibodies were isolated. Finally, three B cell hybridoma lines producing tetrasaccharide specific monoclonal IgG antibodies (MTA1-3) were generated. All three mAbs bound native *B. anthracis* endospores as determined by an indirect immunofluorescence assay (Tamborrini et al. 2006). By contrast, endospores of close relatives of *B. anthracis* including *B. cereus*, *B. subtilis*, and *B. thuringiensis* strains were not bound by the mAbs MTA1-3.

Independently, other research groups generated anti-anthrax-tetrasaccharide antibodies using neoglycoconjugates comprised of synthetic tetrasaccharide **1** and carrier proteins. Kováč et al. as well as Boons et al. produced antibodies in rabbits with a high specificity for *B. anthracis* (Kuehn et al. 2009; Mehta et al. 2006).

Such antibodies that are highly specific for *B. anthracis* spores are excellent tools to detect *B. anthracis*. Efforts to exploit these antibodies to generate *B. anthracis* spore tests have met with success. Such tests once fully developed will ensure that spores will be detected more readily in order to allow for faster, life-saving treatment and to take the necessary measures when *B. anthracis* spores are used as biological weapons.

2.2.3 Analysis of Anthrax Carbohydrate–Antibody Interactions

Interactions of antibodies with the anthrax oligosaccharide antigen were biochemically analyzed in great detail due to the enormous importance and medical potential of this antigen. A combination of synthetic glycan microarray screening, surface plasmon resonance (SPR), and Saturation Transfer Difference (STD) NMR were used to identify crucial antibody-binding positions on the sugar antigen (Oberli et al. 2010). First, mAbs against a truncated structure, the non reducing terminal disaccharide **36**, (designated MTD1-6) were generated as described above in order to investigate and compare the importance of the anthrose moiety for immunogenicity in the following biochemical experiments.

A collection of synthetic oligosaccharides related to the BclA tetrasaccharide were chemically synthesized. The synthetic oligosaccharide analogues and fragments ranged from mono- to tetrasaccharides related to the original anthrax tetrasaccharide **1**. These synthetic glycans were analyzed for their ability to bind the anti-disaccharide mAbs (MTD1-6) and the anti-tetrasaccharide mAbs (MTA1-3) (Fig. 2.2).

To uncover which structural elements of the anthrax carbohydrate influence the selectivity of antibody–carbohydrate interactions, microarray screening was performed using the generated mAbs (MTA1-3 and MTD1-6) and microarrays bearing the collection of synthetic anthrax oligosaccharides. The anti-tetrasaccharide and the anti-disaccharide mAbs exhibited profoundly different binding patterns. The anti-disaccharide mAbs recognized all synthetic structures with an intact anthrose moiety (structures **22–27** and **33–37**), including anthrose monosaccharide

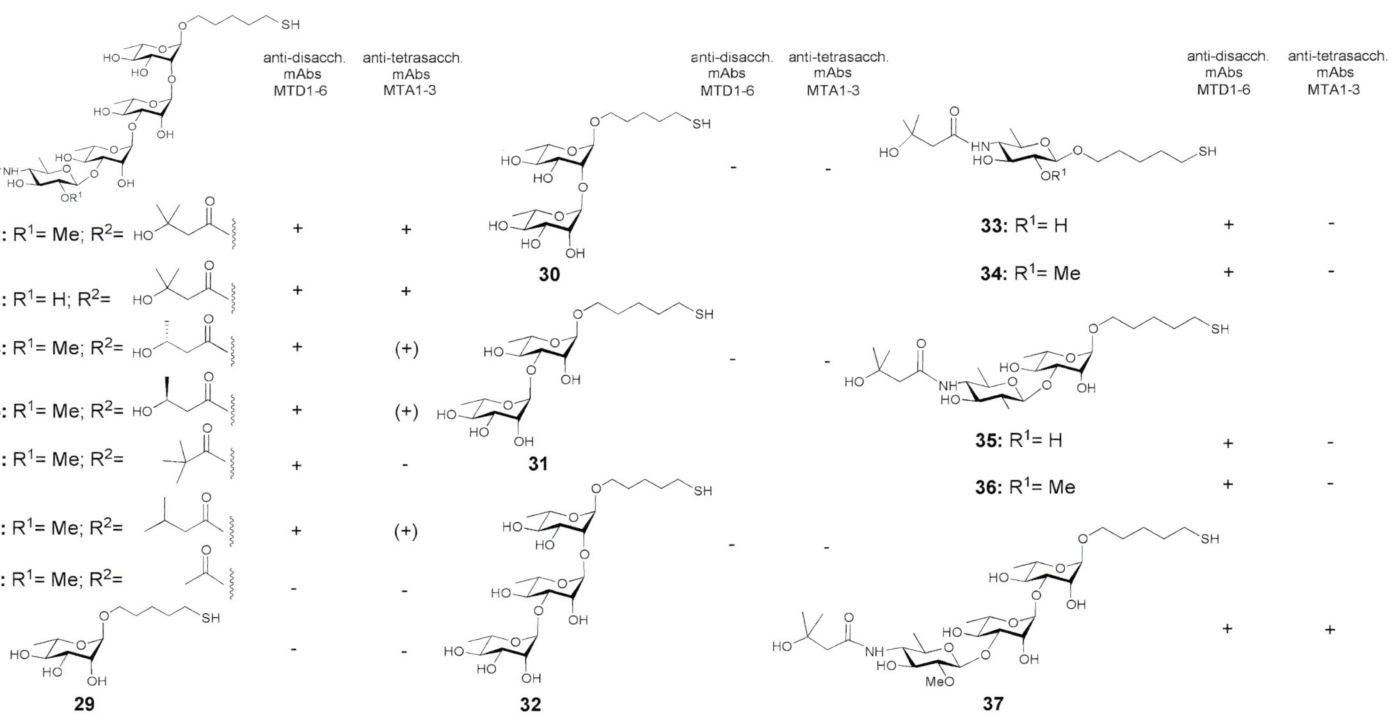

Fig. 2.2 Synthetic glycans related to the *B. anthracis* cell surface tetrasaccharide BclA. The synthetic glycans were used for antibody mapping by microarray screening, SPR and STD NMR analysis. Microarray analysis demonstrates the cross-reactivity of monoclonal antibodies generated against anthrose–rhamnose disaccharide **36** (MTD1–MTD6) and tetrasaccharide **22** (MTA1–MTA3) (Reprinted with permission from Oberli et al. (2010). Copyright© 2010, American Chemical Society)

34. Similarly, the anti-tetrasaccharide mAbs strongly bound tetrasaccharide analogues **22** and **23**, and the trisaccharide **37**. However, the anti-tetrasaccharide antibodies bound tetrasaccharide analogues **24**, **25** and **27** only weakly, and tetrasaccharide analogues **26** and **28** were not bound at all. Notably, each of these structures contained a modified terminal anthrose. No antibody, neither anti-disaccharide nor anti-tetrasaccharide mAbs, recognized mono-, di-, or trirhamnose structures (**29**–**32**). Altogether, these results demonstrate that anthrose is the minimal unit required for binding anti-disaccharide mAbs. Interestingly, while a terminal anthrose is absolutely required for oligosaccharide recognition by the anti-tetrasaccharide mAbs, these mAbs failed to bind the anthrose containing truncated mono- and disaccharide structures (**32**–**36**). Therefore, the anti-tetrasaccharide mAbs require at least two rhamnose units as well as the terminal anthrose for tight oligosaccharide binding.

Anthrose, other than most glycans in mammalian systems contains a side chain appendage other than *N*-acetylation. Since the anthrose unit is essential for antibody binding, its distinctive side chain was investigated in greater detail. A drastic truncation of the chain, produced by reducing 3-hydroxy-3-methylbutyrate to acetate (Fig. 2.2, **28**), resulted in a structure that was not recognized by any of the mAbs that were tested. However, deleting a methyl group within the side chain, by replacing 3-hydroxy-3-methylbutyrate with 3-hydroxybutyrate (Fig. 2.2, carbohydrates **24** and **25**), reduced binding of the anti-tetrasaccharide mAbs dramatically, but had little effect on binding anti-disaccharide mAbs. Similarly, placement of a trimethylacetyl moiety (Fig. 2.2, **26**), or deletion of a 3-hydroxyl group (Fig. 2.2, **27**) only affected anti-tetrasaccharide mAb binding significantly. Therefore, while the anthrose side chain must be present on the glycan to bind both classes of mAbs, only the anti-tetrasaccharide mAbs are affected by altering the specific chemical composition of the side chain, such as removing the C3 methyl group for instance.

A more detailed analysis of the anthrax carbohydrate–antibody interactions relied on SPR experiments (Fig. 2.3). These measurements confirmed and underscored the tight interaction ($K_D = 9.1\ \mu M$) between the anti-tetrasaccharide mAb MTA1 and the tetrasaccharide **1** antigen used to elicit the immune response. Consistent with the microarray results, MTA1 did not bind any other synthetic glycan tested with strong affinity. SPR analysis further demonstrated that the kinetics of the tetrasaccharide **1**-MTA1 interaction are fast and are indeed much faster than the binding kinetics of anti-disaccharide antibodies with any ligand. Notably, the anti-disaccharide mAb MTD6 showed unusually high affinity ($K_D = 0.51\ \mu M$) to its original disaccharide antigen (**36**). Few carbohydrate–antibody interactions with K_Ds below 1 μM have been reported, thus making this discovery particularly significant. Interestingly, K_D values were comparable for interactions between MTD6 and two structurally diverse oligosaccharides, the tetrasaccharide **1** ($K_D = 3.7\ \mu M$) and the anthrose monosaccharide ($K_D = 7.2\ \mu M$). Given this small difference in K_D, we can conclude that the rhamnose units in the tetrasaccharide contribute little to MTD6 binding.

The molecular details of anthrax carbohydrate–antibody interactions were analyzed using STD NMR to determine individual groups and atoms that are important for binding. STD NMR is particularly suited to establish differences in binding to different

	anti-tetrasaccharide mAb MTA1		anti-disaccharide mAb MTD6	
Oligosaccharide	**Affinity K_D[μM]**	**Kinetics (on-/off-Rate)**	**Affinity K_D[μM]**	**Kinetics (on-/off Rate)**
Tetrasaccharide 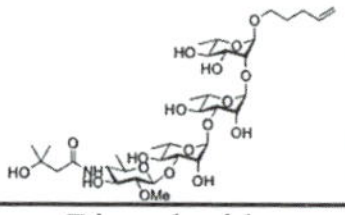	9.1	fast*	3.7	slow (k_a = 19540 $M^{-1}s^{-1}$ k_d = 0.0596 s^{-1} k_d/k_a = 3.05 μM)
Disaccharide 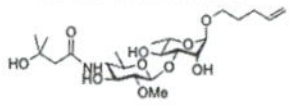	> 1.000	n.a.	0.51	slow (k_a = 46300 $M^{-1}s^{-1}$ k_d = 0.0049 s^{-1} k_d/k_a = 0.11 μM)
Monosaccharide 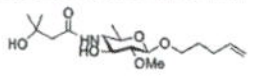	> 1.000	n.a.	7.2	slow (k_a = 8786 $M^{-1}s^{-1}$ k_d = 0.05312 s^{-1} k_d/k_a = 6.0 μM)
Rhamnose-Disaccharide 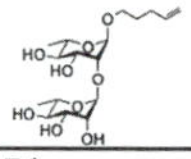	> 1.000	n.a.	> 1.000	n.a.
Rhamnose-Trisaccharide 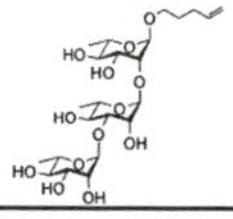	> 1.000	n.a.	> 1.000	n.a.

Fig. 2.3 Determination of affinity and interaction kinetics by surface plasmon resonance. Dissociation constants as determined by steady-state measurements (dilution series), and interaction kinetics as determined by fitting individual binding curves (*The sensorgrams of the tetrasaccharide/MTA1 interaction indicated mass transport-limited association. Kinetic constants could therefore not be determined reliably by SPR)

ligands (discriminating tightly-bound domains from weakly-bound domains) without having to assign the resonance of the macromolecular receptor. Unfortunately, extremely slow dissociation of the MTD6–disaccharide complex prevented further analysis of this antibody–oligosaccharide pair by STD NMR (Meyer and Meyer 1999; Meyer and Peters 2003). Such slow kinetics result in very limited transfer of ligands from the antibody-bound state to the free state, and greatly affect the signal-to-noise ratio of STD NMR experiments. In addition, the increasing antibody–ligand complex lifetime in such cases results in intra-ligand spin diffusion that decreases the discrimination between individual positions of the ligand and prevents detailed mapping.

The complex of MTA1 and tetrasaccharide **1**, however, was a good candidate for further analysis by STD NMR. By assessing antibody binding at a 30:1 ratio of carbohydrate ligand to protein, it was confirmed that MTA1 tightly binds all four sugars of the tetrasaccharide (Fig. 2.4), but had little effect on the non-natural linker at the reducing end of rhamnose D. Strong STD effects indicate that tight-binding sites were located throughout the entire tetrasaccharide on all four sugars, with a cluster of tight-binding sites found within the ß-anthrose-(1→3)-rhamnose substructure. Binding was relatively weaker at the opposite end of the molecule, but STD effects of 12.4% (rhamnose C–H1) and 9.2% (rhamnose D–H2), showed that

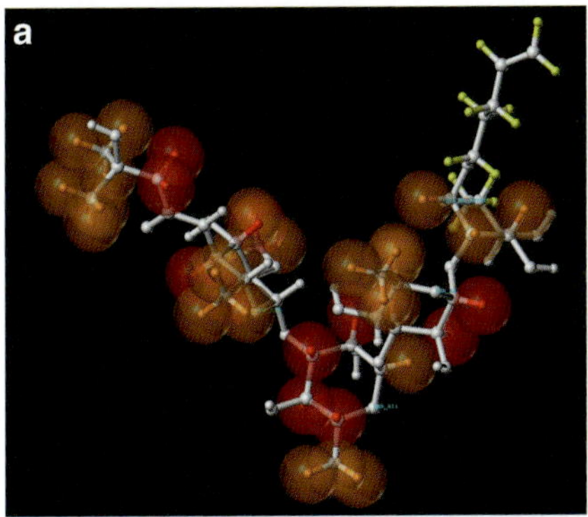

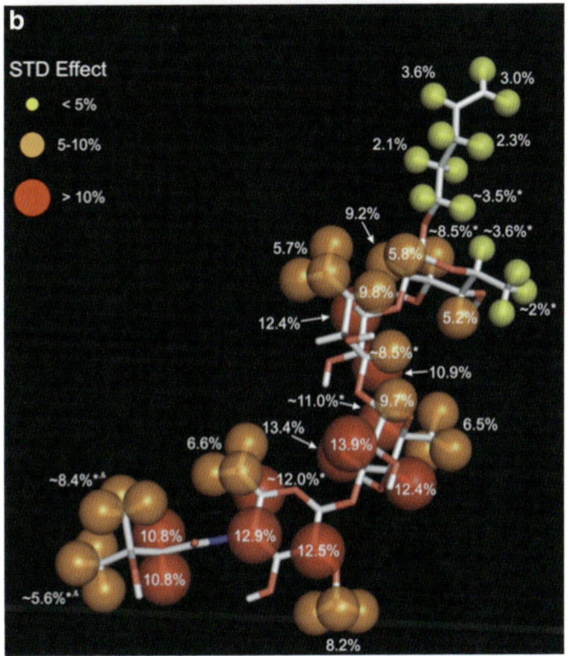

Fig. 2.4 Epitope mapping of the BclA tetrasaccharide **1**/MTA1 interaction by STD NMR spectroscopy. Percent STD effects are shown for individual protons of tetrasaccharide **1**. In addition, strong (>10%), medium (5–10%) and weak (<5%) STD effects are indicated by *red*, *orange*, and *yellow* spheres of decreasing size. Positions marked with an *asterisk* could not be determined to high accuracy due to resonance overlap. The methyl groups marked with *asterisk* were not assigned stereospecifically. Microarray data support the assignment of stronger STD effects to the pro-*S* methyl group, as shown here. The MTA1 antibody recognizes a complex epitope comprising of all four monosaccharide units. Protons of the anthrose moiety and the adjacent rhamnose sugar receive the strongest saturation transfer and are thus most tightly bound by the antibody (Reprinted with permission from Oberli et al. (2010). Copyright© 2010, American Chemical Society)

binding in this region is still significant. Looking at STD effects throughout the structure, it was observed that one face of the trirhamnose chain, (protons H1–H2–H3), was bound more tightly by the antibody than the opposite side (protons H4–H5–H6). Indeed, for rhamnose B, the combined average STD value for protons H1–H2–H3 was 12.3% and 10% for H4–H5–H6, for rhamnose C the average STD values were 10.6% (H1–H2–H3) and 7.8% (H4–H5–H6), and for rhamnose D the average STD values were 7.8% (H1–H2–H3) and 3.6% (H4–H5–H6). The H1–H2–H3 face of the trirhamnose chain is apparently oriented closer to the antibody within the tetrasaccharide–antibody complex. STD NMR analysis indicated that there is a cluster of sites that are tightly bound by MTA1 within the anthrose unit. Specifically, on the anthrose sugar ring, three protons showed strong STD effects. However, the 2-*O*-methyl group is bound less strongly, with an STD effect of 8.2%. This observation agrees with the microarray data that indicated that this side chain appendage is of minor importance for recognition by MTA1. The microarray data also indicated that the anthrose C4 chain, a methylene group, as well as two methyl groups appear to have significant STD values. Interestingly, the two methyl groups have different STD values (8.4% and 5.6%), indicating that one methyl group is oriented closer to MTA1 and this group is bound more tightly (8.4%). It is remarkable that this difference in binding affinity was also detected by microarray screening, where tetrasaccharide **25**, containing a 4-((3*S*)-3-hydroxy-3-methylbutyrate) side chain, showed stronger affinity towards anti-tetrasaccharide mAb MTA2 compared to compound **24** which is decorated with a 4-((3*R*)-3-hydroxy-3-methylbutyrate) side chain. We therefore conclude that the methyl group presented in the (*S*)-configured isomer **25** is proximal to the antibody and thus makes a greater contribution to binding.

The power of combining microarray profiling, SPR, and STD NMR was demonstrated in this study to precisely map the molecular elements of the BclA tetrasaccharide that participate in tight antibody binding. Understanding which structural features of the oligosaccharide are most important for this interaction will enable the design of better carbohydrate-based anthrax vaccines. Furthermore, this approach ultimately aids elucidating general principles of carbohydrate–antibody interactions, enabling guided structure-based design of a broad spectrum of carbohydrate-based antigens and therapeutics thereof.

2.3 The Anthrax Hexasaccharide

In addition to the anthrax carbohydrate present on the surface of spores described above, the structure of the secondary cell wall polysaccharide of *B. anthracis* vegetative cells was elucidated (Choudhury et al. 2006). This capsular polysaccharide of *B. anthracis* vegetative cells mainly consists of hexasaccharide repeating units (hexasaccharide **2**) and is tethered to the *B. anthracis* cell surface S-layer proteins. This structure represents another promising carbohydrate antigen for the development of vaccines and diagnostics, because the β-linked *N*-acetylmannosamine is a pattern that does not occur in mammalian carbohydrates and is therefore presumably a highly immunogenic structure. Following the disclosure of the structure elucidation data, two research groups reported on efforts towards the chemical synthesis of the anthrax hexasaccharide. While the Boons group reported on the synthesis of two trisaccharide fragments (Vasan et al. 2008), we accomplished the synthesis of the complete hexasaccharide repeating unit (Oberli et al. 2008).

2.3.1 Synthesis of the Hexasaccharide Repeating Unit

The retrosynthetic analysis of the fully protected hexasaccharide **39** (Scheme 2.5) dissected the target molecule into two terminal α-galactose building blocks **41**, **42**,

Scheme 2.5 Retrosynthetic analysis of a hexasaccharide repeating unit of the capsular polysaccharide of *B. anthracis*

and two disaccharide parts **A** and **B**. For part **A**, two building blocks **40** and **42** were identified. The *N*-acetyl group of the glucosamine of part **A** was masked as an azide to ensure α-selectivity in the (2 + 2) glycosylation. For part **B,** the trichloroacetyl-protected glucosamine **43** was to be used already attached to the pentenyl handle in order to allow for a facile transformation either into an aldehyde or a thiol. The β-mannosaminic linkage is introduced by inverting the C2-hydroxyl of the glucose moiety after construction of the β-glucosidic bond with **44**.

The synthesis commenced with the union of glucose thioglycoside **44** and glucosamine *n*-pentenyl glucoside **43** to form a β(1→4) glycosidic linkage. The challenging *cis*-β-mannosamine linkage was installed by creating the *trans*-glucosidic bond, readily prepared with the help of the participating fluorenylmethoxycarbonate (Fmoc) group in C2. Subsequently, the Fmoc group was cleaved and the C2 stereocenter was inverted by displacement of the triflate *via* the action of tetrabutylammonium azide to afford the disaccharide **47** that contains the mannosamine motif. Benzylidene protection of the C4 and C6 hydroxyls of the glucose unit proved to be essential for the successful inversion. Selective benzylidene ring opening yielded disaccharide acceptor **48** ready for glycosylation (Scheme 2.6).

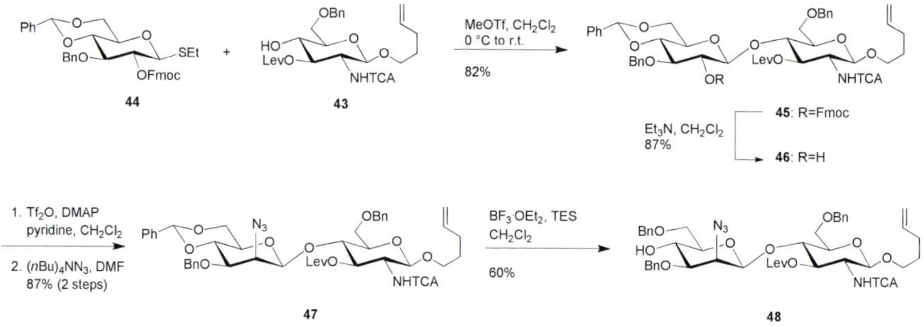

Scheme 2.6 Synthesis of disaccharide **48**

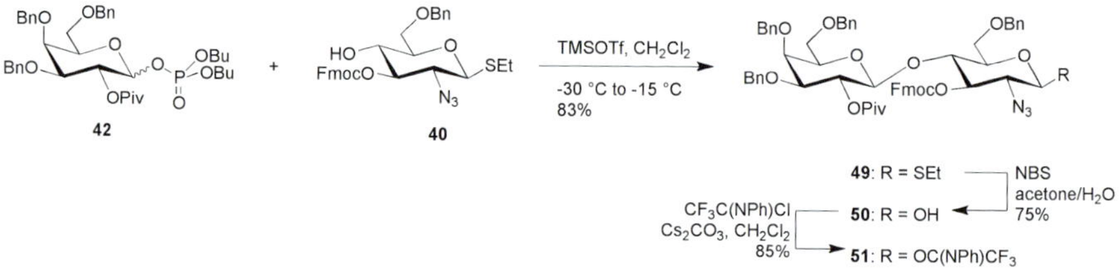

Scheme 2.7 Synthesis of disaccharide building block **51**

The differentially protected lactosamine building block **49** was prepared from galactose phosphate **42** and thioglycoside **40** (Scheme 2.7). The pivaloyl group (Piv) as neighboring-participating group in C2 ensured the selective creation of the β-linkage. In a subsequent step, the C–S bond was cleaved by the action of *N*-bromosuccinimide and water to afford hemiacetal **50**. This hemiacetal was converted into the *N*-phenyltrifluoroacetimidate **51**.

Glycosylation of disaccharide **48** with *N*-phenyltrifluoroacetimidate **51** in a mixture of dichloromethane and diethyl ether selectively afforded tetrasaccharide **52** with the corresponding α-glucosaminic linkage (Scheme 2.8). To complete the synthesis, tetrasaccharide **52** was treated with triethylamine to remove the Fmoc group. A first glycosylation with perbenzylated *N*-phenyltrifluoroacetimidate **41** yielded a pentasaccharide (not shown). Further removal of the levulinoyl ester protecting group by action of hydrazine monohydrate and subsequent glycosylation with the same building block **41** afforded the hexasaccharide **53**. This step-by-step procedure proved superior to a double glycosidation of the tetrasaccharide for the installation of α-galactosidic linkages. Complete deprotection and the transformation of azide moieties into amines were achieved by the action of sodium in liquid ammonia. To reveal NHAc groups – and also to allow for a more facile purification – the completely deprotected carbohydrate was acetylated with a mixture of acetic anhydride, pyridine and DMAP. Final saponification of the completely acetylated structure removed all ester protecting groups leading to target compound **38**. Further functionalization of the *n*-pentenyl moiety allowed for attachment to a carrier protein to yield a neoglycoconjugate that can be readily used in immunization studies.

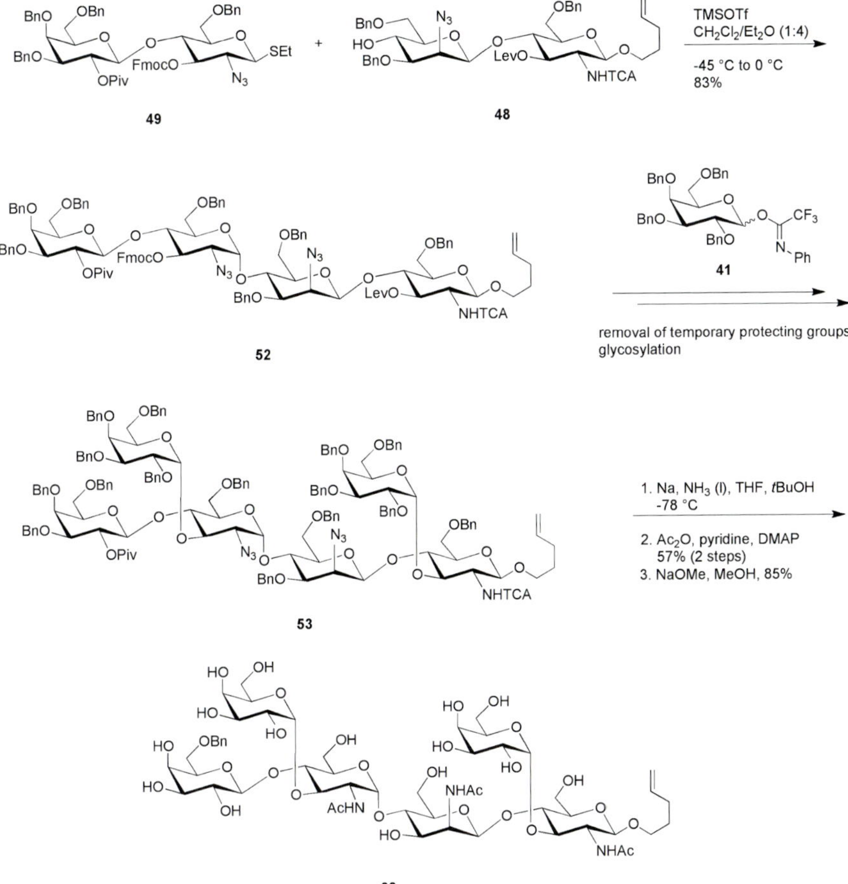

Scheme 2.8 Assembly of the pentenyl hexasaccharide **38**

2.3.2 Immunology

The immunogenicity of the *B. anthracis* cell wall polysaccharide and synthetic carbohydrate antigens were investigated (Vasan et al. 2008). Isolated *B. anthracis* cell wall polysaccharide was coupled to KLH as carrier protein. Rabbits were immunized with this polysaccharide–KLH conjugate or live- or irradiated *B. anthracis* spores. As determined by ELISA, all immunized rabbits elicited IgG antibodies that recognized the isolated polysaccharide, thereby indicating that the polysaccharide structure is also present on the spores. Furthermore, sera from all types of immunized rabbits recognized the synthetic trisaccharide fragments, albeit to a different extent. Whereas both trisaccharides were bound equally well by sera from rabbit immunized with polysaccharide–KLH and irradiated spores, one of the two trisaccharides was bound much better than the other by sera from rabbits that were immunized with live spores. The different recognition of the trisaccharides presumably results from different presentation of the antigens on the polysaccharide chains. Most interesting is the observation that spores can elicit anti-polysaccharide antibodies that also recognize the small synthetic trisaccharides. This observation suggests that not only vegetative cells but also *B. anthracis* spores express the polysaccharide. This finding implies that a subunit vaccine based on the polysaccharide may provide immunity towards vegetative cells as well as spores.

2.4 Conclusion and Outlook

Two carbohydrate structures that were identified on the surface of *Bacillus anthracis* are the focus of this account. The first one, tetrasaccharide **1**, is attached to the major glycoprotein BclA that is present on the exosporium of *B. anthracis* spores. Several groups have reported the chemical synthesis of this target structure and related tri- and pentasaccharide. The second structure, hexasaccharide **2**, is a hexasaccharide repeating unit of the major cell wall capsular polysaccharide of vegetative cells. Again, chemical syntheses of the hexasaccharide and its substructures served as targets of challenging total syntheses, but also provided synthetic antigens to investigate potential vaccine candidates and can be exploited as tools to create diagnostic antibodies.

The history of these two *B. anthracis* antigens illustrates how fast and efficient today's glycoscientists can work. After the terror attack in the US in 2001 where several people died after the exposure to *B. anthracis* spores, research efforts with respect to the underlying mechanisms of this horrible disease and with respect to structure elucidation of relevant target molecules were intensified. Immediately, after disclosure of the oligosaccharide structure, several groups started their synthetic approaches. As soon as the target was assembled by chemical means, conjugation to carrier proteins and immunization studies were performed yielding mAbs able to detect spores. In the meantime, it has been shown that the anti-tetrasaccharide antibodies are not completely selective (Tamborrini et al. 2009), a view that has been confirmed by an analysis of the corresponding anthrose gene cluster that has also been found in a few *B. cereus* strains (Dong et al. 2008). Even though few *B. cereus* strains show cross-reactivity a detection system based on these antibodies is currently under development in Switzerland. The potential of these oligosaccharides as part of a multi-component vaccine is still valid and challenge studies with anthrax tetra- and hexasaccharide structures are ongoing.

References

Adamo R, Saksena R, Kováč P (2005) Synthesis of the beta anomer of the spacer-equipped tetrasaccharide side chain of the major glycoprotein of the *Bacillus anthracis* exosporium. Carbohydr Res 340:2579–2582

Beatty ME, Ashford DA, Griffin PM, Tuxe RV, Sobel J (2003) Gastrointestinal anthrax: review of the literature. Arch Intern Med 163:2527–2531

Brachman PS, Gold H, Plotkin SA, Fekety FR, Werrin M, Ingraham NR (1962) Field evaluation of a human anthrax vaccine. Am J Public Health Nations Health 52:632–645

Carpino LA, El-Faham A (1995) Efficiency in peptide coupling: 1-hydroxy-7-azabenzotriazole vs 3,4-dihydro-3-hydroxy-4-oxo-1,2,3-benzotriazine. J Org Chem 60:3561–3564

Choudhury B, Leoff C, Saile E, Wilkins P, Quinn CP, Kannenberg EL, Carlson RW (2006) The structure of the major cell wall polysaccharide of *Bacillus anthracis* is species-specific. J Biol Chem 281:27932–27941

Crich D, Vinogradova O (2007) Synthesis of the antigenic tetrasaccharide side chain from the major glycoprotein of *Bacillus anthracis* exosporium. J Org Chem 72:6513–6520

Daubenspeck JM, Zeng H, Chen P, Dong S, Steichen CT, Krishna NR, Pritchard DG, Turnbough CL Jr (2004) Novel oligosaccharide side chains of the collagen-like region of BclA, the major glycoprotein of the *Bacillus anthracis* exosporium. J Biol Chem 279: 30945–30953

Dong S, McPherson SA, Tan L, Chesnokova ON, Turnbough CL Jr, Pritchard DG (2008) Anthrose biosynthetic operon of *Bacillus anthracis*. J Bacteriol 190:2350–2359

Food and Drug Administration (2005) 21 CFR Parts 201 and 610. Biological products; bacterial vaccines and toxoids; implementation of efficacy review; anthrax vaccine adsorbed; final order. Federal Register 70:75180–75198

Fürstner A, Müller T (1999) Efficient total synthesis of resin glycosides and analogues by ring-closing olefin methathesis. J Am Chem Soc 121:7814–7821

Golik J, Wong H, Krishnan B, Vyas DM, Doyle TW (1991) Stereochemical studies on esperamicins: determination of the absolute configuration of hydroxyamino sugar fragment. Tetrahedron Lett 32:1851–1854

Guo H, O'Doherty GA (2007a) De Novo asymmetric synthesis of the anthrax tetrasaccharide by a palladium-catalyzed glycosylation reaction. Angew Chem Int Ed 46:5206–5208

Guo H, O'Doherty GA (2007b) De Novo asymmetric synthesis of anthrax tetrrasaccharide and related tetrasaccharide. J Org Chem 73:5211–5220

Kuehn A, Kováč P, Saksena R, Bannert N, Klee SR, Ranisch H, Grunow R (2009) Development of antibodies against anthrose tetrasaccharide for specific detection of *Bacillus anthracis* spores. Clin Vaccine Immunol 16:1728–1737

Lucez D (2005) *Bacillus anthracis* (anthrax). In: Mandell G, Bennett J, Dolin R (eds) Mandell, Douglas, and Bennett's principles and practice of infectious disease. Churchill Livingstone, Philadelphia, pp 2485–2491

Mehta AS, Saile E, Zhong W, Buskas T, Carlson R, Kannenberg E, Reed Y, Quinn CP, Boons GJ (2006) Synthesis and antigenic analysis of the BclA glycoprotein oligosaccharide from the *Bacillus anthracis* exosporium. Chem Eur J 12:9136–9149

Meyer M, Meyer B (1999) Characterization of ligand binding by saturation transfer difference NMR spectroscopy. Angew Chem Int Ed 38:1784–1788

Meyer B, Peters T (2003) NMR spectroscopy techniques for screening and identifying ligand binding to protein receptors. Angew Chem Int Ed 42:864–890

Moayeri M, Leppla SH (2004) The roles of anthrax toxin in pathogenesis. Curr Opin Microbiol 7:19–24

Mock M, Fouet A (2001) Anthrax. Annu Rev Microbiol 55:647–671

Nicholson WL, Munakata N, Horneck G, Melosh HJ, Setlow P (2000) Resistance of *Bacillus* endospores to extrem terrestrial and extraterrestrial environments. Microbiol Mol Biol Rev 64:548–572

Oberli MA, Bindschädler P, Werz DB, Seeberger PH (2008) Synthesis of a hexasaccharide repeating unit from *Bacillus anthracis* vegetative cell walls. Org Lett 10:905–908

Oberli MA, Tamorrini M, Tsai YH, Werz DB, Horlacher T, Adibekian A, Gauss D, Möller HM, Pluschke G, Seeberger PH (2010) Molecular analysis of carbohydrate-antibody interactions: a case study using a *B. anthracis* tetrasaccharide. J Am Chem Soc 132:10239–10241

Pasteur L (1881) De l'attenuation des virus et de leur retour à la virulence. Acad Sci Agric Bulg 92:429–435

Quinn C, Turnbull P (1998) Anthrax. In: Collier L, Balows A, Sussman M (eds) Topley & Wilson's microbiology and microbial infections, 9th edn. Arnold/Oxford University Press, London/New York, pp 799–818

Raguputhi G, Koganty RR, Qiu D, Lloyd KO, Livingston PO (1998) A novel and efficient method for synthetic carbohydrate conjugation vaccine prepapation: synthesis of sialyl Tn-KLH conjugate using a 4-(4-N-maleimidomethyl)-cyclohexane-1-carboxyl hydrazide (MMCCH) linker arm. Glycoconj J 15:217–221

Rotz LD, Khan AS, Lillibridge SR, Ostroff SM, Hughes JM (2002) Public health assessment of potential biological terrorism agents. Emerg Infect Dis 8:225–230

Saksena R, Adamo R, Kováč P (2005) Studies toward a conjugate vaccine for anthrax. Synthesis and characterization of anthrose [4,6-dideoxy-4-(3-hydroxy-3-methylbutanamido)-2-O-methyl-D-glucopyranose] and its methyl glycosides. Carbohydr Res 340:1591–1600

Saksena R, Adamo R, Kováč P (2006) Synthesis of the tetrasaccharide side chain of the major glycoprotein of the *Bacillus anthracis* exosporium. Bioorg Med Chem Lett 16:615–617

Saksena R, Adamo R, Kováč P (2007) Immunogens related to the synthetic tetrasaccharide side chain of the *Bacillus anthracis* exosporium. Bioorg Med Chem 15:4283–4310

Sarkar K, Mukherjee I, Roy N (2003) Synthesis of the trisaccharide repeating unit of the O-antigen related to the enterohemorrhagic *Escherichia coli* type O26:H. J Carbohydr Chem 22:95–107

Seeberger PH, Werz DB (2007) Synthesis and medical application of oligosaccharides. Nature 446:1046–1051

Sterne M (1939) The use of anthrax vaccines prepared from avirulent (uncapsulated) variants of *Bacillus anthracis*. J Vet Sci Anim Ind 13:307–312

Sylvestre P, Couture-Tosi E, Mock M (2002) A collagen-like surface glycoprotein is a structural component of the *Bacillus anthracis* exosporium. Mol Microbiol 45:169–178

Tamborrini M, Werz DB, Frey J, Pluschke G, Seeberger PH (2006) Anti-carbohydrate antibodies for detection of anthrax spores. Angew Chem Int Ed 45:6581–6582

Tamborrini M, Oberli MA, Werz DB, Schürch N, Frey J, Seeberger PH, Pluschke G (2009) Immuno-detection of anthrose containing tetrasaccharide in the exosporium of *Bacillus anthracis* and *Bacillus cereus* strains. JAMA 106:1618–1628

Tigertt WD (1980) William Smith Greenfield, M.D., F.R.C.P, Professor Superintendent, the Brown Animal Sanatory Institution (1878–81) Concerning the priority due to him for the production of the first vaccine against anthrax. J Hyg London:415–420

Vasan M, Rauvolfova J, Wolfert MA, Leoff C, Kannenberg EL, Quinn CP, Carlson RW, Boons GJ (2008) Chemical synthesis and immunological properties of oligosaccharides derived from the vegetative cell wall of *Bacillus anthracis*. Chembiochem 9:1716–1720

Wang ZG, Williams LJ, Zhang XF, Zatorski A, Kudryashov V, Ragupathi G, Spassova M, Bornmann W, Slovin SF, Scher HI, Livingston PO, Lloyd KO, Danishefsky SJ (2000) Polyclonal antibodies from patients immunized with a globo H-keyhole limpet hemocyanin vaccine: isolation, quantification, and characterization of immune responses by using totally synthetic immobilized tumor antigens. Proc Natl Acad Sci USA 97:2719–2724

Werz DB, Seeberger PH (2005) Total synthesis of antigen *Bacillus anthracis* tetrasaccharide-creation of an anthrax vaccine candidate. Angew Chem Int Ed 44:6315–6318

The Role of Sialic Acid in the Formation of Protective Conformational Bacterial Polysaccharide Epitopes

3

Harold J. Jennings

3.1 Introduction

The capsular polysaccharides of human pathogenic bacteria are strong virulence factors and their use as human vaccines are well established (Jennings 1983). Some bacteria have acquired the ability to incorporate sialic acid into their capsules which further enables them to evade the human immune system. For example, the presence of sialic acid enhances the ability of bacteria to mimic human sialylated antigens, which are ubiquitous on normal human cells, giving them the ability to downregulate the human immune system. This deficiency can be overcome however, by using aggressive immunization schedules, by conjugation of the polysaccharide before immunization, or by further modification of the polysaccharide prior to conjugation, but in many cases as detailed in this review, the protective immune response is then mediated through unique length-dependent epitopes (Jennings et al. 1984). This is because the immune system preferentially selects these extended epitopes to produce high affinity protective antibodies, thus avoiding the possible and problematic induction of auto-antibodies against shorter self antigens. This phenomenon is extensively exhibited by the capsular polysaccharides of group B *Neisseria meningitidis* and group B *Streptococcus* and the definition of their extended respective protective epitopes is the subject of this review.

H.J. Jennings (✉)
Institute for Biological Sciences, National Research Council of Canada, 100 Sussex Drive, Ottawa, ON, Canada K1A 0R6,
e-mail: harry.jennings@nrc-cnrc.gc.ca

P. Kosma and S. Müller-Loennies (eds.), *Anticarbohydrate Antibodies*,
DOI 10.1007/978-3-7091-0870-3_3, © Springer-Verlag/Wien 2012

3.2 Group B *Neisseria meningitidis*

3.2.1 Structure of the Group B Meningococcal Polysaccharide

The structure of the group B meningococcal polysaccharide (GBMP) consists of approximately 40 kD chains of $\alpha(2 \rightarrow 8)$ polysialic acid (Bhattacharjee et al. 1975), which for the sake of brevity is designated PSA in the text. Other pathogenic bacteria also produce polysialic acid capsules which are $\alpha(2 \rightarrow 8)$-linked in *E. coli* K1 (Orskov et al. 1979), $\alpha(2 \rightarrow 9)$-linked in group C *N. meningitidis* (GCMP) (Bhattacharjee et al. 1975), and alternate $\alpha(2 \rightarrow 8)$, $\alpha(2 \rightarrow 9)$-linked in *E. coli* K92 (Egan et al. 1977). However when freshly isolated from the culture medium many of these polysaccharides retain, as in the case of the homologous $\alpha(2 \rightarrow 9)$-linked GCMP capsule (Gotschlich et al. 1981), a terminal glycosidic hydrophobic phospholipid residue. The GBMP also has a terminal lipid residue which contains the same components as that of the GCMP (Gotschlich et al. 1981), but its structure is less well defined. Although small, this lipid component has a profound effect on the physical and immune properties of the GBMP. Thus as in the case of the GCMP, it not only causes the individual chains to aggregate, but unique to the GBMP, this aggregation also results in the formation of a potentially important protective epitope on the surface of group B meningococci and *E. coli* K1 (see Sect. 3.3.2).

3.2.2 Immunology of GBMP

Group B *Neisseria meningitidis* is the most prevalent cause of meningococcal meningitis, being responsible for over 60% of all cases in developed countries (Peltola 1998), and *E. coli* K1, which also has a PSA capsule, is the leading cause of neonatal meningitis (Orskov et al. 1979). However, even in its aggregated form PSA is poorly immunogenic in both infants and adults and therefore, unlike the GCMP, cannot be used as a vaccine (Wyle et al. 1972). The reason for its poor immunogenicity is because PSA is recognized as self by the human immune system, which therefore suppresses the production of antibodies having this specificity. PSA was first identified in human cells attached to neural cell adhesion molecules (Finne et al. 1983), and has been identified as a universal mammalian developmental antigen (Troy 1992), which is also expressed on a number of important human tumors (Roth et al. 1993) including small cell lung cancer (Krug et al. 2004).

Although the conjugation of PSA to protein carriers resulted in enhancement of PSA-specific antibody levels, including some antibodies of the IgG isotype, these levels were low and no bactericidal activity associated with these antibodies was reported (Jennings et al. 1981a). Interestingly a similar result was obtained with protein conjugates of the capsular polysaccharide of *E. coli* K92. The K92 polysaccharide is composed of alternate $\alpha(2\rightarrow8)$- and $\alpha(2\rightarrow9)$-linked sialic acid residues which make it a potential vaccine against both groups B and C meningococci. However, conjugates of the K92 polysaccharide only produce a strong and bactericidal antibody response against group C meningococci (Devi et al. 1991; Pon et al. 2002). The above results indicate that the immune system is reluctant to produce antibodies to the $\alpha(2\rightarrow8)$ sialic acid linkage and that it is unlikely that protein conjugates of the GBMP will be useful as vaccines against meningitis caused by group B meningococci.

Fortunately, despite its poor immunogenicity, PSA-specific antibodies can be produced under special circumstances. Hyper-immunization of a horse with *E. coli* K1 produced high levels of PSA-specific IgM antibodies (Orskov et al. 1979), and murine monoclonal antibodies (mAb) with the same specificity, some of which have been shown to be protective, have been produced using similar immunization protocols (Frosch et al. 1985; Rougon et al. 1986), human transformed cell lines producing protective PSA-specific antibodies have been described (Raff et al. 1988), and a human macroglobulin (IgM NOV) having the same specificity has been reported (Kabat et al. 1986). All the above antibodies were of the IgM isotype, with the exception of mAb 735, which was produced in an autoimmune New Zealand black mouse and was of the IgG isotype (Frosch et al. 1985). However, none of the aggressive immunization procedures described above would be acceptable as routine human vaccination protocols.

3.2.3 Extended Helical Epitope of PSA

The presence of a length dependent epitope in PSA was first demonstrated by inhibition experiments, in which the binding of PSA to a polyclonal IgM horse serum (H46) was inhibited by PSA oligomers $(\text{NeuNAc})_n$, where $n = 1$–17 (Jennings et al. 1984, 1985). These experiments indicated that, because they did not maximize, the inhibition curves of PSA were unconventional, and the epitope was therefore considered to be conformational in nature, because it was estimated from the data that the minimum size of oligomer that had the closest resemblance to PSA was ten sialic acid residues. This observation was also confirmed in other studies (Finne and Mäkelä 1985; Hayrinen et al. 1989) and is also consistent with NMR studies (Michon et al. 1987) which demonstrated that the conformation of the linkages of PSA and its shorter oligomers were very different. In contrast, similar experiments on the GCMP using rabbit polyclonal antisera, produced more conventional inhibition curves, which maximized rapidly, indicating that five $\alpha(2\rightarrow9)$-linked residues were sufficient to inhibit its binding to the rabbit antiserum (Jennings et al. 1985). This result is consistent with the proposal made from classic serological studies on linear glucans (Kabat 1976), that the upper limit in size for most antibody combining sites is six glucose units. Because antibodies specific for PSA require an unusually long segment for binding to occur, it has been hypothesized that they recognize an extended helical form of PSA. Support for this hypothesis is based on the identification of a common length dependent epitope responsible for the binding of both PSA and poly(A) to the human macroglobulin IgMNOV (Kabat et al. 1988), and the known propensity of poly(A) to form helices of $n = 8$–10 monomer units. Although PSA and poly(A) share no common structural features, both polymers were able to precipitate an equal quantity of IgMNOV, and this was attributed to them sharing a common epitope, composed of a similar helical arrangement of negative charges.

Further support for the extended helical nature of the PSA epitope was obtained from potential energy calculations and NMR data (Brisson et al. 1992), which showed that although PSA exists predominantly in the random coil form, it can readily adopt extended helical conformations in which $n = 9$. This study also established that the stability of the extended helical conformation is dependent on its carboxylate groups, which interestingly is consistent with immunological studies, in which it was demonstrated that reduction of the carboxylate groups of PSA prevented it from binding to PSA-specific antibodies (Brisson et al. 1992). Furthermore it was established that binding to IgMNOV was not diminished by substituting the *N*-acetyl groups of PSA by larger *N*-propionyl groups (Kabat et al. 1988). Models of the PSA helical epitope where $n = 9$ obtained from the above data, and of the equivalent n = 9 epitope of poly(A), generated from X-ray data (Brisson et al. 1992), are shown in Fig. 3.1a, and illustrate that even though they share no common structural features, the negative charges of both extended helical forms of the linear polymers are superimposable.

To obtain unequivocal evidence for the existence of the extended helical epitope, attempts were made to co-crystallize an α(2→8)-linked oligomer ($n = 10$) of PSA with a Fab fragment obtained from PSA-specific mAb 735, but unfortunately they were not successful. However convincing evidence was obtained when, in the absence of hapten, the Fab fragment was crystallized and subjected to X-ray diffraction analysis (Evans et al. 1995). The binding site consisted of a very long groove, which was bimodal in that it underwent a striking reversal in shape and charge distribution along the interface between heavy and light chains, which

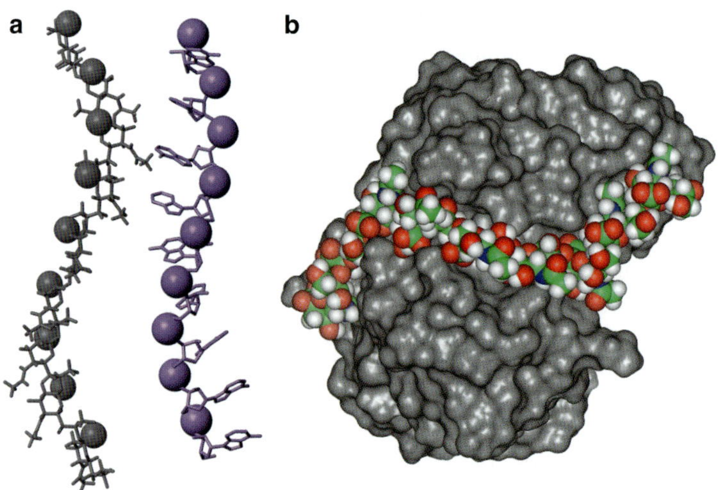

Fig. 3.1 (**a**) Models of the $n = 9$ helices of PSA and polyA. (**b**) Stereoview of the fit of the $n = 10$ helical model of PSA to the binding surface of Fab 735

accounted for the binding of both the carboxylate and *N*-acetyl groups to the binding site. This is consistent with the immunological properties of mAb 735, being different from those of IgMNOV (Kabat et al. 1988), because unlike IgMNOV, substitution of the *N*-acetyl groups of PSA by *N*-propionyl groups negated its binding to mAb 735 (see Table 3.3 in Sect. 3.3.1). With only minor adjustments, the extended helix proposed by Brisson et al. (1992), when modeled into the binding site, had a shape and charge distribution which was complementary to the Fab from mAb 735 as shown in Fig. 3.1b. At least eight α(2→8)-linked sialic acid residues are accommodated in the site, the helical twist of PSA positioning the appropriate functional groups for binding to the bimodal site.

From reported binding studies on different PSA-specific antibodies, all are specific for an extended helical epitope (Jennings et al. 1984, 1985; Finne and Mäkelä 1985; Kabat et al. 1988; Hayrinen et al. 1989). Because conformational studies indicate that this epitope is only a minor contributor to the total number of possible epitopes formed by PSA (Brisson et al. 1992), the dominance of antibodies specific for the less populous epitope must be the result of immunological selection. The reluctance of the immune system to produce antibodies associated with the more populous random coil form of PSA probably occurs because the shorter α(2→8)-linked oligomers of PSA are conformationally similar to structures identified in sialylated human tissue antigens (Finne et al. 1983). Thus the production of antibodies which cross-react with these latter antigens is even more stringently avoided than those induced to the extended helical form of PSA.

3.3 N-Propionylated PSA Conjugate Vaccine

The failure of PSA–protein conjugates to provide satisfactory levels of protective antibody against group B meningococci prompted interest in the chemical modification of PSA prior to its conjugation. One modification that has shown some success was to replace the *N*-acetyl of the sialic acid residues by *N*-propionyl (NPr) groups. Fragments of NPrPSA (10–11 kD), previously treated with sodium metaperiodate to introduce terminal aldehyde groups, were then conjugated to tetanus toxoid by reductive amination (Jennings et al. 1986). The NPrPSA conjugate, when administered to mice with Freunds' complete adjuvant, induced high titers of NPrPSA-specific antibodies which were bactericidal for group B meningococci and passively protective against both group B meningococci and *E. coli* K1 (Jennings et al. 1986, 1987; Ashton et al. 1989). The NPrPSA conjugate was also able to induce much higher levels of cross-reactive PSA antibodies relative to the native PSA conjugate but unfortunately these antibodies were not bactericidal for group B meningococci (Jennings et al. 1987).

While group B meningococci were able to absorb out the bactericidal activity from mouse anti-NPrPSA–TT sera (Ashton et al. 1989), surprisingly none of the bactericidal activity could be removed when PSA was used as adsorbent (Table 3.1). Thus it was demonstrated that NPrPSA-specific antibodies consist of two distinct populations, one of which (minor population) cross-reacts with PSA and is not

Table 3.1 Bactericidal titers of anti-NPrPSA serum absorbed with PSA

Serum	Radioactive antigen binding assay		
	PSA	NPrPSA	Bactericidal titer
Anti-NPrPSA (unabsorbed)	50[a]	77	512
Anti-NPrPSA (absorbed with PSA)[b]	0	73	512
Control	0	0	<4

[a]Percentage of binding to ^{3}H-labeled antigens
[b]500 μl of serum absorbed with 250 μl of 1 mg ml^{-1} PSA (10–11 kDa) for 4 days at 4°C

protective, whereas the larger population of antibodies, which do not cross-react with PSA, surprisingly contain all the bactericidal activity (Jennings et al. 1987, 1989). This evidence indicates that NPrPSA mimics a different epitope on the surface of group B meningococci and *E. coli* K1 than is presented by PSA alone.

These studies suggest that an NPrPSA–protein conjugate would be an excellent vaccine candidate against group B *N. meningitidis*, for which there is currently no efficacious vaccine available, and this has been confirmed in recent pre-clinical studies with these conjugates in mice (Jennings et al. 1986) and primates (Fusco et al. 1997). However preliminary human trials using the NPrPSA–TT conjugate were disappointing because, although found to be safe and immunogenic in human adults, the antisera that it induced lacked bactericidal activity against group B meningococci (Bruge et al. 2004). This was probably because only a mild adjuvant (aluminium hydroxide) was used (Jennings 1997), and support for this explanation was obtained in a recent human trial against small cell lung cancer using an NPrPSA-KLH vaccine in combination with a stronger saponin (QS-21) adjuvant. The desired goal of the trial was to use the induced cross-reactive PSA-specific IgM antibodies to eliminate any residual PSA-expressing small cell lung cancer cells remaining after other radiation and/or surgical treatments (Krug et al. 2004). However, in an assessment of the same patient antisera for protection against *N. meningitidis*, it was shown that the majority of the vaccinees (five out of six), none of whom had bactericidal activity in their preimmune sera, produced antisera which were highly bactericidal for group B meningococci (Table 3.2). The antisera contained antibodies specific for NPrPSA (IgG and IgM) and crossreactive with PSA (IgM), and by analogy with the previously described results of using an NPrPSA–TT conjugate vaccine in mice (Jennings et al. 1987) shown in Table 3.1, it is probable that only the NPrPSA-specific antibodies are bactericidal for group B meningococci.

Currently there is no fully efficacious vaccine against meningitis caused by group B meningococci and *E. coli* K1, and the evidence described above would suggest that an NPrPSA–protein conjugate would be a promising candidate. However, although the above study also demonstrates that this type of vaccine will also induce a subset of PSA-specific human antibodies that bind in vitro to polysialylated human brain glycopeptides (Hayrinen et al. 1995), there is evidence to suggest that they do not bind in vivo (Saukkonen et al. 1986). Furthermore, when pregnant cynomolgus monkeys were hyperimmunized with an adjuvanted NPrPSA–TT conjugate, the induced antibodies, that were bactericidal for group B meningococci and were maintained during the whole gestation period, were shown

Table 3.2 Bactericidal activity of sera from patients vaccinated with NPrPSA–KLH/QS-21 against group B meningococcus

Patient	Week	Bactericidal activity: antisera dilution able to give	
		80% killing	50% killing
1	1	200	500
	4	>10,000	>10,000
	10	3,000	>10,000
2	1	–	200
	4	>10,000	>10,000
3	1	–	200
	4	100	200
4	1	–	200
	4	2,500	7,000
5	1	–	200
	4	1,500	4,500
6	1	–	200
	4	2,000	>10,000

Table 3.3 Biological activity of monoclonal antibodies to NPrPSA

Vaccine	Clone	Isotype	NPrPSA	$(Neu5Pr)_4$	PSA	GBMP[a]	Epitope size	Bactericidal activity
$(Neu5Pr)_4$–TT	11 G1	IgG_{2a}	+	+	+	+	Short	–
NPrPSA–TT	13D9	IgG_{2a}	+	–	–	+	Extended	+
	6B9	IgG_{2a}	+	+	–	–	Short	–
Group B meningococci	735	IgG_{2a}	–	–	+	+	Extended	+

[a]Contains aggregated PSA

to have no harmful consequences on the development of the organs and nervous system of fetuses and sucklings (Bruge et al. 1996).

3.3.1 Extended Helical Epitope of NPrPSA

On the evidence that NPrPSA mimics a protective epitope distinct from PSA on the surface of group B meningococci (Jennings et al. 1989) it must be regarded as a potential vaccine candidate, and it is therefore important to define both the epitope mimic and the mimicked bacterial surface epitope. These epitopes were characterized more fully by producing a series of NPrPSA-specific mAbs, by immunizing Balb/c mice with NPrPSA–TT, which were then screened by a number of PSA antigens (Pon et al. 1997). On the basis of these properties the mAbs could be divided into two distinct types, as represented by the predominant type mAb 13D9, which binds only extended NPrPSA epitopes, and is bactericidal, and the minor type non-bactericidal mAb 6B9, which binds shorter fragments of NPrPSA as shown in Table 3.3. The inability of mAb 6B9 to be bactericidal for group B meningococci can be explained by its failure to bind to PSA or aggregated PSA. However it is interesting to note mAb 11 G1, produced by a vaccine consisting of a short fragment of NPrPSA conjugated to tetanus toxoid $(NeuNPr)_4$–TT, reacted with PSA, aggregated PSA and NPrPSA but was still not bactericidal. This is probably because it binds exclusively to the terminal non-reducing end of both NPrPSA and PSA, as demonstrated by more recent surface plasmon resonance studies (MacKenzie and Jennings 2003).

That mAb 735 is bactericidal for group B meningococci is consistent with the observation that it binds to PSA and not to NPrPSA, while mAb 13D9 is more unusual in that it only binds to NPrPSA, but is still able to provide bactericidal protection in mice challenged with group B meningococci. This it achieves by mimicking a unique PSA-associated intermolecular epitope, which is only found in aggregated PSA.

Interestingly inspection of Table 3.3 indicates that both protective mAbs 735 and 13D9 are immunospecific, in terms of binding only to extended fragments of PSA and NPrPSA respectively, and in previous inhibition experiments (Jennings et al. 1989), a similar length-dependency had also been observed in the binding of NPrPSA to a polyclonal anti-mouse NPrPSA–TT serum. This length-dependency is also consistent with NMR spectroscopic and molecular modeling data (Baumann et al. 1993) that show that the replacement of the *N*-acetyl groups of PSA by *N*-propionyl groups, do not result in major changes of its conformation, and similar to its PSA counterpart, are consistent with the protective extended NPrPSA epitope being situated on an inner helical ($n \sim 9$) segment of NPrPSA. The precise size of the extended NPrPSA epitope was confirmed by surface plasmon resonance, where the binding of a series of protein conjugated NPrPSA oligomers ($n = 7$–11) to a high concentration of mAb 13D9 were studied (MacKenzie and Jennings 2003). As shown in Fig. 3.2a oligomers $n = 7$ and 8 did not bind, whereas oligomer $n = 9$

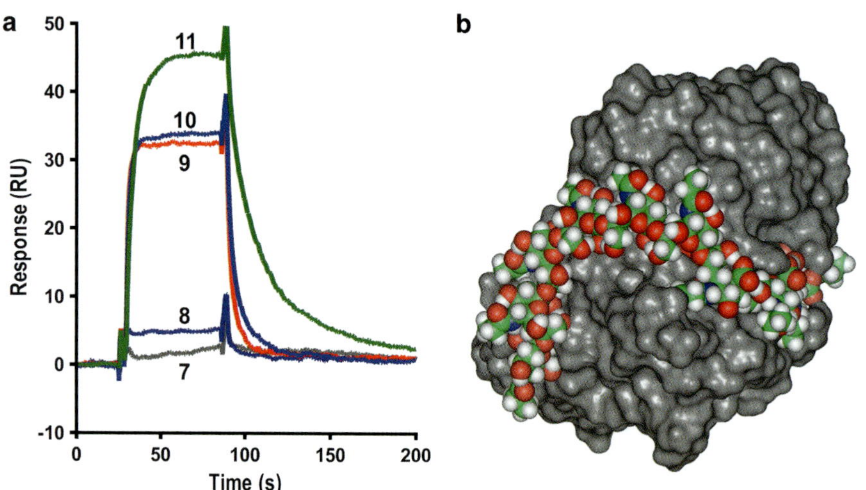

Fig. 3.2 (**a**) Sensorgrams showing Fab 13D9 binding capacities of NPrPSA monomeric units $n = 7$–11. (**b**) Stereoview of the fit of the $n = 10$ helical model of NPrPSA to the binding surface of Fab 13D9

and above bound equally well. The increase in binding is consistent with a minimum size of $n = 9$ for the protective epitope, and the sudden increase in binding from $n = 8$ to $n = 9$ and above is consistent with the formation of a conformational epitope.

The critical importance of the carboxylate group to the stability of the extended helical epitope of both PSA and NPrPSA can be ascertained from NMR spectroscopic studies and potential energy calculations on the carboxyl reduced PSA (Baumann et al. 1993), which indicate that because the extended helical epitope is not stabilized in the reduced polymer it should exhibit conventional immunological properties. This proved to be true, when it was demonstrated that in contrast to PSA, much smaller ($n \sim 5$) reduced oligomers were required to inhibit the binding of reduced PSA to its homologous antiserum. Another structural feature that is critical to the stability of the extended helical epitopes of PSA and NPrPSA is that they require the presence of contiguous α(2→8)-linked residues. Although conjugates of the *N*-propionylated K92 polysaccharide, which consist of alternating α(2→8) and α(2→9) sialic acid residues, were able to induce antibodies that cross react with NPrPSA, they were bactericidal for group C but not group B meningococci. NMR and molecular modeling of the NPrK92 polysaccharide have shown that it cannot form the extended helices required to mimic the bactericidal epitope because of the innate flexibility of its α(2→9)-linkages (Pon et al. 2002).

Confirmation of the existence of this extended helical conformation was obtained by X-ray crystallographic analysis of the crystallized Fab fragment of mAb 13D9 (Patenaude et al. 1998). The binding site, consisting of an unusually long groove was similar to that found for the binding of the Fab fragment of mAb 735 to PSA (Fig. 3.2b), even though mAbs 13D9 and 735 are immunospecific for their homologous antigens, NPrPSA and PSA respectively. An extended helix of NPrPSA modeled into the binding site had a shape and charge distribution complementary to the Fab of mAb 13D9, as shown in Fig. 3.2b. At least eight contiguous α(2→8)-linked NPr-sialic acid residues are accommodated in the site, the helical twist of the residues being necessary to position the appropriate functional groups for binding to the site.

3.3.2 Mimicked Protective Capsular Epitope

That PSA is a component of the mimicked protective capsular epitope can be deduced from the fact that both group B meningococci and *E. coli* K1, which both have PSA capsules, were able to absorb out the bactericidal antibodies from an NPrPSA-specific mouse antiserum (Ashton et al. 1989). In addition, the fact that mAb 13D9 reacts only with PSA in its aggregated form (Table 3.3), confirms the role of PSAs' terminal phospholipid group in the protective epitope. Although the mimicked protective epitope has not yet been fully defined, it has been identified in the capsular layers of both group B meningococci and *E. coli* K1 by electron microscopy using mAb 13D9 and a gold-labeled anti-mouse IgG antibody (Pon et al. 1997), and there is convincing evidence to suggest that it is formed by the interaction of the helical epitopes of PSA with the long hydrophobic chains of its phospholipid component in its native form (Jennings et al. 1989). When a mouse anti-NPrPSA–TT serum was passed through affinity columns in which PSA was linked to the solid support by either long or short aliphatic spacer arms, only the former was able to remove the bactericidal antibodies (Jennings et al. 1989). This implies that the long hydrophobic spacer is functional in binding NPrPSA-specific bactericidal antibodies, and that because of its attachment to a solid support, is able to intermingle with PSA, thus forming a mimic of the intermolecular epitope.

3.4 Group B *Streptococcus*

3.4.1 Structure of the Group B *Streptococcus* (GBS) Polysaccharides

Group B streptococci are Gram-positive organisms which based on their capsular polysaccharides, are classified into nine different serotypes, of which types Ia, Ib, II, III and type V, constitute the major disease isolates (Pon and Jennings 2008). The structures of the group B streptococcal polysaccharides (GBSP), including that of type 7, are shown in Table 3.4.

The structures of the GBSP are unique in that they all have one terminal sialic acid residue per repeating unit, and are composed of sequences of the same constituent sugars, except that they differ in some linkages. Some strain specific *O*-acetylation of terminal sialic acid has been reported (Lewis et al. 2004), but because of base treatment during purification of the GBSP (Wessels et al. 1990), none of the conjugate vaccines discussed below contained *O*-acetylated GBSP (see Sect. 3.4.2). Of even more interest is the high degree of homology that the GBSP have with the oligosaccharides of human glycoproteins (Jennings et al. 1984), and in fact this structural mimicry probably acts as a virulence factor by enabling the bacteria to evade the human immune mechanism. Certainly experiments have confirmed that even the presence of terminal sialic acid alone is able to suppress activation of the alternate complement pathway (Edwards et al. 1982), a potent protective mechanism when levels of type-specific polysaccharide antibodies are low.

3.4.2 Immunology of GBSP

Group B *Streptococcus* (GBS) has become the leading cause of neonatal sepsis and meningitis, which is associated with significant morbidity and mortality (Baker and Kasper 1985), and it was envisioned that infant protection against invasive group B streptococci may be afforded by using their capsular polysaccharides as vaccines in child-bearing women. Thus the protective IgG antibodies induced in the mother would be transferred across the placenta to the neonate. However a significant flaw in this strategy was identified when it was found that a significant number of women

Table 3.4 Structures of the capsular polysaccharides of Group B *Streptococcus*

Type	Structure[a,b]
Ia	→4) βD-Glc*p* (1→4) βD-Gal*p* (1→ 3 ↑ 1 αD-Neu*p*NAc (2→3) βD-Gal*p* (1→4) βD-Glc*p*NAc
Ib	→4) βD-Glc*p* (1→4) βD-Gal*p* (1→ 3 ↑ 1 αD-Neu*p*NAc (2→3) βD-Gal*p* (1→3) βD-Glc*p*NAc
II	→4) βD-Glc*p*NAc(1→3)βD-Gal*p*(1→4)βD-Glc*p*(1→3)βD-Glc*p*(1→2)βD-Gal*p*-(1→ 6 3 ↑ ↑ 1 2 βD-Gal*p* αD-Neu*p*NAc
III	→4) βD-Glc*p* (1→6) βD-Glc*p*NAc (1→3) βD-Gal*p* (1→ 4 ↑ 1 αD-Neu*p*NAc (2→3) βD-Gal*p*
V	→4) αD-Glc*p* (1→4) βD-Gal*p* (1→4) βD-Glc*p* (1→ 6 3 ↑ ↑ 1 1 αD-Neu*p*NAc (2→3) βD-Gal*p* (1→4) βD-Glc*p*NAc βD-Glc*p*
VII	→4) αD-Glc*p* (1→4) βD-Gal*p* (1→4) βD-Glc*p* (1→ 6 ↑ 1 αD-Neu*p*NAc (2→3) βD-Gal*p* (1→4) βD-Glc*p*NAc

[a]Individual references can be found in Pon and Jennings (2008)
[b]Strain-specific *O*-acetylation of Neu5Ac variably at positions 7, 8, or 9 has been reported (Lewis et al. 2004)

did not respond to the polysaccharide vaccines (Baker and Kasper 1985), and therefore a method to enhance the polysaccharide immune response was needed. This was achieved by linking the de-*O*-acetylated GBSP to protein carriers to form conjugate vaccines (Paoletti et al. 1994). With the exception of type V (Guttormsen et al. 2008), the conjugates of GBSP types Ia, Ib, II and III were able to induce strong IgG responses that cross the placenta and persist in the newborn for at least 2 to 3 months, the period of maximum susceptibility (Baker and Kasper 1976). Surprisingly, despite the fact that the former GBSP conjugates share extensive structural homology with human tissue antigens, they are still able to induce in humans strong IgG responses to their respective polysaccharides. This can be explained in the case of types Ia, II and III GBSP because they are able to form length-dependent conformational epitopes (Jennings et al. 1984; Paoletti et al. 1992; Schifferle et al. 1985), similar to those formed by the $\alpha(2\rightarrow8)$-linked PSA (see Sect. 3.2.3). Presumably these conformational epitopes are preferentially selected by the human immune system from a range of alternative conformations present in the flexible polysaccharide, to avoid binding to the shorter oligosaccharides found in human tissue antigens (Jennings et al. 1981b; Jennings et al. 1984). By contrast the types Ib (Schifferle et al. 1985) and V (Guttormsen et al. 2008) GBSP, even though they share similar structural homology, do not form length-dependent epitopes, and in addition the type V GBSP does not even induce a strong IgG response in humans (see Sect. 3.4.4).

3.4.3 Extended Helical Epitope of GBSPIII

While sialic acid controlled conformational epitopes have been identified in types Ia, II (Jennings et al. 1984; Schifferle et al. 1985; Paoletti et al. 1992) and III GBSP (Jennings et al. 1981b), more focused studies aimed at defining these epitopes have concentrated on the latter. The conformational nature of GBSPIII was first demonstrated when rabbits immunized with GBSPIII-TT produced two distinct populations of GBSPIII-specific antibodies (Jennings et al. 1981b). The major population being dependent on the presence of sialic acid, and the minor population reacting only with the desialylated GBSPIII, which is incidentally structurally identical to the capsular polysaccharide of type 14 *S. pneumoniae*. However in human antisera it was found that only antibody directed to the native sialylated type III GBSP correlated highly with protection (Kasper et al. 1979). By using related chemically modified and overlapping saccharides (Jennings et al. 1981b) to inhibit the binding of GBSPIII to anti-rabbit GBSPIII sera, it was not possible to define the epitope responsible for protection, but evidence for its unusual length-dependency, and its conformational control by non-immunogenic terminal sialic acid residues was obtained. It was further established that for the binding of integral GBSPIII repeating units (RU) to the above antisera (Wessels et al. 1987a), 2 RU were required for even suboptimal binding, but a more precise definition of the protective epitope had to await the generation of GBSPIII-specific mAbs.

Inhibition and binding affinities of GBSPIII fragments (nRU) to mAbs 1B1 and 1A6, both representative of protective IgG antibodies, using ELISA and surface plasmon resonance, established that epitope stabilization occurred at 2 RU (decasaccharide), with a small increase from 2 RU to 3 RU, and that further significant epitope stabilization occurred between 6 RU and 20 RU (Zou et al. 1999). These data are consistent with the presence of only one conformational epitope from

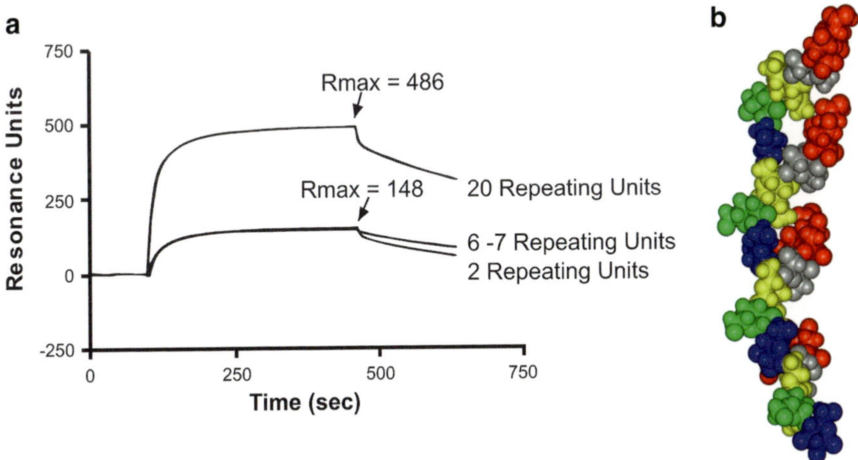

Fig. 3.3 (**a**) Sensorgrams showing the Fab 1B1 binding capacities of 2, 6, 7, and 20 repeating unit of type IIIGBSP. (**b**) Extended helix of 4 repeating units of type III GBSP

2 RU to 7 RU, and this was confirmed when valency effects were eliminated by binding the 2 RU to 7 RU fragments to the 1B1 Fab fragment in surface plasmon resonance experiments (Fig. 3.3a). Further increases in binding with fragments larger than 7 RU were initially attributed to epitope multivalency, but SPR data demonstrated that further optimization of the epitope was still a factor even at this length of saccharide (Zou et al. 1999). Contrary to a previously proposed model of GBSPIII binding (Wessels et al. 1987b) in which the binding of the first antibody propagates a continuum of helical epitopes, binding kinetics obtained from SPR studies (Zou et al. 1999), are consistent only with the discontinuous and infrequent formation of the helical epitope.

Physical evidence of the conformational nature of the GBSPIII protective epitope was first obtained by comparison of the chemical shifts in the ^{13}C NMR spectra of GBSPIII and its desialylated core (Jennings et al. 1981b). Substantial chemical shift differences in the linkage carbons involved in the backbone interchain glucosamine linkages were detected, which are consistent with the hypothesis that terminal GBSPIII sialic acid residues, situated remote from inner core, can influence the overall conformation of its polymeric backbone presumably through sialic acid-backbone interactive forces (Jennings et al. 1981b). This hypothesis was strengthened when the above ^{13}C NMR experiment was repeated at higher resolution (Brisson et al. 1997), and even more interchain chemical shift differences were detected. NMR and molecular dynamics studies (Brisson et al. 1997) on GBSPIII and/or its fragments, confirmed that GBSPIII is capable of forming extended helices (Fig. 3.3b), and that the interaction of terminal sialic acid with its interchain residues is probably a factor in defining its protective conformational epitope. Thus like PSA (see Sect. 3.2.3), GBSPIII exists primarily as a random coil but can spontaneously form infrequent protective extended helices. Unfortunately the acquisition of confirmatory evidence in support of this extended helical epitope has been thwarted by the failure of the Fab 1B1 to crystallize. However, a model of the Fab 1B1 has been constructed from its peptide sequence (Kadirvelraj et al. 2006), demonstrating that it has a long grooved binding site which can accommodate 3 RU of the GBSPIII extended helical epitope.

3.4.4 GBSP Epitopes Independent of Sialic Acid Control

Despite the close structural resemblance of GBSPIb to GBSPIa (Table 3.4), differing only in one side chain linkage, the protective antibodies induced by their conjugates are uniquely type-specific. Furthermore, while terminal sialic acid residues are critical to the formation of the protective epitope in GBSPIa, they do not have the same role in GBSPIb (Schifferle et al. 1985). By analogy with GBSPIII, one could invoke the explanation that only in the former the sialic acid residue is capable of interacting with its backbone to form an extended helical epitope, but evidence is still required to substantiate this. Immunological studies show that for GBSPIb its specificity is not dependent on its terminal sialic acid residues but is dependent on a readily accessible highly immunogenic inner epitope centered on the unique Gal (1→3)GlcNAc linkage in its linear side chain (Schifferle et al. 1985).

Like GBSPIb, the human immunological response to GBSPV conjugates (Guttormsen et al. 2008) indicates that terminal sialic acid residues are not critical to the formation of its protective antibodies, and that therefore it does not form sialic acid-controlled extended helical epitopes. This was confirmed when GBSPV was subjected to ^{13}C NMR spectroscopic analysis (Guttormsen et al. 2008), which demonstrated that, in contrast to GBSPIII (Jennings et al. 1984; Brisson et al. 1997), on removal of terminal sialic acid, the only significant chemical shift displacements were restricted to its neighbouring galactopyranose residue (Fig. 3.4), which is consistent with the absence of a conformational epitope. Interestingly, the ^{13}C NMR spectrum of GBSPVII (Kogan et al. 1995), which has an identical structure to GBSPV, except that GBSPV has an additional branched glucopyranose residue (Fig. 3.4), showed that on removal of terminal sialic acid, chemical shift displacements of substantial magnitude were detected in its inner chain, indicative of the presence of a sialic acid-controlled conformational epitope. This evidence strongly suggests that the additional glucopyranose residue in GBPSV prevents the sialic acid residue from interacting with its inner residues and thus from forming a conformational epitope similar to GBSPVII.

When injected into humans and macaques, the GBSPV conjugate exhibited another unique property in that it induced a predominant IgM response to GBSPV whereas in contrast, the Ia, Ib, II and III GBSP conjugates, induced in humans the IgG response necessary for protection (Paoletti and Kasper 2003). However a desialylated GBSPV conjugate was able to induce the required IgG response in macaques and their antibodies were completely cross-reactive with those induced by the native GBSPV conjugate (Guttormsen et al. 2008). This evidence identifies the desialylated GBSPV conjugate as the preferred vaccine against GBSV infections,

Fig. 3.4 Significant ^{13}C NMR chemical shift displacements (>0.2 ppm) caused by removal of terminal sialic acid from GBSPV and GBSPVII

and also implicates sialic acid, or perhaps the entire branched trisaccharide (NeuNAc(2→3)Gal(1→4)GlcNAc), in modulating the macaques immune system. Of interest is the fact that GBSPIa also contains the same branched trisaccharide, but its conjugates are able to induce protective IgG antibodies in humans. This result is consistent with the hypothesis that in the protective conformational epitope of GBSPIa, the sialic acid interacts with its inner residues, perhaps preferentially shielding it from the immune downregulating mechanism.

3.5 Concluding Remarks

Because of the ubiquity of sialic acid in human tissue antigens, the ability of bacteria to incorporate sialic acid into their surface molecules endows them with another powerful tool to evade the human immune system by mimicking human antigen structures. Examples of this phenomenon are found in the capsular polysaccharides of group B *Neisseria meningitidis* and group B *Streptococcus* as described in this review, however this phenomenon extends to other pathogens as well. The human immune system has adapted to this problem by invoking a unique immune response whereby high affinity protective IgG antibodies are produced exclusively to length-dependent conformational epitopes found on the invasive pathogen, but which are poorly expressed in human tissues. In the case of the α(2→8)-linked polysialic acid capsule of group B *N. meningitidis* and *E. coli* K1, which is a structural homolog of a human neonatal development antigen, induced immune responses are weak, and even when they are enhanced by chemical modification of the PSA capsule, only antibodies to length-dependent epitopes are protective. There is evidence to suggest that these conformational epitopes are more ordered and helical in nature as opposed to the random coil orientations found in shorter mimicked human tissue antigens. Similar sialic acid driven, length-dependent helical epitopes have now been found and described in the protective human immune response to many group B streptococcal polysaccharides. These studies identify the important ability of the human immune system to distinguish polysaccharides through protective recognition of their extended conformations, and lay the groundwork for further elucidation of new immune related conformational dependencies.

Acknowledgements I would like to acknowledge J-R Brisson for the preparation of figures and Robert Pon for helpful critical discussions and preparation of the manuscript.

References

Ashton FE, Ryan JA, Michon F, Jennings HJ (1989) Protective efficacy of mouse serum to the *N*-propionyl derivative of meningococcal group B polysaccharide. Microb Pathog 6:455–458

Baker CJ, Kasper DL (1976) Correlation of maternal antibody deficiency with susceptibility to neonatal group B streptococcal infection. N Engl J Med 294:753–756

Baker CJ, Kasper DL (1985) Group B streptococcal vaccines. Rev Infect Dis 7:458–467

Baumann H, Brisson JR, Michon F, Pon R, Jennings HJ (1993) Comparison of the conformation of the epitope of α(2–8) polysialic acid with its reduced and N-acyl derivatives. Biochemistry 32:4007–4013

Bhattacharjee AK, Jennings HJ, Kenny CP, Martin A, Smith ICP (1975) Structural determination of the sialic acid polysaccharide antigens of *Neisseria meningitidis* serogroups B and C with carbon 13 nuclear magnetic resonance. J Biol Chem 250:1926–1932

Brisson JR, Baumann H, Imberty A, Perez S, Jennings HJ (1992) Helical epitope of the group B meningococcal α(2–8)-linked sialic acid polysaccharide. Biochemistry 31:4996–5004

Brisson JR, Uhrinova S, Woods RJ, van der Zwan M, Jarrell HC, Paoletti LC, Kasper DL, Jennings HJ (1997) NMR and molecular dynamics studies of the conformational epitope of the type III group B *Streptococcus* capsular polysaccharide and derivatives. Biochemistry 36:3278–3292

Bruge J, Moulin JC, Danve B, Dalla Longa N, Valentin C, Goldman C, Rougon G, Herman JP, Coquet B, Thoinet M, Schulz D (1996) Evaluation of the innocuity of a group B meningococcal polysaccharide conjugate in hyperimmunized, pregnant cynomolgus monkeys and their offspring. In: Zollinger W, Frasch CE, Deal CD (eds) Tenth international pathogenic Neisseria conference abstracts, Baltimore, pp 222–223

Bruge J, Bouveret-Le-Cam N, Danve B, Rougon G, Schulz D (2004) Clinical evaluation of a group B meningococcal N-propionylated polysaccharide conjugate vaccine in adult, male volunteers. Vaccine 22:1087–1096

Devi SJN, Robbins JB, Schneerson R (1991) Antibodies to poly [(2–8)-α-N-acetylneuraminic acid] and poly [(2–9)-α-N-acetylneuraminic acid] are elicited by immunization of mice with *Escherichia coli* K92 conjugates: potential vaccines for groups B and C meningococci and *E. coli* K1. Proc Natl Acad Sci USA 88:7175–7179

Edwards MS, Kasper DL, Jennings HJ, Baker CJ, Nicholson-Weller A (1982) Capsular sialic acid prevents activation of the alternative complement pathway by type III, group B streptococci. J Immunol 128:1278–1283

Egan W, Liu TY, Dorow D, Cohen JS, Robbins JD, Gotschlich EC, Robbins JB (1977) Structural studies on the sialic acid polysaccharide antigen of *Escherichia coli* strain Bos-12. Biochemistry 16:3687–3692

Evans SV, Sigurskjold BW, Jennings HJ, Brisson JR, To R, Tse WC, Altman E, Frosch M, Weisgerber C, Kratzin HD, Klebert S, Vaesen M, Bitter-Suermann D, Rose DR, Young NM, Bundle DR (1995) Evidence for the extended helical nature of polysaccharide epitopes. The 2.8 A resolution structure and thermodynamics of ligand binding of an antigen binding fragment specific for α-(2–8)-polysialic acid. Biochemistry 34:6737–6744

Finne J, Finne U, Deagostini-Bazin H, Goridis C (1983) Occurrence of α(2–8) linked polysialosyl units in a neural cell adhesion molecule. Biochem Biophys Res Commun 112:482–487

Finne J, Mäkelä PH (1985) Cleavage of the polysialosyl units of brain glycoproteins by a bacteriophage endosialidase. Involvement of a long oligosaccharide segment in molecular interactions of polysialic acid. J Biol Chem 260:1265–1270

Frosch M, Gorgen I, Boulnois GJ, Timmis KN, Bitter-Suermann D (1985) NZB mouse system for production of monoclonal antibodies to weak bacterial antigens: isolation of an IgG antibody to the polysaccharide capsules of *Escherichia coli* K1 and group B meningococci. Proc Natl Acad Sci USA 82:1194–1198

Fusco PC, Michon F, Tai JY, Blake MS (1997) Preclinical evaluation of a novel group B meningococcal conjugate vaccine that elicits bactericidal activity in both mice and nonhuman primates. J Infect Dis 175:364–372

Gotschlich EC, Fraser BA, Nishimura O, Robbins JB, Liu TY (1981) Lipid on capsular polysaccharides of gram-negative bacteria. J Biol Chem 256:8915–8921

Guttormsen HK, Paoletti LC, Mansfield KG, Jachymek W, Jennings HJ, Kasper DL (2008) Rational chemical design of the carbohydrate in a glycoconjugate vaccine enhances IgM-to-IgG switching. Proc Natl Acad Sci USA 105:5903–5908

Hayrinen J, Bitter-Suermann D, Finne J (1989) Interaction of meningococcal group B monoclonal antibody and its Fab fragment with α 2–8-linked sialic acid polymers: requirement of a long oligosaccharide segment for binding. Mol Immunol 26:523–529

Hayrinen J, Jennings H, Raff HV, Rougon G, Hanai N, Gerardy-Schahn R, Finne J (1995) Antibodies to polysialic acid and its N-propyl derivative: binding properties and interaction with human embryonal brain glycopeptides. J Infect Dis 171:1481–1490

Jennings HJ (1983) Capsular polysaccharides as human vaccines. Adv Carbohydr Chem Biochem 41:155–208

Jennings HJ, Lugowski C (1981a) Immunochemistry of groups A, B and C meningococcal polysaccharide–tetanus toxoid conjugates. J Immunol 127:1012–1018

Jennings HJ, Lugowski C, Kasper DL (1981b) Conformational aspects critical to the immunospecificity of the type III group B streptococcal polysaccharide. Biochemistry 20:4511–4518

Jennings HJ, Katzenellenbogen E, Lugowski C, Michon F, Roy R, Kasper DL (1984) Structure, conformation, and immunology of sialic acid-containing polysaccharides of human pathogenic bacteria. Pure Appl Chem 56:893–905

Jennings HJ, Roy R, Michon F (1985) Determinant specificities of the groups B and C polysaccharides of *Neisseria meningitidis*. J Immunol 134:2651–2657

Jennings HJ, Roy R, Gamian A (1986) Induction of meningococcal group B polysaccharide-specific IgG antibodies in mice by using an N-propionylated B polysaccharide–tetanus toxoid conjugate vaccine. J Immunol 137:1708–1713

Jennings HJ, Gamian A, Ashton FE (1987) N-propionylated group B meningococcal polysaccharide mimics a unique epitope on group B *Neisseria meningitidis*. J Exp Med 165: 1207–1211

Jennings HJ, Gamian A, Michon F, Ashton FE (1989) Unique intermolecular bactericidal epitope involving the homosialopolysaccharide capsule on the cell surface of group B *Neisseria meningitidis* and *Escherichia coli* K1. J Immunol 142:3585–3591

Jennings HJ (1997) N-propionylated group B meningococcal polysaccharide glycoconjugate vaccine against group B meningococcal meningitis. Int J Infect Dis 1:158–164

Kabat EA (1976) Structural concepts in immunology and immunochemistry, 2nd edn. Holt, Rinehart, and Winston, New York, pp 241–267

Kabat EA, Nickerson KG, Liao J, Grossbard L, Osserman EF, Glickman E, Chess L, Robbins JB, Schneerson R, Yang YH (1986) A human monoclonal macroglobulin with specificity for α-(2–8)-linked poly-N-acetylneuraminic acid, the capsular polysaccharide of group B meningococci and *Escherichia coli* K1, which crossreacts with polynucleotides and with denatured DNA. J Exp Med 164:642–654

Kabat EA, Liao J, Osserman EF, Gamian A, Michon F, Jennings HJ (1988) The epitope associated with the binding of the capsular polysaccharide of the group B meningococcus and of *Escherichia coli* K1 to a human monoclonal macroglobulin, IgMNOV. J Exp Med 168:699–711

Kadirvelraj R, Gonzalez OJ, Foley BL, Beckham ML, Jennings HJ, Foote S, Ford MG, Woods RJ (2006) Understanding the bacterial polysaccharide antigenicity of *Streptococcus agalactiae* versus *Streptococcus pneumoniae*. Proc Natl Acad Sci USA 103:8149–8154

Kasper DL, Baker CJ, Baltimore RS, Crabb JH, Schiffman G, Jennings HJ (1979) Immunodeterminant specificity of human immunity to type III group B *Streptococcus*. J Exp Med 149:327–339

Kogan G, Brisson JR, Kasper DL, von Hunolstein C, Orefici G, Jennings HJ (1995) Structural elucidation of the novel type VII group B *Streptococcus* capsular polysaccharide by high resolution NMR spectroscopy. Carbohydr Res 277:1–9

Krug LM, Ragupathi G, Ng KK, Hood C, Jennings HJ, Guo Z, Kris MG, Miller V, Pizzo B, Tyson L, Baez V, Livingston PO (2004) Vaccination of small cell lung cancer patients with polysialic acid or N-propionylated polysialic acid conjugated to keyhole limpet hemocyanin. Clin Cancer Res 10:916–923

Lewis AL, Nizet V, Varki A (2004) Discovery and characterization of sialic acid *O*-acetylation in group B *Streptococcus*. Proc Natl Acad Sci USA 101:11123–11128

MacKenzie CR, Jennings HJ (2003) Characterization of polysaccharide conformational epitopes by surface plasmon resonance. Methods Enzymol 363:340–354

Michon F, Brisson JR, Jennings HJ (1987) Conformational differences between linear α-(2–8)-linked homosialooligosaccharides and the epitope of the group B meningococcal polysaccharide. Biochemistry 26:8399–8405

Orskov F, Orskov I, Sutton A, Schneerson R, Lin W, Egan W, Hoff GE, Robbins JB (1979) Form variation in *Escherichia coli* K1: determined by *O*-acetylation of the capsular polysaccharide. J Exp Med 149:669–685

Paoletti LC, Wessels MR, Michon F, DiFabio JL, Jennings HJ, Kasper DL (1992) Group B *Streptococcus* type II polysaccharide – tetanus toxoid conjugate vaccine. Infect Immun 60:4009–4014

Paoletti LC, Wessels MR, Rodewald AK, Shroff AA, Jennings HJ, Kasper DL (1994) Neonatal mouse protection against infection with multiple group B streptococcal (GBS) serotypes by maternal immunization with a tetravalent GBS polysaccharide–tetanus toxoid conjugate vaccine. Infect Immun 62:3236–3243

Paoletti LC, Kasper DL (2003) Glycoconjugate vaccines to prevent group B streptococcal infections. Expert Opin Biol Ther 3:975–984

Patenaude SI, Vijay SM, Yang QL, Jennings HJ, Evans SV (1998) Crystallization and preliminary X-ray diffraction analysis of antigen-binding fragments which are specific for antigenic conformations of sialic acid homopolymers. Acta Crystallogr D Biol Crystallogr 54:1005–1007

Peltola H (1998) Meningococcal vaccines. Current status and future possibilities. Drugs 55:347–366

Pon RA, Lussier M, Yang QL, Jennings HJ (1997) N-propionylated group B meningococcal polysaccharide mimics a unique bactericidal capsular epitope in group B *Neisseria meningitidis*. J Exp Med 185:1929–1938

Pon RA, Khieu NH, Yang QL, Brisson JR, Jennings HJ (2002) Serological and conformational properties of *E. coli* K92 capsular polysaccharide and its N-propionylated derivative both illustrate that induced antibody does not recognize extended epitopes of polysialic acid:

Implications for a comprehensive conjugate vaccine against groups B and C *N. meningitidis*. Can J Chem 80:1055–1063

Pon RA, Jennings HJ (2008) Carbohydrate-based antibacterial vaccines. In: Guo Z, Boons GJ (eds) Carbohydrate-based vaccines and immunotherapies. Wiley, Hoboken, pp 117–166

Raff HV, Devereux D, Shuford W, Abbott-Brown D, Maloney G (1988) Human monoclonal antibody with protective activity for *Escherichia coli* K1 and *Neisseria meningitidis* group B infections. J Infect Dis 157:118–126

Roth J, Zuber C, Komminoth P, Scheidegger EP, Warhol MJ, Bitter-Suermann D, Heitz PU (1993) Expression of polysialic acid in human tumors and its significance for tumor growth. In: Roth J, Rutishauser U, Troy FA (eds) Polysialic acid: from microbes to man. Birkhauser, Basel, pp 335–348

Rougon G, Dubois C, Buckley N, Magnani JL, Zollinger W (1986) A monoclonal antibody against meningococcus group B polysaccharides distinguishes embryonic from adult N-CAM. J Cell Biol 103:2429–2437

Saukkonen K, Haltia M, Frosch M, Bitter-Suerman D, Leinonen M (1986) Antibodies to the capsular polysaccharide of *Neisseria meningitidis* group B or *E. coli* K1 bind to the brains of infant rats in vitro but not in vivo. Microb Pathog 1:101–105

Schifferle RE, Jennings HJ, Wessels MR, Katzenellenbogen E, Roy R, Kasper DL (1985) Immunochemical analysis of the types Ia and Ib group B streptococcal polysaccharides. J Immunol 135:4164–4170

Troy FA (1992) Polysialylation: from bacteria to brains. Glycobiology 2:5–23

Wessels MR, Munoz A, Kasper DL (1987a) A model of high-affinity antibody binding to type III group B *Streptococcus* capsular polysaccharide. Proc Natl Acad Sci USA 84:9170–9174

Wessels MR, Pozsgay V, Kasper DL, Jennings HJ (1987b) Structure and immunochemistry of an oligosaccharide repeating unit of the capsular polysaccharide of type III group B *Streptococcus*. A revised structure for the type III group B streptococcal polysaccharide antigen. J Biol Chem 262:8262–8267

Wessels MR, Paoletti LC, Kasper DL, DiFabio JL, Michon F, Holme K, Jennings HJ (1990) Immunogenicity in animals of a polysaccharide–protein conjugate vaccine against type III group B *Streptococcus*. J Clin Invest 86:1428–1433

Wyle FA, Artenstein MS, Brandt BL, Tramont EC, Kasper DL, Altieri PL, Berman SL, Lowenthal JP (1972) Immunologic response of man to group B meningococcal polysaccharide vaccines. J Infect Dis 126:514–521

Zou W, MacKenzie R, Therien L, Hirama T, Yang QL, Gidney MA, Jennings HJ (1999) Conformational epitope of the type III group B *Streptococcus* capsular polysaccharide. J Immunol 163:820–825

Antibody Recognition of *Chlamydia* LPS: Structural Insights of Inherited Immune Responses

4

Ryan J. Blackler, Sven Müller-Loennies, Lore Brade, Paul Kosma, Helmut Brade, and Stephen V. Evans

The atomic coordinates and structure factors for all structures discussed have been deposited in the Protein Data Bank, Research Collaboratory for Structural Bioinformatics, Rutgers University, New Brunswick NJ (http://www.rcsb.org). See Table 4.1.

4.1 Overview

The increasing utility of carbohydrate-specific antibodies in diagnostic and therapeutic medicine, in disease bio-marker identification, and in carbohydrate-based vaccine design has underlined the need to understand these important interactions at the molecular level (Holmgren et al. 1984; Hakomori 1984, 1989; Fung et al. 1990; Cygler et al. 1991; Casadevall et al. 1992; MacLean et al. 1992, 1993; Bundle et al. 1994; Pirofski et al. 1995; Fukuda 1996; Mari et al. 1999; van Ree 2000; Hemmer et al. 2001; Kudryashov et al. 2001; Foetisch et al. 2003; Ebo et al. 2004; Lo-Man et al. 2004; Manimala et al. 2005; Müller-Loennies et al. 2006; Ni et al. 2006; Vliegenthart 2006; de Geus et al. 2009; Hecht et al. 2009; Astronomo and Burton 2010; Avci and Kasper 2010; Collot et al. 2010). One of the premiere methods to study the specific recognition of carbohydrates by antibodies is through crystal structure determination *via* X-ray diffraction; however, this requires relatively large quantities of pure proteins and antigens. As well, crystallization of the

R.J. Blackler • S.V. Evans (✉)
Department of Biochemistry and Microbiology, University of Victoria, Victoria, BC, Canada V8P 3P6
e-mail: svevans@uvic.ca

S. Müller-Loennies • L. Brade • H. Brade
Research Center Borstel, Leibniz-Center for Medicine and Biosciences, Parkallee 22, D-23845 Borstel, Germany

P. Kosma
Department of Chemistry, University of Natural Resources and Life Sciences, A-1190 Vienna, Austria

P. Kosma and S. Müller-Loennies (eds.), *Anticarbohydrate Antibodies*,
DOI 10.1007/978-3-7091-0870-3_4,

Table 4.1 PDB codes for antibody structures

Antibody	Antigen	PDB code
S25-2	Unliganded	1Q9K, 1Q9L
	Kdo	3T4Y
	Kdo(2→8)Kdo(2→4)Kdo	3SY0
	Kdo(2→4)Kdo	3T77
	Kdo(2→8)Kdo	3T65
	Kdo(2→4)Kdo(2→4)Kdo	2R2B
	Ko	2R2H
	Ko(2→4)Kdo	2R23
	7-epi-Kdo	2R2E
	Kdo(2→4)KdoC1red	2R1Y
	3,4-Dehydro-3,4,5-trideoxy-Kdo(2→8)Kdo	2R1W
	5-Deoxy-4-epi-2,3-dehydro-Kdo(4→8)Kdo	2R1X, 3BPC
S67-27	Ko	3IJH
	Kdo(2→8)Kdo	3IJY
	Kdo(2→8)-7-O-Me-Kdo	3IKC
	Kdo(2→4)Kdo(2→6)GlcN4*P*(1→6)GlcN1*P*	3IJS
S73-2	Kdo	3HZM
	Kdo(2→4)Kdo	3HZK
	Kdo(2→4)Kdo(2→4)Kdo	3HZY
	Kdo(2→8)Kdo(2→4)Kdo	3HZV
S54-10	Kdo(2→4)Kdo(2→4)Kdo	3I02
S25-39	Unliganded	3OKM
	Kdo	3OKD
	Ko	3OKE
	Kdo(2→4)Kdo	3OKK
	Kdo(2→8)Kdo	3OKL
	Kdo(2→4)Kdo(2→4)Kdo	3OKN
	Kdo(2→8)Kdo(2→4)Kdo	3OKO
S45-18	Unliganded	1Q9O
	Kdo(2→4)Kdo(2→4)Kdo(2→6)GlcN4*P*(1→6)GlcN1*P*	1Q9W
S64-4	Kdo	3PHQ
	Kdo(2→4)Kdo(2→4)Kdo(2→6)GlcN4*P*(1→6)GlcN1*P*	3PHO

relevant complexes is often hindered by the relatively low affinity of antibodies for carbohydrate antigens, which is generally much weaker than for proteins or peptides, and so there are limited structural data available.

A major antigenic feature on the surface of Gram-negative bacteria is lipopolysaccharide (LPS), and it is not surprising that the bulk of reported structural studies of antibody recognition of carbohydrates correspond to antibodies specific for and in complex with antigens based on carbohydrate structures found in LPS. Together with accurate assays of avidity to a range of antigens, these structures reveal not only specific mechanisms of recognition, but insight into how the immune system has evolved to balance the ability to recognize common pathogens (i.e. inherited immunity) with the need to adapt to new ones.

4.2 The Antibody Response to Carbohydrate Antigens

The diversity of the antibody response arises from V(D)J recombination in developing B-cells, in which a limited number of germline immunoglobulin (Ig) gene segments are rearranged and expressed to yield mature B-cells bearing Ig surface receptors (Fig. 4.1) (for a review see Alt and Baltimore 1982; Bonilla and Oettgen 2010; Chaudhuri and Alt 2004; Cook and Tomlinson 1995; Dudley et al. 2005; Foote and Milstein 1994; Gearhart 1982; Jacob et al. 1991; James et al. 2003; Kindt et al. 2007; Levinson 1992; Li et al. 2004; Manis et al. 2002; Muramatsu et al. 2000; Oettinger et al. 1990; Tonegawa 1983). Each circulating B-cell undergoes a single variable region Ig rearrangement, with the result that all B-cell receptors (BCR) of that cell are identical and so have the same specificity. Any B-cells that recognize self-antigens normally undergo apoptosis (Han et al. 1995; Janeway et al. 2001; Melamed and Nemazee 1997; Tsubata et al. 1993), and the remainder is therefore primed to recognize foreign antigens.

Circulating B-cells are normally dormant, but can be activated upon stimulation by cognate non-self antigen and co-stimulation by T-helper cells. Activated B-cells migrate to peripheral lymphoid organs where they undergo somatic hypermutation (SHM) of their Ig locus to produce slightly mutated daughter cells of altered affinity. Successive rounds of selection and clonal expansion of mutant daughter cells that bind antigen (a process known as affinity maturation) produces B-cells that display antibody receptors with significantly increased affinity for the stimulating antigen (Alt and Baltimore 1982; Cook and Tomlinson 1995; Gearhart 1982; Oettinger et al. 1990; Tonegawa 1983). Additional utility of the antibody response is generated during this process through class-switching to replace the heavy chain constant region of some B-cells to alter their effector functions and/or produce soluble circulating antibodies (Chaudhuri and Alt 2004; Li et al. 2004; Muramatsu et al. 2000).

In special circumstances, B-cell activation can occur without co-stimulation of T-helper cells upon stimulation by thymus-independent (TI) antigens. TI antigens, including the bacterial cell-wall components LPS and capsular polysaccharides or polymeric protein antigens (Bonilla and Oettgen 2010; Kindt et al. 2007; Mond et al. 1995a, b; Snapper and Mond 1996; Stein 1992; Vos et al. 2000), activate B-cells either by the cross-linking of BCRs or through concomitant stimulation of the BCR and the Myeloid differentiation factor-2 (MD2)/Toll-like Receptor 4 (TLR-4) receptor complex (Fig. 4.2). However, the overall humoral response to TI antigens is typically weaker than that to thymus-dependent (TD) antigens, with no generation of memory cells, affinity maturation or class-switching.

The majority of carbohydrate antigens are TI, and therefore do not by themselves induce significant affinity maturation (Mond et al. 1995b; Snapper and Mond 1996; Vos et al. 2000). As there is a limited number of germline gene segments available

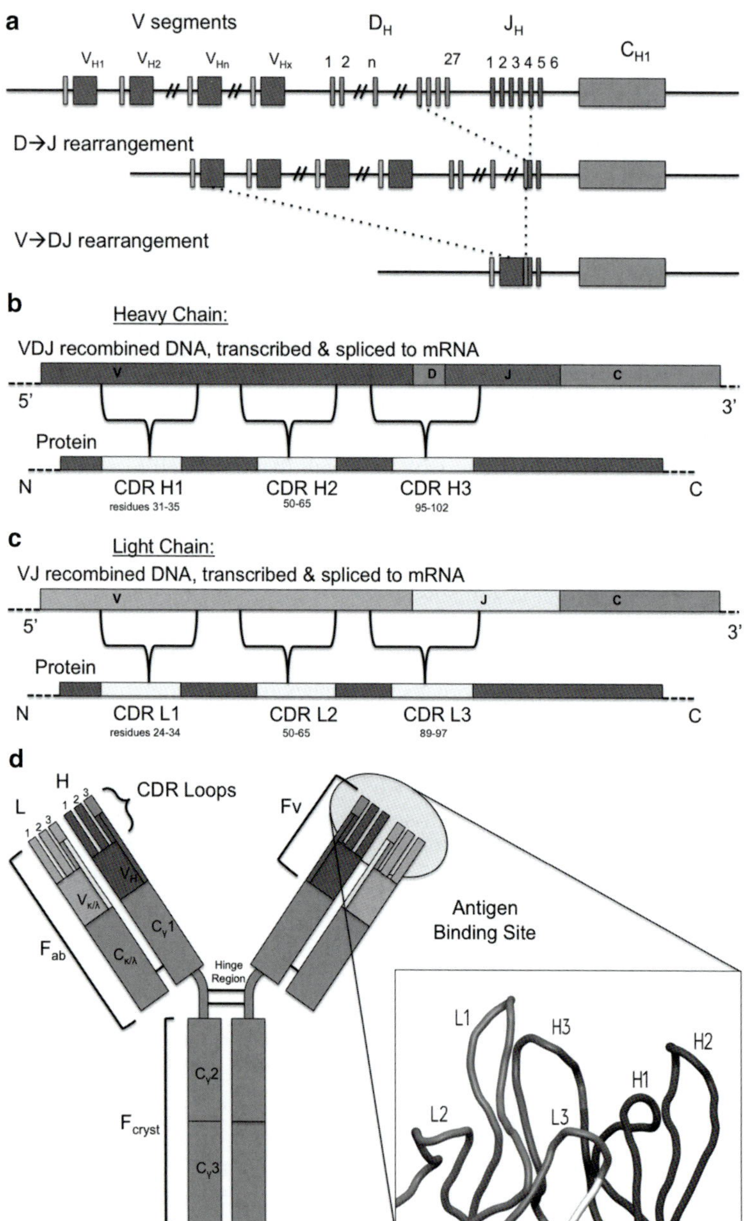

Fig. 4.1 Antibodies are generated in developing B-cells by V(D)J recombination of germline immunoglobulin gene segments (**a**). This recombined DNA is transcribed to RNA and processed and spliced with C gene segments to yield mRNA, which is translated to yield complete antibody heavy chain (**b**) or light chain (**c**), which is generated by the VJ recombination of a unique set of gene segments. The heavy and light chains are then assembled (in various orders and locations depending on the immunoglobulin class) to yield intact antibody which are directed to their final locations. An IgG molecule (**d**) is composed of two heavy chains and two light chains and is the most abundant type of serum Ig

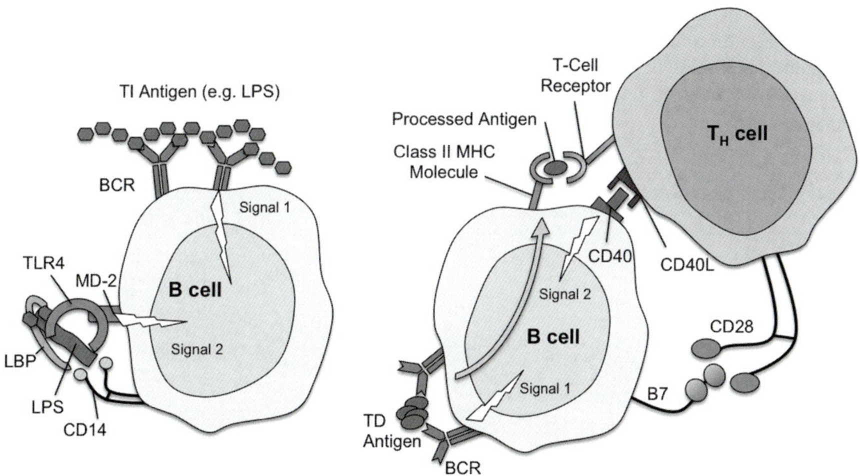

Fig. 4.2 B-cell activation, proliferation and differentiation occur in response to antigen and may occur in a T-cell independent (TI) or T-cell dependant (TD) manner. Most responses are TD and involve the processing and presentation of antigen by B-cells to T-cells and require direct contact between the two. Some antigens however, such as LPS or capsular polysaccharide, may activate B-cells in a TI manner through the cross-linking of the BCR or through both interaction with the BCR and complex formation of TLR-4 and MD-2 with acylated LPS

for the generation of antibodies to all potential antigens, evolutionary pressure would select for those gene segments that both protect against common pathogens and remain able to respond to novel threats.

Despite the large number of possible antibodies generated by combinatorial diversity through SHM (Table 4.2), the number of potential antigens the immune system may encounter has been postulated to be much larger (Sherwood 2010). Given that every antibody produced by affinity maturation to a foreign molecule must descend from a germline antibody, germline antibodies in general would be expected to display significant cross-reactivity or polyspecificity (Foote and Milstein 1994; James et al. 2003; James and Tawfik 2003; Levinson 1992; Manivel et al. 2000, 2002; Marchalonis et al. 2001; Nguyen et al. 2003; Pinilla et al. 1999).

The general inability of carbohydrate antigens to stimulate T-cell help would indicate that some portion of the germline antibody response would have evolved toward immediate recognition of carbohydrate epitopes from common pathogens. This means that carbohydrate antigens could be useful probes for the characterization of antibody cross-reactivity and polyspecificity in the germline response.

4.3 The Specificity of Anti-Carbohydrate Antibodies

Proteoglycans, glycolipids and glycoproteins are the most prominent types of cell-surface molecule (Bucior and Burger 2004; Tauber et al. 2001), as they are integral to cell-signaling, cell trafficking (Kansas et al. 1993; Ley et al. 1991), cell adhesion

Table 4.2 The diversity of the antibody response in humans and mice is generated by the recombination of a limited number of germline gene segments to produce a much larger number of unique antibodies than the germline could code for individually. This diversity is further increased by events such as somatic mutation and class-switch recombination but still does not appear great enough to match the number of possible antigens the immune system may encounter, suggesting additional means of generating diversity such as antibody cross-reactivity and polyspecificity

	Human	Mouse
Heavy chain		
V gene families	7	15
V gene segments	37	101
D gene segments	23	9
Potential reading frames	6	6
J gene segments	6	4
H chain combinations	30,636	32,724
κ light chain		
V gene families	5	18
V gene segments	35	93
J gene segments	5	3
κ light chain combinations	175	372
λ light chain		
V gene families	11	3
V gene segments	35	3
J gene segments	4	2
λ light chain combinations	140	8
Combined variable region diversity	9.6×10^6	1.2×10^7

(Jiménez et al. 2005; Kaltner and Stierstorfer 2000; Misevic and Burger 1993), cell differentiation (Cao et al. 2001; Panjwani et al. 1995; Yoshida-Noro et al. 1999), embryogenesis (Haslam et al. 2002; Schachter et al. 2002), spermatogenesis (Fenderson et al. 1984; Fukuda and Akama 2004; Scully et al. 1987), angiogenesis (Iivanainen et al. 2003; Kannagi et al. 2004; Madri and Pratt 1986), and fertilization (Ahuja 1982; Brandley and Schnaar 1986; Glabe et al. 1982). Each of these glycoconjugates is generated by glycosylation pathways of varying complexity involving one or more glycosyltransferases (Joziasse 1992; Paulson and Colley 1989; Zhao et al. 2008), and the breakdown of any of these pathways can lead to a disruption of cellular homeostasis. One mechanism credited with the prevention of associated disease is B-cell surveillance of these cell surface oligosaccharides and elimination of abnormal cells (Cohen 2007; Hakomori 1984, 1989; Hecht et al. 2009; Lang et al. 2007; Lutz 2007; Vliegenthart 2006; Vollmers and Brändlein 2007).

Neoplastic transformation often results in breakdown of the regulation of glycosylation pathways, which in turn can lead to advanced transformation and metastasis through manipulation of receptor activation, cell adhesion or cell motility (Freire et al. 2006). Some of these aberrant glycosylations are known tumor-associated-antigens (TAA) and have been well-studied for a variety of cancers (Fukuda 1996; Fung et al. 1990; Hakomori 1984, 1989, 1991, 2001; Lo-Man et al. 2004; Ramsland et al. 2004). Human antibodies are known to be capable of recognizing many of these unusual TAAs, and there is a substantial research focus in the generation of TAA-conjugate vaccines to stimulate immune responses to various cancers (Buskas et al. 2009; Danishefsky and Allen 2000; Ouerfelli et al. 2005; Roy 2004; Slovin et al. 2005).

The prevalence of carbohydrate structures on the surfaces of healthy cells leads to a degree of immune tolerance, and infectious agents can sometimes use these same structures to mask their antigenic surface proteins to evade immune surveillance (Benz and Schmidt 2002; Bhavsar et al. 2007; Sansonetti 2002; Schmidt et al. 2003). However, many antibodies to carbohydrate antigens are remarkably specific and a significant protective response against most pathogenic bacteria is still achieved through the generation of antibodies to LPS or capsular polysaccharide (Astronomo and Burton 2010; Berry et al. 2005; Casadevall et al. 1992; Cordero et al. 2011; Pirofski et al. 1995; Raetz 1990; Raetz and Dowhan 1990; Raetz and Whitfield 2002; Shaw et al. 1995).

The ability of antibodies to distinguish between closely-related antigens is exemplified in some transfusion mismatches of the human ABO(H) blood group. The antibody response to the foreign blood group antigen is often so severe as to result in fatality (Storry and Olsson 2009), yet the human A and B blood group trisaccharide antigens are nearly identical (Fig. 4.3) (Kabat 1956) and differ only in the substitution of a hydroxyl group for an acetamido group on the terminal sugar (i.e. the substitution of galactosyl for *N*-acetylgalactosaminyl). It is this potential to distinguish between closely related antigens that drives the development of carbohydrate-specific antibodies in diagnostic medicine (Holmgren et al. 1984; Manimala et al. 2005; Schellekens et al. 2000; van Ree 2000).

Although many antibodies do display high-specificity, others are known to display cross-reactivity, where antibodies raised against one antigen are able to

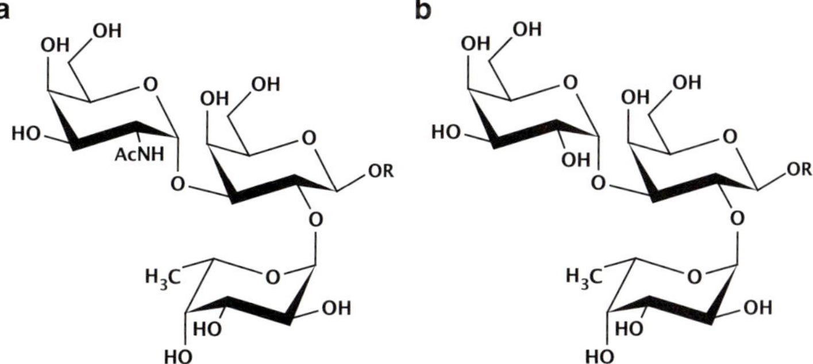

Fig. 4.3 A and B blood group trisaccharides (**a**) αGalNAc(1→3)[αFuc(1→2)]Gal and (**b**) αGal (1→3)[αFuc(1→2)]Gal differ only in the substitution of a hydroxyl group for an acetamido group on the terminal sugar, yet a transfusion mismatch is potentially fatal due to the specificity of the antibody response to these antigens

bind to chemically-related antigens or, more rarely, polyspecificity, where antibodies raised against one antigen are able to bind antigens that are not related.

This can pose serious problems, as the cross-reactivity of some antibodies is associated with certain autoimmune disorders that are triggered when antibodies are developed against infectious organisms that display an immunogen with structural similarities to self-antigens (Albert and Inman 1999; Narayanan 2000; Oldstone 2005).

Cross-reactivity and polyspecificity are postulated to take a key role in the expansion of the potential of the humoral immune system to recognize a variety of antigens (Foote and Milstein 1994; James et al. 2003; Manivel et al. 2002; Marchalonis et al. 2001) and, as we shall see, are intimately associated with the success of the antibody response to carbohydrates.

4.4 Structural Studies with Immunoglobulin Fragments

Many fundamentals of antibody structure and function were elucidated in early studies by Rodney Porter and Gerald Edelman, for which they shared the Nobel Prize in medicine in 1972 (Edelman 1991; Porter 1991; Steiner and Fleishman 2008). Following in the footsteps of Petermann and Landsteiner, who discovered that an intact immunoglobulin is not required for antigen specificity (Landsteiner 1990; Petermann 1946; Petermann and Pappenheimer 1941; Rothen and Landsteiner 1942), Porter's work on the digestion of IgG with papain revealed the multivalent nature of the immunoglobulin and established the existence of the fragments that were 'antigen binding' (Fab) and 'crystallizable' (Fc) (Fig. 4.1d) (Ceppellini et al. 1964). Edelman discovered that antibodies were composed of multiple chains cross-linked by disulfide bridges (Edelman 1959; Edelman and Poulik 1961). Further research established the 'four peptide chain structure' (two light chains and two heavy chains) of the IgG (Fleischman et al. 1963) and a more precise mapping of disulfide bridges (O'Donnell et al. 1970). In a landmark paper, Kabat showed that immunoglobulins as a group possessed six regions of hyper-variable sequence (three on the light chain and three on the heavy chain), which he hypothesized to lie at the basis of individual antibody specificity (Kabat et al. 1977).

The first antibody Fab crystal structures verified this model of the immunoglobulin, and showed that the six hypervariable regions were clustered at the terminus of each antigen-binding fragment (Poljak et al. 1973). Scores of subsequent crystallographic studies have shown the same fundamental structure (Allcorn and Martin 2002). The six regions of hypervariable sequence confirmed to be responsible for antibody specificity are now commonly referred to as 'complementarity determining regions' or CDRs, and named L1, L2, and L3, and H1, H2, and H3, corresponding to their location on the light and heavy chains, respectively (Fig. 4.1b–d). In the germline, the light chain V gene codes for CDRs L1, L2 and part of L3, with the light chain J gene also contributing to CDR L3. The coding of the heavy chain is more complex. While the heavy chain V gene codes for CDRs H1 and H2, CDR H3 is coded by the VDJ junction, which provides for an even higher level of variability that turns out to be key to the recognition of LPS.

The large database of structures of Fabs specific for a variety of antigens has made possible the characterization and classification of CDR loop conformations, and there exist methodologies for predicting the approximate conformation of each CDR based on sequence (Abhinandan and Martin 2008; Al-Lazikani et al. 1997, 2000; Chothia and Lesk 1987; Chothia et al. 1992; Nakouzi and Casadevall 2003; North et al. 2010; Tomlinson et al. 1995); however, methods to accurately predict the conformation of the entire antigen combining site have remained elusive (North et al. 2010).

While the large database of structures of Fabs in complex with proteins and peptides has allowed the molecular basis of antibody recognition of these antigens to be extensively characterized and reviewed (Davies and Cohen 1996; Davies et al. 1990; Sheriff et al. 1987; Slootstra et al. 1996; Sundberg and Mariuzza 2002; Wilson et al. 1991), there has been no corresponding exploration of the structural basis of antibody recognition of carbohydrate antigens until relatively recently.

4.5 Early Structural Studies of Carbohydrate-Specific Antibodies

In retrospect, many of the key features of antibody recognition of carbohydrate antigens were identified in the first structurally-characterized example from David Bundle's work, which was antibody Se155-4 in complex with a fragment of *Salmonella* O-antigen dodecasaccharide (Cygler et al. 1991). Previously, the structures of carbohydrate binding proteins such as enzymes and lectins (reviewed here (Quiocho 1986)) revealed extensive hydrogen bonding networks between sugar hydroxyl groups and side chains of asparagine, glutamine, arginine, glutamic and aspartic acid and lysine residues (including coordination by buried water molecules and some bifurcated hydrogen bonds), with significant contributions from van der Waals interactions and surface complementarity.

The structure of antibody Se155-4 revealed that the anti-carbohydrate antibodies could utilize additional strategies. While intricate hydrogen bond networks remained a significant force mediating the interaction, Se155-4 showed a lack of binding utilizing amino acid residues with amide or acidic/basic amino acid side chains, with the possible exception of some histidine residues. Instead, the combining site was formed almost exclusively by aromatic residues tyrosine, tryptophan, and phenylalanine, along with histidine (Fig. 4.4), and showed that an antibody can achieve relatively high affinity for carbohydrate using neutral amino acid hydrogen bonding partners.

The few crystal structures that appeared in the literature in subsequent years reinforced this general binding scheme, including antibodies against the Lewis-X blood-group (van Roon et al. 2004) and Lewis-Y tumor antigens (Ramsland et al. 2004), HIV-1 oligomannoses of GP120 (Calarese et al. 2003, 2005) and *Shigella flexneri* serotype Y O-polysaccharides (Vyas et al. 2002). All tended to display

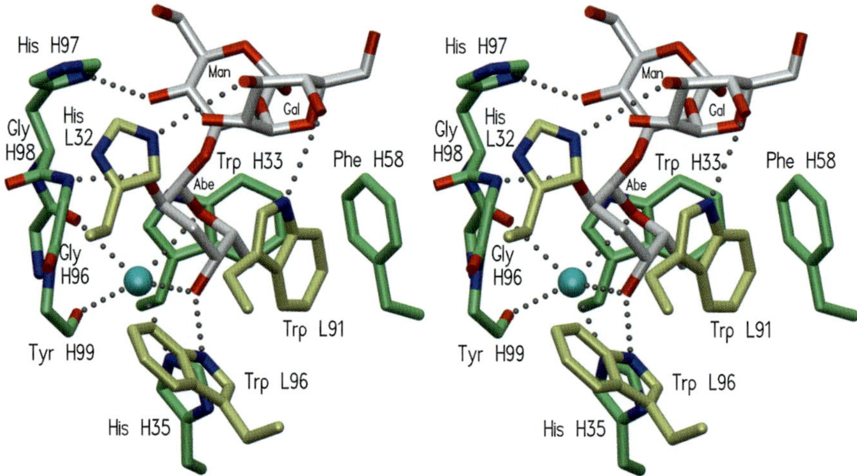

Fig. 4.4 The binding site of mAb Se155-4 (PDB code 1MFD) in complex with *Salmonella* cell-surface oligosaccharide fragment was the first structurally-characterized carbohydrate–antibody complex and revealed many of the key features of antibody recognition of carbohydrate antigens (Cygler et al. 1991)

a binding theme similar to that observed for Se155-4 (Bundle and Young 1992; Cygler et al. 1991; de Geus et al. 2009; Murase et al. 2009). In time, a few structures began to appear with some polar side chains contributing hydrogen bonds to the antigen like those seen in other carbohydrate binding proteins.

Unfortunately, the small number of structures of antibodies in complex with carbohydrate antigens and the disparate nature of their respective antigens still precluded a detailed analysis.

4.6 LPS as a Probe of the Antibody Response

Lipopolysaccharide is a highly immunogenic conserved building block of the Gram-negative outer membrane, and can be exploited as an excellent probe of the antibody response to TI carbohydrate antigens (Fig. 4.2) (Brabetz et al. 1997; Kawahara et al. 1987; Klena et al. 1993; Raetz and Whitfield 2002; Rietschel et al. 1994; Schnaitman and Klena 1993). It is present in the order of 10^6 copies per bacterium, and is crucial for the structural integrity of the membrane and for blocking serum components such as the membrane attack complex (Figueroa and Densen 1991; Kochi et al. 1991; Müller-Eberhard 1984; Podack and Tschopp 1984). Lipopolysaccharides from Enterobacteria are the prototypical example of bacterial endotoxin, and are large molecules generally divided into three components: The lipid A anchor is an acylated glucosamine disaccharide embedded in the bacterial outer membrane and is the causative agent of septic shock. Attached to the GlcN disaccharide of lipid A is a short chain of sugars called the core oligosaccharide, which is subdivided into the inner and outer core and which can vary significantly between bacterial species (Lüderitz et al. 1982; Raetz 1990; Raetz and Whitfield 2002). Last is the 'O-antigen' or the 'O-polysaccharide', which is a repeating oligosaccharide attached to the outer core that varies among bacterial strains (Brabetz et al. 1997; Heine et al. 2003; Kawahara et al. 1987; Klena et al. 1993; Lüderitz et al. 1982; Osborn 1963; Raetz 1990; Raetz and Whitfield 2002; Rietschel et al. 1994; Schnaitman and Klena 1993; Susskind et al. 1995). Under natural conditions, a functional outer membrane in Gram-negative bacteria contains atleast a (2→4) linked disaccharide of 3-deoxy-α-D-*manno*-oct-2-ulosonic acid (Kdo) or a single Kdo phosphorylated in position 4 or 5. In some species such as *Burkholderia cepacia* and certain strains of *Acinetobacter*, one of the Kdo residues may be substituted with the isosteric D-*glycero*-D-*talo*-oct-2-ulosonic acid (Ko) (Holst et al. 1995; Isshiki et al. 1998; Süsskind et al. 1995).

4.7 Antibodies to *Chlamydiaceae* LPS

Chlamydiaceae is a bacterial family containing two genera, *Chlamydia* and *Chlamydophila*, with a total of nine species representing a range of human and animal pathogens that cause a variety of diseases. The LPS of this family displays an unusual truncated LPS based on the sugar Kdo, consisting of the family-specific oligosaccharide Kdo(2→8)Kdo(2→4)Kdo, with *Chlamydophila psittaci* also displaying Kdo(2→4)Kdo(2→4)Kdo and the species-specific branched oligosaccharide Kdo(2→4)[Kdo(2→8)]Kdo(2→4)Kdo (Fig. 4.5a–c) (Brade et al. 1987; Kosma et al. 1990, 2008; Müller-Loennies et al. 2000, 2006).

The antibody response against the family-specific antigen is the basis of a diagnostic test for *Chlamydophila pneumoniae* infection in humans (Medac GmbH, Wedel, Germany). In this ELISA test glycoconjugates of oligosaccharides containing various chlamydial Kdo-based LPS epitopes are used as antigens. Such antigens have also proved useful in the immunization of BALB/c mice for generating a range of antibodies with varying specificities and affinities for Kdo and Ko containing antigens (Brade et al. 2000, 2002; Kosma et al. 1988, 1989, 1990, 1999, 2000, 2008; Maaheimo et al. 2000; Müller et al. 1997; Müller-Loennies et al. 2000, 2002, 2006). An example of the glycoconjugates used to generate these antibodies is shown in Fig. 4.5d.

4.8 Chlamydial LPS as a Probe of the Antibody Response to Carbohydrates

The germline antibody response is generally IgM, and a germline antibody (by definition) having not undergone affinity maturation is of generally lower affinity. Further, IgM itself is difficult to work with in the laboratory as enzyme digest will produce the Fv fragment in low yield, and so most studies of antibody recognition are carried out using affinity-matured IgG. Although this may seem counterintuitive, much useful information about the germline response can be obtained through these studies. First, the higher affinity of the IgG will better allow co-crystallization with the antigen of interest. Second, the class-switching that accompanies affinity maturation allows the production of large quantities of IgG that can be digested to yield the Fab fragment in high yield. Third, murine germline genes are well defined, and analysis of the antibody sequence of a successful structure determination of an antibody–antigen complex will still reveal the likely germline interactions.

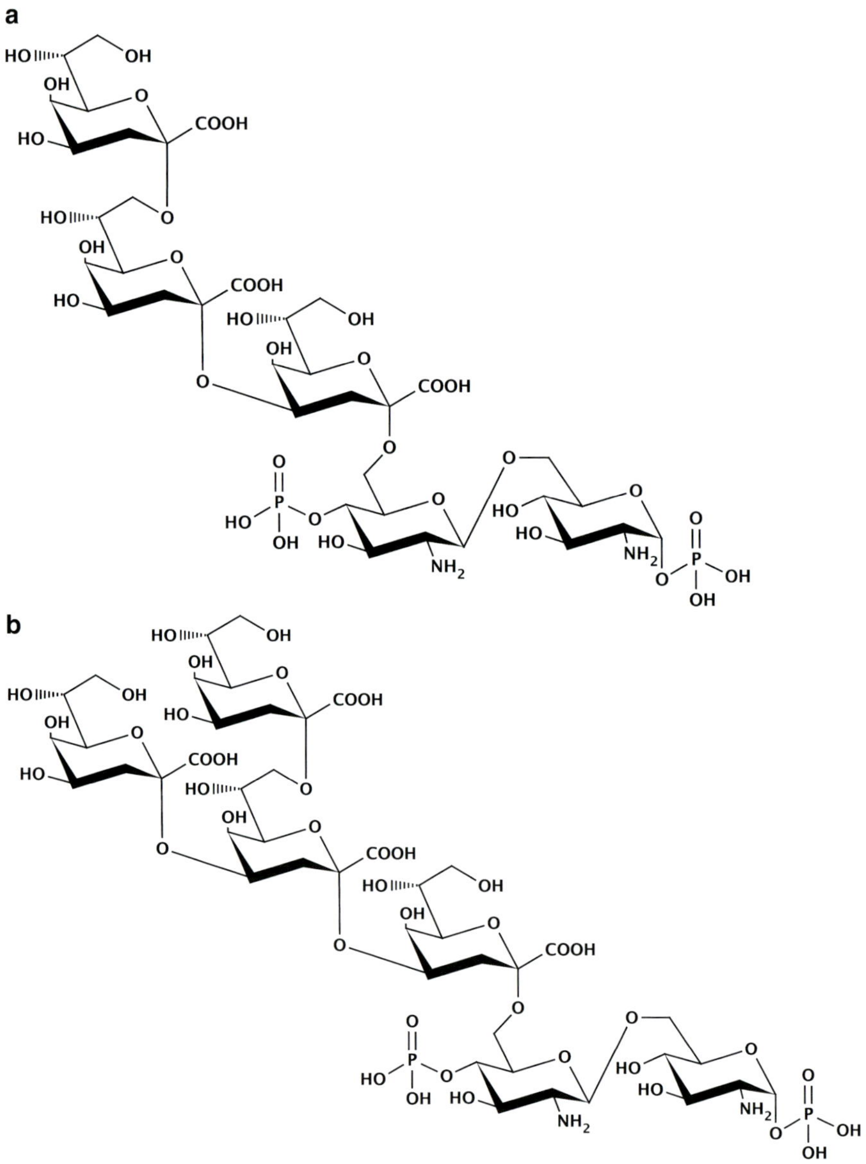

a

HO OH OH O HO COOH HO O OH O HO COOH HO OH OH O O COOH O O O P HO O OH HO O NH2 HO HO O NH2 O P O OH OH

b

HO OH OH O COOH HO OH OH O HO COOH HO O HO OH O O COOH HO OH OH O O COOH O O O P HO O OH HO O NH2 HO HO O NH2 O P O OH OH

Fig. 4.5 (continued)

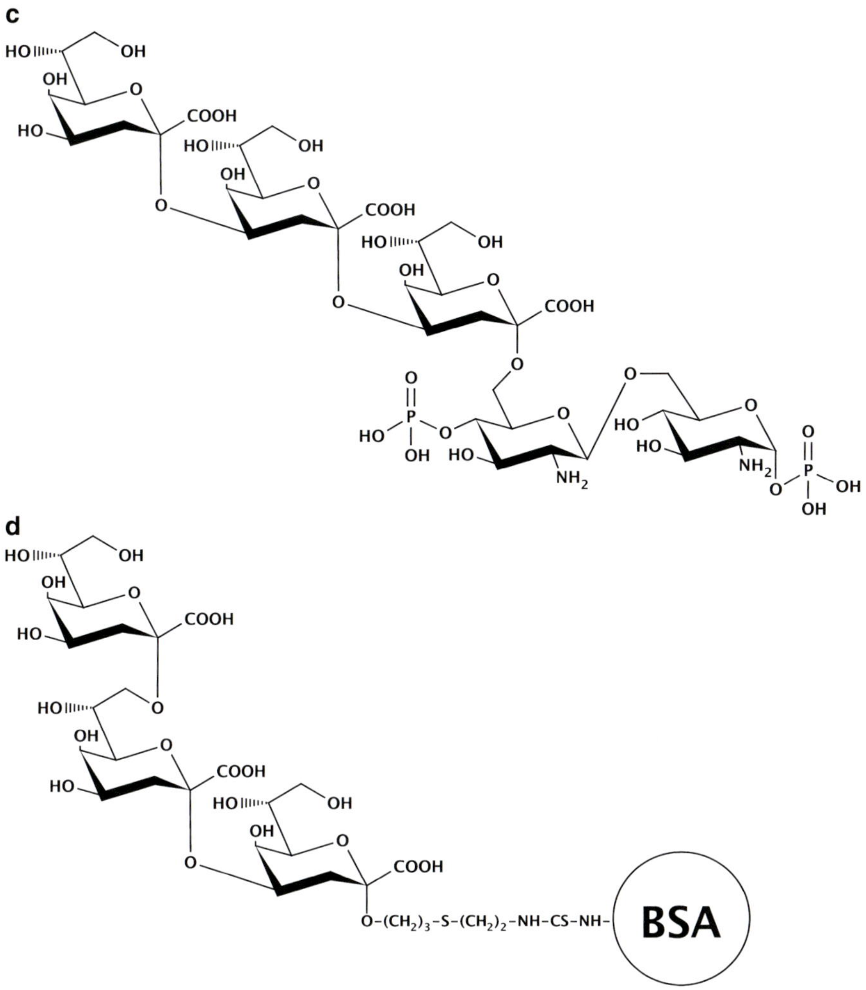

Fig. 4.5 The bacterial family *Chlamydiaceae* displays an unusual truncated LPS of (**a**) Kdo(2→8)Kdo(2→4)Kdo, (**b**) Kdo(2→4)[Kdo(2→8)]Kdo(2→4)Kdo and (**c**) Kdo(2→4)Kdo (2→4)Kdo. BSA glycoconjugates were used for murine immunization to generate large quantities of high-affinity IgG, an example being (**d**) Kdo(2→8)Kdo(2→4)Kdo–$(CH_2)_3$–S–$(CH_2)_2$–NH–CS–NH–BSA

Although carbohydrate antigens are generally T-cell independent, a T-cell response can be induced by conjugating the antigen to a protein or peptide carrier (Fung et al. 1990; Guttormsen et al. 1998; Kudryashov et al. 2001; Lo-Man et al. 2004; MacLean et al. 1992, 1993; Ni et al. 2006). This method produces a large number of soluble IgG antibodies from various germline origins with different relative avidities and specificities for antigen. The relative ease of generating Fab fragments from high-affinity IgG greatly improves the chance of co-crystallization.

A representative list of the antigens and immunogens used to raise antibodies and to test their specificity to chlamydial LPS is presented in Tables 4.3 and 4.4. A full range of natural and analogue structures were tested to investigate antibody specificity, including synthetic antigens not found in nature that could probe their cross-reactive potential (Fig. 4.6) (Foote and Milstein 1994; James et al. 2003; James and Tawfik 2003; Levinson 1992; Manivel et al. 2000, 2002; Marchalonis et al. 2001; Nguyen et al. 2003; Pinilla et al. 1999).

The sizeable panel of antibodies that was developed displayed a range of specificities. Some bound the Kdo(2→4)Kdo glycosidic linkage preferentially over the Kdo(2→8)Kdo linkage and *vice versa*. Some would only bind antigens of one or two carbohydrate residues, while others exclusively bound those greater than two residues in size. Some were highly specific for a single epitope, while some cross-reactive antibodies displayed avidity for several distinct Kdo epitopes. Together, these antibodies have provided an unparalleled opportunity to explore germline recognition of carbohydrate antigens in general (and specifically *Chlamydia* LPS antigens), and to analyze the effects of specific mutations on binding (Brooks et al. 2008a, b, 2010a, b; Gerstenbruch et al. 2010; Nguyen et al. 2001).

4.9 Related Carbohydrate Antigens Induce the Same Germline Response

The germline genes from which an affinity-matured antibody has descended can almost always be elucidated by a comparison of the nucleotide sequence of the antibody with those of the germline genes (for example, see Brochet et al. 2008). The structure of the antibody in complex with antigen can then show which conserved residues in contact with antigen were likely responsible for the germline interaction, and which residues have been mutated to increase antigen affinity.

The repeated utilization of a particular set of germline genes in response to a particular class of carbohydrate antigen is common and known as 'V-region restriction'. It has been observed for both the human and murine antibody response to capsular polysaccharides from *Haemophilus influenzae* (Adderson et al. 1991; Senn et al. 2003), *Streptococcus pneumoniae* (Shaw et al. 1995), *Cryptococcus neoformans* (Casadevall and Scharff 1991; Pirofski et al. 1995), *Neisseria meningitidis* (Berry et al. 2005), and *C. neoformans* glucuronoxylomannan (Nakouzi and Casadevall 2003). V-region restriction has been hypothesized to be a result of the limited epitope diversity of polysaccharides, being repeating units of short oligosaccharide epitopes (Zhou et al. 2002). A large proportion of antibodies raised against chlamydial LPS display V-region restriction as demonstrated by their shared germline gene segment usage (Table 4.5). Remarkably, this is true even for those antibodies raised using chemically and stereochemically distinct immunogens.

This redundant usage of germline gene segments in response to Kdo-based immunogens suggests an evolutionary conservation of a combining site predisposed

Table 4.3 Antibodies generated by immunization of BALB/c mice with LPS glycoconjugates displayed a variety of binding profiles with varying specificities when tested by ELISA with immobilized glycoconjugates of LPS antigens; some mimics of naturally occurring chlamydial LPS oligosaccharides and other unnatural variations of these epitopes

Antigen	mAb conc. (ng/mL) yielding OD_{405} >0.2 using 2 pmol/well							
	S25-2	S25-39	S45-18	S54-10	S69-4	S73-2	S67-27	S64-4
Ko	>1,000	>1,000	>1,000	>1,000	>1,000	>1,000	500	>1,000
Ko(2→4)Kdo	>1,000	>1,000	63	500	>1,000	250	63	>1,000
Kdo	500	500	16	150	>1,000	250	16	>1,000
Kdo(2→4)Kdo	500	125	2	63	>1,000	8	16	>1,000
Kdo(2→4)Kdo(2→4)Kdo	1,000	63	0.5	4	16	4	16	>1,000
Kdo(2→4)Kdo(2→4)Kdo(2→6)βGlcNAc	1,000	32	1	4	16	4	16	>1,000
Kdo(2→4)Kdo(2→4)Kdo(2→6)βGlcN4*P*(1→6)αGlcN	>1,000	63	1	8	250	8	16	500
Kdo(2→8)Kdo	250	16	4	250	>1,000	250	16	>1,000
Kdo(2→8)Kdo(2→4)Kdo	32	8	8	250	>1,000	16	16	1,000
Kdo(2→8)Kdo(2→4)Kdo(2→6)βGlcNAc	63	8	125	1,000	>1,000	500	63	>1,000
Kdo(2→8)Kdo(2→4)Kdo(2→6)βGlcN4*P*(1→6)αGlcN1*P*	63	16	1,000	>1,000	>1,000	1,000	1,000	2
Kdo(2→8)[Kdo(2→4)]Kdo(2→4)Kdo	>1,000	32	0.5	4	16	4	16	>1,000
Kdo(2→8)[Kdo(2→4)]Kdo(2→4)Kdo(2→6)βGlcN4*P*(1→6)α GlcN	>1,000	125	1	8	1,000	16	32	250
Kdo(2→8)[Kdo(2→4)]Kdo(2→4)Kdo(2→6)βGlcN4*P*(1→6)α GlcN1*P*	>1,000	32	0.5	4	63	4	16	>1,000

Table 4.4 The antibodies S25-2 and S67-27 were tested against various synthetic unnatural Kdo- and Ko-based antigens to probe the cross-reactive potential of this antibody family. Binding of Fab fragments to synthetic allyl glycoside Kdo antigens representing natural and unnatural variations of LPS epitopes were determined by SPR. S25-2 and S67-27 showed appreciable avidity for several of these antigens, and S67-27 displayed avidity for an unnatural antigen that was higher than for any natural antigen or even its cognate immunogen

Antibody/antigen	K_d (x10^{-6} M) determined by SPR
S25-2	
Kdo	15[a]
Kdo(2→8)Kdo	1.8[a]
Kdo(2→8)Kdo(2→4)Kdo	0.6[a]
Kdo(2→4)Kdo	1.1[a]
Kdo(2→4)Kdo(2→4)Kdo	63[b]
Kdo(2→4)KdoC1red	31[b]
Ko(2→4)Kdo	190[b]
KdoC1red(2→4)Kdo	290[b]
3,4-Dehydro-3,4,5-trideoxy-Kdo(2→8)Kdo	25[b]
5-Deoxy-4-epi-2,3-dehydro-Kdo(4→8)Kdo	16[b]
S67-27	
Kdo	35[b]
Kdo(2→8)Kdo	9.1[b]
7-*O*-Me-Kdo(2→8)Kdo	0.35[b]

[a]Immobilized BSA glycoconjugates
[b]Solution affinity

to the recognition of these epitopes, accentuating their importance as antigenic markers with which the immune system has co-evolved to provide 'inherited immunity'.

Interestingly, several studies have concluded that extensive somatic hypermutation can generate a large measure of paratope diversity even from a limited gene usage (Lucas et al. 2001; Reason and Zhou 2004; Zhou et al. 2002, 2004). V-region restriction appears to be an evolved strategy to provide a mechanism of broad recognition of important related carbohydrate antigens that places minimal strain on the size of the germline gene repertoire, and acts as a starting point that can mature towards specific recognition of particular epitopes of these related antigens.

4.10 V-Region Restriction to Chlamydial Antigens

One particular combination of heavy and light chain V genes repeatedly appears in response to different chlamydial LPS immunogens (Table 4.5), and results in antibodies that display a wide range of specificities and cross reactivities. As the V genes provide a largely common L1, L2, L3, H1 and H2, it can be postulated that the differences in avidity and specificity shown by these antibodies can be attributed first to the different D and J genes that code for H3, and second to mutations arising through affinity maturation.

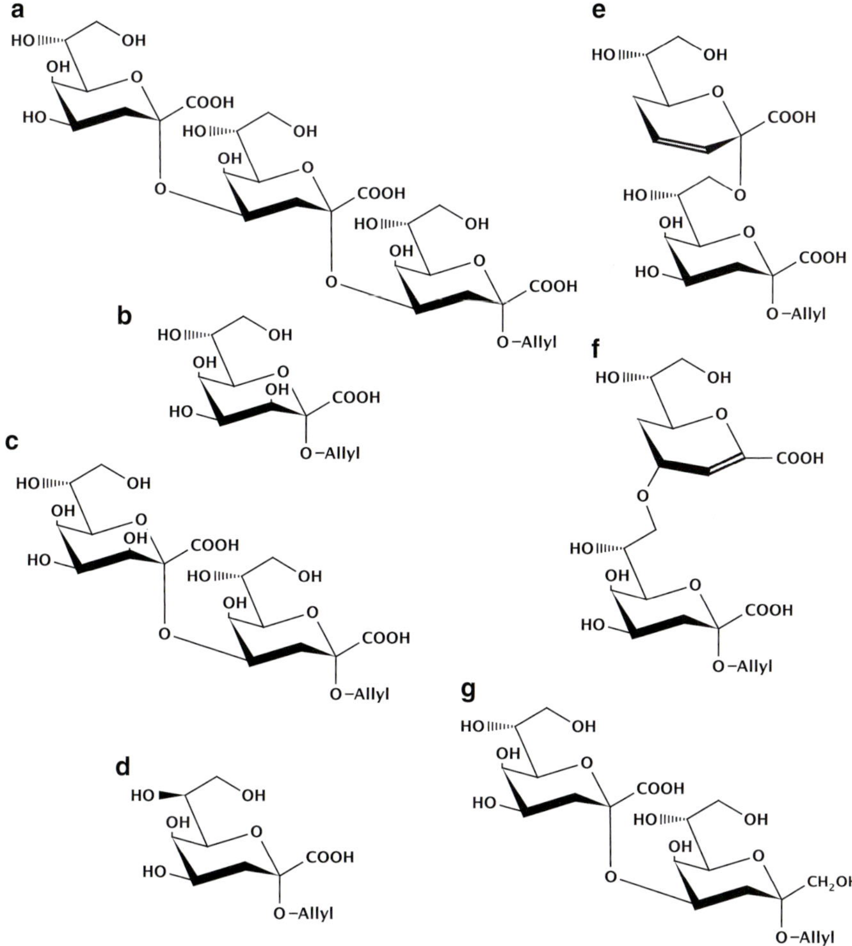

Fig. 4.6 Various natural and synthetic antigens were used to probe the cross-reactive potential of the S25-2 binding mechanism: (**a**) Kdo(2→4)Kdo(2→4)Kdo, (**b**) Ko, (**c**) Ko(2→4)Kdo, (**d**) 7-epi-Kdo, (**e**) 3,4-dehydro-3,4,5-trideoxy-Kdo(2→8)Kdo, (**f**) 5-deoxy-4-epi-2,3-dehydro-Kdo(4→8)Kdo, and (**g**) Kdo(2→4)KdoC1red

The first of this group of antibodies to be structurally characterized was the archetypical S25-2 (Brooks et al. 2008b; Nguyen et al. 2003), which is the closest of the group to germline in sequence with only three amino acid mutations (Table 4.6). This antibody was raised against Kdo(2→8)Kdo(2→4)Kdo(2→6)β GlcNAc-BSA and displays the highest avidity for Kdo antigens with a (2→8)-terminal linkage. However, S25-2 also showed weak cross-reactivity for a range of other antigens, which was exploited to generate co-crystal structures by high concentration antigen soaks. These structures provided the first indication of the versatility of the S25-2 combining site.

Table 4.5 Antibodies generated towards Ko- and Kdo-based LPS antigens display a conserved germline gene segment usage despite their generation against (sometimes significantly) distinct antigens, evidencing the presence of a Kdo/Ko binding motif evolutionary conserved in the germline

Clone	Immunogen (conjugated to BSA)	Light chain (κ)		Heavy chain		
		V gene	J gene	V gene	D gene	J gene
S25-2	Kdo(2→8)Kdo(2→4)Kdo(2→6)βGlcNAc	IGKV8-21*01	IGKJ2*02	IGHV7-3*02	IGHD2-9*01	IGHJ3*01
S25-39	Kdo(2→8)Kdo(2→4)Kdo(2→6)βGlcNAc	IGKV8-21*01	IGKJ1*01	IGHV7-3*02	IGHD2-3*01	IGHJ3*01
S45-18	Kdo(2→4)Kdo(2→4)Kdo	IGKV8-21*01	IGKJ2*02	IGHV7-3*02	IGHD1-1*01	IGHJ4*01
S54-10	Kdo(2→8)[Kdo(2→4)]Kdo(2→4)Kdo(2→6)βGlcNAc(1→6)αGlcNAc	IGKV8-21*01	IGKJ1*01	IGHV7-3*02	IGHD2-14*01	IGHJ4*01
S69-4	Kdo(2→8)[Kdo(2→4)]Kdo(2→4)Kdo	IGKV8-21*01	IGKJ1*01	IGHV7-3*02	IGHD2-4*01	IGHJ4*01
S67-27	Ko(2→4)Kdo	IGKV8-21*01	IGKJ1*01	IGHV7-3*02	IGHD1-1*02	IGHJ3*01
S73-2	Kdo(2→8)[Kdo(2→4)]Kdo	IGKV8-21*01	IGKJ1*01 or IGKJ5*01	IGHV7-3*02	IGHD2-3*01	IGHJ4*01
S64-4	Kdo(2→8)Kdo(2→4)Kdo(2→6)βGlcNAc4*P*(1→6)αGlcNAc	IGKV3-12*01	IGKJ1*01	IGHV7-3*02	IGHD2-9*01	IGHJ3*01

Table 4.6 Amino acid sequences of antibody CDR regions illustrate the high similarity of these antibodies to each other and the putative germline sequence. These antibodies have undergone varying degrees of affinity maturation and deviations from expected germline sequence are shown here in bold. It is also clear that these antibodies have their largest source of sequence diversity in the CDR H3 region, suggesting that this loop is largely responsible for antibody specificity

Clone	CDR L1	CDR L2	CDR L3		CDR H1	CDR H2	CDR H3	
	IGKV8-21*01			J gene	IGHV7-3*02			D/J genes
Germline	QSLLNSRTRKNYLA	WASTRES	CKQSYNL		GFTFTDYYMS	FIRNKANGYTTEYSAS	ARD	
S25-2	QSLLNSRTRKNYLA	WASTRES	CKQSYNL	RTF	GFTFTDYYMS	FIRNKANGYTTEYS**P**S	ARD	HDGYYE
S25-39	QSLLNSRTRKNYLA	WASTRES	CKQSYNL	RTF	GFTFTDYYMS	FIRNKA**K**GYTTEYSAS	ARD	HDGYYE
S45-18	QSLLNSRTRK**S**YLA	WAATRES	CKQSYNL	RTF	GFTFTDYYMS	FIRNK**PK**GYTTEYSAS	**V**RD	IYSFGSRD
S54-10	QSLLNSRTRKNYLA	WASTRES	CKQSYNL	RTF	GFTFTDYYMS	FIRNK**VK**GYT**ID**YSAS	ARD	MRRFDDGD
S69-4	QSLLNSRTRKNYLA	WASTRES	CKQSYNL	RTF	GFTFTDYYM**G**	FIRNKA**K**GYTTEYSAS	ARD	LIYFDYDD
S73-2	QSLLNSRTRKNYLA	WASTRES	CKQSYNL	RTF	GFTFTDYYMS	FIRNKA**K**GYTTEYSAS	ARD	INPGSDGYYD
S67-27	QSLLNSRTRKNYLA	WASTRES	CKQS**N**NL	RTF	GFTFTDYYMS	FIRNKA**K**GYTTEYSAS	ARD	ISPSYGVYYE
S64-4[a]	KSVSSSVNSYMH	LASNLES	CQHSREL	RTF	GFTFIDYYMS	FIRNK**G**NGYTTEYS**T**S	ARD	IGYGNS

[a]Deviations of S64-4 from germline light chain not shown owing to different gene usage

S25-2 was first solved in complex with ligands representing the natural chlamydial epitopes Kdo(2→8)Kdo(2→4)Kdo, Kdo(2→8)Kdo and Kdo(2→4)Kdo (Fig. 4.5), as well as with the simple Kdo monosaccharide which was placed in the crystallization drop in high concentration. In all of these structures, the terminal Kdo residue or Kdo monosaccharide was observed bound in a pocket composed almost exclusively of residues corresponding to germline sequence from CDRs H1, H2 and L3. The single residue that could not be traced to the germline sequence was Arg L96 of CDR L3 (residues are numbered according to the KabatMan numbering scheme for antibodies (Abhinandan and Martin 2008)), which is found at the VJ junction of gene segments and would therefore be prone to mutation (Chaudhuri and Alt 2004; Li et al. 2004; Muramatsu et al. 2000; Oettinger et al. 1990). The remainder of each of the antigens was bound in S25-2 by interactions with residues with flexible side chains in the remainder of the combining site (Fig. 4.7a).

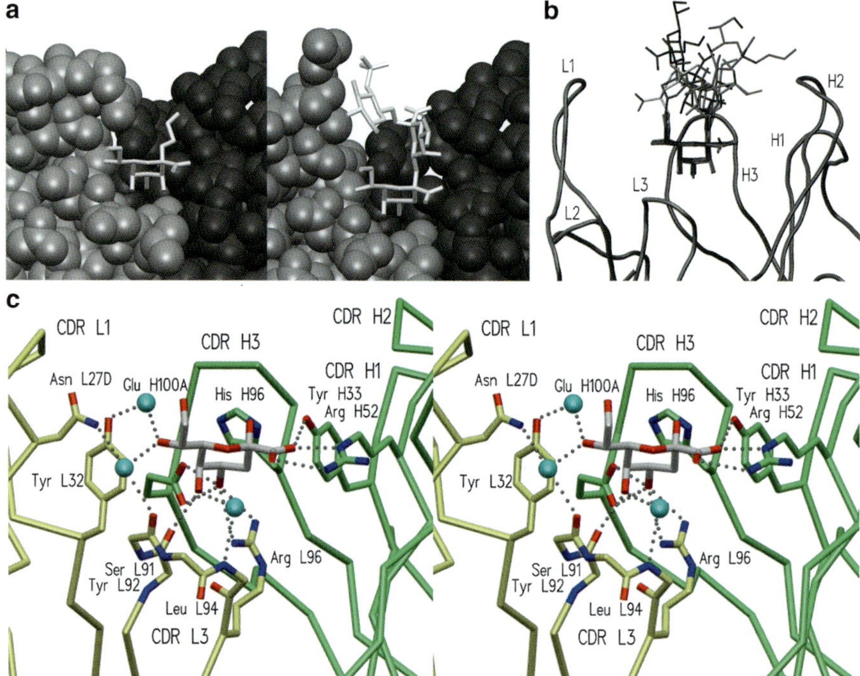

Fig. 4.7 (**a**) The S25-2 type antibody family utilizes a conserved monosaccharide pocket (*left panel*) and a flexible binding groove (*right panel*) to accommodate antigens of various size (light chain in *light grey* and the heavy chain in *dark grey*). (**b**) MAb S25-2 bound a range of natural and unnatural antigens by utilizing the conserved pocket to bind a terminal sugar and the flexible groove to accommodate the remainder of the antigens: Kdo(2→4)Kdo(2→4)Kdo, Kdo(2→8)Kdo (2→4)Kdo, Ko, Ko(2→4)Kdo, 3,4-dehydro-3,4,5-trideoxy-Kdo(2→8)Kdo, 5-deoxy-4-epi-2,3-dehydro-Kdo(4→8)Kdo, and Kdo(2→4)KdoC1red. (**c**) The S25-2 monosaccharide binding pocket uses a variety of molecular interactions to bind Kdo. The light chain is shown in *yellow* and the heavy chain in *green*. Hydrogen bonds are represented by *dashed grey* spheres. Protein backbone is displayed as an alpha-carbon trace unless other groups take part in binding. Water molecules are represented by *cyan spheres*

These structures provided the first glimpse of a recurring theme for the recognition of Kdo-containing antigens by S25-2 type antibodies, which combined a highly conserved monosaccharide binding pocket specific for a Kdo residue, with grooves that varied in sequence, shape, and flexibility surrounding the pocket capable of accommodating a range of antigens.

4.11 The Germline Pocket Binds Kdo Using Multiple Molecular Interactions

The mechanisms of recognition of the terminal sugar residue by the Kdo binding pocket in S25-2 is utilized in every antigen that it was observed to bind (Fig. 4.7b), with largely the same set of hydrogen bonds (Fig. 4.7c) despite significant shifts in relative ligand position (up to 0.7 Å).

The interactions formed with ligand by this binding pocket consist largely of hydrogen bonds and van der Waals forces as observed in previous carbohydrate–antibody complexes (Bundle et al. 1994; Calarese et al. 2003, 2005; Cygler et al. 1991; Jeffrey et al. 1995; Ramsland et al. 2004; van Roon et al. 2004; Vyas et al. 2002). Specifically, Kdo sits with the O4 hydroxyl in the base of the binding pocket where it forms hydrogen bonds to Arg L95 and Glu H100, and O5 is observed to form a hydrogen bond to the main chain oxygen of Ser L91.

Significantly, the interactions consistently included charged residue interactions with the Kdo carboxyl group (Fig. 4.7c), which forms a bidentate salt bridge with Arg H52 in addition to a hydrogen bond with Tyr H33. S25-2 was the first structurally-characterized carbohydrate-specific antibody observed to exchange charged residue interactions with the antigen (Cygler et al. 1991; Nguyen et al. 2001, 2003).

As in other antibody–antigen complexes, a limited number of coordinated water molecules also play a role in maximizing surface complementarity in the S25-2 structures, and while O7 and O8 of the terminal Kdo residue never make direct interactions with the antibody they are bridged by water molecules to Asn L27D, Arg L27F, Tyr L32 and Tyr L92. Lastly, there is an additional water molecule that sits partially under the monosaccharide and bridges O5 and ring O6 to Leu L94 main chain nitrogen. Although buried water molecules have been observed in other carbohydrate–antibody complexes (Bundle and Young 1992), none of the waters described above are completely isolated from the solvent shell.

4.12 A Flexible Groove Accommodates Additional Carbohydrate Residues

While the ability of S25-2 to cross-react with a range of chlamydial LPS antigens stems partly from the binding of a terminal Kdo residue in the conserved monosaccharide recognition pocket, its increased (and differential) affinity for the di- and trisaccharide ligands is due to their recognition by flexible side chains in the

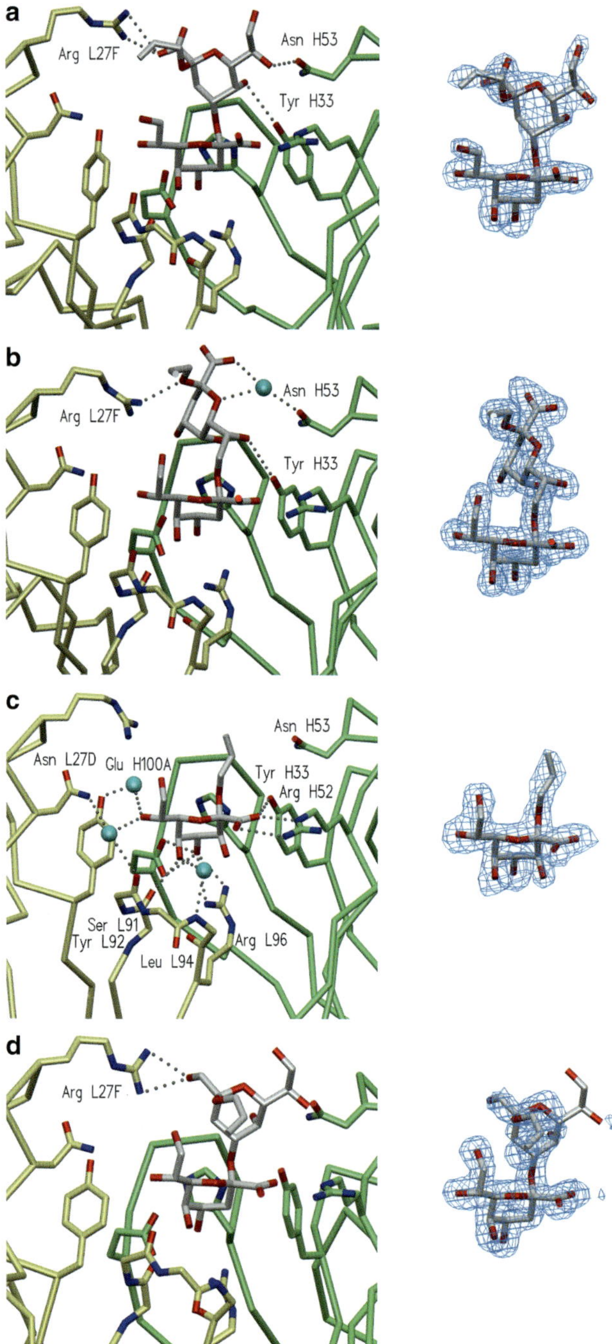

Fig. 4.8 (continued)

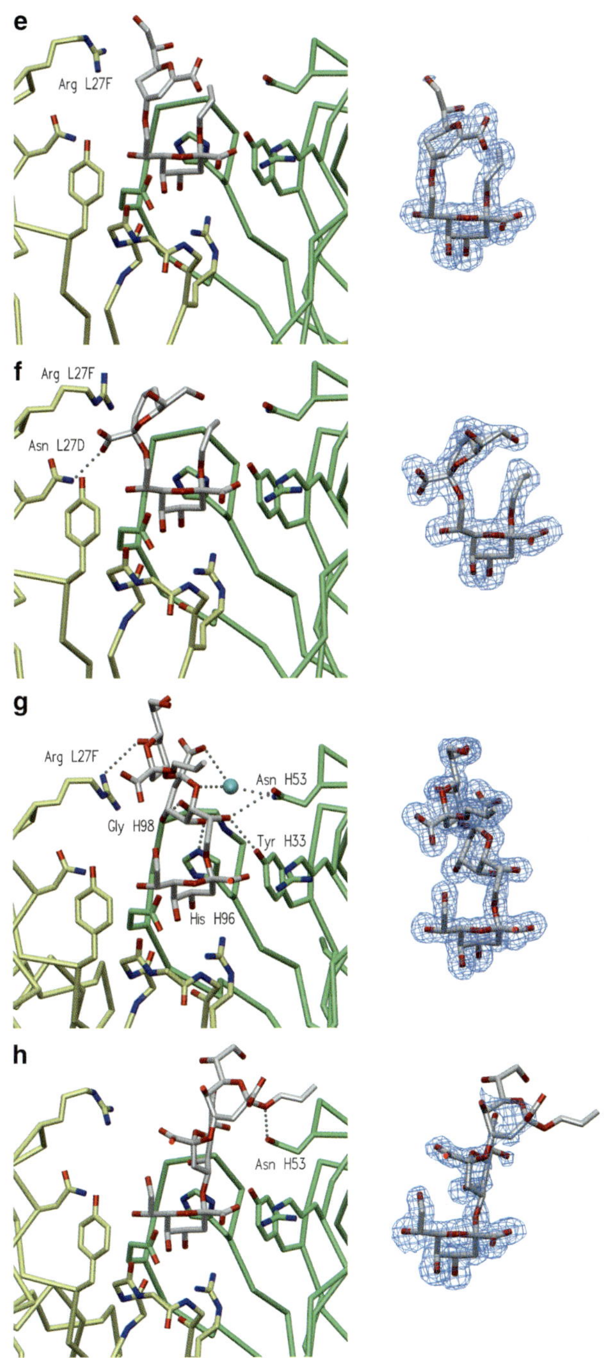

Fig. 4.8 (continued)

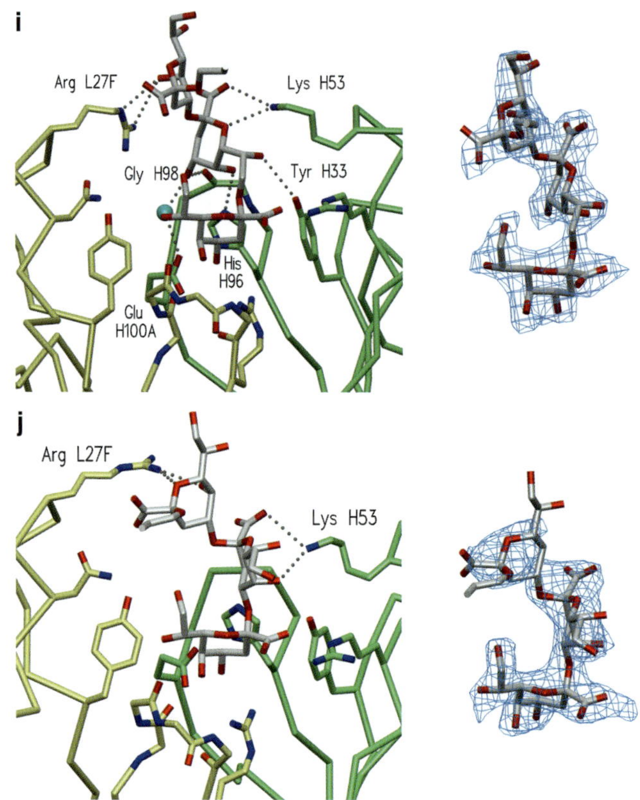

Fig. 4.8 Binding of various antigens is achieved through conserved interactions with the monosaccharide pocket and differential binding by the flexible groove. Interactions of select antibodies and antigens are shown with corresponding 2Fo-Fc σA-weighted electron density maps for antigens contoured to 1.0σ: (**a**) S25-2 and Kdo(2→4)Kdo, (**b**) S25-2 and Kdo(2→8)Kdo, (**c**) S25-2 and Ko, (**d**) Kdo(2→4)KdoC1red, (**e**) S25-2 and 5-deoxy-4-epi-2,3-dehydro-Kdo(4→8)Kdo, (**f**) S25-2 and 3,4-dehydro-3,4,5-trideoxy-Kdo(2→8)Kdo, (**g**) S25-2 and Kdo(2→8)Kdo(2→4)Kdo, (**h**) S25-2 and Kdo(2→4)Kdo(2→4)Kdo, (**i**) S25-39 and Kdo(2→8)Kdo(2→4)Kdo, and (**j**) S25-39 and Kdo(2→4)Kdo(2→4)Kdo

remainder of the combining site. Key to recognition of all of the antigens are residues Arg L27F of CDR L1 and Asn H53 of CDR H2, which interact with almost all of the antigens in different ways.

The differing glycosidic linkages of the disaccharide and trisaccharide ligands require them to lie in distinct conformations in the combining site (Figs. 4.7b and 4.8). In the case of the (2→8) linkage, the second Kdo is bound by hydrogen bonds from Asn H53 and Tyr H33 to Kdo O7, His H96 to Kdo O5, and Gly H98 to Kdo O4, with interactions to a number of bridging water molecules. The (2→4) linkage is much less favorably oriented (Table 4.3), and shows many fewer interactions (Fig. 4.8a, b).

Interestingly, while the second sugar residue of the Kdo(2→8)Kdo(2→4)Kdo trisaccharide is accommodated in much the same fashion as the (2→8) disaccharide ligand, the second residue of the Kdo(2→4)Kdo(2→4)Kdo trisaccharide adopts a significantly different position than the corresponding residue of the (2→4) disaccharide (Fig. 4.8). These different conformations are each stabilized by specific interactions, where the third Kdo residue of the Kdo(2→8)Kdo(2→4)Kdo trisaccharide interacts with the flexible side chain of Arg L27F of CDR L1 through both a hydrogen bonding and a stacking interaction, while the Kdo(2→4)Kdo(2→4)Kdo trisaccharide has a simple hydrogen bond to Asn H53.

ELISA data show that S25-2 has higher avidity for the (2→8) linked sugars over the (2→4), and much higher avidity for Kdo(2→8)Kdo(2→4)Kdo over the Kdo (2→4)Kdo(2→4)Kdo trisaccharide (Table 4.3). This is also evident in the quality of the electron density maps for the two trisaccharides in the combining site, where the Kdo(2→4)Kdo(2→4)Kdo trisaccharide clearly shows some disorder (Fig. 4.8).

Despite these observations of cross-reactivity, it is important to note that the comparison of binding to ligands as they occur in nature with the lipid A backbone reveals exclusive binding of the Kdo(2→8)Kdo(2→4)Kdo trisaccharide (Table 4.3). This is due to the bulky lipid A backbone sterically hindering the entry of smaller ligands into the binding pocket (Brooks et al. 2008b). While this is obviously very important in biological recognition scenarios, the study of cross-reactivity to the smaller ligands discussed here is still quite relevant in the examination of molecular carbohydrate–antibody recognition.

4.13 S25-2 is Permissive to Modified Epitopes and Unnatural Antigens

The ability of the near germline antibody S25-2 to cross-react with distinct epitopes primarily through the action of a monosaccharide binding pocket of conserved sequence (Nguyen et al. 2003) appears to be an evolved strategy for general recognition of Kdo-containing foreign antigens, and indicates that antibodies like S25-2 can serve as a starting point for affinity maturation for many Kdo-containing and Kdo-like antigens. This is apparent in the power of this pocket to recognize modified and unnatural Kdo ligands like those in Fig. 4.6 (Brooks et al. 2008b).

Remarkably, the S25-2 Kdo pocket was observed to accommodate significant alterations of its cognate immunogen. Slightly modified monosaccharide ligands that bound S25-2 included Ko, a natural carbohydrate differing from Kdo by an additional hydroxyl at carbon 3 (Fig. 4.8c), and the 7-epi-Kdo diastereomer. Both of these ligands showed slight changes in binding mode albeit with slight (7-epi-Kdo) or significant (Ko) decreases in avidity (Table 4.3).

Disaccharides with modifications of non-terminal Kdo residues such as Kdo (2→4)KdoC1red displayed appreciable avidity (Table 4.4), and structural analysis showed that flexible side chains lining the combining site groove could accommodate the unnatural antigens as long as a terminal Kdo was present on the antigen to bind in the monosaccharide pocket (Fig. 4.8d). Compounds with significantly altered terminal sugar residues were observed to bind in an "upside-down" orientation, so instead of the terminal modified Kdo analogue occupying the monosaccharide binding pocket the second Kdo residue was observed bound (Fig. 4.8e, f).

Although the Kdo monosaccharide binding pocket observed in the first structures of S25-2 bound to the natural antigens was initially hypothesized to offer specific recognition by a germline antibody of a single sugar residue on a foreign antigen from which highly-specific antibodies could be developed by affinity maturation (Nguyen et al. 2003), the pocket turned out to be surprisingly adaptable and would recognize modified and non-terminal Kdo residues (Brooks et al. 2008b).

4.14 S25-2 Utilizes an Unusual CDR L3 Canonical Conformation

The conformations of the CDRs of the first antibody structures were organized by Chothia and Lesk into approximately 25 canonical classes in 1987 (Al-Lazikani et al. 1997, 2000; Chothia and Lesk 1987; Chothia et al. 1992; Tomlinson et al. 1995). These classifications have been expanded and revised as the number of antibody structures solved increased (Decanniere et al. 1999, 2000; Favre et al. 1999; Guarné et al. 1996; Harmsen et al. 2000; Kuroda et al. 2009; Shirai et al. 1996; Vargas Madrazo and Paz 2002). A new 'clustering' scheme for CDR conformations has recently been developed that increases the classic 25 canonical conformations to 72 clusters (North et al. 2010). The CDR conformations found in the S25-2 type antibodies generally fall into the original canonical structures with the exception of CDR L3, which adopts a somewhat unusual form. The CDR H3 loops have not been analyzed for canonical forms due to their diversity among these structures, and the difficulty in doing so due to the hypervariable nature of CDR H3. That being said, there has been progress in the classification of CDR H3 conformations and there exist many resources for their determination (Morea et al. 1998; North et al. 2010; Shirai et al. 1996, 1999).

This unusual CDR L3 conformation arises from a nucleotide mutation at the junction of light chain V and J genes, causing the germline proline to be replaced by arginine in every antibody of the S25-2 family (Fig. 4.9). Interestingly, the

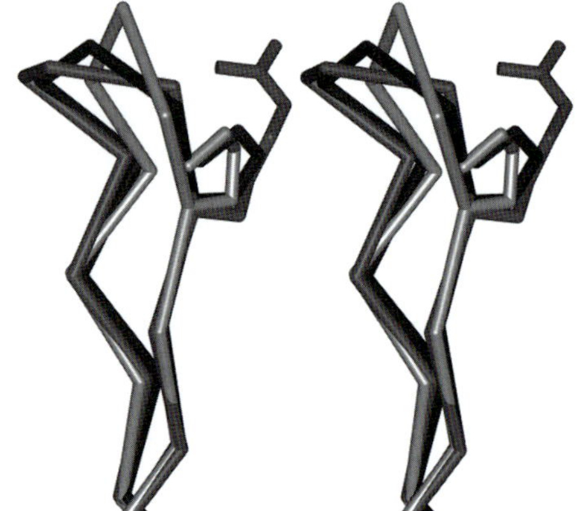

Fig. 4.9 The S25-2 type antibodies make use of an unusual CDR L3 canonical structure, Class 6, to bind Kdo ligands; displayed here is a superposition of CDR L3 canonical structures Chothia Class 3 Subtype A (*light grey*; PDB: 1YQV), Subtype B (*dark grey*; PDB: 1EO8) and Class 6, or Cluster L3-8-1 (*medium grey*; PDB 3IJY, S67-27 of S25-2 family)

mutation of proline to arginine that is key to forming the Kdo monosaccharide binding site also lies at the center of efforts to refine the classification of the canonical conformations. As the canonical forms of CDR L3 are largely based on the presence and location of key proline residues (Guarné et al. 1996), their absence can profoundly affect loop conformations (North et al. 2010). CDR L3 of all S25-2 type antibodies lies in a canonical family deemed Class 6, in which this key proline is absent (Guarné et al. 1996; Vargas Madrazo and Paz 2002).

4.15 Modest Levels of Somatic Mutation can Significantly Improve Binding

All of the S25-2 type antibodies sequenced to date are further from germline than S25-2 itself, but the range of specificities they display stems not only from affinity maturation of the heavy and light chain V regions, but from different D and J genes that code for alternate CDR H3 loops.

MAb S25-39 has the same heavy and light chain V genes as well as the same heavy chain J gene as S25-2. Although the two antibodies utilize different D genes, the resulting CDRs H3 are identical in sequence. The result is an antibody-combining site that is nearly identical to that of S25-2 with a single mutation that corresponds to a change from germline of asparagine H53 to lysine (Table 4.6). Interestingly, this single mutation does not significantly affect the specificity of S25-39, but is associated with a general increase in avidity across a range of antigens (Table 4.3). The terminal (2→8) linked ligands show an increase in avidity of 15-fold for the disaccharide and fourfold for the trisaccharide, while the (2→4) linked ligands show an increase in avidity of fourfold for the disaccharide and 16-fold for the trisaccharide (Table 4.3).

The structures of the various antibody–antigen complexes reveal that Lys H53 in S25-39 forms additional strong hydrogen bonds and/or charged residue interactions with the second Kdo residue of every oligosaccharide antigen (Fig. 4.8i, j). The increased avidity of binding is consistent with the quality of electron density for corresponding (2→4) ligands (Fig. 4.8g–j). In addition, S25-39 binds the (2→4) trisaccharide in the expected conformation, with Kdo2 bound by Lys H53 and Kdo3 by Arg L27F. In contrast, S25-2 showed no significant interaction with Kdo2 and Kdo3 of this antigen, which was observed in an unusual conformation with Kdo2 and Kdo3 rotated approximately 180° from their positions in complex with S25-39 and bending towards Asn H53 of CDR H2.

An important aspect of antigen binding by these antibodies stems from the differing conformational freedom of the (2→4) and (2→8) glycosidic linkages, and the ability of the antibody binding grooves to accommodate low-energy conformations of these flexible antigens (Bock et al. 1992; Haselhorst et al. 1999; Maaheimo et al. 2000). The germline residue Asn H53 of S25-2 was not long enough to stabilize Kdo2 in a position that would also allow optimal positioning of Kdo3 for interaction with Arg L27F of CDR L1 on the other side of the binding groove. However, the longer and more flexible Lys H53 of S25-39 does allow for this optimal positioning of both Kdo2 and Kdo3, and this is reflected in the 16-fold increase in avidity and improved observed electron density (Table 4.3 and Fig. 4.8).

The NH53K mutation is the result of a single nucleotide substitution in the germline sequence of T→A that alters the codon from AAU (Asn) to AAA (Lys). Given the ease with which it can be achieved and the resulting significant increases in binding avidities, it is interesting that this particular mutation was found to be common among the antibodies raised against glycoconjugates containing carbohydrate epitopes of chlamydial LPS, where 11 of the 21 antibodies of this group with known sequence contain this mutation.

It is significant that this single mutation in the combining site of the weakly cross-reactive S25-2 results in clear cross-reactivity of S25-39 toward a range of Kdo-containing antigens (Table 4.3), which emphasizes the potential of the germline monosaccharide pocket as a starting point for affinity maturation.

There are a few other common mutations observed among the S25-2 group of antibodies, but none so prominent or with such apparent effect on binding as lysine at H53. The key residues of the Kdo monosaccharide binding pocket are highly conserved in the germline, suggesting that this site is already optimized for the recognition of Ko or Kdo-containing antigens. Mutation of the remainder of the antigen binding site through affinity maturation would provide a clear path for the development of antibodies of higher affinity and altered specificity; however, this does not take into account the equally evolved response found in the D and J genes that codes for CDR H3.

4.16 CDR H3 Significantly Affects Specificity

The conserved monosaccharide pocket is the defining feature of S25-2 antibodies as it provides specific recognition of a common epitope of the chlamydial LPS. The pocket makes up a portion of the combining site coded by the V genes and the remainder of the site certainly contributes to and modulates antigen binding; however, it is CDR H3 that is largely responsible for S25-2 type antibody specificity.

CDR H3 is generally well known to strongly influence the specificity of antibodies, as unique loops arise from the hypervariable nature of the VDJ interface (Fig. 4.1) (Alt and Baltimore 1982; Brooks et al. 2010a; Gearhart 1982; Li et al. 2004; Oettinger et al. 1990; Webster et al. 1994; Wedemayer et al. 1997; Xu and Davis 2000). One landmark study revealed that switching the CDR H3 of otherwise identical IgM molecules can dramatically alter their specificities for haptens and protein antigens (Xu and Davis 2000).

The study of the S25-2 type antibodies reveals that not only are the unique interactions *via* CDR H3 important in most antigen recognition scenarios, but the shape of CDR H3 has a significant influence in directing the antigen binding site towards specificity or cross-reactivity. The importance of combining site architecture in actual antigen recognition scenarios of these pathogens cannot be understated due to the context-dependent presentation of these antigens linked to the bulky lipid A backbone. We will see that this also comes into consideration with alternate light chain V genes.

4.17 An Inward CDR H3 Tilt Precludes Binding of Certain Epitopes

S45-18 is an S25-2 type antibody and so shares the same heavy and light chain V genes, but possesses D and J genes that code for a different CDR H3 (Tables 4.5 and 4.6). Whereas S25-2 was raised against an antigen with a (2→8) terminal linkage, this antibody was raised against the Kdo(2→4)Kdo(2→4)Kdo trisaccharide and it shows high avidity for (2→4) terminal ligands. The differences in binding specificities between S45-18 and S25-2 (Table 4.3) can be attributed to the different CDR H3 sequence and conformation.

The structure of S45-18 in complex with the Kdo(2→4)Kdo(2→4)Kdo trisaccharide shows that the terminal Kdo residue is recognized by the same monosaccharide binding pocket as in S25-2. However, while S25-2 has a comparatively short CDR H3 and an open combining site, the longer CDR H3 of S45-18 bends inwards and forms a more restricted pocket (Figs. 4.10a and 4.11). Further, it possesses a key phenylalanine residue at position H99 that protrudes into the combining site to form favorable stacking interactions with the Kdo(2→4)Kdo(2→4)Kdo trisaccharide antigen (Fig. 4.10a). These interactions are not available with the Kdo(2→8)Kdo(2→4) Kdo trisaccharide due to the alternate length and conformational freedom of the (2→8) linkage, and so binding of this antigen is less favored (Table 4.3).

The S25-2 type antibodies S54-10, S73-2 and S67-27 also contain longer CDR H3 loops (Table 4.6). Interestingly, S54-10 showed strikingly similar specificity to S45-18, but with a different CDR H3. The structure of S54-10 in complex with the Kdo(2→4)Kdo(2→4)Kdo trisaccharide antigen again showed a CDR H3 with an inward bend (Fig. 4.11). Remarkably, the similarity of the binding profile could be traced to the protrusion of a phenylalanine residue into the combining site at the same position as observed in S45-18 to form similar stacking interactions with (2→4) ligands and again impede the binding of (2→8) ligands.

The presence in the germline of multiple DJ combinations that give rise to similar binding motifs indicates that there must be a survival advantage conferred by a redundant repertoire specific for pathogens displaying these Kdo-based markers.

4.18 An Outward Tilt to CDR H3 Encourages Cross-Reactivity

S73-2 and S67-27 possess CDR H3 loops that are both longer and with different sequence than S45-18 or S54-10 (Table 4.6). Structural studies show that they lean away from the Kdo specificity pocket in both antibodies (Fig. 4.11). Interestingly, these antibodies both adopt a backward leaning CDR H3 despite their being raised with different immunogens; S73-2 with a sterically-challenging branched Kdo trisaccharide, and S67-27 with the comparatively small Ko(2→4)Kdo disaccharide

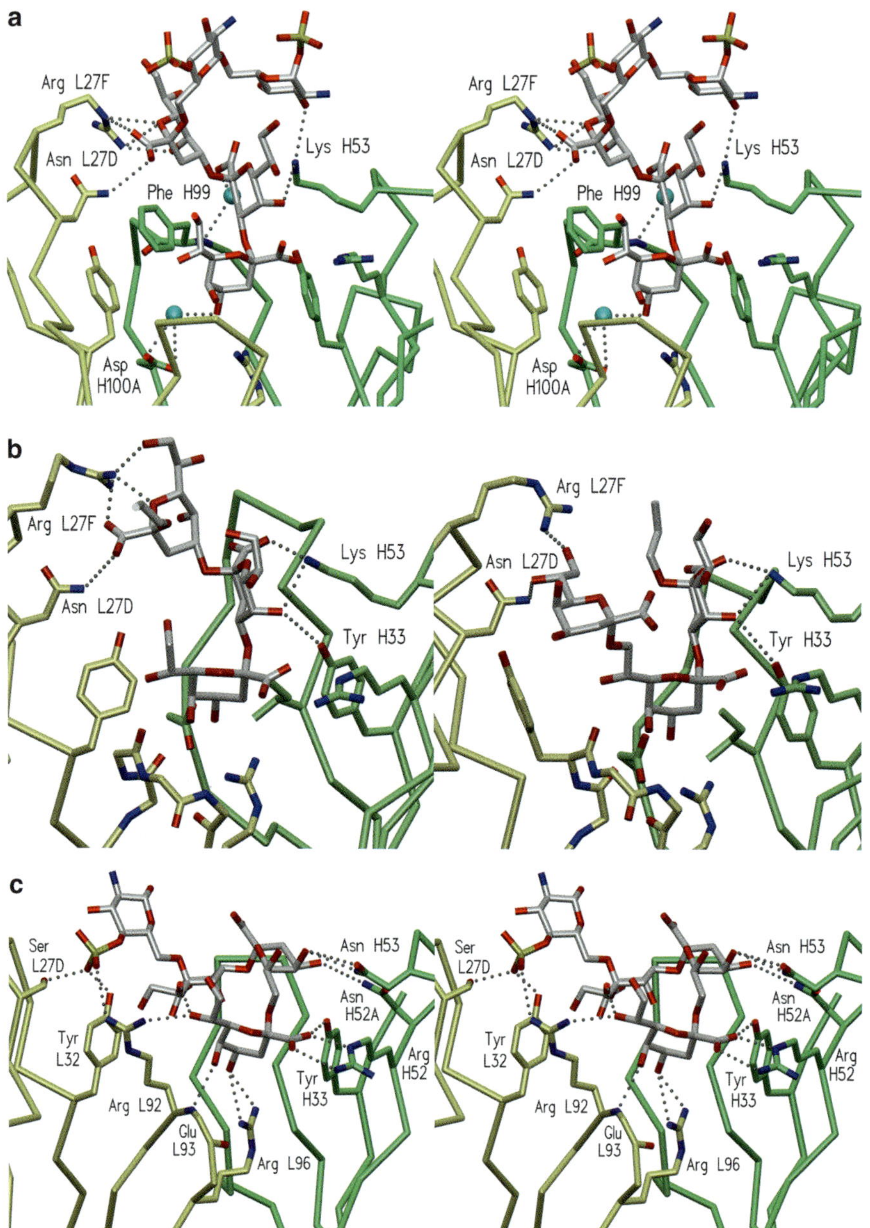

Fig. 4.10 The antibodies raised against Kdo-based glycoconjugates show various specificities and cross-reactivites for certain epitopes. (**a**) S45-18 binds the antigen Kdo(2→4)Kdo(2→4)Kdo (2→6)βGlcN4*P*(1→6)αGlcN in an 'upright' position similar to the binding of other antigens by S25-2 type antibodies. (**b**) S73-2 binds Kdo(2→4)Kdo(2→4)Kdo (*left panel*) in the expected 'upright' position, but displays cross-reactivity for an unusual bent epitope of Kdo(2→8)Kdo (2→4)Kdo (*right panel*) by recognizing an internal Kdo in the conserved pocket. (**c**) S64-4 binds the same antigen as S45-18; Kdo(2→8)Kdo(2→4)Kdo(2→6)βGlcN4*P*(1→6)αGlcN1*P*, but uses a different light chain V gene to recognize a different 'flattened' epitope (only four sugars modeled here)

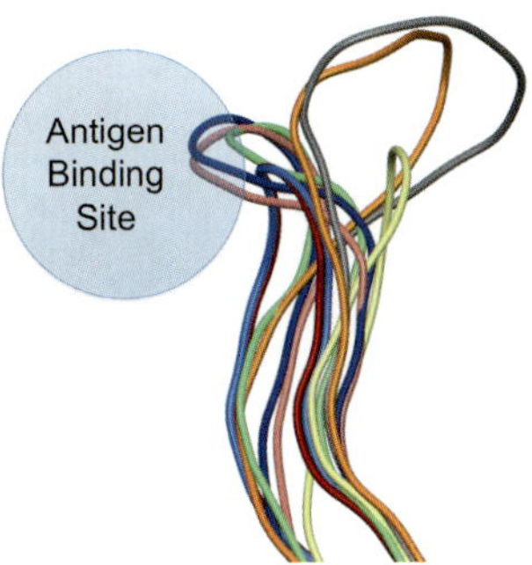

Fig. 4.11 The greatest source of diversity among these antibodies is in the sequences of CDR H3, and differential binding interactions and modulation of antigen binding site architecture directs their respective binding profiles. A CDR H3 overlap of all antibodies with the antigen binding site indicated displays the differences in loop conformations: S67-27 (*grey*), S73-2 (*orange*), S64-4 (*yellow*), S54-10 (*light green*), S69-4 (*dark blue*), S45-18 (*salmon*), S25-2 (*light blue*) and S25-39 (*red*)

(Table 4.5). Unlike S45-18 and S54-10, S73-2 uses CDR H3 only to interact with the terminal Kdo residue, and this CDR forms no other interactions with antigen (Figs. 4.10b and 4.11). S73-2 binds Kdo(2→4)Kdo(2→4)Kdo in an orientation similar to that observed with S25-39, but remarkably the Kdo(2→8)Kdo(2→4)Kdo trisaccharide antigen adopts a bent conformation with the internal second Kdo residue bound in the specificity pocket (Fig. 4.10b). This is probably due to the fact that the outward bending CDR H3 in S73-2 would not facilitate interactions with the second and third residues of the Kdo(2→8)Kdo(2→4)Kdo trisaccharide antigen if it were bound in the previously observed fashion. By locating the central residue of the antigen in the specificity pocket, the terminal Kdo forms interactions with CDRs L1 and L3 resulting in all three residues forming interactions with the antibody.

S73-2 also contains the common somatic mutation NH53K described earlier for S25-39 that allows for strong interactions with the second Kdo residue of the oligosaccharide antigens, but in the case of Kdo(2→8)Kdo(2→4)Kdo it is the carboxylic acid group of the third Kdo residue with which it forms a strong charged residue interaction. It is evident that the CDR H3 of S73-2 does not provide enough stabilization for a linear conformation of Kdo(2→8)Kdo(2→4)Kdo with the terminal Kdo in the conserved binding pocket, and therefore cross-reacts with this alternate folded epitope to maximize antibody–antigen contacts.

4.19 An Unusual CDR H3 Conformation Exposes Hydrophobic Residues

S67-27 was an antibody that cross-reacted with most Kdo-based epitopes tested with comparable avidity (Table 4.3). Of great interest was one synthetic unnatural antigen, 7-*O*-methyl-Kdo(2→8)Kdo disaccharide, which bound to S67-27 with

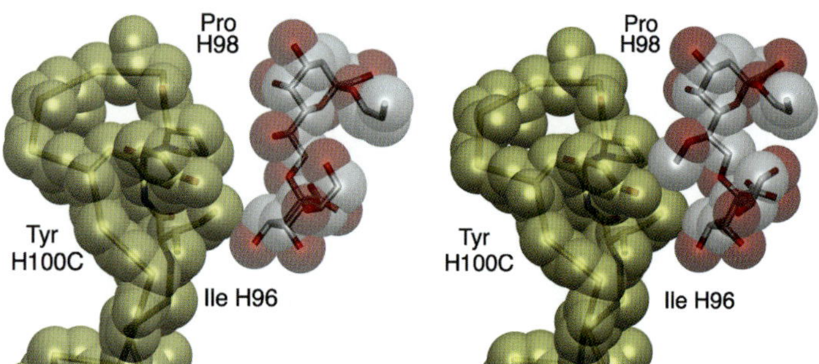

Fig. 4.12 The CDR H3 of S67-27 forms additional surface contacts with the synthetic antigen 7-O-Me-Kdo(2→8)Kdo (*right panel*) that are not present with Kdo(2→8)Kdo (*left panel*), resulting in an increased avidity for this unnatural ligand

a 30-fold higher avidity than any other antigen tested, including the immunogen against which the antibody was raised (Table 4.4).

The structure of S67-27 in complex with a number of antigens showed that, like S73-2, it possessed a CDR H3 several residues longer than those previously seen. However, while it too was oriented away from the combining site (Figs. 4.11 and 4.12) the bend was more pronounced than that in S73-2. This resulted in a relatively 'open' combining site that allowed recognition of many antigens with (2→4) and (2→8) linked terminal Kdo residues.

Interestingly, the high avidity of the unnatural 7-*O*-Me-Kdo(2→8)Kdo analog can be traced to its methoxy group, which is directed toward the base of CDR H3 where it is buried in the hydrophobic residues Ile H96, Pro H98 and part of Tyr H100C that were exposed by a backward tilt of the CDR (Fig. 4.12). S67-27 represents another demonstration of the adaptability of the germline gene segments to antigens it is unlikely to have encountered.

4.20 Antibody Specificity and Affinity Maturation

It has been proposed that germline antibodies have a greater tendency toward cross-reactivity, and that the specificity of an antibody tends to increase as affinity maturation progresses (James and Tawfik 2003; Manivel et al. 2000). There is structural evidence that specificity can be modulated through conformational diversity, such as one study where an affinity-matured antibody and its putative germline precursor were each crystallized in the presence and absence of the antigen. While the germline antibody showed significant induced fit, the matured antibody did not (James et al. 2003).

It is difficult to draw comparisons with the antibodies specific for chlamydial LPS as many of them utilize D and J genes that code for unrelated CDRs H3; however, it can be said that some architectures of some CDRs H3 seem to be predisposed for selective antibodies while others are predisposed to being more cross-reactive, before any consideration of the changes brought by affinity maturation.

4.21 Induced Fit of CDR H3 in Antigen Recognition

It has been proposed that conformational flexibility of germline CDRs H3 can generate additional diversity in the antibody response by adopting alternate conformations that are able to recognize distinct antigens. In theory, these different conformations could recognize unique antigens and subsequently undergo structural rigidification *via* affinity maturation to generate a specific lock-and-key type receptor for each antigen (Babor and Kortemme 2009; James et al. 2003; James and Tawfik 2003; Jiménez et al. 2004; Manivel et al. 2000, 2002; Marchalonis et al. 2001; Nguyen et al. 2003; Pinilla et al. 1999). However, induced fit of the antibody combining site upon antigen binding is thermodynamically unfavorable as it introduces an 'entropic penalty' by causing a flexible polypeptide loop to become ordered. Structurally-observable induced fit in antibodies is rare (Debler et al. 2007; Rini et al. 1992; Stanfield et al. 1993; Stanfield and Wilson 1994; van den Elsen et al. 1999), but some of the most dramatic examples in the literature have been observed in antibodies S25-2 and S25-39, two antibodies binding their ligands with nanomolar affinity.

The homologous antibodies S25-2 and S25-39 share an identical CDR H3 sequence (Table 4.6), and while all liganded structures of both antibodies have a common conformation of the combining site, the unliganded structures of S25-2 and S25-39 together show three different conformations that are each different from that seen in the liganded structures (Fig. 4.13).

Most reported instances of induced fit are simple side chain rotamers, although there are a few reports of major rearrangement of backbone configuration (James et al. 2003; James and Tawfik 2003; Rini et al. 1992; Stanfield et al. 1993; Stanfield

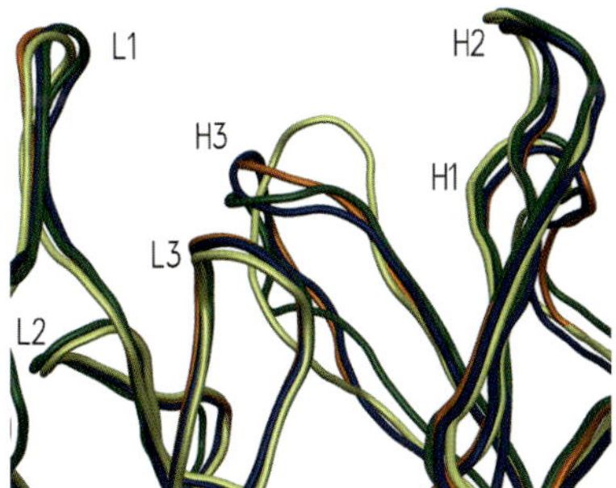

Fig. 4.13 The antibodies S25-2 and S25-39 share an identical CDR H3 sequence and utilize a common conformation for the recognition of Kdo antigens. However, each of these antibodies display unique, well-ordered, unliganded conformations different than that induced by antigen binding. A superposition is shown of the combining sites of unliganded S25-2 (two forms; *orange* and *blue*), unliganded S25-39 (*green*), and the liganded conformation shared by both (*yellow*)

and Wilson 1994; van den Elsen et al. 1999; Webster et al. 1994). Two unliganded crystal forms of S25-2 and one of S25-39 yield three distinct conformations for the CDR H3, each with appropriate electron density that all fold in towards the combining site with respect to the liganded conformation (Fig. 4.13). The level of induced fit is remarkable, with a Cα RMSD difference as large as 3.31 Å (calculated for the 15 residues from Cys H92 to Tyr H102; equal to CDR H3 plus one residue on either side), indicating that the CDR H3 shared by S25-2 and S25-39 is conformationally variable in solution, but assumes a specific conformation when induced by any Kdo-based antigen with which it has been crystallized.

Interestingly, the observation of appropriate electron density for these alternate conformations indicates that the CDR H3 of S25-2 and S25-39 is not completely labile, but possesses a small number of low energy conformers that may each allow for the recognition of a unique class of ligand. Such a strategy would allow multiple combining sites from a single gene segment combination, and offset an entropic penalty by the strategic advantage of expanding the repertoire of bound antigens without the need to increase the germline repertoire of BCRs. Also, an entropic penalty in this case would likely be less significant than that associated with the immobilization of a completely labile loop (Rini et al. 1992).

4.22 Different V Gene Combinations Recognize Kdo-Based Antigens

The examples of V-region restriction discussed so far utilize the same combination of heavy and light chain V genes with a number of D and J genes; however, the antibody response to chlamydial LPS produces a number of V gene combinations. Most intriguing was a smaller subset that displays V-region restriction using the same heavy chain V gene in combination with a different light chain V gene (Table 4.5). One antibody of this group that has been crystallized in the presence of antigen is S64-4 (Evans et al. 2011).

Remarkably, although the new light chain V gene is not homologous with the S25-2 type antibodies, S64-4 displays a similar Kdo monosaccharide binding site. Arg L96 at the light chain V–J interface in S25-2 is maintained in S64-4, and also interacts with Kdo O4. In the S25-2 type antibodies, Ser L91 of CDR L3 hydrogen bonds with O5 of Kdo, and this interaction is replaced by Glu L93 in S64-4. The interactions from the ligand to the heavy chain correspond to those in S25-2, with the exception of Glu H100E in CDR H3 which does not participate in binding by S64-4 (Fig. 4.10c).

Although S64-4 is so far unique among these antibodies in that it shows no interaction between antigen and CDR H3, the antibody still displays a conserved Kdo binding pocket. This would appear to be at odds with observations that CDR H3 tends to dominate antigen binding and define specificity (Trinh et al. 1997); however, in a narrow sense this is still true in S64-4 as it is critical that CDR H3 bend away from the pocket to allow its utilization by a novel conformation of the antigen.

Despite the conservation of these interactions in the Kdo pocket, this antibody does not show any observable binding to anything less than a Kdo trisaccharide antigen with a (2→6) linked GlcN4*P*(1→6)GlcN1*P* of the lipid A backbone attached (Table 4.3). This can be traced to the change in architecture of the antigen binding site given by the different light chain V gene, where CDR L1 bends away from the monosaccharide pocket to yield an open combining site. This effect is enhanced by an outward-leaning CDR H3 (Figs. 4.10c and 4.11), and the result is a combining site that cannot form extensive interactions with smaller ligands. This antibody has been crystallized with Kdo(2→8)Kdo(2→4)Kdo(2→6)GlcN4*P* (1→6)GlcN1*P*, which is accommodated by Arg L92 of CDR L3 and by Tyr L32 and Ser L27D of CDR L1.

S64-4 achieves its length requirement by binding the antigen in a conformation different from that observed with the S25-2 type antibodies (Fig. 4.10a–c). This alternate conformation arranges the saccharide residues along the open antigen binding site, which results in a large number of interactions and surface complementarity. The phosphate moiety of GlcN4*P* is key to recognition, as it forms extensive interactions with the antibody.

S64-4 binds Kdo(2→8)Kdo(2→4)Kdo(2→6)GlcN4*P*(1→6)GlcN1*P* with at least eight times higher avidity than any S25-2 type antibody, most of which show very poor binding (Table 4.3), which demonstrates the value of this particular V-region combination. The presence in the germline of a redundant strategy for the generation of a Kdo-specific site that can recognize this antigen is offset by the concomitant changes to CDR L1 that allow for tighter binding to longer ligands, and the general expansion of the recognition potential of the germline repertoire (Stanfield and Wilson 1994; van den Elsen et al. 1999; Webster et al. 1994).

Conclusions

Structural studies of a group of related antibodies raised against chlamydial LPS structures have allowed an examination of the mechanisms of carbohydrate recognition by germline antibodies. By combining a simple Kdo recognition pocket coded into the germline in at least one heavy and two light chain V genes with differential CDR H3 loops and the power of somatic hypermutation and affinity maturation, it is possible to glimpse how the humoral response can balance adaptability and specificity in the anti-carbohydrate response.

First, these structures show a remarkable mechanism for the recognition of Kdo-containing antigens that combines a conserved monosaccharide binding pocket that recognizes a Kdo residue through an amalgamation of hydrogen bonds, charged residue interactions, bridging water molecules and hydrophobic interactions, with a groove above this pocket on the remainder of the combining site that is composed of flexible (usually charged) amino acid side chains able to accommodate the remainder of a range of different antigens. Simple mutations accrued though affinity maturation may significantly improve binding, as accomplished by the NH53K mutation by forming interactions with the second

Kdo residue. The combination of two different light chain V genes with a single heavy chain V gene revealed how this simple strategy could expand the range of Kdo-based antigens that could be effectively and specifically recognized.

A critical factor in determining specificity is CDR H3, which can modulate the specificity by forming unique interactions with certain epitopes. As well, CDR H3 strongly influences combining site architecture, which may either be constricted for the sake of specificity, or expanded for the sake of cross-reactivity. Unique CDR H3 loops can recognize the same antigen in a similar manner, as with S45-18 and S54-10, or in a completely different conformation, as seen with S73-2, revealing how the germline has evolved to be both redundant and adaptable in providing protection against conserved antigens and defending against new threats.

Acknowledgments This work was supported in part by grants from the Natural Sciences and Engineering Research Council of Canada (SVE), the Deutsche Forschungsgemeinschaft grant SFB 470/C1 (SML and HB) and from the Austrian Science Fund FWF-grants P17407 and P19295 (PK). SVE is the recipient of Senior Scholarship from the Michael Smith Foundation for Health Research. The technical assistance of U. Agge, N. Harmel, Ch. Schneider and V. Susott is gratefully acknowledged.

References

Abhinandan KR, Martin ACR (2008) Analysis and improvements to Kabat and structurally correct numbering of antibody variable domains. Mol Immunol 45:3832–3839

Adderson EE, Shackelford PG, Quinn A, Carroll WL (1991) Restricted Ig H chain V gene usage in the human antibody response to *Haemophilus influenzae* type b capsular polysaccharide. J Immunol 147:1667–1674

Ahuja KK (1982) Fertilization studies in the hamster: the role of cell-surface carbohydrates. Exp Cell Res 140:353–362

Albert LJ, Inman RD (1999) Molecular mimicry and autoimmunity. N Engl J Med 341:2068

Al-Lazikani B, Lesk AM, Chothia C (1997) Standard conformations for the canonical structures of immunoglobulins. J Mol Biol 273:927–948

Al-Lazikani B, Lesk AM, Chothia C (2000) Canonical structures for the hypervariable regions of T cell αβ receptors. J Mol Biol 295:979–995

Allcorn LC, Martin ACR (2002) SACS – self-maintaining database of antibody crystal structure information. Bioinformatics 18:175–181

Alt FW, Baltimore D (1982) Joining of immunoglobulin heavy chain gene segments: implications from a chromosome with evidence of three D-JH fusions. Proc Natl Acad Sci USA 79:4118–4122

Astronomo RD, Burton DR (2010) Carbohydrate vaccines: developing sweet solutions to sticky situations? Nat Rev Drug Discov 9:308–324

Avci FY, Kasper DL (2010) How bacterial carbohydrates influence the adaptive immune system. Annu Rev Immunol 28:107–130

Babor M, Kortemme T (2009) Multi constraint computational design suggests that native sequences of germline antibody H3 loops are nearly optimal for conformational flexibility. Proteins 75:846–858

Benz I, Schmidt MA (2002) Never say never again: protein glycosylation in pathogenic bacteria. Mol Microbiol 45:267–276

Berry JD, Boese DJ, Law DK, Zollinger WD, Tsang RS (2005) Molecular analysis of monoclonal antibodies to group variant capsular polysaccharide of Neisseria meningitidis: recurrent heavy chains and alternative light chain partners. Mol Immunol 42:335–344

Bhavsar AP, Guttman JA, Finlay BB (2007) Manipulation of host-cell pathways by bacterial pathogens. Nature 449:827–834

Bock K, Thomsen JU, Kosma P, Christian R, Holst O, Brade H (1992) A nuclear magnetic resonance spectroscopic investigation of Kdo-containing oligosaccharides related to the genus-specific epitope of *Chlamydia* lipopolysaccharides. Carbohydr Res 229:213–224

Bonilla FA, Oettgen HC (2010) Adaptive immunity. J Allergy Clin Immunol 125:S33–S40

Brabetz W, Müller-Loennies S, Holst O, Brade H (1997) Deletion of the heptosyltransferase genes rfaC and rfaF in *Escherichia coli* K-12 results in an Re-type lipopolysaccharide with a high degree of 2-aminoethanol phosphate substitution. Eur J Biochem 247:716–724

Brade H, Brade L, Nano FE (1987) Chemical and serological investigations on the genus-specific lipopolysaccharide epitope of *Chlamydia*. Proc Natl Acad Sci USA 84:2508–2512

Brade L, Rozalski A, Kosma P, Brade H (2000) A monoclonal antibody recognizing the 3-deoxy-D-manno-oct-2-ulosonic acid (Kdo) trisaccharide Kdo(2→4)Kdo(2→4)Kdo of *Chlamydophila psittaci* 6BC lipopolysaccharide. J Endotoxin Res 6:361–368

Brade L, Gronow S, Wimmer N, Kosma P, Brade H (2002) Monoclonal antibodies against 3-deoxy-α-D-manno-oct-2-ulosonic acid (Kdo) and D-glycero-α-D-talo-oct-2-ulosonic acid (Ko). J Endotoxin Res 8:357–364

Brandley BK, Schnaar RL (1986) Cell-surface carbohydrates in cell recognition and response. J Leukoc Biol 40:97–111

Brochet X, Lefranc MP, Giudicelli V (2008) IMGT/V-QUEST: the highly customized and integrated system for IG and TR standardized V–J and V–D–J sequence analysis. Nucleic Acids Res 36:W503–W508

Brooks CL, Blackler RJ, Gerstenbruch S, Kosma P, Müller-Loennies S, Brade H, Evans SV (2008a) Pseudo-symmetry and twinning in crystals of homologous antibody Fv fragments. Acta Crystallogr D Biol Crystallogr 64:1250–1258

Brooks CL, Müller-Loennies S, Brade L, Kosma P, Hirama T, MacKenzie CR, Brade H, Evans SV (2008b) Exploration of specificity in germline monoclonal antibody recognition of a range of natural and synthetic epitopes. J Mol Biol 377:450–468

Brooks CL, Blackler RJ, Sixta G, Kosma P, Müller-Loennies S, Brade L, Hirama T, MacKenzie CR, Brade H, Evans SV (2010a) The role of CDR H3 in antibody recognition of a synthetic analog of a lipopolysaccharide antigen. Glycobiology 20:138–147

Brooks CL, Müller-Loennies S, Borisova SN, Brade L, Kosma P, Hirama T, Mackenzie CR, Brade H, Evans SV (2010b) Antibodies raised against chlamydial lipopolysaccharide antigens reveal convergence in germline gene usage and differential epitope recognition. Biochemistry 49:570–581

Bucior I, Burger MM (2004) Carbohydrate–carbohydrate interactions in cell recognition. Curr Opin Struct Biol 14:631–637

Bundle DR, Young NM (1992) Carbohydrate–protein interactions in antibodies and lectins. Curr Opin Struct Biol 2:666–673

Bundle DR, Eichler E, Gidney MA, Meldal M, Ragauskas A, Sigurskjold BW, Sinnott B, Watson DC, Yaguchi M, Young NM (1994) Molecular recognition of a *Salmonella* trisaccharide epitope by monoclonal antibody Se155-4. Biochemistry 33:5172–5182

Buskas T, Thompson P, Boons GJ (2009) Immunotherapy for cancer: synthetic carbohydrate-based vaccines. Chem Commun 36:5335–5349

Calarese DA, Scanlan CN, Zwick MB, Deechongkit S, Mimura Y, Kunert R, Zhu P, Wormald MR, Stanfield RL, Roux KH (2003) Antibody domain exchange is an immunological solution to carbohydrate cluster recognition. Science 300:2065–2071

Calarese DA, Lee HK, Huang CY, Best MD, Astronomo RD, Stanfield RL, Katinger H, Burton DR, Wong CH, Wilson IA (2005) Dissection of the carbohydrate specificity of the broadly neutralizing anti-HIV-1 antibody 2G12. Proc Natl Acad Sci USA 102:13372–13377

Cao Z, Zhao Z, Mohan R, Alroy J, Stanley P, Panjwani N (2001) Role of the Lewis x glycan determinant in corneal epithelial cell adhesion and differentiation. J Biol Chem 276: 21714–21723

Casadevall A, Scharff MD (1991) The mouse antibody response to infection with *Cryptococcus neoformans:* VH and VL usage in polysaccharide binding antibodies. J Exp Med 174:151–160

Casadevall A, Mukherjee J, Devi SJ, Schneerson R, Robbins JB, Scharff MD (1992) Antibodies elicited by a *Cryptococcus neoformans*–tetanus toxoid conjugate vaccine have the same specificity as those elicited in infection. J Infect Dis 165:1086–1093

Ceppellini R, Dray S, Edelman G, Fahey J, Franek F, Franklin E, Goodman HC, Grabar P, Gurvich AE, Heremans JF (1964) Nomenclature for human immunoglobulins. Immunochemistry 1:145–149

Chaudhuri J, Alt FW (2004) Class-switch recombination: interplay of transcription, DNA deamination and DNA repair. Nat Rev Immunol 4:541–552

Chothia C, Lesk AM (1987) Canonical structures for the hypervariable regions of immunoglobulins. J Mol Biol 196:901–917

Chothia C, Lesk AM, Gherardi E, Tomlinson IM, Walter G, Marks JD, Llewelyn MB, Winter G (1992) Structural repertoire of the human VH segments. J Mol Biol 227:799–817

Cohen IR (2007) Biomarkers, self-antigens and the immunological homunculus. J Autoimmun 29: 246–249

Collot M, Wilson IB, Bublin M, Hoffmann-Sommergruber K, Mallet JM (2010) Synthesis of cross-reactive carbohydrate determinants fragments as tools for in vitro allergy diagnosis. Bioorg Med Chem 19:1306–1320

Cook GP, Tomlinson IM (1995) The human immunoglobulin VH repertoire. Immunol Today 16: 237–242

Cordero RJ, Frases S, Guimaraes AJ, Rivera J, Casadevall A (2011) Evidence for branching in cryptococcal capsular polysaccharides and consequences on its biological activity. Mol Microbiol 79(4):1101–1117

Cygler M, Rose DR, Bundle DR (1991) Recognition of a cell-surface oligosaccharide of pathogenic *Salmonella* by an antibody Fab fragment. Science 253:442–445

Danishefsky SJ, Allen JR (2000) From the laboratory to the clinic: a retrospective on fully synthetic carbohydrate-based anticancer vaccines. Angew Chem Int Ed Engl 39:836–863

Davies DR, Padlan EA, Sheriff S (1990) Antibody–antigen complexes. Annu Rev Biochem 59: 439–473

Davies DR, Cohen GH (1996) Interactions of protein antigens with antibodies. Proc Natl Acad Sci USA 93:7–12

de Geus DC, van Roon AM, Thomassen EA, Hokke CH, Deelder AM, Abrahams JP (2009) Characterization of a diagnostic Fab fragment binding trimeric Lewis X. Proteins 76:439–447

Debler EW, Kaufmann GF, Kirchdoerfer RN, Mee JM, Janda KD, Wilson IA (2007) Crystal structures of a quorum-quenching antibody. J Mol Biol 368:1392–1402

Decanniere K, Desmyter A, Lauwereys M, Ghahroudi MA, Muyldermans S, Wyns L (1999) A single-domain antibody fragment in complex with RNase A: non-canonical loop structures and nanomolar affinity using two CDR loops. Structure 7:361–370

Decanniere K, Muyldermans S, Wyns L (2000) Canonical antigen-binding loop structures in immunoglobulins: more structures, more canonical classes? J Mol Biol 300:83–91

Dudley DD, Chaudhuri J, Bassing CH, Alt FW (2005) Mechanism and control of V(D)J recombination versus class switch recombination: similarities and differences. Adv Immunol 86:43–112

Ebo DG, Hagendorens MM, Bridts CH (2004) Sensitization to cross reactive carbohydrate determinants and the ubiquitous protein profilin: mimickers of allergy. Clin Exp Allergy 34: 137–144

Edelman GM (1959) Dissociation of γ-globulin. J Am Chem Soc 81:3155–3156

Edelman GM, Poulik MD (1961) Studies on structural units of the γ-globulins. J Exp Med 113: 861–884

Edelman GM (1991) Antibody structure and molecular immunology. Scand J Immunol 34:4–22

Evans DW, Müller-Loennies S, Brooks CL, Brade L, Kosma P, Brade H, Evans SV (2011) Structural insights into parallel strategies for germline antibody recognition of lipopolysaccharide from *Chlamydia*. Glycobiology 21(8):1049–1059

Favre M, Moehle K, Jiang L, Pfeiffer B, Robinson JA (1999) Structural mimicry of canonical conformations in antibody hypervariable loops using cyclic peptides containing a heterochiral diproline template. J Am Chem Soc 121:2679–2685

Fenderson BA, O'Brien DA, Millette CF, Eddy EM (1984) Stage-specific expression of three cell surface carbohydrate antigens during murine spermatogenesis detected with monoclonal antibodies. Dev Biol 103:117–128

Figueroa JE, Densen P (1991) Infectious diseases associated with complement deficiencies. Clin Microbiol Rev 4:359–395

Fleischman JB, Porter RR, Press EM (1963) The arrangement of the peptide chains in γ-globulin. Biochem J 88:220–228

Foetisch K, Westphal S, Lauer I, Retzek M, Altmann F, Kolarich D, Scheurer S, Vieths S (2003) Biological activity of IgE specific for cross-reactive carbohydrate determinants. J Allergy Clin Immunol 111:889–896

Foote J, Milstein C (1994) Conformational isomerism and the diversity of antibodies. Proc Natl Acad Sci USA 91:10370–10374

Freire T, Bay S, Vichier-Guerre S, Lo-Man R, Leclerc C (2006) Carbohydrate antigens: synthesis aspects and immunological applications in cancer. Mini Rev Med Chem 6:1357–1373

Fukuda M (1996) Possible roles of tumor-associated carbohydrate antigens. Cancer Res 56: 2237–2244

Fukuda MN, Akama TO (2004) The role of N-glycans in spermatogenesis. Cytogenet Genome Res 103:302–306

Fung P, Madej M, Koganty RR, Longenecker BM (1990) Active specific immunotherapy of a murine mammary adenocarcinoma using a synthetic tumor-associated glycoconjugate. Cancer Res 50:4308–4314

Gearhart PJ (1982) Generation of immunoglobulin variable gene diversity. Immunol Today 3: 107–112

Gerstenbruch S, Brooks CL, Kosma P, Brade L, MacKenzie CR, Evans SV, Brade H, Müller-Loennies S (2010) Analysis of cross-reactive and specific anti-carbohydrate antibodies against lipopolysaccharide from *Chlamydophila psittaci*. Glycobiology 20:461–472

Glabe CG, Grabel LB, Vacquier VD, Rosen SD (1982) Carbohydrate specificity of sea urchin sperm binding: a cell surface lectin mediating sperm–egg adhesion. J Cell Biol 94:123–128

Guarné A, Bravo J, Calvo J, Lozano F, Vives J, Fita I (1996) Conformation of the hypervariable region L3 without the key proline residue. Protein Sci 5:167–169

Guttormsen HK, Wetzler LM, Finberg RW, Kasper DL (1998) Immunologic memory induced by a glycoconjugate vaccine in a murine adoptive lymphocyte transfer model. Infect Immun 66: 2026–2032

Hakomori S (1984) Tumor-associated carbohydrate antigens. Annu Rev Immunol 2:103–126

Hakomori S (1989) Aberrant glycosylation in tumors and tumor-associated carbohydrate antigens. Adv Cancer Res 52:257–331

Hakomori S (1991) Possible functions of tumor-associated carbohydrate antigens. Curr Opin Immunol 3:646–653

Hakomori S (2001) Tumor-associated carbohydrate antigens defining tumor malignancy: basis for development of anti-cancer vaccines. Adv Exp Med Biol 491:369–402

Han S, Zheng B, Dal Porto J, Kelsoe G (1995) In situ studies of the primary immune response to (4-hydroxy-3-nitrophenyl) acetyl. IV. Affinity-dependent, antigen-driven B cell apoptosis in germinal centers as a mechanism for maintaining self-tolerance. J Exp Med 182:1635–1644

Harmsen MM, Ruuls RC, Nijman IJ, Niewold TA, Frenken LGJ, de Geus B (2000) Llama heavy-chain V regions consist of at least four distinct subfamilies revealing novel sequence features. Mol Immunol 37:579–590

Haselhorst T, Espinosa JF, Jimenez-Barbero J, Sokolowski T, Kosma P, Brade H, Brade L, Peters T (1999) NMR experiments reveal distinct antibody-bound conformations of a synthetic disaccharide representing a general structural element of bacterial lipopolysaccharide epitopes. Biochemistry 38:6449–6459

Haslam SM, Gems D, Morris HR, Dell A (2002) The glycomes of *Caenorhabditis elegans* and other model organisms. Biochem Soc Symp 69:117–134

Hecht ML, Stallforth P, Silva DV, Adibekian A, Seeberger PH (2009) Recent advances in carbohydrate-based vaccines. Curr Opin Chem Biol 13:354–359

Heine H, Müller Loennies S, Brade L, Lindner B, Brade H (2003) Endotoxic activity and chemical structure of lipopolysaccharides from *Chlamydia trachomatis* serotypes E and L2 and *Chlamydophila psittaci* 6BC. Eur J Biochem 270:440–450

Hemmer W, Focke M, Kolarich D, Wilson IBH, Altmann F, Wöhrl S, Götz M, Jarisch R (2001) Antibody binding to venom carbohydrates is a frequent cause for double positivity to honeybee and yellow jacket venom in patients with stinging-insect allergy. J Allergy Clin Immunol 108: 1045–1052

Holmgren J, Lindholm L, Persson B, Lagergård T, Nilsson O, Svennerholm L, Rudenstam CM, Unsgaard B, Yngvason F, Pettersson S (1984) Detection by monoclonal antibody of carbohydrate antigen CA 50 in serum of patients with carcinoma. Br Med J (Clin Res Ed) 288: 1479–1482

Holst O, Bock K, Brade L, Brade H (1995) The structures of oligosaccharide bisphosphates isolated from the lipopolysaccharide of a recombinant *Escherichia coli* strain expressing the gene gseA [3-deoxy-D-manno-octulopyranosonic acid (Kdo) transferase] of *Chlamydia psittaci* 6BC. Eur J Biochem 229:194–200

Iivanainen E, Kähäri VM, Heino J, Elenius K (2003) Endothelial cell–matrix interactions. Microsc Res Tech 60:13–22

Isshiki Y, Kawahara K, Zähringer U (1998) Isolation and characterisation of disodium (4-amino-4-deoxy-β-L-arabinopyranosyl)-(1→8)-(D-glycero-α-D-talo-oct-2-ulopyranosylonate)-(2→4)-(methyl 3-deoxy-D-manno-oct-2-ulopyranosid)onate from the lipopolysaccharide of *Burkholderia cepacia*. Carbohydr Res 313:21–27

Jacob J, Kelsoe G, Rajewsky K, Weiss U (1991) Intraclonal generation of antibody mutants in germinal centres. Nature 354:389–392

James LC, Tawfik DS (2003) Conformational diversity and protein evolution – a 60-year-old hypothesis revisited. Trends Biochem Sci 28:361–368

James LC, Roversi P, Tawfik DS (2003) Antibody multispecificity mediated by conformational diversity. Science 299:1362–1367

Janeway CA, Travers P, Walport M, Capra JD (2001) Immunobiology: the immune system in health and disease, 5th edn. Garland Science, New York

Jeffrey PD, Bajorath J, Chang CYY, Yelton D, Hellström I, Hellström KE, Sheriff S (1995) The X-ray structure of an anti-tumour antibody in complex with antigen. Nat Struct Mol Biol 2: 466–471

Jiménez R, Salazar G, Yin J, Joo T, Romesberg FE (2004) Protein dynamics and the immunological evolution of molecular recognition. Proc Natl Acad Sci USA 101:3803–3808

Jiménez D, Roda-Navarro P, Springer TA, Casasnovas JM (2005) Contribution of N-linked glycans to the conformation and function of intercellular adhesion molecules (ICAMs). J Biol Chem 280:5854–5861

Joziasse DH (1992) Mammalian glycosyltransferases: genomic organization and protein structure. Glycobiology 2:271–277

Kabat EA (1956) Blood group substances: their chemistry and immunochemistry. Academic, New York

Kabat EA, Wu TT, Bilofsky H (1977) Unusual distributions of amino acids in complementarity-determining (hypervariable) segments of heavy and light chains of immunoglobulins and their possible roles in specificity of antibody-combining sites. J Biol Chem 252:6609–6616

Kaltner H, Stierstorfer B (2000) Animal lectins as cell adhesion molecules. Cells Tissues Organs 161: 162–179

Kannagi R, Izawa M, Koike T, Miyazaki K, Kimura N (2004) Carbohydrate mediated cell adhesion in cancer metastasis and angiogenesis. Cancer Sci 95:377–384

Kansas GS, Ley K, Munro JM, Tedder TF (1993) Regulation of leukocyte rolling and adhesion to high endothelial venules through the cytoplasmic domain of L-selectin. J Exp Med 177: 833–838

Kawahara K, Brade H, Rietschel ET, Zähringer U (1987) Studies on the chemical structure of the core-lipid A region of the lipopolysaccharide of *Acinetobacter calcoaceticus* NCTC 10305. Detection of a new 2-octulosonic acid interlinking the core oligosaccharide and lipid A component. Eur J Biochem 163:489–495

Kindt TJ, Goldsby RA, Osborne BA, Kuby J (2007) Kuby immunology, 6th edn. W.H. Freeman, New York

Klena JD, Pradel E, Schnaitman CA (1993) The rfaS gene, which is involved in production of a rough form of lipopolysaccharide core in *Escherichia coli* K-12, is not present in the rfa cluster of *Salmonella typhimurium* LT2. J Bacteriol 175:1524–1527

Kochi SK, Johnson RC, Dalmasso AP (1991) Complement-mediated killing of the Lyme disease spirochete *Borrelia burgdorferi*. Role of antibody in formation of an effective membrane attack complex. J Immunol 146:3964–3970

Kosma P, Schulz G, Brade H (1988) Synthesis of a trisaccharide of 3-deoxy-D-manno-2-octulopyranosylonic acid (KDO) residues related to the genus-specific lipopolysaccharide epitope of *Chlamydia*. Carbohydr Res 183:183–199

Kosma P, Schulz G, Unger FM, Brade H (1989) Synthesis of trisaccharides containing 3-deoxy-D-manno-2-octulosonic acid residues related to the KDO-region of enterobacterial lipopolysaccharides. Carbohydr Res 190:191–201

Kosma P, Bahnmüller R, Schulz G, Brade H (1990) Synthesis of a tetrasaccharide of the genus-specific lipopolysaccharide epitope of *Chlamydia*. Carbohydr Res 208:37–50

Kosma P, Reiter A, Zamyatina A, Wimmer N, Glück A, Brade H (1999) Synthesis of inner core antigens related to *Chlamydia*, *Pseudomonas* and *Acinetobacter* LPS. J Endotoxin Res 5:157–163

Kosma P, Reiter A, Hofinger A, Brade L, Brade H (2000) Synthesis of neoglycoproteins containing Kdo epitopes specific for *Chlamydophila psittaci* lipopolysaccharide. J Endotoxin Res 6:57–69

Kosma P, Brade H, Evans SV (2008) Lipopolysaccharide antigens of *Chlamydia*. In: ACS symposium series. ACS Publications, pp 239–257

Kudryashov V, Glunz PW, Williams LJ, Hintermann S, Danishefsky SJ, Lloyd KO (2001) Toward optimized carbohydrate-based anticancer vaccines: epitope clustering, carrier structure, and adjuvant all influence antibody responses to Lewis y conjugates in mice. Proc Natl Acad Sci USA 98:3264–3269

Kuroda D, Shirai H, Kobori M, Nakamura H (2009) Systematic classification of CDR L3 in antibodies: implications of the light chain subtypes and the VL-VH interface. Proteins 75: 139–146

Landsteiner K (1990) The specificity of serological reactions. Dover Publications, New York

Lang KS, Burow A, Kurrer M, Lang PA, Recher M (2007) The role of the innate immune response in autoimmune disease. J Autoimmun 29:206–212

Levinson SS (1992) Antibody multispecificity in immunoassay interference. Clin Biochem 25: 77–87

Ley K, Gaehtgens P, Fennie C, Singer MS, Lasky LA, Rosen SD (1991) Lectin-like cell adhesion molecule 1 mediates leukocyte rolling in mesenteric venules in vivo. Blood 77:2553–2555

Li Z, Woo CJ, Iglesias-Ussel MD, Ronai D, Scharff MD (2004) The generation of antibody diversity through somatic hypermutation and class switch recombination. Genes Dev 18(1): 1–11

Lo-Man R, Vichier-Guerre S, Perraut R, Dériaud E, Huteau V, BenMohamed L, Diop OM, Livingston PO, Bay S, Leclerc C (2004) A fully synthetic therapeutic vaccine candidate targeting carcinoma-associated Tn carbohydrate antigen induces tumor-specific antibodies in nonhuman primates. Cancer Res 64:4987–4994

Lucas AH, Moulton KD, Tang VR, Reason DC (2001) Combinatorial library cloning of human antibodies to *Streptococcus pneumoniae* capsular polysaccharides: variable region primary structures and evidence for somatic mutation of Fab fragments specific for capsular serotypes 6B, 14, and 23 F. Infect Immun 69:853–864

Lüderitz O, Freudenberg MA, Galanos C, Lehmann V, Rietschel ET, Shaw DH (1982) Lipopolysaccharides of gram-negative bacteria. Curr Top Membr Transp 17:79–151

Lutz HU (2007) Homeostatic roles of naturally occurring antibodies: an overview. J Autoimmun 29:287–294

Maaheimo H, Kosma P, Brade L, Brade H, Peters T (2000) Mapping the binding of synthetic disaccharides representing epitopes of chlamydial lipopolysaccharide to antibodies with NMR. Biochemistry 39:12778–12788

MacLean GD, Bowen-Yacyshyn MB, Samuel J, Meikle A, Stuart G, Nation J, Poppema S, Jerry M, Koganty R, Wong T (1992) Active immunization of human ovarian cancer patients against a common carcinoma (Thomsen-Friedenreich) determinant using a synthetic carbohydrate antigen. J Immunother 11:292–305

MacLean GD, Reddish M, Koganty RR, Wong T, Gandhi S, Smolenski M, Samuel J, Nabholtz JM, Longenecker BM (1993) Immunization of breast cancer patients using a synthetic sialyl-Tn glycoconjugate plus Detox adjuvant. Cancer Immunol Immunother 36:215–222

Madri JA, Pratt BM (1986) Endothelial cell–matrix interactions: in vitro models of angiogenesis. J Histochem Cytochem 34:85–91

Manimala JC, Li Z, Jain A, VedBrat S, Gildersleeve JC (2005) Carbohydrate array analysis of anti Tn antibodies and lectins reveals unexpected specificities: implications for diagnostic and vaccine development. Chembiochem 6:2229–2241

Manis JP, Tian M, Alt FW (2002) Mechanism and control of class-switch recombination. Trends Immunol 23:31–39

Manivel V, Sahoo NC, Salunke DM, Rao KV (2000) Maturation of an antibody response is governed by modulations in flexibility of the antigen-combining site. Immunity 13:611–620

Manivel V, Bayiroglu F, Siddiqui Z, Salunke DM, Rao KV (2002) The primary antibody repertoire represents a linked network of degenerate antigen specificities. J Immunol 169:888–897

Marchalonis JJ, Adelman MK, Robey IF, Schluter SF, Edmundson AB (2001) Exquisite specificity and peptide epitope recognition promiscuity, properties shared by antibodies from sharks to humans. J Mol Recognit 14:110–121

Mari A, Iacovacci P, Afferni C, Barletta B, Tinghino R, Di Felice G, Pini C (1999) Specific IgE to cross-reactive carbohydrate determinants strongly affect the in vitro diagnosis of allergic diseases. J Allergy Clin Immunol 103:1005–1011

Melamed D, Nemazee D (1997) Self-antigen does not accelerate immature B cell apoptosis, but stimulates receptor editing as a consequence of developmental arrest. Proc Natl Acad Sci USA 94: 9267–9272

Misevic GN, Burger MM (1993) Carbohydrate–carbohydrate interactions of a novel acidic glycan can mediate sponge cell adhesion. J Biol Chem 268:4922–4929

Mond JJ, Lees A, Snapper CM (1995a) T cell-independent antigens type 2. Annu Rev Immunol 13: 655–692

Mond JJ, Vos Q, Lees A, Snapper CM (1995b) T cell independent antigens. Curr Opin Immunol 7: 349–354

Morea V, Tramontano A, Rustici M, Chothia C, Lesk AM (1998) Conformations of the third hypervariable region in the VH domain of immunoglobulins. J Mol Biol 275:269–294

Müller R, Brade H, Kosma P (1997) Synthesis of deoxy analogues of (2→8)-linked 3-deoxy-α-D-manno-oct-2-ulopyranosylonic acid (Kdo) disaccharides for binding studies with *Chlamydia* specific monoclonal antibodies. J Endotoxin Res 4:347–355

Müller-Eberhard HJ (1984) The membrane attack complex. Springer Semin Immunopathol 7: 93–141

Müller-Loennies S, MacKenzie CR, Patenaude SI, Evans SV, Kosma P, Brade H, Brade L, Narang S (2000) Characterization of high affinity monoclonal antibodies specific for chlamydial lipopolysaccharide. Glycobiology 10:121–130

Müller-Loennies S, Grimmecke D, Brade L, Lindner B, Kosma P, Brade H (2002) A novel strategy for the synthesis of neoglycoconjugates from deacylated deep rough lipopolysaccharides. J Endotoxin Res 8:295–305

Müller-Loennies S, Gronow S, Brade L, MacKenzie R, Kosma P, Brade H (2006) A monoclonal antibody against a carbohydrate epitope in lipopolysaccharide differentiates *Chlamydophila psittaci* from *Chlamydophila pecorum, Chlamydophila pneumoniae*, and *Chlamydia trachomatis*. Glycobiology 16:184–196

Muramatsu M, Kinoshita K, Fagarasan S, Yamada S, Shinkai Y, Honjo T (2000) Class switch recombination and hypermutation require activation-induced cytidine deaminase (AID), a potential RNA editing enzyme. Cell 102:553–563

Murase T, Zheng RB, Joe M, Bai Y, Marcus SL, Lowary TL, Ng KK (2009) Structural insights into antibody recognition of mycobacterial polysaccharides. J Mol Biol 392:381–392

Nakouzi A, Casadevall A (2003) The function of conserved amino acids in or near the complementarity determining regions for related antibodies to *Cryptococcus neoformans* glucuronoxylomannan. Mol Immunol 40:351–361

Narayanan S (2000) Molecular mimicry: basis for autoimmunity. Indian J Clin Biochem 15:78–82

Nguyen HP, Seto NOL, Brade L, Kosma P, Brade H, Evans SV (2001) Crystallization and preliminary X-ray diffraction analysis of two homologous antigen-binding fragments in complex with different carbohydrate antigens. Acta Crystallogr Sect D Biol Crystallogr 57:1872–1876

Nguyen HP, Seto NO, MacKenzie CR, Brade L, Kosma P, Brade H, Evans SV (2003) Germline antibody recognition of distinct carbohydrate epitopes. Nat Struct Biol 10:1019–1025

Ni J, Song H, Wang Y, Stamatos NM, Wang LX (2006) Toward a carbohydrate-based HIV-1 vaccine: synthesis and immunological studies of oligomannose-containing glycoconjugates. Bioconjugate Chem 17:493–500

North B, Lehmann A, Dunbrack RL Jr (2010) A new clustering of antibody CDR loop conformations. J Mol Biol 406:228–256

O'Donnell IJ, Frangione B, Porter RR (1970) The disulphide bonds of the heavy chain of rabbit immunoglobulin G. Biochem J 116:261–268

Oettinger MA, Schatz DG, Gorka C, Baltimore D (1990) RAG-1 and RAG-2, adjacent genes that synergistically activate V (D) J recombination. Science 248:1517–1523

Oldstone MBA (2005) Molecular mimicry, microbial infection, and autoimmune disease: evolution of the concept. Curr Top Microbiol Immunol 296:1–17

Osborn MJ (1963) Studies on the Gram-negative cell wall. I. Evidence for the role of 2-keto-3-deoxyoctonate in the lipopolysaccharide of *Salmonella typhimurium*. Proc Natl Acad Sci USA 50:499–506

Ouerfelli O, Warren JD, Wilson RM, Danishefsky SJ (2005) Synthetic carbohydrate-based antitumor vaccines: challenges and opportunities. Expert Rev Vaccines 4:677–685

Panjwani N, Zhao Z, Ahmad S, Yang Z, Jungalwala F, Baum J (1995) Neolactoglycosphingolipids, potential mediators of corneal epithelial cell migration. J Biol Chem 270:14015–14023

Paulson JC, Colley KJ (1989) Glycosyltransferases. Structure, localization, and control of cell type-specific glycosylation. J Biol Chem 264:17615–17618

Petermann ML, Pappenheimer AM Jr (1941) The ultracentrifugal analysis of Diphtheria proteins. J Phys Chem 45:1–9

Petermann ML (1946) The splitting of human gamma globulin antibodies by papain and bromelin. J Am Chem Soc 68:106–113

Pinilla C, Martin R, Gran B, Appel JR, Boggiano C, Wilson DB, Houghten RA (1999) Exploring immunological specificity using synthetic peptide combinatorial libraries. Curr Opin Immunol 11:193–202

Pirofski L, Lui R, DeShaw M, Kressel AB, Zhong Z (1995) Analysis of human monoclonal antibodies elicited by vaccination with a *Cryptococcus neoformans* glucuronoxylomannan capsular polysaccharide vaccine. Infect Immun 63:3005–3014

Podack ER, Tschopp J (1984) Membrane attack by complement. Mol Immunol 21:589–603

Poljak RJ, Amzel LM, Avey HP, Chen BL, Phizackerley RP, Saul F (1973) Three-dimensional structure of the Fab fragment of a human immunoglobulin at 2.8 Å resolution. Proc Natl Acad Sci USA 70:3305–3310

Porter RR (1991) Structural studies of immunoglobulins. Scand J Immunol 34:382–388

Quiocho FA (1986) Carbohydrate-binding proteins: tertiary structures and protein–sugar interactions. Annu Rev Biochem 55:287–315

Raetz CR (1990) Biochemistry of endotoxins. Annu Rev Biochem 59:129–170

Raetz CR, Dowhan W (1990) Biosynthesis and function of phospholipids in *Escherichia coli*. J Biol Chem 265:1235–1238

Raetz CR, Whitfield C (2002) Lipopolysaccharide endotoxins. Annu Rev Biochem 71:635–700

Ramsland PA, Farrugia W, Bradford TM, Mark Hogarth P, Scott AM (2004) Structural convergence of antibody binding of carbohydrate determinants in Lewis Y tumor antigens. J Mol Biol 340:809–818

Reason DC, Zhou J (2004) Correlation of antigenic epitope and antibody gene usage in the human immune response to *Streptococcus pneumoniae* type 23 F capsular polysaccharide. Clin Immunol 111:132–136

Rietschel ET, Kirikae T, Schade FU, Mamat U, Schmidt G, Loppnow H, Ulmer AJ, Zähringer U, Seydel U, Di Padova F et al (1994) Bacterial endotoxin: molecular relationships of structure to activity and function. FASEB J 8:217–225

Rini JM, Schulze-Gahmen U, Wilson IA (1992) Structural evidence for induced fit as a mechanism for antibody–antigen recognition. Science 255:959–965

Rothen A, Landsteiner K (1942) Serological reactions of protein films and denatured proteins. J Exp Med 76:437–450

Roy R (2004) New trends in carbohydrate-based vaccines. Drug Discov Today Technol 1:327–336

Sansonetti P (2002) Host–pathogen interactions: the seduction of molecular cross talk. Gut 50: 1112–1118

Schachter H, Chen S, Zhang W, Spence AM, Zhu S, Callahan JW, Mahuran DJ, Fan X, Bagshaw RD, She YM (2002) Functional post-translational proteomics approach to study the role of N-glycans in the development of *Caenorhabditis elegans*. Biochem Soc Symp 69:1–21

Schellekens GA, Visser H, De Jong BAW, Van Den Hoogen FHJ, Hazes JMW, Breedveld FC, Van Venrooij WJ (2000) The diagnostic properties of rheumatoid arthritis antibodies recognizing a cyclic citrullinated peptide. Arthritis Rheum 43:155–163

Schmidt MA, Riley LW, Benz I (2003) Sweet new world: glycoproteins in bacterial pathogens. Trends Microbiol 11:554–561

Schnaitman CA, Klena JD (1993) Genetics of lipopolysaccharide biosynthesis in enteric bacteria. Microbiol Rev 57:655–682

Scully NF, Shaper JH, Shur BD (1987) Spatial and temporal expression of cell surface galactosyltransferase during mouse spermatogenesis and epididymal maturation. Dev Biol 124:111–124

Senn BM, Lopez-Macias C, Kalinke U, Lamarre A, Isibasi A, Zinkernagel RM, Hengartner H (2003) Combinatorial immunoglobulin light chain variability creates sufficient B cell diversity to mount protective antibody responses against pathogen infections. Eur J Immunol 33: 950–961

Shaw DR, Kirkham P, Schroeder HW Jr, Roben P, Silverman GJ (1995) Structure-function studies of human monoclonal antibodies to pneumococcus type 3 polysaccharide. Ann N Y Acad Sci 764:370–373

Sheriff S, Silverton EW, Padlan EA, Cohen GH, Smith-Gill SJ, Finzel BC, Davies DR (1987) Three-dimensional structure of an antibody–antigen complex. Proc Natl Acad Sci USA 84: 8075–8079

Sherwood L (2010) Human physiology: from cells to systems, 7th edn. Brooks/Cole, Cengage Learning, Australia/United States

Shirai H, Kidera A, Nakamura H (1996) Structural classification of CDR-H3 in antibodies. FEBS Lett 399:1–8

Shirai H, Kidera A, Nakamura H (1999) H3-rules: identification of CDR-H3 structures in antibodies. FEBS Lett 455:188–197

Slootstra JW, Puijk WC, Ligtvoet GJ, Langeveld JPM, Meloen RH (1996) Structural aspects of antibody–antigen interaction revealed through small random peptide libraries. Mol Divers 1: 87–96

Slovin SF, Keding SJ, Ragupathi G (2005) Carbohydrate vaccines as immunotherapy for cancer. Immunol Cell Biol 83:418–428

Snapper CM, Mond JJ (1996) Commentary: a model for induction of T cell-independent humoral immunity in response to polysaccharide antigens. J Immunol 157:2229–2233

Stanfield RL, Takimoto-Kamimura M, Rini JM, Profy AT, Wilson IA (1993) Major antigen-induced domain rearrangements in an antibody. Structure 1:83–93

Stanfield RL, Wilson IA (1994) Antigen-induced conformational changes in antibodies: a problem for structural prediction and design. Trends Biotechnol 12:275–279

Stein KE (1992) Thymus-independent and thymus-dependent responses to polysaccharide antigens. J Infect Dis 165(suppl 1):S49–52

Steiner LA, Fleishman JB (2008) RR Porter and the structure of antibodies. In: Reid KBM, Sim RBS (eds.) Molecular aspects of innate and adaptive immunity. Royal Society of Chemistry, Cambridge, UK, pp 3–10

Storry JR, Olsson ML (2009) The ABO blood group system revisited: a review and update. Immunohematology 25:48–59

Sundberg EJ, Mariuzza RA (2002) Molecular recognition in antibody–antigen complexes. Adv Protein Chem 61:119–160

Süsskind M, Müller-Loennies S, Nimmich W, Brade H, Holst O (1995) Structural investigation on the carbohydrate backbone of the lipopolysaccharide from *Klebsiella pneumoniae* rough mutant R20/O1. Carbohydr Res 269:C1–7

Tauber R, Reher K, Helling K, Scherer H (2001) Complex carbohydrates – structure and function with respect to the glycoconjugate composition of the cupula of the semicircular canals. Biol Sci Space 15:362–366

Tomlinson IM, Cox JP, Gherardi E, Lesk AM, Chothia C (1995) The structural repertoire of the human V kappa domain. EMBO J 14:4628–4638

Tonegawa S (1983) Somatic generation of antibody diversity. Nature 302:575–581

Trinh CH, Hemmington SD, Verhoeyen ME, Phillips SEV (1997) Antibody fragment Fv4155 bound to two closely related steroid hormones: the structural basis of fine specificity. Structure 5:937–948

Tsubata T, Wu J, Honjo T (1993) B-cell apoptosis induced by antigen receptor crosslinking is blocked by a T-cell signal through CD40. Nature 364:645–648

van den Elsen J, Vandeputte-Rutten L, Kroon J, Gros P (1999) Bactericidal antibody recognition of meningococcal PorA by induced fit. J Biol Chem 274:1495–1501

van Ree R (2000) Carbohydrate epitopes and their relevance for the diagnosis and treatment of allergic diseases. Int Arch Allergy Immunol 129:189–197

van Roon AMM, Pannu NS, de Vrind JPM, van der Marel GA, van Boom JH, Hokke CH, Deelder AM, Abrahams JP (2004) Structure of an anti-Lewis X Fab fragment in complex with its Lewis X antigen. Structure 12:1227–1236

Vargas Madrazo E, Paz GE (2002) Modifications to canonical structure sequence patterns: analysis for L1 and L3. Proteins: Struct, Funct, Bioinform 47:250–254

Vliegenthart JF (2006) Carbohydrate based vaccines. FEBS Lett 580:2945–2950

Vollmers HP, Brändlein S (2007) Natural antibodies and cancer. J Autoimmun 29:295–302

Vos Q, Lees A, Wu ZQ, Snapper CM, Mond JJ (2000) B-cell activation by T-cell-independent type 2 antigens as an integral part of the humoral immune response to pathogenic microorganisms. Immunol Rev 176:154–170

Vyas NK, Vyas MN, Chervenak MC, Johnson MA, Pinto BM, Bundle DR, Quiocho FA (2002) Molecular recognition of oligosaccharide epitopes by a monoclonal Fab specific for *Shigella flexneri* Y lipopolysaccharide: X-ray structures and thermodynamics. Biochemistry 41:13575–13586

Webster DM, Henry AH, Rees AR (1994) Antibody–antigen interactions. Curr Opin Struct Biol 4:123–129

Wedemayer GJ, Patten PA, Wang LH, Schultz PG, Stevens RC (1997) Structural insights into the evolution of an antibody combining site. Science 276:1665–1669

Wilson IA, Stanfield RL, Rini JM, Arevalo JH, Schulze-Gahmen U, Fremont DH, Stura EA (1991) Structural aspects of antibodies and antibody–antigen complexes. Ciba Found Symp 159: 13–28

Xu JL, Davis MM (2000) Diversity in the CDR3 region of V(H) is sufficient for most antibody specificities. Immunity 13:37–45

Yoshida-Noro C, Heasman J, Goldstone K, Vickers L, Wylie C (1999) Expression of the Lewis groupcarbohydrate antigens during Xenopus development. Glycobiology 9:1323–1330

Zhao YY, Takahashi M, Gu JG, Miyoshi E, Matsumoto A, Kitazume S, Taniguchi N (2008) Functional roles of N-glycans in cell signaling and cell adhesion in cancer. Cancer Sci 99: 1304–1310

Zhou J, Lottenbach KR, Barenkamp SJ, Lucas AH, Reason DC (2002) Recurrent variable region gene usage and somatic mutation in the human antibody response to the capsular polysaccharide of *Streptococcus pneumoniae* type 23 F. Infect Immun 70:4083–4091

Zhou J, Lottenbach KR, Barenkamp SJ, Reason DC (2004) Somatic hypermutation and diverse immunoglobulin gene usage in the human antibody response to the capsular polysaccharide of *Streptococcus pneumoniae* Type 6B. Infect Immun 72:3505–3514

5 Designing a *Candida albicans* Conjugate Vaccine by Reverse Engineering Protective Monoclonal Antibodies

David R. Bundle, Casey Costello, Corwin Nycholat, Tomasz Lipinski, and Robert Rennie

5.1 Introduction

Candida albicans is a human commensal fungus typically found in the vulvovaginal and gastrointestinal tracts, and the oropharyngeal cavity. Under opportunistic conditions, the interaction between host and fungus can become pathogenic leading to candidiasis (Mochon and Cutler 2005). Cutaneous/mucocutaneous and hematogenously disseminated candidiasis are the two main forms in which the disease manifests. The most common forms of mucocutaneous candidiasis are vulvovaginitis and oral thrush, neither of which is considered life-threatening. Candida infections have the potential to significantly compromise the health of immunocompromised patients (Dreizen 1984), including cancer patients with myelosuppression (Bodey 1986), a condition involving decreased bone marrow activity, T-cell deficient individuals (Mochon and Cutler 2005), women with chronic or recurring vulvovaginitis (Foxman et al. 2000), and HIV/AIDS patients with esophageal candidiasis (Dreizen 1984). Hematogenously disseminated

D.R. Bundle (✉) • C. Costello
Department of Chemistry, University of Alberta, Edmonton, AB, Canada, T6G 2G2
e-mail: dave.bundle@ualberta.ca

C. Nycholat
Department of Chemistry, University of Alberta, Edmonton, AB, Canada, T6G 2G2

The Scripps Research Institute, 10550 North Torrey Pines Road, MEM-L71, La Jolla, CA 92037 USA

T. Lipinski
Department of Chemistry, University of Alberta, Edmonton, AB, Canada, T6G 2G2

Institute of Immunology and Experimental Therapy, Polish Academy of Sciences, ul. Rudolfa Weigla 12, 53-114 Wroclaw, Poland

R. Rennie
The Department of Laboratory Medicine & Pathology, University of Alberta Hospitals, Edmonton, AB, Canada, T6G 2G2

P. Kosma and S. Müller-Loennies (eds.), *Anticarbohydrate Antibodies*,
DOI 10.1007/978-3-7091-0870-3_5,

candidiasis is the life-threatening form of the disease (Anttile et al. 1994; Komshian et al. 1989), and may involve the kidney, liver, spleen, heart, lung, and central nervous system (Mochon and Cutler 2005).

C. albicans is the most frequently encountered fungal disease in humans (Mochon and Cutler 2005; Schaberg et al. 1991). On an annual basis, up to two million patients in the USA are affected by nosocomial infections (Banerjee et al. 1991; Emori and Gaynes 1993). Hospital acquired bacteremia or fungemia numbered 250,000, leading to death in up to 50% of cases (Pittet et al. 1997; Reimer et al. 1997; Weinstein et al. 1997). Patient groups most at risk from *Candida* bloodstream infections include those that undergo immunosuppression (88% of patients), antibiotic treatment (95% of patients), and the presence of a central venous line (93% of patients) (Mochon and Cutler 2005). Of the patients with candidiasis, 52% died, with 23% of those patients' deaths attributed to *Candida* (Karlowsky et al. 1997). In a study involving HIV positive men, 48.9% of individuals developed oral candidiasis (Sangeorzan et al. 1994). In addition to bloodstream infection, another site commonly infected is the urinary tract (Jarvis and Martone 1992; Richards et al. 1998, 1999a, 2004).

The development of an opportunistic candidal infection is most likely associated with alterations in the balance of host immunity and normal microflora rather than the acquisition of hypervirulent factors associated with *C. albicans*. Neutropenia is considered a significant risk factor for development of hematogenously disseminated candidiasis (Martino et al. 1989; Nucci et al. 1997; Colovic et al. 1999), and experimental studies in animal models support this conclusion (Han and Cutler 1997; Baghian and Lee 1989; Jensen et al. 1993; Jones-Carson et al. 1995; Walsh et al. 1990a,b). T-cell deficiency or dysfunction is not an obvious risk factor in humans (Fidel and Sobel 1995) but in animals T-cell dependent cell-mediated immunity is responsible for host defense against this form of candidiasis (Kagaya et al. 1981; Netea et al. 2002). In humans with HIV/AIDS and chronic mucocutaneous candidiasis (CMC) there is no correlation with moderate or severe T-cell deficiency and the development of disseminated candidiasis (Kirkpatrick et al. 1971; Brawner and Hovan 1995). Although cell-mediated immunity against disseminated disease is generally considered to be an important factor in humans it has not been unambiguously established. It seems most likely that defense mechanisms are a composite of innate and acquired specific immunity acting in concert including phagocytic cells, cell mediated immune responses, specific antibodies and a range of associated humoral factors such as complement and cytokines.

Disseminated candidiasis is a significant public health problem with high morbidity and mortality rates amongst at risk groups. Therapeutics such as amphotericin B (Lopez-Bernstein et al. 1989), azole derivatives (Ruhnke et al. 1997; Sanati et al. 1997; Hazen et al. 2003), and cell wall inhibitors (Naider et al. 1983; Denning 2003) are effective but invasive candidiasis continues to proliferate as a result of diagnostic challenges (Bodey 1986), drug resistance (Sangeorzan et al. 1994; Odds 1993; Johnson and Warnock 1995), and poor immunologic status (Meunier et al. 1992). The cost of treatment has therefore increased dramatically (Jouault et al. 1997). These factors have encouraged the search for alternative forms of treatment and the development of preventative strategies, such as a vaccine (Han and Cutler 1995; Mochon and Cutler

2005). Amongst several candidates fungal cell wall carbohydrate epitopes figure prominently. One promising conjugate vaccine based on β-glucan glycoconjugates is being developed (Torosantucci et al. 2005; Bromuro et al. 2010). Extensive studies suggest that the *C. albicans* β(1→2)-linked mannan is a protective antigen. This unique antigen is a minor component of the cell wall phosphomannan, which has been the subject of considerable interest as the most exposed cell wall antigen.

5.2 Cell Wall Carbohydrate Antigens

Branched β(1→3) and β(1→6) glucans, chitin, and phosphomannan glycoconjugates are the three major glycans of the *C. albicans* cell wall (Chaffin et al. 1998; Bishop et al. 1960). The phosphomannan has been the subject of detailed structural analysis and immunological studies.

The structural elucidation of the phosphomannan represents a major achievement since unlike the bacterial cell wall polysaccharide this glycoconjugate lacks a regular repeating unit motif and as with most glycoproteins its glycan component possesses marked microheterogeneity across serotypes and different *Candida* species.

A composite structure of the mannan component of *Candida albicans* (Fig. 5.1) has been proposed based on acetolysis and partial hydrolysis in conjunction with

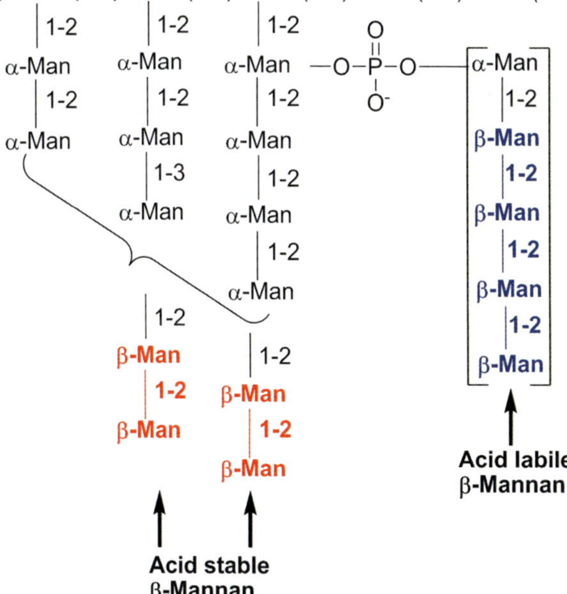

Fig. 5.1 Composite structure of the *Candida albicans* phosphomannan. Three distinct β-mannan epitopes can be distinguished based on their mode of attachment to the α-mannan backbone. The phosphodiester linked β-mannan is referred to as acid labile

NMR and mass spectrometry (Shibata et al. 1992a,b, 1995; Kobayashi et al. 1990). Less than 10% of the mannan is *O*-linked, consisting largely of short α(1→2)- and α(1→3)-D-mannopyranan (Cassone 1989). The complex *N*-linked components are composed of an extended α(1→6)-D-mannopyranan backbone containing α(1→2)-D-mannopyranan branches, some of which may contain α(1→3)-D-mannopyranose residues. Furthermore β(1→2)-mannopyranan oligomers are attached to these side chains in two ways either glycosidically or through a phosphodiester bridge. The position of attachment of this phosphodiester has yet to be determined. The mannan is heterogeneous and differences in mannan chain length have been shown to be nutrient and environment dependent (Chaffin et al. 1988).

The precise antigenic epitopes of the β-mannan exist in three different forms. Two forms of the β(1→2)-linked oligosaccharides exist as extensions of the α(1→2)-mannose and α(1→3)-mannose residues (Kobayashi et al. 1992). The former corresponds to the serotype-A specific epitope of *C. albicans*. The third structural form is the β(1→2)-D-mannopyranan attached via the phosphodiester (Shibata et al. 1992a,b).

Candida albicans strains can be assigned to either of two major serogroups, A or B (Kobayashi et al. 1992; Shibata et al. 1992a,b, 1995). The acid labile β-mannan (linked through a phosphodiester) to the phosphomannan side chains is said to be a major epitope of both serotypes A and B. *Candida albicans* of serotype A also has β-mannose residues attached *via* a glycosidic bond to α(1→2) mannose side chain residues. The phosphomannan of serogroup B cells lacks β-mannan attached *via* a glycosidic bond and possesses only phosphodiester linked β-mannan. Antisera that recognize serogroups A are said to have factors 1, 4, 5, and 6, while antisera recognizing serotype B strains have factors 1, 4, 5 and 13b. Factor 5 is said to correspond to the phosphodiester and glycosidically linked β-mannan. Factor 6 is limited to β-mannan glycosidically attached to α-mannose residues. With β-mannan epitopes of such closely related structures it is not surprising that antibodies recognizing factors 5 and 6 can show a wide range of cross reactivity. The results of inhibition data with oligomers isolated from acid stable and acid labile β-mannan components reflect these close structural similarities (Kobayashi et al. 1992). The β-mannan epitopes are also found in *Candida tropicalis* and in *Candida guilliermondii*, where this epitope is attached via a (1→3)-linkage to an α-mannose residue (Kobayashi et al. 1994; Shibata et al. 1996a,b). Although β-mannan epitopes larger than a tetrasaccharide are reported it appears that (1→2)-β-mannopyranan oligomers are predominantly present as di-, tri and tetrasaccharides (Shibata et al. 1986; Kobayashi et al. 1991; Faille et al. 1991). Goins and Cutler (2000) have also reported that tri- and disaccharide epitopes are most abundant in the β(1→2)-mannopyranan oligomers released from the phosphomannan by β elimination.

During structural studies of several *Candida* species Shibata et al. employed detailed multidimensional NMR studies and inferred from nuclear Overhauser enhancement data that the β(1→2) linked mannose oligosaccharides possessed a "distorted" structure (Shibata et al. 1992b). Faille et al. (1992) also reported a complete assignment of both ^{1}H and ^{13}C NMR spectra for D-mannooligosaccharides of the β(1→2)-linked series. Following the successful synthesis of such oligosaccharides as allyl glycosides (Nitz and Bundle 2001), a detailed NMR investigation of the solution conformation in conjunction with unrestrained molecular dynamics generated a discrete model suggesting that these β-mannans are rather well ordered (Nitz et al. 2002). In solution a family of low energy conformations are expected to be in a dynamic equilibrium but the range of sampled glycosidic torsional angles suggest a helical repeat approximately every three mannose residues. It is of interest to note that a crystal structure of a tetrasaccharide with attached organic protecting groups also adopts a conformation with similar gross features (Crich et al. 2004).

5.3 Protection by Vaccines and Monoclonal Antibodies

Immunization of mice with *C. albicans* cell wall mannans administered as a liposomal preparation produced two monoclonal antibodies capable of conferring passive protection (Han and Cutler 1995, 1997; Han et al. 1998, 2000). Each was specific for the β(1→2) mannan epitope (Mabs B6.1, an IgM and C3.1, an IgG3) and binding studies were consistent with the recognition of a trisaccharide (Han et al. 1997; Nitz et al. 2002) (Fig. 5.2). Immunization with liposomal mannan vaccine and a mannan extract conjugated to bovine serum albumin induced

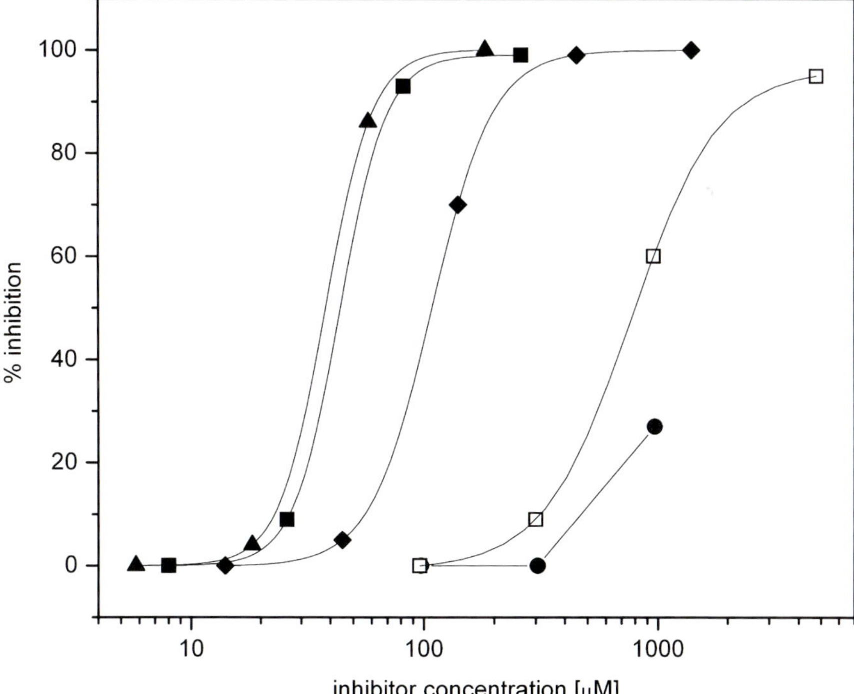

Fig. 5.2 Inhibition by synthetic oligosaccharides of mouse IgG monoclonal antibody C3.1 binding to β-mannan. *Filled square* propyl β(1→2)-D-mannopyranobioside, *triangle* propyl β(1→2)-D-mannopyranotrioside, *diamond* propyl β(1→2)-D-mannopyranotetroside, *open square* propyl β(1→2)-D-mannopyranopentoside, *filled circle* propyl β(1→2)-D-mannopyranohexoside

protective responses that could be passively transferred to naïve mice (Han and Cutler 1997; Han et al. 1998, 1999). The protection afforded by antibodies B6.1 and C3.1 was correlated with their ability to rapidly and efficiently fix complement to the fungal surface (Caesar-TonThat and Cutler 1997; Han et al. 2001).

5.3.1 Recognition Epitope

The work of Cutler's group had established that di- and trisaccharides of β(1→2)-linked mannose were effective inhibitors of both B6.1 and C3.1 antibodies (Han et al. 1997). The chemical synthesis of a panel of β(1→2)-linked oligomannosides provided a more detailed and surprising definition of the specificity of both antibodies (Nitz et al. 2002).

Methyl β-D-mannopyranoside **1** gave no inhibition but disaccharide methyl glycoside **2** and trisaccharide methyl glycoside **3** exhibited the highest affinity. Most surprising was the observation that inhibitory power decreased rapidly as the chain length of the methyl glycosides of synthetic β-mannans increased from tetrasaccharide **4** through pentasaccharide **5** up to hexasaccharide **6** (Nitz et al. 2002). In fact the activity of the latter was so low with C3.1 it was not possible to reach the 50% inhibition level at a concentration of 1 mM (Fig. 5.2). An identical trend was observed for the IgM B6.1 although the intrinsic affinities were lower (Nitz et al. 2002).

This decrease of activity with increasing chain length is in sharp contrast to the paradigm of anti-carbohydrate antibodies first reported by Kabat (1956, 1960). His results with human polyvalent sera raised against the homopolymeric dextran antigen showed that the inhibitory power of oligosaccharides steadily increased as the size of an inhibitor increased and reached a plateau at about the size of tetra to hexamer. Over the intervening years the generality of this observation has been confirmed by numerous solved crystal structures of carbohydrate antigen–antibody complexes (Cygler et al. 1991; Zdanov et al. 1994; Müller-Loennies et al. 2000; Nguyen et al. 2003; Vyas et al. 2002; van Roon et al. 2004). Even though the crystal structures of the binding sites of several antibodies with bound ligands suggest the binding site is essentially filled by tri- and tetrasaccharide epitopes, there is no precedence for loss of inhibitory power with increasing chain length. One crystal structure and binding study demonstrates that nearly all the binding energy derives from recognition of a terminal non-reducing saccharide (Villeneuve et al. 2000). While the majority of antibody crystal structures with bound oligosaccharide and associated binding studies show the binding site filled by a relatively small oligosaccharide, there are fewer reports of larger epitopes (Vulliez-Le Normand et al. 2008), and in one special case for α(2→8)-polysialic acid the binding site appeared to be exceptionally long (Evans et al. 1995). Anti-carbohydrate binding sites can vary significantly in the size of epitope they accommodate. It is surprising that both protective antibodies B6.1 (Han and Cutler 1995; Han et al. 1997) and C3.1 (Han et al. 2000) an IgM and an IgG, each derived from a separate cell fusion experiment, show a similar trend of lower affinities with increased size of the synthetic oligomers (Nitz et al. 2002). This may imply that amongst the relatively well ordered family of solution conformations sampled by β(1→2)-mannopyranan oligomers there exists a preferred epitope surface capable of inducing protective antibodies. It further suggests and is consistent with the observation already cited that a preponderance of β-mannan chains are relatively short (Shibata et al. 1986; Kobayashi et al. 1991; Faille et al. 1991; Goins and Cutler 2000).

5.3.2 Epitope Mapping

Synthesis of monodeoxy and mono-*O*-methyl derivatives **7–21** (Fig. 5.3) of the minimum disaccharide recognition epitope and subsequent assay of inhibitory power permitted the identification of oligosaccharide hydroxyl groups involved in

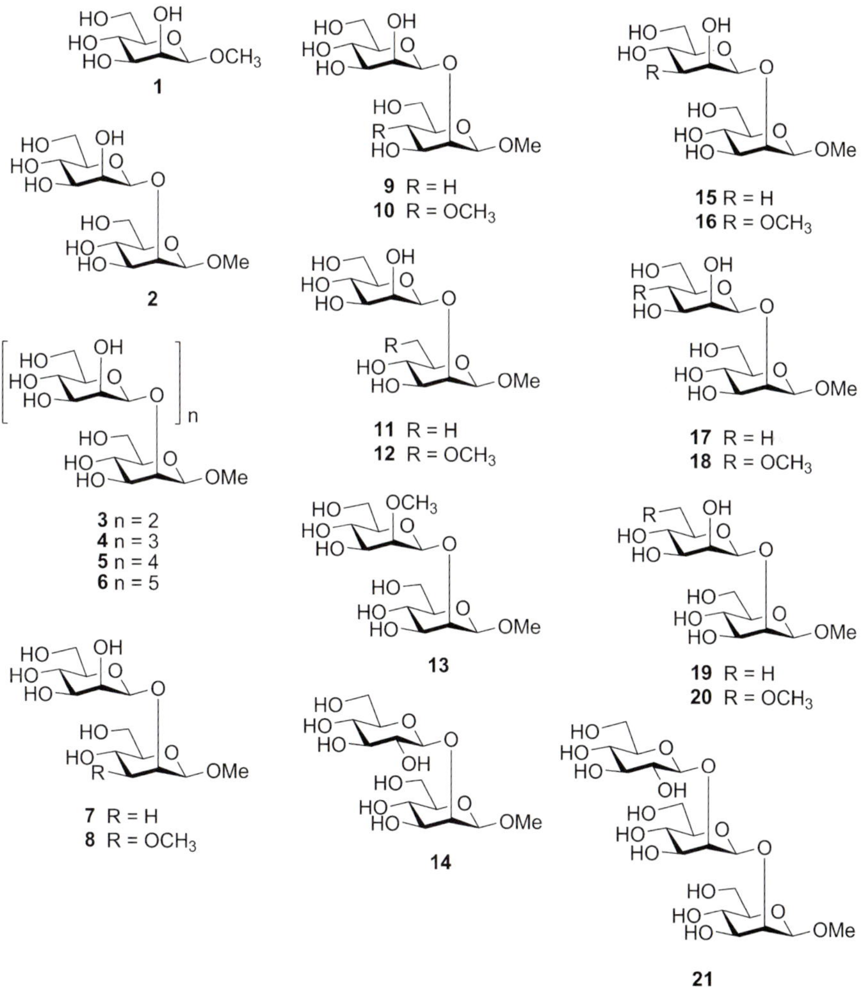

Fig. 5.3 Synthetic congeners **1–21** of the native β-mannan disaccharide used to map the binding site of the monoclonal antibody, C3.1

intermolecular hydrogen bonds with antibody (Nikrad et al. 1992; Lemieux 1993). When hydroxyl groups in contact with the aqueous phase are modified in this way observed changes in inhibitor activity are minimal. However, monodeoxygenation of hydroxyl groups involved in hydrogen bonds with protein at the periphery of the binding site results in derivatives that exhibit a range of activity changes, while the corresponding *O*-methyl congeners exhibit a strong decrease in activity due to the steric bulk of the *O*-methyl group and loss of complementarity. Hydroxyl groups that are involved in hydrogen bonds within the binding site can neither be deoxygenated nor *O*-methylated without virtually complete loss of activity. This strategy was employed to map the binding site of the C3.1 monoclonal antibody (Nycholat and Bundle 2009; Nycholat Ph.D. thesis U of A). Representative schemes are shown of the synthesis of the respective 4-deoxy **9**, 4-methyl **10**,

Scheme 5.1a Reagents and conditions: (a) BzCl, pyridine, quant.; (b) $NaCNBH_3$, HCl, Et_2O, 81%; (c) thiocarbonyl diimidazole, toluene, 60%; (d) *n*-Bu_3SnH, AIBN, toluene, 68%; (e) MeI, NaH, DMF, 0 °C then AcOH, 97%; (f) $NaOCH_3$, CH_3OH, 89% (for **28**), 95% (for **29**)
Scheme 5.1b Reagents and conditions: (a) **28**, TMSOTf, CH_2Cl_2, 0 °C, 83%; (b) **29**, TMSOTf, CH_2Cl_2, 0 °C, 97%; (c) $NaOCH_3$, CH_3OH, 78% (for **32**), 97% (for **35**); (d) Me_2SO, Ac_2O, then L-Selectride, THF, -78 °C, 65% (for **33** over two steps), 61% (for **36** over two steps); (e) H_2, Pd/C, CH_3OH, CH_2Cl_2, 52% (for **9**), 88% (for **10**)

4′-deoxy **17** and 4′-methyl **18** disaccharide congeners modified in the reducing and non-reducing mannose residues (Schemes 5.1 and 5.2).

Congeners modified in the terminal reducing residue were synthesized by first performing selective protection of a methyl β-D-mannopyranoside. For example the 3-*O*-benzyl derivative **22** was benzoylated to give **23** and reductive cleavage of the benzylidene acetal afforded the selectively deprotected alcohol **24**, which could be subjected to a Barton–McCombie deoxygenation sequence **24** → **25** → **26** (Barton and McCombie 1975), or directly methylated to give **27**. Transesterification of **26** and **27** gave the two glycosyl acceptors **28** and **29** for disaccharide synthesis. The selectively protected glucosyl imidate **30** was employed to glycosylate **28** and **29**. The participating acetyl group at *O*-2 ensured stereocontrolled installation of a β-glucopyranosyl residue, and following a transesterification, oxidation–reduction sequence (Ekborg et al. 1972) **31** → **32** → **33** and **34** → **35** → **36** β-mannobioside congeners **9** and **10** could be obtained by a hydrogenolysis step (Scheme 5.1).

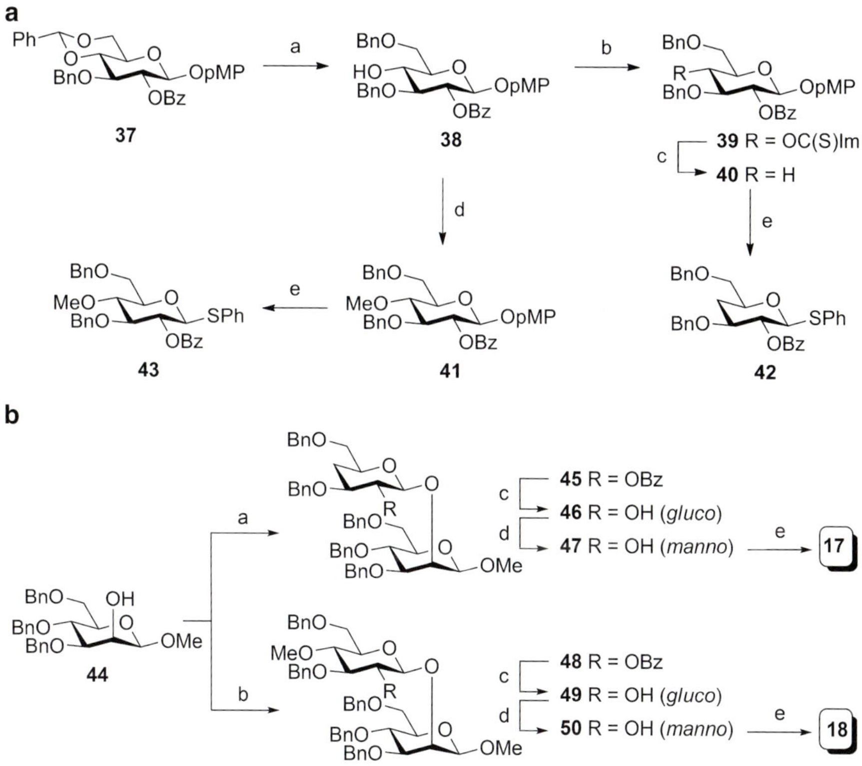

a

37 → (a) → 38 → (b) → 39 R = OC(S)Im → (c) → 40 R = H → (e) → 42; 38 → (d) → 41 → (e) → 43

b

44 → (a) → 45 R = OBz → (c) → 46 R = OH (*gluco*) → (d) → 47 R = OH (*manno*) → (e) → 17

44 → (b) → 48 R = OBz → (c) → 49 R = OH (*gluco*) → (d) → 50 R = OH (*manno*) → (e) → 18

Scheme 5.2a Reagents and conditions: (a) $NaCNBH_3$, HCl, Et_2O, 0 °C, 82%; (b) thiocarbonyl diimidazole, toluene, 89%; (c) *n*-Bu_3SnH, AIBN, toluene, 80%; (d) MeI, NaH, DMF, 0 °C then AcOH, 88%; (e) PhSH, $BF_3{\cdot}OEt_2$, CH_2Cl_2, 0 °C, 92% (for **42**), 68% (for **43**)

Scheme 5.2b Reagents and conditions: (a) **42**, TMSOTf, CH_2Cl_2, 0 °C, 75%; (b) **43**, TMSOTf, CH_2Cl_2, 0 °C, 85%; (c) $NaOCH_3$, CH_3OH, 77% (for **34**), 94% (for **37**); (d) Me_2SO, Ac_2O, then L-Selectride, THF, -78 °C, 73% (for both **47** and **50** over two steps); (e) H_2, Pd/C, CH_3OH, CH_2Cl_2, 72% (for **17**), 62% (for **18**)

Disaccharides **17** and **18** modified in the terminal non-reducing residue were synthesized from glucosyl donors possessing the requisite monodeoxy or mono-*O*-methyl functionality. For example, reductive cleavage of the benzylidene acetal of *p*-methoxyphenyl glucopyranoside **37** gave **38**. A Barton–McCombie deoxygenation sequence **38** → **39** → **40** (Barton and McCombie 1975), or a direct methylation **38** → **41** gave the 4-deoxy- and 4-*O*-methyl *p*-methoxyphenyl glucopyranosides **40** and **41**. Both derivatives were readily converted to the corresponding thiophenyl glucopyranosides **42** and **43**. The methyl β-mannopyranoside **44** was glycosylated by either of the glucosyl donors **42** or **43** to yield disaccharides bearing a terminal β-glucopranosyl residue. The transesterification, oxidation–reduction sequence (Ekborg et al. 1972) described for the synthesis of **9** and **10** was employed to accomplish the conversions to β-mannobioside; **45** → **46** → **47** and **48** → **49** → **50**. Congeners **17** and **18** were obtained from **47** to **50** by a hydrogenolysis step.

The activities of these disaccharides in an inhibition assay as well as the activity of relevant trisaccharides are reported in Table 5.1. The data provide unambiguous identification of three disaccharide hydroxyl groups that are important for recognition by the monoclonal antibody. The inactivity of the 3-deoxy (**7**), 3-*O*-methyl (**8**)

Table 5.1 The effects of functional group and related modifications on the inhibition of mouse monoclonal antibody C3.1 (IgG3) binding to ELISA plates coated with β(1→2)-D-mannan trisaccharide-BSA conjugate

Compound	Inhibitor name	IC_{50} (μmol/L)	Relative potency	ΔΔG kcal/mol
2	Disaccharide	31	100	0
3	Trisaccharide	17	182	−0.4
4	Tetrasaccharide	84	37	0.57
5	Pentasaccharide	421	7	1.8
6	Hexasaccharide	>1,000	<3	>2
7	3-Deoxy	Inactive[a]	<1	>2.7
8	3-*O*-Methyl	Inactive[b]	<1	>2.6
9	4-Deoxy	Inactive[a]	<1	>2.7
10	4-*O*-Methyl	Inactive[b]	<1	>2.6
11	6-Deoxy	14	221	−0.47
12	6-*O*-Methyl	81	38	0.57
13	2′-*O*-Methyl	33	94	0.04
14	2′-*Gluco*-	47	66	0.25
15	3′-Deoxy	na	na	na
16	3′-*O*-Methyl	62	50	0.41
17	4′-Deoxy	Inactive[a]	<1	>2.7
18	4′-*O*-Methyl	670	5	1.8
19	6′-Deoxy	426	7	1.6
20	6′-*O*-Methyl	588	5	1.7
21	2″-*Gluco*	52	60	0.3

[a]No inhibition at 2,938 μmol/L
[b]No inhibition at 2,700 μmol/L

as well as the 4-deoxy (**9**), 4-*O*-methyl (**10**) congeners requires that these are buried hydroxyl groups that make essential hydrogen bonds to the antibody binding site. By comparison, the inactivity of the 4′-deoxy analogue **17** and the weak activity of the 4′-*O*-methyl disaccharide **18** are consistent with this hydroxyl being relatively exposed and also a hydrogen bond acceptor. The sterically demanding *O*-methyl group could not be accommodated if this hydroxyl group were buried in the site, and its activity suggests that 4′-OH lies in an exposed position at the periphery of the site where it likely accepts a hydrogen bond from the protein and perhaps donates a hydrogen bond to water. Since elaboration of the β-mannan requires substitution at O-2′, it is not surprising to observe that methylation at this position, disaccharide **13**, shows little change in activity suggesting that this is a solvent exposed region. In support of this the neighbouring 3′ deoxy **15** and 3′-*O*-methyl **16** derivatives exhibit relatively small changes in binding energy, consistent with the location of 3′-OH in a solvent exposed region of the epitope. The weaker activities of the 6′ congeners **19** and **20** suggest that the 6′-OH makes weak hydrogen bonds at or close to the periphery of the binding site. Based on the free energy changes for functional group modifications on the non-reducing residue it is concluded that this hexose is less involved in the binding site than the reducing mannopyranose. Consistent with this inference is the relatively high activity of congener **14** with a terminal β-glucopyranosyl residue, which indicates that the steric demands for accommodating the second *manno*-configuration are quite relaxed. Of interest is the only slightly higher activity ($\Delta(\Delta G) = -0.4$ kcal/mol) of trisaccharide **3** relative to disaccharide **2**. The trisaccharide analogue **21** with a terminal non-reducing *gluco* residue is only slightly less active than native disaccharide **2**. The inference from inhibition data points to an epitope certainly no bigger than a trisaccharide and more likely a disaccharide with the primary polar recognition element confined to the reducing-terminal mannose (Fig. 5.4). Since the monosaccharide methyl glycoside **1** exhibits no activity it seems likely that the second

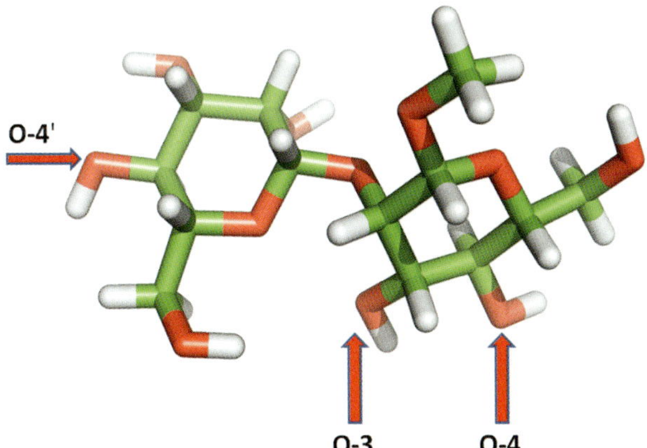

Fig. 5.4 The key polar contacts of the β-mannan disaccharide epitope recognized by the C3.1 monoclonal antibody

residue of the disaccharide must make important non polar complementary contacts with the binding site.

5.3.3 Location of the Disaccharide Epitope

These data are decisive with respect to the involvement of the terminal reducing residue of the disaccharide as the primary recognition element. This is surprising since many protective antibodies bind to the most exposed residues at the distal end of cell surface antigens (Carlin et al. 1987; Lind and Lindberg 1992). These results pose an important question. When the β-mannan of the cell wall antigen is larger than a disaccharide, which disaccharide element is bound by the antibody? Does the antibody always bind to the terminal reducing disaccharide or can it frame shift and bind a non-reducing disaccharide? Furthermore, is the recognized β-mannan part of the acid labile phosphodiester linked β-mannan or the β-mannan linked glycosidically to the α(1→2) mannose residues? These issues are illustrated for the two types of β-mannan oligosaccharides (Fig. 5.5).

By constructing trisaccharides that incorporate 4-deoxy or 4-*O*-methyl groups that epitope mapping established as inactive (Nycholat, PhD thesis) we were able to investigate the possibility that C3.1 could bind frame shifted disaccharide epitopes (Costello, MSc thesis). Chemical synthesis of trisaccharides **51**–**53** incorporate functional group replacements that abrogate binding to alternate terminal disaccharide elements (Fig. 5.6). For example by introducing a 4-deoxy or 4-*O*-methyl group on a hydroxyl group essential for binding compound **51** would only permit recognition of a terminal reducing disaccharide, whereas compounds **52** and **53** prevent binding of the reducing disaccharide and require the non-reducing disaccharide to be recognized.

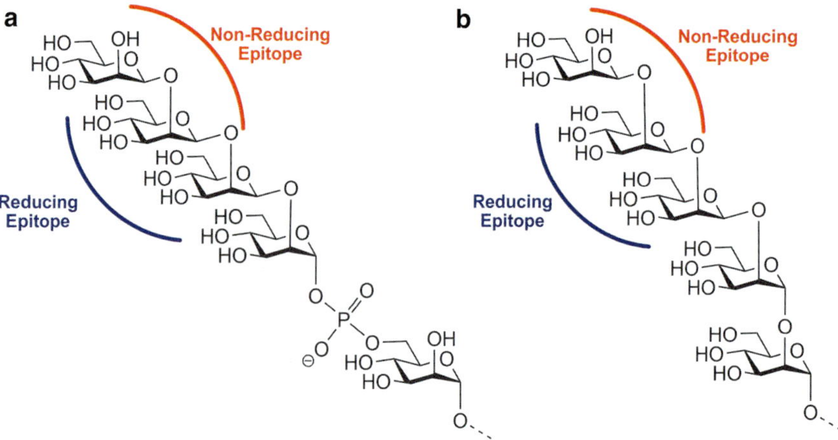

Fig. 5.5 Acid labile and acid stable β-mannan disaccharide epitopes as presented by two forms of β-mannan trisaccharide present in the *Candida albicans* cell wall phosphomannan. 5.5a shows the phosphodiester linked β-mannan and 5.5b the related glycosidically linked epitope

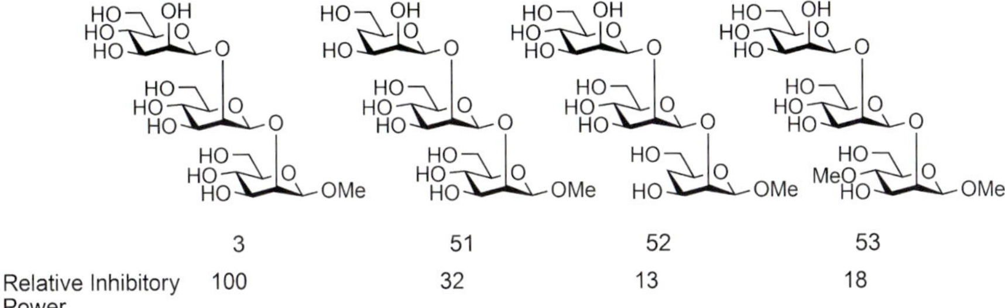

Fig. 5.6 The relative activities of native **3** and trisaccharide congeners designed to direct binding of either terminal reducing **51** or terminal non-reducing disaccharides **52** and **53**

Measurement of the activity of these compounds by solid phase inhibition showed there was a preference towards binding the reducing disaccharide element, as compound **51** was the most active of the three trisaccharide analogues **51**–**53**. However, since compounds **52** and **53** were only twofold to threefold less active than **51**, these data are consistent with a frame shift to bind the non-reducing end disaccharide element of a trisaccharide. When the terminal non-reducing disaccharide is bound, it appears that the residue at the reducing end of the trisaccharide likely makes some unfavourable contacts at the periphery of the binding site but these are not decisive in preventing binding.

5.4 Designing a Conjugate Vaccine

The nearly equivalent inhibitory activity of disaccharide and trisaccharide for C3.1 suggests that a conjugate vaccine consisting of a trisaccharide or perhaps even a disaccharide could result in protective antibody. Initial attempts to synthesize and evaluate a conjugate vaccine focused on a trisaccharide (Nitz and Bundle 2001; Wu and Bundle 2005; Bundle et al. 2007; Lipinski et al. 2011a,b), because we reasoned that the larger epitope would allow for the development of antibodies that could accommodate a disaccharide epitope, yet still allow the binding of larger epitopes. The trisaccharide immunogen should evoke antibodies that would allow both the entry and exit of larger structures when a disaccharide epitope is accepted in a binding site. In published crystal structures of a *Salmonella* specific antibody we showed that if larger oligosaccharides bind but are unable to adopt low energy conformations for those segments exiting and entering the binding site, then a significant energy penalty may result (Milton and Bundle 1998).

5.4.1 Preparation of glycoconjugates

The β(1→2)-mannose trisaccharide was synthesized as its allyl glycoside and photochemical addition of cysteamine and removal of saccharide protecting groups provided a tether derivative **54** (Nitz and Bundle 2001), which was derivatized with

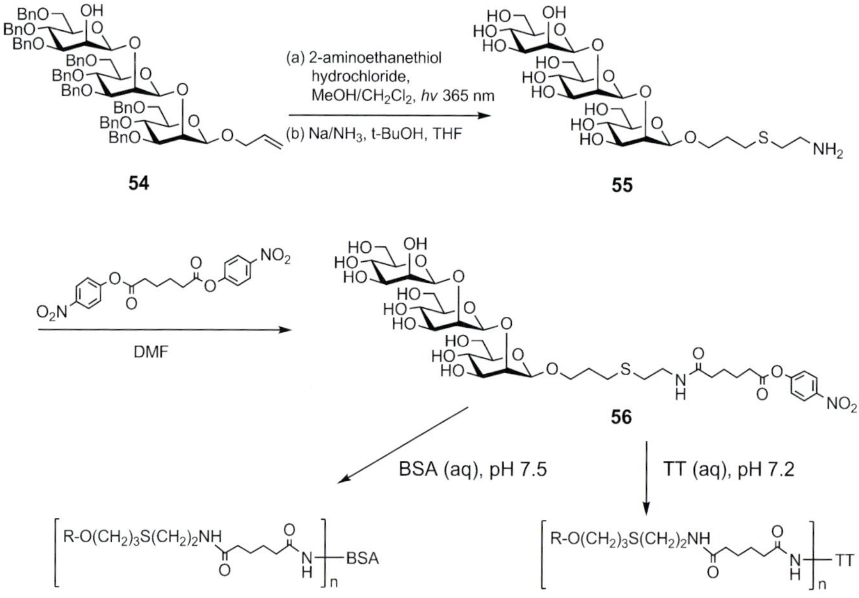

Scheme 5.3 Preparation of trisaccharide bovine serum albumin (BSA) and trisaccharide tetanus toxoid (TT) glycoconjugates

the homobifunctional reagent, di-*p*-nitrophenyl adipate (Wu et al. 2004) to give **55** for conjugation to protein (Scheme 5.3) (Wu and Bundle 2005a,b). Conjugation to BSA and tetanus toxoid via the adipic acid tether provided a BSA glycoconjugate bearing from 9 to 13 residues of the trisaccharide hapten and a tetanus toxoid conjugate vaccine with 8 to 12 attached trisaccharide epitopes (Scheme 5.3) as determined by MALDI-TOF analysis (Wu and Bundle 2005a,b).

5.4.2 Induction of Anti-β-Mannan Antibodies

To test the immunogenicity of the trisaccharide conjugate vaccine three rabbits were immunized with tetanus toxoid glycoconjugates adsorbed on alum. Each rabbit received 300 μg of glycoconjugates per injection corresponding to ~11 to 12 μg of saccharide. On day 21 each rabbit received an identical injection of the antigen/adjuvant. Ten days later sera were collected and antibody titres were determined using trisaccharide-BSA coated ELISA plates and also against plates coated with native *C. albicans* cell wall preparation (Wu and Bundle 2005a,b). Antibody titers against synthetic trisaccharide BSA conjugate were significantly higher than those measured against plates coated with native *C. albicans* cell wall antigen. Average titers were 166,000 (geomean) and 40,000 respectively. Sera from the control group showed no reactivity towards either antigen. This observation is consistent with a population of antibodies that recognized portions of the

Fig. 5.7 The chicken serum albumin (CSA) disaccharide glycoconjugate employed to immunize rabbits

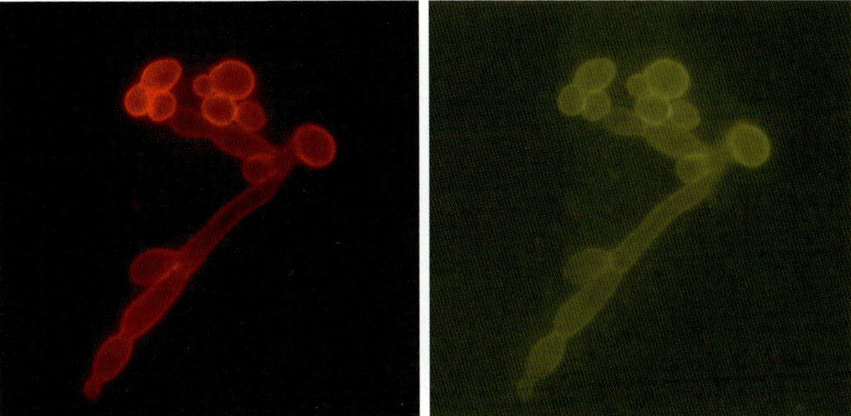

Fig. 5.8 Immunofluorescent staining of *Candida albicans* cells. Rabbit immune sera was diluted 1/1,000 and slides were stained with Rhodamine labeled goat anti-rabbit antibody (*red*) or *green* with fungi-fluor staining reagent. Staining by sera from rabbits immunized with tetanus toxoid did not give noticeable fluorescence (not shown)

trisaccharide plus tether as well as a significant proportion that are able to recognize the native β-mannan when it is part of the cell wall antigen complex. Similar results were observed when a disaccharide conjugate was synthesized and used to hyperimmunize rabbits (Fig. 5.7). In this case rabbits received five injections of conjugate over 6 months and the geomean of the titres of sera from six rabbits measured against the native cell wall mannan was 88,000 (Lipinski et al. 2011b).

Immunofluorescent staining experiment of *C. albicans* cells was performed with immune and preimmune sera diluted 1:100, 1:1,000 and 1:10,000 and this experiment confirmed that the antibodies induced by the conjugate vaccine were able to recognize the β-mannan when displayed on the *C. albicans* cell wall. Serum diluted 1/1,000 gave good staining of *Candida* cell wall in both hyphae and budding cells (Fig. 5.8) (Lipinski et al. unpublished results).

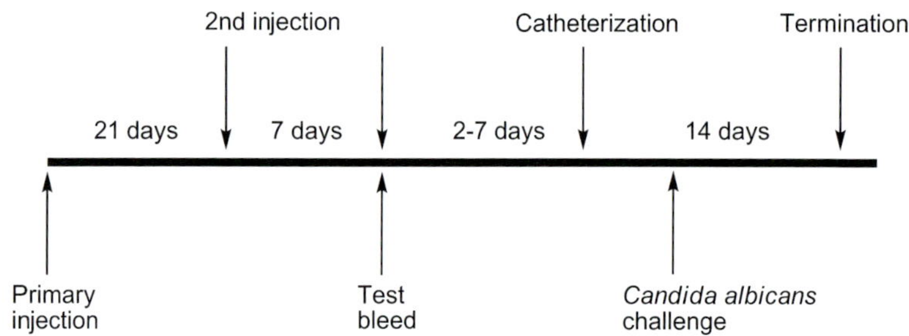

Fig. 5.9 Time lines for vaccination, serum collection, immunosuppresions and *Candida albicans* challenge

5.4.3 Protection Experiments

Having established that a trisaccharide conjugate vaccine induced antibodies that bound the native cell wall phosphomannan when coated on ELISA plates and as a constituent of live *C. albicans* cells, we investigated the potential of these antibodies to confer protection in live *C. albicans* challenge experiments.

Protection experiments were conducted to simulate the clinical situation of immunosuppression, for example the situation of patients expected to undergo solid organ transplant. We anticipated that a protocol could be envisioned where vaccination can be performed before a patient is treated with immunosuppressive drugs (Fig. 5.9). An immunization protocol similar to that used above was followed and blood was taken 7 days after the second injection. Then to simulate the immunocompromised state and to render rabbits susceptible to disseminated candidiasis while avoiding bacterial infections, rabbits were catheterized to aid administration of cytostatic and antimicrobial maintenance drugs. At day 1 after catheter insertion 200 mg of cyclophosphamide was injected and repeated on days 4 and 8. The applied regime resulted in a reduction of WBC counts to approximately 2×10^9/L.

Due to limitations in the number of animals that could be handled at one time, protection/challenge experiments were performed on successive groups of 4–6 rabbits. Rabbits in the experimental group were immunized with the glycoconjugate vaccine according to the protocol described above, while a control group received identically spaced injections of tetanus toxoid.

On day 6 after catheterization animals were challenged with 1×10^3 live *Candida* cells administered via the catheter and euthanized 8 days later. Accumulated data were collected for 16 rabbits in the vaccinated group and 13 rabbits in the control group.

5.4.4 Vaccination Reduces Candida Burden in Vital Organs

Vaccination resulted in a reduction of fungal burden in different organs after challenge with live fungal cells (Figs. 5.10 and 5.11). Kidney and liver appeared

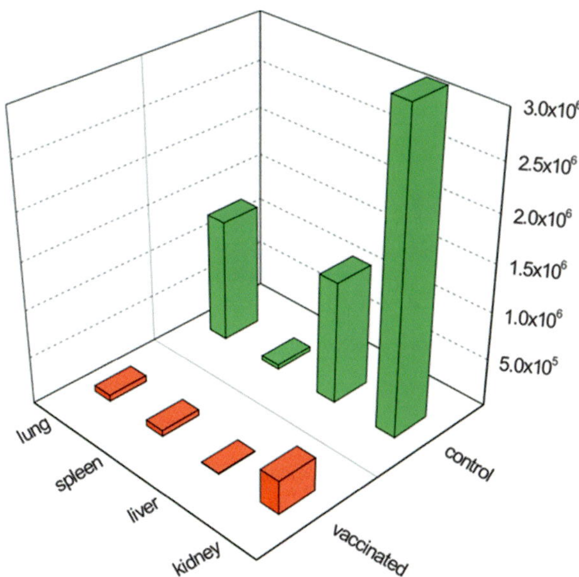

Fig. 5.10 Bar graph representing mean values of C. *albicans* CFU counts in four vital organs. CFU was estimated per gram of a tissue. Values for vaccinated and control group respectively: kidney – 3.5×10^5, 3.3×10^6; liver – 6.6×10^3, 1.3×10^6; lungs – 6.3×10^4, 6.3×10^5; spleen – 6.2×10^4, 4.5×10^4

to be predestined for fungal colonization in our model. Vaccinated animals showed significantly reduced CFU at the 75th percentile for kidney, liver, lungs, and spleen with observed 24-, 626-, 145- and 15-fold reductions. Median values for the group show a smaller reduction rate in the kidney and liver, about fivefold and threefold respectively but also a small increase in lungs and spleen. Vaccination also correlates with a significant compression in the range of CFU counts in all analyzed organs, which is especially pronounced in the liver.

The statistical treatment of data with the Generalized Estimating Equation (GEE) method revealed that the reduction of Candida CFU was statistically significant in the kidney (average reduction in log counts 4.4, $p = 0.016$) and liver (average reduction in log counts 3.6, $p = 0.033$). The effect of vaccination was not observed in lungs and spleen (increase in log counts 0.002, $p = 0.99$; 0.411, $p = 0.80$ respectively).

A challenge experiment that followed a similar post-immunization protocol with rabbits hyperimmunized with the disaccharide-CSA (chicken serum albumin) conjugate gave a similar outcome to that reported for the trisaccharide (Lipinski et al. 2011b). The two sets of findings support the contention that antibody mediated immunity plays a role in combating *C. albicans* infections and suggests that a synthetic conjugate vaccine may have therapeutic potential. Surprisingly, it appears that a disaccharide epitope may suffice to induce protective antibody. If this is the case a fully synthetic conjugate vaccine becomes an attractive target since

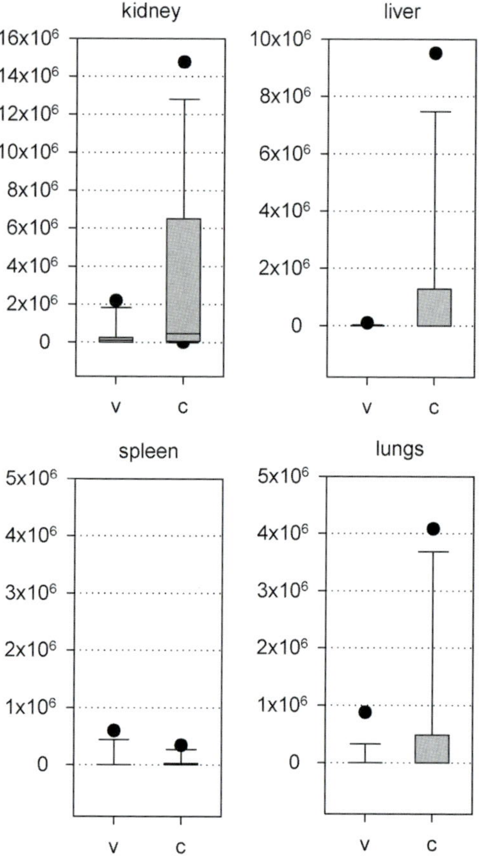

Fig. 5.11 (continued)

the methodology and costs for producing disaccharide and even trisaccharide conjugates will be relatively inexpensive.

5.5 Efficacy of Trisaccharide Conjugate Vaccine in Mice

Candida challenge experiments are expensive and time consuming to conduct in rabbits. However all of the conjugates described above as well as others reported in our published work failed to induce sufficiently high antibody titres in mice that could afford protection (Lipinski et al. 2011a; Wu et al. 2007, 2008). In general titres against the native cell wall phosphomannan complex were modest to weak.

With Cutler's group we have reported a successful approach to protect mice (Dziadek et al. 2008; Xin et al. 2008). This work employed T-cell peptides that are found in cell wall proteins of *C. albicans*. A synthetic method was developed to

category	*Candida* CFU in vaccine group kidney	liver	spleen	lungs
min	0	0	0	0
max	2.19×10^6	9.33×10^4	5.99×10^5	8.76×10^5
median	1.00×10^5	3.90×10^2	2.97×10^2	2.95×10^2
25th %	0	0	0	0
75th %	2.6×10^5	1.96×10^3	1.20×10^3	1.70×10^3

category	*Candida* CFU in control group kidney	liver	spleen	lungs
min	0	0	0	0
max	1.48×10^7	9.52×10^6	3.48×10^5	4.08×10^6
median	4.61×10^5	1.20×10^3	0	0
25th %	7.09×10^4	52	0	0
75th %	6.22×10^6	1.23×10^6	1.90×10^4	2.48×10^5

Fig. 5.11 (**a**) Distribution of CFU values in different organs. Bars represent range of 25–75th percentile. Median values are shown as *vertical lines*. (**b**) Tables show values of statistical categories

conjugate the β-mannan trisaccharide to the *N*-terminus of these T-cell peptides. Six peptides were selected and conjugated to the trisaccharide.

Employing an intensive schedule of *ex vivo* dendritic cell stimulation followed by *in vivo* transfer and further conventional immunization mice could be protected from challenge with *C. albicans*. This approach suggests that a potential cause of the poor immune response in mice is the absence of an effective presentation of the glycoconjugate vaccine. We have investigated alternative ways to achieve this goal. One approach (Xin et al. unpublished) used the protective glycopeptide described in the preceding paragraph. If these glycoconjugates were synthesized with a tether attached to the C-terminus of the peptide, a conjugate of the glycopeptide with tetanus toxoid could be prepared. Preliminary data with this antigen suggest: that tetanus toxoid can serve as a suitable secondary carrier as it induces robust antibody responses and protective immunity even when administered without adjuvant. In separate experiments we have investigated alternative and simple approaches to target glycoconjugate vaccines to dendritic cells (DC). Again preliminary data suggest that with appropriate DC target the glycoconjugate vaccine that worked so well in rabbits can also be effective at inducing protective antibodies in mice.

Conclusions

Current dogma suggests that the oligosaccharide component of glycoconjugate vaccines should possess a certain minimal size if protective antibodies are to be generated. This size usually ranges from an octasaccharide (Lindberg et al. 1983) to as large as a hexadecasaccharide (Phalipon et al. 2006, 2009; Pozsgay et al. 2007). In *Candida albicans* where the protective antigen is a cell wall glycoprotein, it appears that a disaccharide or trisaccharide epitope can afford protective antibody. When combined with a T-cell peptide that is capable of inducing cell mediated immunity we can envisage a fully synthetic conjugate vaccine that engages both arms of the adaptive immune response. Since disaccharide and trisaccharide epitopes should be cost effective to produce at scale a chemically defined conjugate vaccine against *Candida albicans* may become an attractive prospect.

References

Anttile VJ, Ruutu P, Bondestam S, Jansson SE, Nordling S, F'arkkil'a M, Sivonen A, Castren M, Ruutu T (1994) Hepatosplenic yeast infection in patients with acute leukemia: a diagnostic problem. Clin Infect Dis 18:979–981

Baghian A, Lee KW (1989) Systemic candidosis in beige mice. J Med Vet Mycol 27:51–55

Banerjee SN, Emori TG, Culver DH, Gaynes RP, Jarvis WR, Horan T, Edwards JR, Tolson JS, Henderson T, Martone WJ (1991) Secular trends in nosocomial primary bloodstream infections in the United States, 1980–1989. national nosocomial infections surveillance system. Am J Med 91(3B):86S–89S

Barton DHR, McCombie SW (1975) A new method for the deoxygenation of secondary alcohols. J Chem Soc Perkin Trans 1:1574–1585

Bishop CT, Blank F, Gardner PE (1960) The cell wall polysaccharides of *Candida albicans*: glucan, mannan, and chitin. Can J Chem 38:869–881

Bodey GP (1986) Infection in cancer patients. A continuing association. Am J Med 81:11–26

Brawner DL, Hovan AJ (1995) Oral candidiasis in HIV-infected patients. Curr Top Med Mycol 6:113–25

Bromuro C, Romano M, Chiani P, Berti F, Tontini M, Proietti D, Mori E, Torosantucci A, Costantino P, Rappuoli R, Cassone A (2010) Beta-glucan-CRM197 conjugates as candidates antifungal vaccines. Vaccine 28:2615–2623

Bundle DR, Nitz M, Wu X, Sadowska JM (2007) A uniquely small, protective carbohydrate epitope may yield a conjugate vaccine for *Candida albicans*. Amer Chem Soc Symp Ser 989:163–183

Caesar-TonThat TC, Cutler JE (1997) A monoclonal antibody to Candida albicans enhances mouse neutrophil candidacidal activity. Infect Immun 65:5354–5357

Carlin NIA, Bundle DR, Lindberg AA (1987) Characterization of five *Shigella flexneri* variant Y – specific monoclonal antibodies using defined saccharides and glycoconjugate antigens. J Immunol 138:4419–4427

Cassone A (1989) Cell wall of *Candida albicans*: its functions and its impact on the host. Curr Top Med Mycol 3:248–314

Chaffin WL, Skudlarek J, Morrow KJ (1988) Variable expression of a surface determinant during proliferation of *Candida albicans*. Infect Immun 56:302–309

Colovic M, Lazarevic V, Colovic R, Janković G, Suvajdzić N, Bogdanović A, Bila J (1999) Hepatosplenic candidiasis after neutropenic phase of acute leukemia. Med Oncol 16:139–142

Costello C (2011) The preferred recognition epitope of the *Candida albicans* β-mannan. MSc thesis, University of Alberta

Crich D, Banerjee A, Yao Q (2004) Direct chemical synthesis of the β-D-mannans: the β-(1→2) and β-(1→4) series. J Am Chem Soc 126:14930–14934

Cygler M, Rose DR, Bundle DR (1991) Recognition of a cell surface oligosaccharide epitope of pathogenic *Salmonella* by an antibody Fab fragment. Science 253:442–446

Denning DW (2003) Echinocandin antifungal drugs. Lancet 362:1142–1151

Dreizen S (1984) Oral candidiasis. Am J Med 30:28–33

Dziadek S, Jacques S, Bundle DR (2008) A novel linker methodology for the synthesis of tailored conjugate vaccines composed of complex carbohydrate antigens and specific T_H-cell peptide epitopes. Chem Eur J 14:5908–5917

Ekborg G, Lindberg B, Lonngren J (1972) Synthesis of β-D-mannopyranosides. Acta Chem Scand 26:3287–3292

Emori TG, Gaynes RP (1993) An overview of nosocomial infections, including the role of the microbiology laboratory. Clin Microbiol Rev 6:428–442

Evans SV, Sigurskjold BW, Jennings HJ, Brisson J-R, To R, Altman E, Frosch M, Weisgerber C, Kratzin H, Klebert S, Vaesen M, Bitter-Suermann D, Rose DR, Young NM, Bundle DR (1995) The 2.8 Å resolution structure, and thermodynamics of ligand binding, of an Fab specific for α(2 → 8)-polysialic acid. Biochemistry 34:6737–6744

Faille C, Wieruszeski JM, Lepage G, Michalski JC, Poulain D, Strecker G (1991) ^{1}H-NMR spectroscopy of manno-oligosaccharides of the β-1,2-linked series released from the phosphopeptidomannan of *Candida albicans* VW-32 (serotype A). Biochem Biophys Res Commun. 181:1251–1258

Faille C, Wieruszeski JM, Michalski JC, Poulain D, Strecker G (1992) Complete ^{1}H- and ^{13}C-resonance assignments for D-mannooligosaccharides of the β-D-(1–2)-linked series released from the phosphopeptidomannan of *Candida albicans* VW.32 (serotype A). Carbohydr Res 236:17–27

Fidel PL Jr, Sobel JD (1995) The role of cell-mediated immunity in candidiasis. Trends Microbiol 2:202–206

Foxman B, Barlow R, D'Arcy H, Gilespie B, Sobel J (2000) Candida vaginitis: self-reported incidence and associated costs. Sex Transm Dis 27:230–235

Goins TL, Cutler JE (2000) Relative abundance of oligosaccharides in *Candida* species as determined by fluorophore-assisted carbohydrate electrophoresis. J Clin Microbiol 38:2862–2869

Han Y, Cutler JE (1995) Antibody response that protects against disseminated candidiasis. Infect Immun 63:2714–2719

Han Y, Cutler JE (1997) Assessment of a mouse model of neutropenia and the effect of an anti-candidiasis monoclonal antibody in these animals. J Infect Dis 175:1169–1175

Han Y, Kanbe T, Cherniak R, Cutler JE (1997) Biochemical characterization of *Candida albicans* epitopes that can elicit protective and nonprotective antibodies. Infect Immun 65:4100–4107

Han Y, Morrison RP, Cutler JE (1998) A vaccine and monoclonal antibodies that enhance mouse resistance to *Candida albicans* vaginal infection. Infect Immun 66:5771–5776

Han Y, Ulrich MA, Cutler JE (1999) *Candida albicans* mannan extract-protein conjugates induce a protective immune response against experimental candidiasis. J Infect Dis 179:1477–1484

Han Y, Riesselman M, Cutler JE (2000) Protection against candidiasis by an immunoglobulin G3 (IgG3) monoclonal antibody specific for the same mannotriose as an IgM protective antibody. Infect Immun 68:1649–1654

Han Y, Kozel TR, Zhang MX, MacGill RS, Carroll MC, Cutler JE (2001) Complement is essential for protection by an IgM and an IgG3 monoclonal antibody against experimental, hematogenously disseminated candidiasis. J Immunol 167:1550–7

Hazen KC, Baron EJ, Colombo AL, Girmenia C, Sanchez-Sousa A, del Palacio A, de Bedout C, Gibbs DL (2003) Global Antifungal Surveillance Group. Comparison of the susceptibilities of *Candida* spp. to fluconazole and voriconazole in a 4-year global evaluation using disk diffusion. J Clin Microbiol 41:5623–5632

Pozsgay V, Kubler-Kielb J, Schneerson R, Robbins JB (2007) Effect of the nonreducing end of *Shigella dysenteriae* type 1 O-specific oligosaccharides on their immunogenicity as conjugates in mice. Proc Natl Acad Sci USA 104:14478–14482

Reimer LG, Wilson ML, Weinstein MP (1997) Update on detection of bacteremia and fungemia. Clin Microbiol Rev 10:444–465

Richards MJ, Edwards JR, Culver DH (1998) Nosocomial infections in coronary care units in the United States. National Nosocomial Infections Surveillance System. Am J Cardiol 82:789–793

Richards MJ, Edwards JR, Culver DH (1999) Nosocomial infections in medical intensive care units in the United States. National Nosocomial Infections Surveillance System. Crit Care Med 27:887–892

Richards MJ, Edwards JR, Culver DH, Gaynes RP (2004) Nosocomial infections in pediatric intensive care units in the United States. National Nosocomial Infections Surveillance System. Pediatrics 103:1–7

Ruhnke M, Schmidt-Westhausen A, Trautmann M (1997) In vitro activities of voriconazole (UK-109,496) against fluconazole-susceptible and -resistant *Candida albicans* isolates from oral cavities of patients with human immunodeficiency virus infection. Antimicrob Agents Chemother 41:575–577

Sanati H, Belanger P, Fratti R, Ghannoum M (1997) A new triazole, voriconazole (UK-109,496), blocks sterol biosynthesis in *Candida albicans* and *Candida krusei*. Antimicrob Agents Chemother 41:2492–2496

Sangeorzan JA, Bradley SF, He X (1994) Epidemiology of oral candidiasis in HIV-infected patients: colonization, infection, treatment, and emergence of fluconazole resistance. Am J Med 97:339–346

Schaberg DR, Culver DH, Gayner RP (1991) Major trends in the microbial etiology of nosocomial infection. Am J Med 91(3B):72S–75S

Shibata N, Kobayashi H, Tojo M, Suzuki S (1986) Characterization of phosphomannan protein complexes isolated from viable cells of yeast and mycelial forms of *Candida-albicans* NIH-B-792 strain by the action of zymolyase-100 T. Arch Biochem Biophys 251:697–708

Shibata N, Arai M, Haga E, Kikuchi T, Najima M, Satoh T, Kobayashi H, Suzuki S (1992a) Structural identification of epitope of antigenic factor 5 in mannans of *Candida albicans* NIH B-792 (serotype B) and C. albicans J-1012 (serotype A) strains as β-1,2-linked oligomannosyl residues. Infect Immun 60:4100–4110

Shibata N, Hisamichi K, Kikuchi T, Kobayashi H, Okawa Y, Suzuki S (1992b) Sequential nuclear magnetic resonance assignment of β1,2-linked mannooligosaccharides isolated from the phosphomannan of the pathogenic yeast *Candida albicans* NIH B-792 strain. Biochemistry 31:5680–5686

Shibata N, Ikuta K, Imai T, Satoh Y, Richi S, Suzuki A, Kojima C, Kobayashi H, Hisamichi K, Suzuki S (1995) Existence of branched side chains in the cell wall mannan of pathogenic yeast, *Candida albicans*. Structure–antigenicity relationship between the cell wall mannans of *Candida albicans* and *Candida parapsilosis*. J Biol Chem 270:1113–1122

Shibata N, Akagi R, Hosoya T, Kawahara K, Suzuki A, Ikuta K, Kobayashi H, Hisamichi K, Okawa Y, Suzuki S (1996a) Existence of novel branched side chains containing β-1,2 and α-1,6 linkages corresponding to antigenic factor 9 in the mannan of *Candida guilliermondii*. J Biol Chem 271:9259–9266

Shibata N, Onosawa M, Tadano N, Hinosawa Y, Suzuki A, Ikuta K, Kobayashi H, Suzuki S, Okawa Y (1996b) Structure and antigenicity of the mannans of *Candida famata* and *Candida saitoana*: comparative study with the mannan of *Candida guilliermondii*. Arch Biochem Biophys 336:49–58

Torosantucci A, Bromuro C, Chiani P, De Bernardis F, Berti F, Galli C, Norelli F, Bellucci C, Polonelli L, Costantino P, Rappuoli R, Cassone A (2005) A novel glyco-conjugate vaccine against fungal pathogens. J Exp Med 202:597–606

van Roon AMM, Pannu NS, de Vrind JPM, van der Marel GA, van Boom JH, Hokke CH, Deelder AM, Abrahams JP (2004) Structure of an anti-Lewis X Fab fragment in complex with its Lewis X antigen. Structure 12:1227–1236

Villeneuve S, Souchon H, Riottot M-M, Mazié J-C, P-s L, Glaudemans CPJ, Kováč P, Fournier J-M, Alzari PM (2000) Crystal structure of an anti-carbohydrate antibody directed against *Vibrio cholerae* O1 in complex with antigen: molecular basis for serotype specificity. Proc Natl Acad Sci USA 97:8433–8438

Vulliez-Le Normand B, Saul FA, Phalipon A, Bélot F, Guerreiro C, Mulard LA, Bentley GA (2008) Structures of synthetic O-antigen fragments from serotype 2a *Shigella flexneri* in complex with a protective monoclonal antibody. Proc Natl Acad Sci USA 105(29):9976–81, Epub 2008 Jul 10

Vyas NK, Vyas MN, Chervenak MC, Johnson MA, Pinto BM, Bundle DR, Quiocho FA (2002) Molecular recognition of oligosaccharide epitopes by a monoclonal Fab specific for *Shigella flexneri* Y lipopolysaccharide: X-ray structures and thermodynamics. Biochemistry 41:13575–13586

Walsh TJ, Lee JW, Lecciones J, Kelly P, Peter J, Thomas V, Bacher J, Pizzo PA (1990a) SCH-39304 in prevention and treatment of disseminated candidiasis in persistently granulocytopenic rabbits. Antimicrob Agents Chemother 34:1560–1564

Walsh TJ, Lee JW, Lecciones J, Kelly P, Peter J, Thomas V, Bacher J, Pizzo PA (1990b) Effects of preventive, early, and late antifungal chemotherapy with fluconazole in different granulocytopenic models of experimental disseminated candidiasis. J Infect Dis 161:755–760

Weinstein MP, Towns ML, Quartey SM, Mirrett S, Reimer LG, Parmigiani G, Reller LB (1997) The clinical significance of positive blood cultures in the 1990s: a prospective comprehensive evaluation of the microbiology, epidemiology, and outcome of bacteremia and fungemia in adults. Clin Infect Dis 24:584–602

Wu X, Ling CC, Bundle DR (2004) A new homobifunctional p-nitro phenyl ester coupling reagent for the preparation of neoglycoproteins. Org Lett 6:4407–4410

Wu X, Bundle DR (2005) Synthesis of glycoconjugate vaccines for *Candida albicans* using novel linker methodology. J Org Chem 70:7381–7388

Wu X, Lipinski T, Carrel FR, Bailey JJ, Bundle DR (2007) Synthesis and immunochemical studies on a *Candida albicans* cluster glycoconjugate vaccine. Org Biomol Chem 5:3477–3485

Wu X, Lipinski T, Paszkiewicz E, Bundle DR (2008) Synthesis and immunochemical characterization of S-linked glycoconjugate vaccines against *Candida albicans*. Chem Eur J 14:6474–6482

Xin H, Dziadek S, Bundle DR, Cutler JE (2008) Synthetic glycopeptide vaccines combining β-mannan and peptide epitopes induce protection against candidiasis. Proc Natl Acad Sci USA 105:13526–13531

Zdanov A, Li Y, Bundle DR, Deng S-J, MacKenzie CR, Narang SA, Young NM, Cygler M (1994) Structure of a single-chain Fv fragment complexed with a carbohydrate antigen at 1.7 Å resolution. Proc Natl Acad Sci USA 91:6423–6427

The Neutralizing Anti-HIV Antibody 2G12

6

Renate Kunert

6.1 The Anti HIV-1 Neutralizing Antibody 2G12 and It's Neutralizing Activity

The human monoclonal antibody (mAb) 2G12 was isolated from an asymptomatic HIV-1 infected patient in 1990. In 1994, its neutralizing activity against HIV-1 strains and binding to the glycoprotein 120 (gp120) was described for the first time (Buchacher et al. 1994; Purtscher et al. 1994; Trkola et al. 1995). At that time a recombinantly expressed 2G12 IgG1 protein was already available (see below) and characterization was exclusively done with this recombinant molecule so that a confusion between hybridoma derived and recombinantly expressed 2G12 could be precluded.

In principle, mAbs possess different ways to counteract HIV-1, (a) cell free neutralization, (b) complement mediated activities and (c) antibody dependent cellular cytotoxicity (ADCC), all of which have been shown to be employed by mAb 2G12 and seem to be responsible for its broad reactivity against primary and T-cell line adapted strains of HIV-1 (Trkola et al. 1996). Due to its broad biological activities, mAb 2G12 is able to defend against infection with primary HIV isolates from various clades, either by direct virus neutralization or in combination with other effector cells and complement activation. This was shown impressively with the HIV-1-MN strain (Trkola et al. 1996) which is not neutralized in a cell free assay. However, in combination with activated human complement, HIV-1-MN was unable to form syncytia of AA-2 lymphoblastoid cells, indicator cells with syncytia formation upon HIV infection. The specific effect of complement activation was confirmed by deposition of complement factor C3 on infected cells.

ADCC activity was evaluated with different HIV-1 infected cell lines in a ^{51}Cr release assay (Klein et al. 2010; Trkola et al. 1996). In this assay, the infected target

R. Kunert (✉)
University of Natural Resources and Life Sciences, Muthgasse 18, 1190 Vienna, Austria
e-mail: renate.kunert@boku.ac.at

P. Kosma and S. Müller-Loennies (eds.), *Anticarbohydrate Antibodies*,
DOI 10.1007/978-3-7091-0870-3_6, © Springer-Verlag/Wien 2012

cells were labelled with $Na_2{}^{51}CrO_4$ and in addition to mAb 2G12, peripheral blood mononuclear cells (PBMCs) isolated from healthy HIV-1 negative donors, were added as effector cells. The percentage of released ^{51}Cr was then calculated relative to the total amount of ^{51}Cr released by 1% Triton X-100 treatment. This test revealed that 2G12 is a potent mediator of ADCC and induces specific lysis of various infected cells (recombinant gp120/IIIB CEM.NKR cells, HIV-1 IIIB infected CEM.NKR cells, HIV-1 MN infected CEM.NKR cells).

6.2 Binding of mAb 2G12 to gp120

Already in the early 1990s the specificity of mAb 2G12 for *N*-linked glycans in the domains C2, C3, V4 and C4 of the HIV-1 gp120 became evident from binding studies. The combination of glycan trees on different constant and variable regions of gp120 forms a unique structure in a special arrangement allowing mAb 2G12 to efficiently bind the isolated protein and also primary HIV-1 isolates, leading to the very broad neutralizing activity. A molecular understanding of the binding to this peculiar envelope epitope should facilitate rational design of a HIV-1 vaccine and the performed structural and biochemical studies will be described below.

6.2.1 Glycans of HIV-1 gp120

The envelope protein gp120 of HIV is highly glycosylated with nearly 50% of the mass contributed by carbohydrates. In general, glycoproteins may possess various forms of *N*-linked carbohydrates categorized as high-mannose, hybrid and complex glycans. It is known that the choice of host cell line has an impact on the glycosylation pattern of secreted proteins. After expression of HTLV-III B gp120 in CHO cells and lymphoblastoid H9 cells high-mannose, hybrid and complex *N*-glycan structures were found to be present (Mizuoch et al. 1988; Mizuochi et al. 1990). By contrast, gp120 produced in insect cells were shown to contain mainly high-mannose glycans after purification on Con-A sepharose (Yeh et al. 1993) which were processed to different extents depending on the site of glycosylation. The glycosylation pattern of gp120 has been analyzed in detail by Leonard et al. (1990) who identified 11 high-mannose- and/or hybrid, and 13 complex type oligosaccharides. The combination of different methods, like the use of different enzymatic digestions, HPLC separation, matrix-assisted laser desorption/ionization (MALDI) and nanoelectrospray MS/MS led to the identification of glycans found on 26 consensus glycosylation sites on recombinant gp120 of HIV-1 strain SF2 expressed in mammalian CHO cells. Based on known crystal structures and the carbohydrate analyses structural models were developed for the completely glycosylated intact protein (Zhu et al. 2000; Chen et al. 2005). Such models indicated that the high-mannose glycans are clustered on the surface of gp120 while the complex glycans form an additional cluster which do not overlap. This clustering might have biological implications for, e.g., the interaction with cellular glycans and also the mannose binding lectin.

6.2.2 Analysis of the 2G12 Epitope

In the first experiments to clarify the nature of the 2G12 epitope, 2G12 binding was characterized in different preparations of recombinant gp120 expressed in mammalian and insect cells. While binding was identified in both preparations and even in urea-denatured forms of mammalian and insect cell-derived gp120, binding was completely abolished when the mammalian protein was in the reduced state. These findings imply that the 2G12 epitope is discontinuous in nature or otherwise sensitive to the gp120 conformation (Moore et al. 1994). Afterwards it was shown that 2G12 could not bind any longer to deglycosylated forms of gp120. These first investigations made clear that 2G12 binds to a conformational epitope generated by sugar moieties. More detailed information was given by site directed mutagenesis experiments affecting glycosylation sites in the C2 and C3 domains near the base of the V3 loop, and in the C4 region giving evidence that the discontinuous epitope is centred around the C3/V4 domain of gp120 and is clearly sensitive to the presence of *N*-linked glycosylation in this part of the molecule (Trkola et al. 1996). Cross-competition experiments with 45 human and rodent mAbs to continuous and discontinuous gp120 epitopes demonstrated that 2G12 binds to a distinctive epitope that is recognized by no other known anti-gp120 mAb.

More detailed information was collected a couple of years later after the neutralizing potential of 2G12 was approved in SCID-mice and macaque challenging studies (Mascola et al. 1999; Mascola et al. 2000; Baba et al. 2000; Zwick et al. 2001; Ruprecht et al. 2001; Stiegler et al. 2002; Gauduin et al. 1997).

At that time it was already known that only very few antibodies are naturally made against the carbohydrate moiety of gp120, possibly due to its large size and potential conformational flexibility. The protein backbone under the glycan surface forms the scaffold for the glycans but is not accessible to immune recognition and therefore this region of gp120 is called the “silent face” of the viral envelope. To elucidate further the molecular nature of the 2G12 epitope site directed alanine scanning mutagenesis was performed on gp120 (Scanlan et al. 2002). In this study, recombinant gp120 was expressed with asparagine (N) to alanine (A) mutations at positions N295, N332, N339, N386, and N392 that eliminated the *N*-linked carbohydrate attachment sites assumed to be of significant importance for the 2G12 binding affinity (HIV-1 isolate JR-CSF). By using these mutants in ELISA tests it became evident that the affinity for the 2G12 interaction decreased significantly for all mutants.

The assumption that all five glycan residues are involved in antibody binding was further tested by alternative mutations showing that the carbohydrates assigned to positions 339 and 386 are not crucial for 2G12 binding. Figure 6.1(a) shows a model of gp120 in the C4-V4 face of gp120 viewed from the perspective of the V4 loop and Fig. 6.1(b) the spatial location of the V3 and V4 loops. The additional

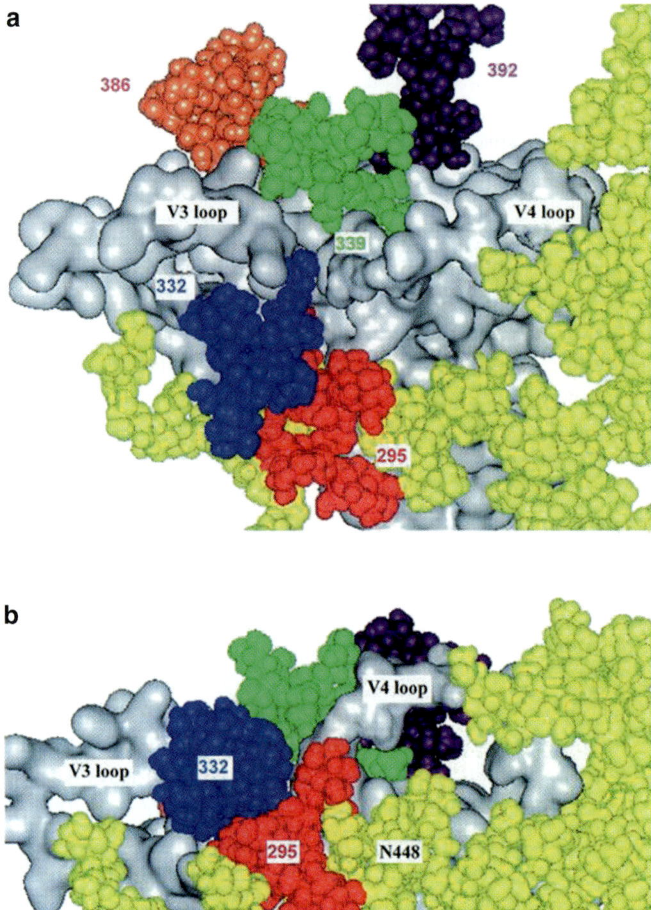

Fig. 6.1 Location of gp120 N-linked glycans involved in 2G12 binding. The *N*-glycans which are likely to be primarily involved in 2G12 binding are shown in *red* (*N*-glycan of N295), *blue* (*N*-glycan of N332), and *purple* (*N*-glycan of N392). *N*-glycans which influence 2G12 binding but which are not directly involved in binding are shown in *green* (*N*-glycan of N339) and *orange* (*N*-glycan of N386). Other carbohydrate chains are shown in *yellow*. (**a**) Surface of the C4-V4 face of gp120 viewed from the perspective of the V4 loop. (**b**) Spatial location of the V3 and V4 loops, which are proposed to extend from the protein surface in the region of the 2G12 epitope. Glycans were modelled onto the core structure of gp120 according to highest population types and lineages, based on results of mass spectrometry (Zhu et al. 2000) (From: J Virol. 2002 July; 76(14): 7306–7321. doi: 10.1128/JVI.76.14.7306-7321.2002. Copyright© 2002, American Society for Microbiology)

carbohydrate in this cluster in position N448 was identified to be unnecessary for 2G12 binding at least in isolate HIV-FR-CSF.

Calculation of the surface area of *N*-glycans involved in 2G12 binding makes clear that the epitope recognized by the antibody can be only a fractional amount of the solvent-accessible surface surrounding the Man residues at glycosylation sites 295, 332, 386, 392 and 448. Thus the actual 2G12 epitope must represent only a small portion of this surface.

In order to elucidate the epitope of mAb 2G12 binding was investigated after enzymatic digest of *N*-glycans. Treatment of gp120 with NgF, Endo F1, Endo H, or α-mannosidase abolished 2G12 binding completely. By contrast, digestion with glycosidases specific for complex glycans like neuraminidase or endo-β-galactosidase had no significant impact on 2G12 binding (Sanders et al. 2002). Control experiments showed that the structure of gp120 was not substantially altered by most glycosidases except NgF. The treatment of gp120 with this enzyme reduced binding of a polyclonal anti-HIV-1 serum significantly. Affinity measurements between 2G12 and different gp120 preparations treated with endoglycosidases revealed that 2G12-gp120 binding was lost when gp120 was treated with *Aspergillus saitoi* mannosidase (cleaving only αMan(1→2)αMan linkages) and also Jack Bean mannosidase (specifically releasing terminal Man residues from α(1→2), α(1→3), and α(1→6)-linked sugars) indicating that the α(1→2)-linked Man disaccharides of oligomannose glycans on gp120 are required for 2G12 binding (Sanders et al. 2002).

Consistent with this finding, the binding of mAb 2G12 to gp120 could be prevented by high concentrations of monomeric Man but not by Gal, Glc, or GlcNAc. The inability of 2G12 to bind to gp120 expressed in the presence of the Glc analogue *N*-butyl-deoxynojirimycin (Sanders et al. 2002) similarly implicated terminal αMan(1→2)αMan in 2G12 binding since this analogue inhibits glucosidase I and II in the endoplasmic reticulum leaving Glc capped sugars on the gp120 high-mannose glycans.

With this information further studies with typical high-mannose type oligosaccharides, namely $Man_5GlcNAc$, $Man_6GlcNAc$ and $Man_9GlcNAc$, isolated from ovalbumin and soybean agglutinin, were performed. $Man_9GlcNAc$ bound with much higher affinity to 2G12 leading to the conclusion that the terminal α(1→2)-linked Man disaccharide is the most important since $Man_9GlcNAc$ contains three accessible disaccharide bonds in contrast to $Man_6GlcNAc$ with only one and $Man_5GlcNAc$ with no α(1→2)-linked Man (Wang et al. 2004). The interaction of 2G12 with different oligomannose derivatives was investigated in greater detail using synthetic mono-, di- and triantennary oligomannosides displaying the original structure of a high-mannose glycan on a glycoprotein (Calarese et al. 2005). The study combined solution-phase ELISA, carbohydrate microcarrier analysis and co-crystallization of distinct oligomannosides with 2G12 Fab. Thereby it became evident that 2G12 can bind to the αMan(1→2)αMan residues at the termini of both arms, D1 and D3, of a high mannose structure.

6.3 Structural Peculiarities of mAb 2G12

The first indication of an unusual structure of 2G12 came from gel filtration analysis of 2G12 Fab papain digests in comparison to other IgG1 antibodies because the 2G12 Fab eluted from a size exclusion column at a molecular mass of approx. 100 kDa, instead of the expected 50 kDa. This suggested that 2G12 Fab exists almost entirely as dimers in solution. The second evidence for the presence of 2G12 Fab dimers in solution was given by a sedimentation coefficient analysis indicating a higher $S_{20,W}$ value for 2G12 as compared to other IgG1 Fabs pointing to a more compact structure of the mAb 2G12 than other IgG with a Y-shaped configuration (Calarese et al. 2003).

The visualization by electron microscopy (Schülke et al. 2002) elucidated that the two Fab arms of 2G12 IgG1 extended in a vertical Y configuration in such a way that the Fab arms were parallel and adjacent to each other. This configuration was found in unreacted 2G12 (Fig. 6.2) as well as in complexes of 2G12 IgG1 with gp120. This so called I-shaped configuration is realized by an unusual non covalent tight interaction of two independent Fab arms observed in each single IgG1 and also in papain digests thereof where the Fab arms form dimers. Moreover, purified 2G12

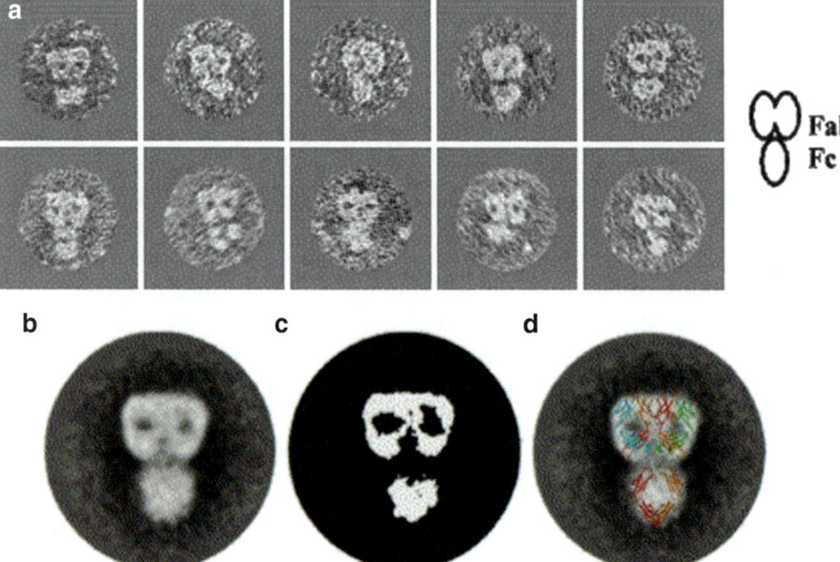

Fig. 6.2 Electron microscopy of 2G12. (**a**) Representative images of individual 2G12 molecules and interpretive diagram. × 500,000. (**b**) Computationally averaged electron micrographs ($n = 123$) of 2G12. (**c**) Averaged image subjected to threshold cutoff analysis emphasizing the portions of the image with greater density. (**d**) Averaged image with superimposed atomic structures of 2G12 Fab dimer (PDB 1om3, Calarese et al. 2003), B–D × 1,000,000 and human Fc fragment (PDB 1fc1, Deisenhofer 1981). *Blue* and *green*: light chains, *red* and *gold*: heavy chains (From: Molecular Immunology 41 (2004) 1001–1011. doi:10.1016/j.molimm.2004.05.008)

heavy and light chains re-associate to form molecules with 2G12 morphology even in the absence of inter-chain disulfide bond formation leading to the assumption that no significant torsional force upon the elbow junction between constant and variable regions is necessary for the extended I-shaped configuration (Roux et al. 2004).

The first crystal structure of Fab 2G12 was reported in 2003 (Calarese et al. 2003). The VH domains form a two-fold symmetry axis with a 178.5° angle due to the variable heavy and light chain interaction forming the regular combining site. The second axis is generated in the same direction by interaction of the two VH domains with an angle of 35°. Thereby two Fabs are arranged side by side (compare Figs. 6.2(d) and 6.3) as a domain-swapped dimer which is able to assemble a novel

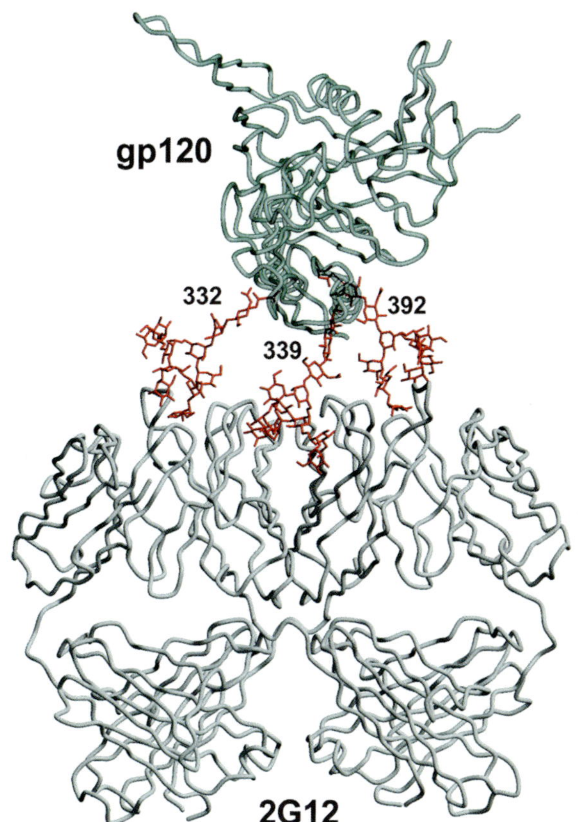

Fig. 6.3 Model of 2G12 glycan recognition of gp120. Three separate Man9GlcNAc2 moieties, shown in *red* (two in the primary combining sites and one in the VH/VH' interface) potentially mediate the binding of 2G12 to gp120. The glycans at the primary combining sites originate from N332 and N392 (labelled) in gp120, whereas the carbohydrate located at the VH/VH' interface would arise from N339 (labelled). *N*-linked glycans occurring at N332 and N392 have previously been implicated as critical for 2G12 binding (Scanlan et al. 2002). The *N*-linked glycan at N339 is not as critical for 2G12 binding, although this glycan could potentially interact with the VH/VH' interface (From: Science, 2003, 300: 2065–2071)

and additional antigen binding site at the VH/VH' interface in addition to the two conventional VH/VL binding sites. Such structures with similar function are also known from Cyanovirin-N, a lectin binding mannose rich glycans (Barrientos and Gronenborn 2002; Barrientos et al. 2003; Botos and Wlodawer 2005).

In 2G12, 3 factors have been identified with potential responsibility for the unusual domain exchange predominantly induced by somatic mutations in VH (Calarese et al. 2005; Kwong and Wilson 2009), (a) the interface contact of VH/VL is rather weak, (b) the connection between VH and CH1, the elbow region, is more flexible and (c) the VH/VH' is favourably created. The somatic mutations were predicted by means of the crystal structure and comparison to germline motifs (Calarese et al. 2003). Thereby five amino acids were identified belonging to the JH region and some additional VH and VL amino acids seemed to be responsible for the generation of the new antigen binding site. For proof of concept recombinant 2G12 like antibodies were expressed in recombinant CHO cells to determine if predominantly changes in the hinge loop or a combination of somatic mutations distributed over the entire variable region are responsible for dimerization of mAb 2G12 Fabs (Gach et al. 2010). Characterization of the structure by circular dichroism spectrometry indicated rather similar structures when only amino acids in the hinge region were exchanged but significant changes in the tertiary structure appeared by introducing additional back mutations to germline genes. In parallel a successive decreasing predominance of the I-shaped conformations was observed in electron microscopy and also dimerization was lost. Moreover, binding to recombinant HIV1-MN envelope protein was nearly abolished. Further investigations of factors responsible for the domain exchange revealed how single amino acids located at the VH/VH' interface interact with the elbow region (Huber et al. 2010) and recently a non-domain-exchanged 2G12 antibody was obtained by exchange of a single amino acid in the framework 1 region of the 2G12 heavy chain. Interestingly, this newly generated antibody was not able to bind to the envelope glycoprotein on HIV-transfected cells and did not neutralize HIV-1 pseudoviruses, despite of the fact that this 2G12 variant was able to bind gp120 in an ELISA test after complexation with anti-Fc antibodies (Doores et al. 2010).

Additionally, the crystallographic data showed that the unusual domain swapped structure of 2G12 is able to bind either two D1 arms from different sugars or a combination of D1 and D3 of a single oligoglycan or even different molecules. This mode of recognition seems to enhance binding avidity to the multivalent clustered carbohydrate surface of gp120, leaving some space for carbohydrate inaccuracies and finally increasing the neutralizing potency significantly. No significant binding of mAb 2G12 to self proteins has been observed.

6.4 Binding of Lectins

The proof of HIV neutralization by mAb 2G12 via a carbohydrate epitope stimulated studies to test the ability of lectins to defend against HIV infections. Subsequently, Griffithsin (GRFT), a lectin isolated from red algae with a 121 amino acid dimeric protein with a domain-swapped structure (Ziółkowska and Wlodawer 2006), and other lectins like Cyanovirin-N (CV-N) or Scytovirin (SVN) have been shown being able to neutralize HIV-1 by binding to mannose-rich glycans found on gp120. The CV-N lectin binds to $\alpha(1{\rightarrow}2)$-linked Man residues and has been shown to inhibit the binding of mAb 2G12 to gp120 (Bewley and Otero-Quintero 2001), providing further indirect evidence for the specificity of 2G12. These competition experiments revealed that 2G12 only interacts with a subset of the available αMan($1{\rightarrow}2$)αMan disaccharides. Consideration of all binding data and a molecular model of gp120 suggests that the most likely epitope for 2G12 is formed by Man residues of glycans attached to N295 and N332, while the other glycans play an indirect role in maintaining the epitope conformation (Scanlan et al. 2002).

Based on their ability to block HIV-1 entry, distinct lectins have been proposed (François and Balzarini 2011; Alexandre et al. 2010) as potential microbicides to prevent the sexual transmission of HIV, despite the fact that these lectins are not HIV specific. The occurrence of high-mannose glycans on mammalian cells, despite rare, leave a low risk of toxicity upon application in humans.

6.5 Expression and Large Scale Production of mAb 2G12 for Clinical Studies

Peripheral blood mononuclear cells (PBMC) were isolated from fresh blood samples and fused with myeloma cells (CB-F7) by electroporation in a hypotonic PEG-containing buffer system (Buchacher et al. 1994). Primary hybridomas were stabilized in hypoxanthine, amenopterin and thymidine (HAT) containing medium and plated with an initial number of 100,000 lymphocytes per well. Growing clones were screened for binding to recombinant vaccinia virus-derived gp160/IIIB (a gift from Immuno AG) and clones with positively reacting culture supernatants were further subcloned by the limiting dilution method to eliminate non producing clones. Thereby the productivity of the 2G12 expressing hybridomas was increased to 10 pg per cell and day.

Of 2G12 hybridoma cells mRNA was isolated and transcribed into cDNA with random hexamer primers and reverse transcriptase (Kunert et al. 1998). From the purified cDNA preparation heavy and light chains were amplified using family specific antibody sense and antisense primers. Amplicons with common heavy and light chain signal regions were inserted into eukaryotic expression vectors (pRC/RSV). The host cell line, CHO-DUKX-B11 (Urlaub and Chasin 1980), was co-transfected with three plasmids, the two for heavy and light chain and one containing the dihydrofolate-reductase gene for amplification of gene copy number with methotrexate (MTX). Clone isolation was done with standard procedures and final screening of the producer clone was done after adaptation to protein free cultivation conditions.

For *in vivo* studies and clinical trials 2G12 IgG1 was manufactured by Polymun Immunbiologische Forschung GmbH (Vienna, Austria) according to current GMP guidelines. One ampoule of the recombinant CHO cell line expressing 2G12 working cell bank is thawed in a protein-free growth medium. For inoculum preparation, cell expansion is performed afterwards in Roux-bottles and spinner flasks to a volume of approximately 2 l. The bioreactor cultivation system for cell propagation to production scale consists of three stirred tank reactors (bioreactor F1 with 15 l working volume, bioreactor F3 with 260 l working volume and bioreactor F5 with 1,750 l working volume). The stirred tank reactors are equipped with axial flow marine type impellers which are used for liquid mixing. Aeration is achieved via gas mixing of air, nitrogen and oxygen. The gas mixture is sparged into the culture fluid. The pH is controlled via CO_2 gas flow and by addition of base solution.

An industrial process-management system (TDC 3000, Honeywell) is used for process control and the fermentation is carried out at set-point 37°C, pH 7.0, pO_2 30% of air saturation. For production of approx. 1,500 l raw supernatant the fermentation procedure contains a three step scale-up procedure, whereas in the third bioreactor a fed-batch process is performed by addition of a nutrient concentrate. Every 8–12 days the total bioreactor volume (up to 1,700 l) with a cell density of 1–5 $\times$ 10^6 cells/ml and cell viability of at least 30% is harvested. The production harvest is transferred into sterile storage vessels and cooled down to 25 $\pm$ 5°C.

The clarification process is carried out in a closed system. A continuous hydrohermetic disk-stack centrifuge (Westfalia CSA-1, Germany) is used for cell separation. Further clarification is achieved by depth filtration using a depth filter (Seitz, Germany, Type Bio or Cuno, USA, Type ZetaPlus) followed by a 0.2 μm filtration (Pall, UK). The clarified supernatant is stored in a sterile plastic bag (Stedim, France) at 5 $\pm$ 3°C.

The clarified supernatant is applied by expanded bed adsorption technology onto the sanitized and equilibrated Streamline® rProtein-A Column (Amersham Biosciences, Sweden). The antibody is adsorbed on the affinity column. After adsorption, unbound proteins and impurities are washed out. DNA-removal and virus inactivation/removal is achieved by incubation with Benzonase® detergent buffer in the expanded bed over night (12–18 h) at room temperature, which is washed out thereafter. The antibody is then eluted in settled bed mode. An additional robust step contributing to the inactivation of potential viral contaminations is the incubation of the eluate of the rProtein A affinity chromatography for at least 2 h at a pH of 3.4–3.9. Q-Sepharose anion exchange chromatography is performed for further DNA and HCP removal afterwards at neutral pH where the antibody passes through the column. Finally, cross flow filtration is used for the buffer exchange to the final formulation buffer (acetic acid/maltose) and concentration to about 9–15 mg/ml.

6.6 Natural Development of mAb 2G12 and the Implications for Vaccine Design

Much effort has been undertaken to elicit 2G12 like antibodies which are neutralizing HIV by binding to an immunologically almost silent site of gp120.

The numerous mutations in the variable regions and the rare occurrence of 2G12 like antibodies suggest that this antibody has undergone intensive somatic maturation. If such antibodies are generally generated in response to HIV infection, it should have been possible to isolate or detect antibodies with 2G12 specificity more frequently. This is clearly not the case, and therefore it seems likely that 2G12 maturation was only possible by a immunological costimulation by different antigens (Doores et al. 2010). Testing 2G12 binding to various mannan rich pathogens revealed that a large number of fungi especially various *Candida* species are recognized by 2G12 (Dunlop et al. 2008). These pathogens are often found associated in immunodeficient patients. The mannose branches on the cellular surface of yeasts would give plausibility for the lost tolerance to self-oligomannose structures which are determined by human cells in HIV infection. With these findings the use of anti-mannan antibodies as components of immune strategies can thereby be re-evaluated. However, it remains to be investigated further at which stage these 2G12 maturation mutations occurred in the evolution of this very unique antibody.

Taken together it is generally accepted that for the development of a carbohydrate recognizing antibody such as 2G12 the viral replication of HIV must be maintained in the patient for years (Sather et al. 2009). Additionally and most likely such antibodies can only be elicited by the immune system if the HIV infection is accompanied by concomitant high antigen load rendering a high degree of somatic mutations to the developing antibody and in case of 2G12 leading to the exceptional I-shaped structure of 2G12 (Kwong and Wilson 2009).

Acknowledgement I want to thank all scientists and technicians at the Institute of Applied Microbiology and at Polymun Scientific who have contributed to the development and production for providing high quality material of 2G12.

References

Alexandre KB, Gray ES, Lambson BE, Moore PL, Choge IA, Mlisana K, Karim SS, McMahon J, O'Keefe B, Chikwamba R, Morris L (2010) Mannose-rich glycosylation patterns on HIV-1 subtype C gp120 and sensitivity to the lectins, Griffithsin, Cyanovirin-N and Scytovirin. Virology 402:187–196

Baba TW, Liska V, Hofmann-Lehmann R, Vlasak J, Xu W, Ayehunie S, Cavacini LA, Posner MR, Katinger H, Stiegler G, Bernacky BJ, Rizvi TA, Schmidt R, Hill LR, Keeling ME, Lu Y, Wright JE, Chou TC, Ruprecht RM (2000) Human neutralizing monoclonal antibodies of the IgG1 subtype protect against mucosal simian-human immunodeficiency virus infection. Nat Med 6:200–206

Barrientos LG, Gronenborn AM (2002) The domain-swapped dimer of cyanovirin-N contains two sets of oligosaccharide binding sites in solution. Biochem Biophys Res Commun 298:598–602

Barrientos LG, Louis JM, Ratner DM, Seeberger PH, Gronenborn AM (2003) Solution structure of a circular-permuted variant of the potent HIV-inactivating protein cyanovirin-N: structural basis for protein stability and oligosaccharide interaction. J Mol Biol 325:211–223

Bewley CA, Otero-Quintero S (2001) The potent anti-HIV protein cyanovirin-N contains two novel carbohydrate binding sites that selectively bind to Man(8) D1D3 and Man(9) with nanomolar affinity: implications for binding to the HIV envelope protein gp120. J Am Chem Soc 123:3892–3902

Botos I, Wlodawer A (2005) Proteins that bind high-mannose sugars of the HIV envelope. Prog Biophys Mol Biol 88:233–282

Buchacher A, Predl R, Strutzenberger K, Steinfellner W, Trkola A, Purtscher M, Gruber G, Tauer C, Steindl F, Jungbauer A (1994) Generation of human monoclonal antibodies against HIV-1 proteins; electrofusion and Epstein-Barr virus transformation for peripheral blood lymphocyte immortalization. AIDS Res Hum Retroviruses 10:359–369

Calarese DA, Scanlan CN, Zwick MB, Deechongkit S, Mimura Y, Kunert R, Zhu P, Wormald MR, Stanfield RL, Roux KH, Kelly JW, Rudd PM, Dwek RA, Katinger H, Burton DR, Wilson IA (2003) Antibody domain exchange is an immunological solution to carbohydrate cluster recognition. Science 300:2065–2071

Calarese DA, Lee HK, Huang CY, Best MD, Astronomo RD, Stanfield RL, Katinger H, Burton DR, Wong CH, Wilson IA (2005) Dissection of the carbohydrate specificity of the broadly neutralizing anti-HIV-1 antibody 2G12. Proc Natl Acad Sci USA 102:13372–13377

Chen B, Vogan EM, Gong H, Skehel JJ, Wiley DC, Harrison SC (2005) Structure of an unliganded simian immunodeficiency virus gp120 core. Nature 433:834–841

Deisenhofer J (1981) Crystallographic refinement and atomic models of a human Fc fragment and its complex with fragment B of protein A from *Staphylococcus aureus* at 2.9- and 2.8-A resolution. Biochemistry 20:2361–2370

Doores KJ, Fulton Z, Huber M, Wilson IA, Burton DR (2010) Antibody 2G12 recognizes di-mannose equivalently in domain- and nondomain-exchanged forms but only binds the HIV-1 glycan shield if domain exchanged. J Virol 84:10690–10699

Dunlop DC, Ulrich A, Appelmelk BJ, Burton DR, Dwek RA, Zitzmann N, Scanlan CN (2008) Antigenic mimicry of the HIV envelope by AIDS-associated pathogens. AIDS 22:2214–2217

François KO, Balzarini J (2011) Potential of carbohydrate-binding agents as therapeutics against enveloped viruses. Med Res Rev doi: 10.1002/med.20216

Gach JS, Furtmüller PG, Quendler H, Messner P, Wagner R, Katinger H, Kunert R (2010) Proline is not uniquely capable of providing the pivot point for domain swapping in 2G12, a broadly neutralizing antibody against HIV-1. J Biol Chem 285:1122–1127

Gauduin MC, Parren PW, Weir R, Barbas CF, Burton DR, Koup RA (1997) Passive immunization with a human monoclonal antibody protects hu-PBL-SCID mice against challenge by primary isolates of HIV-1. Nat Med 3:1389–1393

Huber M, Le KM, Doores KJ, Fulton Z, Stanfield RL, Wilson IA, Burton DR (2010) Very few substitutions in a germ line antibody are required to initiate significant domain exchange. J Virol 84:10700–10707

Klein JS, Webster A, Gnanapragasam PN, Galimidi RP, Bjorkman PJ (2010) A dimeric form of the HIV-1 antibody 2G12 elicits potent antibody-dependent cellular cytotoxicity. AIDS 24:1633–1640

Kunert R, Rüker F, Katinger H (1998) Molecular characterization of five neutralizing anti-HIV type 1 antibodies: identification of nonconventional D segments in the human monoclonal antibodies 2G12 and 2F5. AIDS Res Hum Retroviruses 14:1115–1128

Kwong PD, Wilson IA (2009) HIV-1 and influenza antibodies: seeing antigens in new ways. Nat Immunol 10:573–578

Leonard CK, Spellman MW, Riddle L, Harris RJ, Thomas JN, Gregory TJ (1990) Assignment of intrachain disulfide bonds and characterization of potential glycosylation sites of the type 1 recombinant human immunodeficiency virus envelope glycoprotein (gp120) expressed in Chinese hamster ovary cells. J Biol Chem 265:10373–1038

Mascola JR, Lewis MG, Stiegler G, Harris D, VanCott TC, Hayes D, Louder MK, Brown CR, Sapan CV, Frankel SS, Lu Y, Robb ML, Katinger H, Birx DL (1999) Protection of Macaques against pathogenic simian/human immunodeficiency virus 89.6PD by passive transfer of neutralizing antibodies. J Virol 73:4009–4018

Mascola JR, Stiegler G, VanCott TC, Katinger H, Carpenter CB, Hanson CE, Beary H, Hayes D, Frankel SS, Birx DL, Lewis MG (2000) Protection of macaques against vaginal transmission of a pathogenic HIV-1/SIV chimeric virus by passive infusion of neutralizing antibodies. Nat Med 6:207–210

Mizuoch T, Spellman MW, Larkin M, Solomon J, Basa LJ, Feizi T (1988) Structural characterization by chromatographic profiling of the oligosaccharides of human immunodeficiency virus (HIV) recombinant envelope glycoprotein gp120 produced in Chinese hamster ovary cells. Biomed Chromatogr 2:260–270

Mizuochi T, Matthews TJ, Kato M, Hamako J, Titani K, Solomon J, Feizi T (1990) Diversity of oligosaccharide structures on the envelope glycoprotein gp 120 of human immunodeficiency virus 1 from the lymphoblastoid cell line H9. Presence of complex-type oligosaccharides with bisecting N-acetylglucosamine residues. J Biol Chem 265:8519–8524

Moore JP, Sattentau QJ, Wyatt R, Sodroski J (1994) Probing the structure of the human immunodeficiency virus surface glycoprotein gp120 with a panel of monoclonal antibodies. J Virol 68:469–484

Purtscher M, Trkola A, Gruber G, Buchacher A, Predl R, Steindl F, Tauer C, Berger R, Barrett N, Jungbauer A (1994) A broadly neutralizing human monoclonal antibody against gp41 of human immunodeficiency virus type 1. AIDS Res Hum Retroviruses 10:1651–1658

Roux KH, Zhu P, Seavy M, Katinger H, Kunert R, Seamon V (2004) Electron microscopic and immunochemical analysis of the broadly neutralizing HIV-1-specific, anti-carbohydrate antibody, 2G12. Mol Immunol 41:1001–1011

Ruprecht RM, Hofmann-Lehmann R, Smith-Franklin BA, Rasmussen RA, Liska V, Vlasak J, Xu W, Baba TW, Chenine AL, Cavacini LA, Posner MR, Katinger H, Stiegler G, Bernacky BJ, Rizvi TA, Schmidt R, Hill LR, Keeling ME, Montefiori DC, McClure HM (2001) Protection of neonatal macaques against experimental SHIV infection by human neutralizing monoclonal antibodies. Transfus Clin Biol 8:350–358

Sanders RW, Venturi M, Schiffner L, Kalyanaraman R, Katinger H, Lloyd KO, Kwong PD, Moore JP (2002) The mannose-dependent epitope for neutralizing antibody 2G12 on human immunodeficiency virus type 1 glycoprotein gp120. J Virol 76:7293–7305

Sather DN, Armann J, Ching LK, Mavrantoni A, Sellhorn G, Caldwell Z, Yu X, Wood B, Self S, Kalams S, Stamatatos L (2009) Factors associated with the development of cross-reactive neutralizing antibodies during human immunodeficiency virus type 1 infection. J Virol 83:757–769

Scanlan CN, Pantophlet R, Wormald MR, Ollmann SE, Stanfield R, Wilson IA, Katinger H, Dwek RA, Rudd PM, Burton DR (2002) The broadly neutralizing anti-human immunodeficiency virus type 1 antibody 2G12 recognizes a cluster of $\alpha 1 - > 2$ mannose residues on the outer face of gp120. J Virol 76:7306–7321

Schülke N, Vesanen MS, Sanders RW, Zhu P, Lu M, Anselma DJ, Villa AR, Parren PW, Binley JM, Roux KH, Maddon PJ, Moore JP, Olson WC (2002) Oligomeric and conformational properties of a proteolytically mature, disulfide-stabilized human immunodeficiency virus type 1 gp140 envelope glycoprotein. J Virol 76:7760–7776

Stiegler G, Armbruster C, Vcelar B, Stoiber H, Kunert R, Michael NL, Jagodzinski LL, Ammann C, Jäger W, Jacobson J, Vetter N, Katinger H (2002) Antiviral activity of the neutralizing antibodies 2F5 and 2G12 in asymptomatic HIV-1-infected humans: a phase I evaluation. AIDS 16:2019–2025

Trkola A, Pomales AB, Yuan H, Korber B, Maddon PJ, Allaway GP, Katinger H, Barbas CF, Burton DR, Ho DD (1995) Cross-clade neutralization of primary isolates of human immunodeficiency virus type 1 by human monoclonal antibodies and tetrameric CD4-IgG. J Virol 69:6609–6617

Trkola A, Purtscher M, Muster T, Ballaun C, Buchacher A, Sullivan N, Srinivasan K, Sodroski J, Moore JP, Katinger H (1996) Human monoclonal antibody 2G12 defines a distinctive neutralization epitope on the gp120 glycoprotein of human immunodeficiency virus type 1. J Virol 70:1100–1108

Urlaub G, Chasin LA (1980) Isolation of Chinese hamster cell mutants deficient in dihydrofolate reductase activity. Proc Natl Acad Sci USA 77:4216–4220

Wang LX, Ni J, Singh S, Li H (2004) Binding of high-mannose-type oligosaccharides and synthetic oligomannose clusters to human antibody 2G12: implications for HIV-1 vaccine design. Chem Biol 11:127–134

Yeh JC, Seals JR, Murphy CI, van Halbeek H, Cummings RD (1993) Site-specific N-glycosylation and oligosaccharide structures of recombinant HIV-1 gp120 derived from a baculovirus expression system. Biochemistry 32:11087–11099

Zhu X, Borchers C, Bienstock RJ, Tomer KB (2000) Mass spectrometric characterization of the glycosylation pattern of HIV-gp120 expressed in CHO cells. Biochemistry 39:11194–11204

Ziółkowska NE, Wlodawer A (2006) Structural studies of algal lectins with anti-HIV activity. Acta Biochim Pol 53:617–626

Zwick MB, Wang M, Poignard P, Stiegler G, Katinger H, Burton DR, Parren PW (2001) Neutralization synergy of human immunodeficiency virus type 1 primary isolates by cocktails of broadly neutralizing antibodies. J Virol 75:12198–12208

Immune Recognition of Parasite Glycans

7

Rick M. Maizels and James P. Hewitson

7.1 Introduction

Glycan antigens have a long and detailed history in parasite immunology, dating back to identification of an allergenic polysaccharide from the nematode roundworm *Ascaris* by Campbell in 1936 (Campbell 1936). In the intervening 75 years, an extraordinary array of carbohydrate structures have emerged from both of the major biological groups of parasite, the unicellular protozoa and the multicellular (metazoan) helminth worms. Parasite glycans are represented in a full range of carrier molecules, including glycoproteins through *O*- and *N*-linkages, unusual glycolipid structures, and polysaccharides.

Many of the glycan determinants are novel and unique moieties, readily recognised as foreign by host antibodies, and which can dominate the antigenic profile of the parasite as a result. Importantly, protective immunity is not necessarily conferred by antibodies to immunodominant glycan epitopes, suggesting that in some cases they represent decoy specificities that distract the immune system. In addition, there are also many parasite glycans, particularly where core structures are not greatly modified, which replicate host carbohydrates. These may represent instances of molecular mimicry, allowing parasites to escape antibody targeting, or even "glycan gimmickry" in which parasites produce glycan ligands of host lectin receptors that may dampen immune responsiveness (van Die and Cummings 2010).

A chapter contributed to:
Anticarbohydrate Antibodies – from Molecular Basis to Clinical Applications
Editor : Paul Kosma; Pub : Springer New York Vienna, 2011

R.M. Maizels (✉) • J.P. Hewitson
Institute of Immunology and Infection Research, University of Edinburgh, West Mains Road, Edinburgh EH9 3JT, UK
e-mail: rick.maizels@ed.ac.uk

P. Kosma and S. Müller-Loennies (eds.), *Anticarbohydrate Antibodies*,
DOI 10.1007/978-3-7091-0870-3_7, © Springer-Verlag/Wien 2012

In this chapter, we will review the major immunogenic parasite glycans, and summarise the studies available on the specificity and nature of anti-carbohydrate antibodies in the principal parasite infections. Earlier work, much of which is still instructive, measured responsiveness to global glycan compartments, but more recent studies have resulted in fully-defined glycan structures with corresponding specific monoclonal antibodies. An important aspect is the degree to which isotype switching (e.g. from IgM to IgG) occurs in anti-carbohydrate responses, because the absence of switching may indicate a deficiency in B–T lymphocyte collaboration, and result in poor functional characteristics of the antibody. Immunity, in its broadest sense, also involves the recognition of parasite glycans to other immune system receptors (van Die and Cummings 2010), in particular innate pathogen pattern recognition receptors (PRRs), such as toll-like receptors (TLR), and in the case of glycans, C-type lectin receptors (CTL) and galectins (Robinson et al. 2006; Vasta 2009). In addition, certain parasite glycans are known to act as immunomodulators of the host, again interacting with non-antibody components of the immune system (Harn et al. 2009). Where appropriate, we also comment on these facets.

Parasites are infectious eukaryotic organisms which depend for part or all of their life cycle on a host species, and live at the expense of their host. The two principal biological groups of parasites are protozoa and helminths, which are separated by such substantial phylogenetic distances and utilise sufficiently different cellular pathways that we have chosen to discuss them separately (in Sects. 7.2 and 7.3 below). Parenthetically, it should be noted that in the broader sense, parasitism also embraces groups of ectoparasitic arthropods, but as relatively few studies are available on the glycans of these species, we will not describe them further in this article.

7.2 Trypanosomatids

The trypanosomatids include intracellular protozoa (*Leishmania* spp. and the American trypanosome, *Trypanosoma cruzi*) as well as organisms choosing an extracellular habitat (e.g. *T. brucei*). The trypanosomatids are generally transmitted by arthropod vectors (such as the sandfly for *Leishmania* spp.), and share many cellular and molecular features, including extensive use of glycosylphosphatidylinositol (GPI) membrane anchors in multiple classes of cell surface glycoconjugate antigens (Guha-Niyogi et al. 2001).

There are six species of *Leishmania* which cause serious disease (e.g. mucocutaneous or visceral leishmaniasis) in humans (Handman 2001), and they differ significantly in their glycan structures and antigenicity. In each species, however, the surface is coated with a unique lipophosphoglycan (LPG) which is expressed at the plasma membrane at 1–5 × 10^6 copies per cell. The LPGs share a similar architecture of a GPI tail, a $(Gal)_3(Man)_2(Glc)GlcNAc$ linker oligosaccharide, a repeating phosphodisaccharide (e.g. $\rightarrow 6\beta Gal(1\rightarrow 4)\alpha Man(1P\rightarrow)_{10-40}$), and a small cap (e.g. Gal_2Man), as summarised in Fig. 7.1 (Moody et al. 1991; Descoteaux

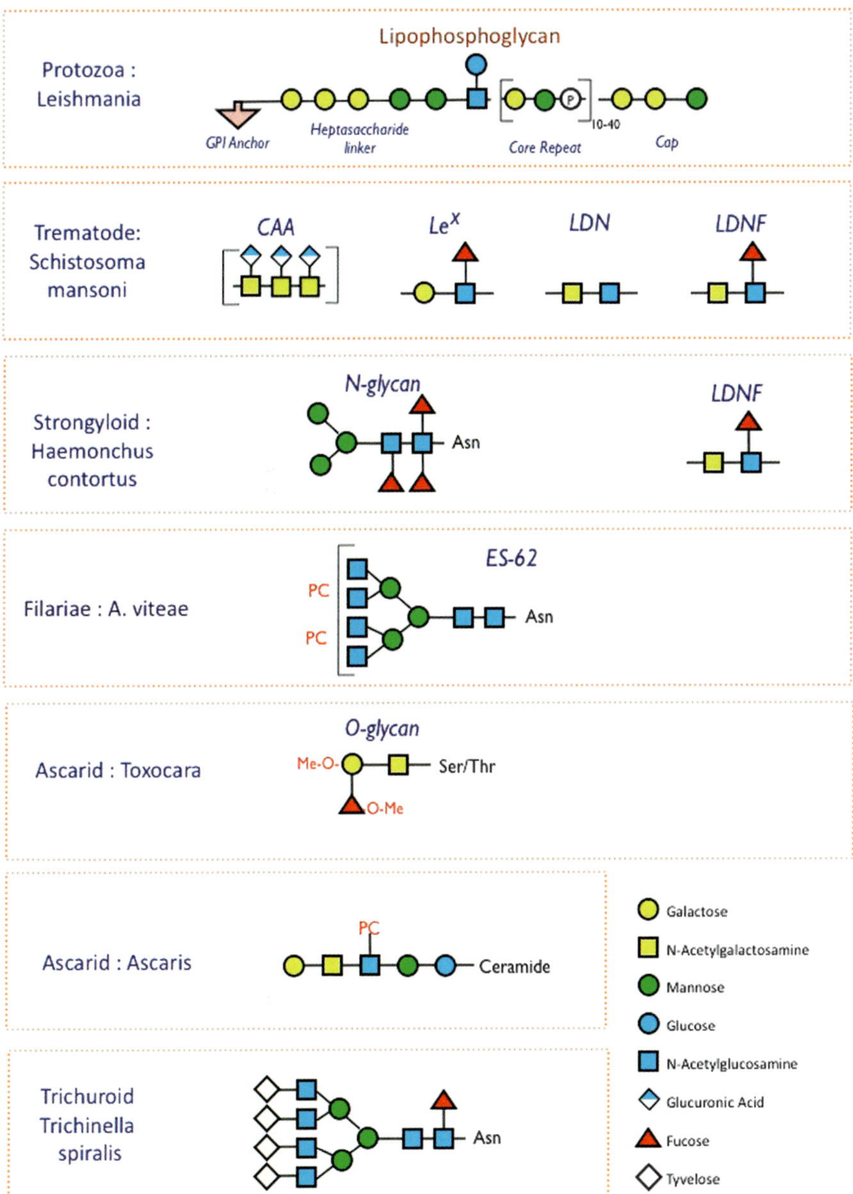

Fig. 7.1 Examples of parasite glycan structures from protozoa (*Leishmania*) and helminth species. Many elaborations of the structures presented are found, as detailed in the text. For example, the core repeat of the *Leishmania* lipophosphoglycan may bear galactose (Gal) side chains, and in Schistosomes there is a high degree of additional fucosylation on the basic LDN structure shown. Unusual modifications include the addition of phosphorylcholine (PC) in filarial and ascarid glycans, the presence of *O*-methylation in *Toxocara*, and the capping of *Trichinella* *N*-glycans with Tyvelose (Tyv) residues

and Turco 1999). The prominence of phosphorylated conjugates reflects their functional importance throughout the complex parasite life cycle (Ilg 2000; Naderer et al. 2004). Species-specific elaborations of this structure play important biological roles: for example, in *L. major*, the core repeat carries β(1→3)Gal substitutions that allow the parasite to bind to the midgut of the sandfly vector for its transmission cycle; once ready to infect a new host, the side chains are extended by addition of an Ara residue in α(1→2)-linkage, allowing the organisms to detach in preparation for invasion. This change may account for the stage-specificity of monoclonal antibodies to LPG from promastigote and amastigote forms (Glaser et al. 1991). Capping the galactosyl side chains may also protect invading parasites from the natural immunity of anti-Gal antibodies in humans. Hence, even with a single species, the structure and therefore antigenicity of LPG will alter around the developmental cycle. Notably, despite the prominence of LPG, it is generally reported to be poorly immunogenic in natural infections, yet is an strong immunogen when presented in a vaccine setting, implying that the live parasite is able to interfere with effective immune priming (McConville et al. 1987).

Leishmania species also express other abundant molecules bearing the same or similar glycan specificities, namely GIPLs (glycosylinositolphospholipids) and PPGs (proteophosphoglycans) (McConville and Bacic 1989; Ilg 2000). While GIPLs contain the (Gal-Man-PO_4) repeat and thus resemble LPG without the linker or cap saccharides, the mucin-like PPGs differ in substituting similar glycans through *O*-linkages to abundant serine residues. Ilg et al. (1993) have described a set of monoclonal antibodies against several different antigens present in the phosphosaccharide repeat, including the terminal Man cap as well as both modified and unmodified phosphorylated repeats. The poor natural immunogenicity of the phosphoglycans (Aebischer et al. 1999) may be explained by their direct immunomodulatory effects, for example on antigen-presenting macrophages.

In African trypanosomes, the building blocks for glycoconjugates are similar to *Leishmania*, but the surface antigen organisation is dramatically different. In *T. brucei*, the entire plasma membrane is a densely packed glycocalyx of one individual product, the Variable Surface Glycoprotein or VSG (Borst and Rudenko 1994). This is GPI-linked, and carries only a modest level of *N*-glycosylation.

The American trypanosome *T. cruzi* is very different from its African congener. Rather than a single uniform *N*-linked gycoprotein, *T. cruzi* expresses a range of *O*-linked glycosylated mucins and GIPLs (Previato et al. 2004). The *O*-linkages are generally through *O*-GlcNAc rather than *O*-GalNAc (Previato et al. 1998), and the overall composition favours GlcNAc and Gal residues (Todeschini et al. 2001). A further intriguing aspect of *T. cruzi* glycans is that the parasite sialylates exposed Gal residues by capturing host sialic acid as a substrate; as with *Leishmania* LPG this modification may protect the parasite from the natural immunity of anti-Gal antibodies in humans. The most prominent resultant sialoglycoproteins are surface-located GPI-linked threonine-rich mucins (Todeschini et al. 2009).

7.2.1 Plasmodium (Malaria)

Plasmodium proteins certainly show a much lower overall level of glycosylation than the trypanosomatids, with the few examples of *N*- or *O*-glycosylation remaining somewhat controversial (Macedo et al. 2010). The glycan structures that have been identified are rudimentary and no specialised modifications have yet been reported in these parasites. The only prominent glycan expressed in malaria is the GPI anchor, similar to other protozoa, but there is little evidence that this is either recognised by host antibody or that antibody plays a protective role. However, release of GPI during processing or degradation of malaria proteins is thought to activate innate inflammatory cells, contributing to the pathogenesis of malaria through glycan-reactive PRRs (Schofield and Hackett 1993).

In contrast to the low profile of parasite glycosylation, malaria organisms rely primarily on interactions with host glycans for the propagation of their life cycle. For example, the ability of parasites to invade host red blood cells involves interactions with sialylated glycans on erythrocyte glycophorin A, while the ability of malaria sexual stages to attach to the mosquito vector midgut requires interaction with a complex insect oligosaccharide (Dinglasan et al. 2003).

7.2.2 *Entamoeba* and Other Protozoa

Entamoeba histolytica is an intestinal protozoon which causes ameobic dysentery and will opportunistically invade the liver. The trophozoite stage in the intestine produces both a *Leishmania*-like LPG and a prominent lipopeptidophosphoglycan (LPPG), also known as PPGs similar in structure to the trypanosomatids, in which the serine residues are coupled to Glc residues (Moody-Haupt et al. 2000). Monoclonal antibody EH5 directed against the LPPG confers protective immunity in experimental mouse infection (Marinets et al. 1997) although the epitope recognised by this antibody has yet to be defined.

7.3 Helminths

Helminths are multicellular worms which are members of the invertebrate phyla Nematoda (roundworms) and Platyhelminthes (flatworms). All have prominent glycoconjugates in their surface structures, such as the glycocalyx of schistosomes and the surface coat of nematodes (Dell et al. 1999). In most species, female worms release eggs which are relatively glycan-rich, and in many cases parasites actively secrete a high level of carbohydrate-containing molecules. Some glycan determinants are found in multiple groups, for example the α(1→3)-linked core fucosylation of LacdiNAc (βGalNAc(1→4)GlcNAc) found in *Schistosoma mansoni*, *Haemonchus contortus* (Haslam et al. 1996) and *Trichinella spiralis* (Fig. 7.1). This structure is not known in vertebrates and may be restricted to invertebrates and plants (Fournet et al. 1987; Wisnewski et al. 1993; Wilson et al. 1998; van Die et al. 1999), and most significantly may be the target of cross-reactive IgE antibodies that were found to bind both honeybee venom and pineapple bromelain in a fucose-dependent manner (Tretter et al. 1993, see also Chap. 8).

A different example is the Tn antigen (truncated GalNAc-*O*-Ser/Thr) which is well-known in mammalian structures and is present (and reactive with the monoclonal antibody 83D4) in multiple cestodes (*Taenia hydatigena*, *Mesocestoides corti*), trematodes (*Fasciola hepatica*) and nematodes (*Nippostrongylus brasiliensis*, *Toxocara canis*) (Casaravilla et al. 2002). Similarly, PC is expressed in most parasitic helminths, in particular as part of *N*-glycan structures of filarial nematodes (Haslam et al. 1999). As one of the objectives of helminth glycoimmunology is specific diagnosis and prophylaxis, the major focus of our discussion will be on species-restricted glycans and the antibodies recognising them.

7.3.1 Schistosomes and Other Trematodes

Several convergent research approaches have provided detailed information on *S. mansoni* glycobiology (Hokke et al. 2007). First, the presence of a thick external glycocalyx around the larval and adult worms revealed by histochemical and lectin staining demonstrated the importance of carbohydrate components in this parasite (Collins et al. 2011). Secondly, it was shown that host antibody responses are dominated by anti-glycan specificities (Norden and Strand 1985; Cummings and Nyame 1999; Hokke and Deelder 2001), and that animals vaccinated with radiation-attentuated cercariae (larvae) generated anti-glycan antibodies (Richter et al. 1996). Thirdly, studies on circulating antigens in *S. mansoni* infections identified two macromolecular carbohydrates present in the serum of infected mice, with contrasting electrophoretic mobility, CAA (circulating anodic antigen, a glycosaminoglycan structure with multiple *O*-linked β(1→6)-linked GalNAc polymers, each with glucuronic acid side chains) and CCA (circulating cathodic antigen, with a shared fucosylated polylactosamine as discussed below) (Cummings and Nyame 1996). Fourthly, a glycomics approach focussing on egg and cercarial secretions has highlighted a suite of complex and novel structures of interest (Jang-Lee et al. 2007). The systematic glycomics also confirmed the structure and reactivity of the major schistosome glycan antigens elucidated in earlier work, including α(1→3)-linked fucosylated derivatives of the basic LacdiNAc (LDN, βGalNAc (1→4)GlcNAc) disaccharide. The three major forms are LDNF (in which GlcNAc is substituted), LDN-DF (in which the side chain on GlcNAc contains a second Fuc) and FLDN (in which the Fuc is linked to GalNAc). In addition, some LDN remains unmodified; this and the presence of fucosylated LDN structures in several other helminth species, such as *F. hepatica* (Kang et al. 1993), and *H. contortus* (see below) is revealed by the binding of *Wistereria floribunda* lectin (to the LDN core) and of the αFuc(1→3)GlcNAc-specific *Lotus tetragonolobus* agglutinin (Nyame et al. 1998).

A further schistosome glycan, and one which appears to be largely expressed only by schistosomes among helminths (Nyame et al. 1998) is the Le^X antigen (βGal(1→4)[αFuc(1→3)]GlcNAc); this is represented for example in the Circulating Cathodic Antigen (Van Dam et al. 1994). The Le^X antigen represents the terminal trisaccharide of the larger lacto-*N*-fucopentaose (LNFPIII) product present in schistosomes. The Le^X structure, along with LDN and LDNF, make up much of the parasite glycocalyx, and monoclonal antibodies to each of these glycans bind strongly to the surface of different parasite stages. Moreover, mAb SMLDN1.1 (specific for LDN) was able to mediate complement-dependent killing of the infective stage (the schistosomula), implying that this determinant could represent an attractive vaccine target (Nyame et al. 2003).

The fucosylated LDN glycans are also highly immunogenic in animal models of infection; over 10% of monoclonal antibodies generated from infected mice recognised fucosylated epitopes, and were also reactive with various tegumental, secretory and/or gut structures of the parasite (van Remoortere et al. 2000). While infected chimpanzees responded with antibodies to αFuc(1→3)GalNAc and αFuc(1→2)αFuc(1→3)GlcNAc, but not to the fucosylated LDN structures (van Remoortere et al. 2003b), human studies indicated the opposite pattern with strong antibody responses to LDN-DF in particular (van Remoortere et al. 2001; Naus et al. 2003), and antibodies to LDN, LDNF and Le^X are all present in chronic human schistosomiasis patients (Nyame et al. 2003).

While Le^X is widely distributed in nature, including the human host, schistosomes present oligomers of this trisaccharide in a species-specific manner; hence while a monoclonal antibody (291-2G3-A) to monomeric Le^X is widely reactive, antibody 54-5C10-A is specific both for schistosome CCA in a diagnostic circulating antigen assay and for ≥ 3 oligmers (de Geus et al. 2009). The sequence and structure of this antibody have been determined and a structural model of the binding site developed which accounts for its selective specificity for the oligomeric form (de Geus et al. 2009).

Schistosome eggs are also heavily glycosylated, and detailed structures of glycans from total egg glycoproteins (Khoo et al. 1997b), egg secretions (Jang-Lee et al. 2007), and individual prominent egg glycoproteins (Wuhrer et al. 2006a; Meevissen et al. 2010, 2011) have been determined. The dominant secreted glycoproteins of schistosome eggs are α-1 and ω-1 (designated by their opposite migration in immunoelectrophoresis). These two proteins share a predominant *N*-glycan structure composed of a diantennary Le^X and a 3,6-difucosylated innermost GlcNAc residue of the *N*-glycan core (Meevissen et al. 2010). In contrast, another important egg glycoprotein, the κ-5 antigen, is modified with a triantennary LDN structure and has a difucosylated and xylosylated core (Meevissen et al. 2011). Human IgG from *Sm*-infected individuals binds to α-1 ω-1, and κ-5, whereas IgE only binds to κ-5, which appears to be the dominant IgE target in human schistosome infection (Schramm et al. 2009). Since recombinant κ-5, lacking schistosome-specific post-translational modifications, failed to bind human IgE, yet was recognised by human IgG, it was suggested that glycans were the immunodominant IgE target. This was confirmed as periodate treatment of native κ-5 ablated IgE recognition, with the specific antigen likely including the β(1→2)-xylosylated core, since neither enzmyatic LDN or core Fuc removal inhibited antibody binding (Meevissen et al. 2011). Despite its lack of immunogenicity in this particular instance, LDN and its carrier κ-5 antigen remain immunologically important given the role of both egg glycans in general and LDN in particular in stimulating the host granulomatous reaction (van de Vijver et al. 2004, 2006). Eggs also release a highly fucosylated schistosome-specific free oligosaccharide (DF-LDN-DF) which is recognised by the monoclonal antibody 114-4D12, and is found in the urine of infected individuals and may be used as a diagnostic tool (Robijn et al. 2007b).

The *N*-glycans of both cercariae (Khoo et al. 2001), and eggs (Khoo et al. 1997b) show a remarkable degree of xylosylation; indeed these Schistosome *N*-glycans may be unique in their configuration of core Fuc and Xyl components. However, xylosylation varies with stage and species, being absent from the adult worms, and present only in cercarial larvae of *S. mansoni* and not *S. japonicum* (Khoo et al. 2001). In the absence of xylosylation, the Le^x structure predominates. Le^x is also the prime determinant of cercarial glycolipids, accompanied by a pseudo-Le^Y structure which is α(1→3) fucosylated on both Gal and GlcNAc residues (Wuhrer et al. 2000). While adult worms do not express the xylosylated structures, there are also interesting differences between male and female worms in both the composition and complexity of *N*-linked antennae (Wuhrer et al. 2006b).

7.3.1.1 Anti-Glycan Antibody Responses in Schistosomes: Host or Parasite Protective?

The role of anti-glycan antibody responses in schistosome infection is hotly debated. Carbohydrate-based vaccines may be advantageous where they are expressed by multiple life-cycle stages, including infective larval parasites thought to be more susceptible to immune attack, both in the secreted material and on the surface of the parasite (Nyame et al. 2004). Several studies have shown that passive immunisation with anti-glycan mAbs (Omer Ali et al. 1988) can confer protection against cercarial challenge, with antibodies IPL-Sm1 reducing worm loads by 50–60% (Grzych et al. 1982), E1 by 40% (Harn et al. 1984), and 3AF12-D6 by 48% (Zodda and Phillips 1982). Because the glycans of keyhole limpet hemocyanin (KLH) are cross-reactive with *S. mansoni*, KLH immunization elicited 50–70% reductions in worm burden in a non-permissive rat model (Grzych et al. 1987), although passive immunisation with rabbit anti-KLH polyclonal antibodies failed to protect more susceptible mice from challenge infection (Mangold and Dean 1992).

An alternative perspective is that anti-glycan immune responses in fact represent a "smokescreen" that benefits the parasite, potentially blocking the binding of more protective anti-peptide antibodies (Eberl et al. 2001). Such blocking anti-glycan antibodies have been demonstrated *in vitro* (Dunne et al. 1987), and non-protective immunisation regimes (e.g. egg immunisation) induce high levels of anti-glycan antibody in baboons, consistent with a non-protective role (Kariuki et al. 2008).

An important consideration is that the isotype of antibody (e.g. the IgG subclass) imparts immunological functions such as complement binding and cell recruitment, and the protective ability of anti-glycan antibodies (which are frequently IgM or IgG3 in humans) may only be conferred by particular immunoglobulin isotypes. Moreover, with increasing evidence that schistosome glycans can be strongly immunomodulatory (discussed in Sect. 4.1 below), the protective potential of such glycans must also be considered in the context of their ability to actually modulate immunity.

7.3.2 Cestodes

Cestodes are a phylum of parasitic helminths which includes tapeworms (such as *Taenia solium*, which causes neurocysticercosis) and *Echinococcus* species which cause two forms of hydatid disease. *T. solium* has two isomeric fucosylated *N*-glycans, one bearing core fucosylation and the other only fucose substitution on peripheral antennae (Lee et al. 2005). Interestingly, among the *O*-glycans of these parasites is a specificity previously associated with mammalian tumors, the Tk antigen, βGlcNAc(1→6)[βGlcNAc(1→3)]Gal, as demonstrated by reactivity with the monoclonal antibody LM389 (Ubillos et al. 2007).

Echinococcus larval stages are encapsulated in a laminated layer, composed of Gal-rich mucins and calcium hexakisphosphate (Diaz et al. 2009, 2011), which induces a suite of immune reactions including IgG antibody production even in the absence of T cell help (Dai et al. 2001). Hydatid protoscoleces, taken from tissue cysts of *Echinococcus granulosus* unusually include some sialic acid content in the *N*-linked glycans, which may well be derived from host sources (Khoo et al. 1997a). Infection of mice generates a strong anti-carbohydrate immune response including antibody to αGal(1→4)Gal as represented by the monoclonal antibody E492/G1 (Dematteis et al. 2001). A βGal(1→6)Gal structure has also been reported in parasite glycosphingolipids to cause antibody cross-reaction between not only the two *Echinococcus* species found in humans, but also more distantly related helminths (Yamano et al. 2009).

7.3.3 Nematodes

Nematode roundworms are both the most numerically prevalent helminth parasites in humans, and the most diverse in terms of the range of different species found in man and animals. The most relevant taxa are Ascarids, Filarial nematodes, Strongylids (including human hookworms), and Trichuroids, and we summarise information available on these groups below.

7.3.3.1 Ascarids

Ascarids include the human and porcine round worms *Ascaris*, and the related intestinal roundworm of animals *Toxocara*. Like many other helminths, the glycoconjugates of *A. suum* from pigs show core fucosylation, but also substitution with phosphorylcholine (PC) (Pöltl et al. 2007). Larval stages of *Toxocara canis* (which cause visceral larva migrans in humans) produce an unusual *O*-linked glycan (Khoo et al. 1991) which is substituted onto multiple polypeptides (Maizels et al. 1987), including a set of secreted mucins (Loukas et al. 2000). The *T. canis* glycan structure is a blood group H-like trisaccharide with 1 or 2 additional *O*-methylated groups on the terminal Fuc and/or central Gal; interestingly, in the closely related feline parasite *T. cati* only the di-methylated form is found. Monoclonal antibodies to the *O*-methylated glycans bind the surface coat as well as large internal secretory glands likely to be the source of mucin synthesis in this organism (Page et al. 1992a,b). Following synthesis of the mono- and di-*O*-methyl substituted structures (Amer et al. 2001), it was shown that mAb Tcn-2 which does not recognise the *T. cati* glycan, binds the mono-*O*-methylated target, while the cross-reactive mAb Tcn-8 that recognises both *Toxocara* species binds to the di-*O*-methylated structure (Schabussova et al. 2007). In addition, human serum antibodies to these glycans are found in infected patients.

7.3.3.2 Filarial Parasites

These parasites are vector-borne and cause lymphatic filariasis and onchocerciasis in humans, estimated to represent 120 million cases worldwide. Although one of the human-infective species, *Brugia malayi*, can be maintained in laboratory animals, most glycobiological research has focussed on two rodent parasites, *Acanthcheilonema viteae* and *Litomosoides sigmodontis*. In *A. viteae*, a significant structure is the *N*-glycan of the secreted protein ES-62, which is prominently substituted with PC on a trimannosyl core (Haslam et al. 1997); similar structures were subsequently found in *Onchocerca* species, one of which causes river blindness in man (Haslam et al. 1999). Curiously, in *B. malayi* the protein homologue of ES-62 (a leucine aminopeptidase) is not conjugated to PC, which is instead linked to a distinct secreted product, GlcNAc transferase (Hewitson et al. 2008).

A further variation on this theme is found in *L. sigmodontis*, in which a mucin-like ES antigen of young female worms (Juv-p120) is conjugated not with PC but with the related dimethylaminoethanol (DMAE) (Hintz et al. 1996). In this instance, the side chain is coupled to *O*-linked Gal and GalNAc residues (Hirzmann et al. 2002; Wagner et al. 2011). The role of antibodies to DMAE remains to be resolved: such antibodies cross-react with the subsequent transmission stage of the parasite, the microfilariae (MF), but expression of DMAE by the female worm does not appear to compromise survival of the MF stage.

7.3.3.3 Strongylid Parasites

Strongylids encompass the human hookworms (*Ancylostoma* and *Necator*) as well as nematodes of veterinary importance (e.g. *Haemonchus contortus*) and widely studied experimental model systems (e.g. *Heligmosomoides polygyrus*). Of these, the most detailed information is available on *H. contortus*, the "barber's pole" worm of ruminant animals, and which is similar to Schistosomes in the degree of core glycan fucosylation.

Excretory–secretory (ES) antigens from *H. contortus* can successfully be used to vaccinate lambs against infection, resulting in almost 90% reduction in egg burden and greater than 50% reduction in worm burden (Vervelde et al. 2003). Significantly, the dominant antibody responses in protected animals were directed against glycan epitopes, particularly LDNF. However, the expression of this determinant does not correlate well with the protective ability of different vaccine fractions; while a native antigen termed H-gal-GP (for *Haemonchis* galactose-containing glycoprotein) elicits protection and high anti-LDNF antibodies, denatured H-gal-P drives antibody responses without immunity; moreover, an MEP3 metalloendopeptidase antigen is protective while not including LDNF among its glycan epitopes (Geldhof et al. 2005).

The nature of the protective glycan in *H. contortus* was more recently studied by van Die and colleagues (van Stijn et al. 2010). These investigators showed that while protection by ES vaccination correlates with high titres of IgG to LDNF, protected lambs also have high levels of IgG to a novel αGal(1→3)GalNAc structure. Using the lectin GSI-B4 that binds terminal α-Gal, and not β-Gal, it appears that this terminal sugar is absent from species such as *D. viteae*, *T. spiralis*, *F. hepatica* or *S. mansoni* and may represent a species-specific glycan with vaccine potential.

A related parasite is *Dictyocaulus vivparus*, the bovine lungworm. In a parallel to the filarial nematode *A. viteae*, this species produces a PC-decorated glycoprotein, although the carrier in this case is a thrombospondin-like ~300-kDa product which can also be found with PC linkages in *H. contortus* (Kooyman et al. 2009). Studies from this group have shown that infection elicits antibody responses against the PC-modified *N*-glycans and that anti-PC antibodies cross-react with host PC-modified platelet activating factor (PAF), which led the authors to suggest that suppression of eosinophilia may result (Kooyman et al. 2007a). In the same system, PNGase-deglycosylated ES proteins proved to elicit a stronger memory response than untreated material, indicating that natural exposure to immunodominant glycans may detract from the generation of a protective immune response to the key protein antigens (Kooyman et al. 2007b).

In our own studies in the model system of *H. polygyrus*, two major glycans antigens were defined (Glycans A and B) that stimulate rapid and strong antibody responses in infected mice. Glycan A, but not Glycan B, is expressed on the outermost surface of the worm, but monoclonal antibodies to these specificities were unable to confer protection following passive transfer (Hewitson et al. 2011). Hence, in this particular parasite, a "smokescreen" model for immunogenic glycans seems more appropriate.

7.3.3.4 The Trichuroid Group of Nematodes

This group includes *Trichinella spiralis*, the pork worm, and *Trichuris trichiura*, the human intestinal whipworm. A novel and important glycan antigen in the *T. spiralis* is a terminal tyvelose (3,6-dideoxy-D-*arabino*-hexose, Tyv) group (Wisnewski et al. 1993; Reason et al. 1994; Ellis et al. 1997). This residue caps the *N*-linked antennary glycans present on the larval surface antigen TSL-1 and specific antibodies confer protective immunity (Ellis et al. 1994). Monoclonal antibodies

9H and 18E to Tyv inhibit *T. spiralis* infection at the level of invasion of epithelial cells, a necessary step in the life cycle, as well as inhibiting larval migration and development (McVay et al. 1998, 2000). Because of the specific expression of Tyv by this parasite, the presence of anti-Tyv antibody is diagnostic of *Trichinella* infection which can be measured on a laboratory synthesized saccharide (Bruschi et al. 2001).

Relatively little data are available on glycans from *Trichuris* species. Excretory–secretory ES products collected in vitro from mouse-derived parasites of *T. muris* contains glycans which bind host Man receptor (MR) although this interaction does not appear to trigger protective immunity, which is normal in MR-deficient mice (deSchoolmeester et al. 2009).

7.4 General Implications of Parasite Glycans

7.4.1 Immunomodulatory Effects of Helminth Glycans

The expression of many of the interesting helminth glycan structures is linked not only to the generation of host antibody responses, but also direct modulation of immune signalling and/or development (Hokke and Yazdanbakhsh 2005). This has been most thoroughly investigated with schistosome associated glycans such as the LNFP-III/Le^X structure, which both stimulates murine B cells to produce the immunoregulatory cytokine IL-10 (Velupillai and Harn 1994; Velupillai et al. 1997) and can drive host macrophages into the down-regulatory "alternative activation" status associated with chronic infection (Atochina et al. 2008). Lectin-mediated internalisation of total schistosome egg antigen (SEA) into human dendritic cells results in suppression of innate responses to microbial ligands of TLRs (van Liempt et al. 2007). Further, the prominent schistosome glycan LDN-DF induces both immunoregulatory (IL-10) and inflammatory (IL-6, TNF-α) cytokine production by human monocytes (Van der Kleij et al. 2002). Glycans may also drive responses which attack the parasite. For example, schistosome glycans trigger granulomatous reaction (van de Vijver et al. 2004, 2006) and core $\alpha(1\rightarrow3)$-fucose and $\beta(1\rightarrow2)$-xylose containing *N*-glycans, as well as LNFP-III/Le^X, can trigger Th2 differentiation (Faveeuw et al. 2003). These immunomodulatory effects of schistosome glycans presumably involve the triggering of a variety of host lectin receptors. In this regard, schistosome extracts have been shown to bind the C-type lectin Dectin-2 (Ritter et al. 2010), Le^X in SEA is recognised by human DC-SIGN (Van Die et al. 2003), a mouse DC-SIGN homolog (SIGNR1) binds schistosome egg and adult worm glycans (Saunders et al. 2009) and host galectin-3 acts as a PRR for LDN (van den Berg et al. 2004). Despite these interactions, the host ligands which result in Th2 differentiation have yet to be defined: whilst SIGNR1 binds glycans from the Th2-promoting schistosome life cycle stages, SIGNR1-deficient mice mount normal Th2 responses during infection (Saunders et al. 2009). Similarly, galectin-3-deficient mice make normal Th2 responses following schistosome infection (Bickle and Helmby

2007), although their Th1 responses may be elevated (Breuilh et al. 2007). Immunomodulation by parasite glycans has also been demonstrated for *Taenia*, although the precise structures of the glycans have yet to be elucidated (Gomez-Garcia et al. 2005).

7.4.2 Diagnostic Applications for Helminth Glycans

CAA is a polymeric polysaccharide made up of a chain of GalNAc residues each of which is joined through a $\beta(1\rightarrow3)$ linkage to a GlcNAc side group (Bergwerff et al. 1994). Monoclonal antibodies to this target have been developed successfully for the diagnosis of infection, taking advantage of the repetitive nature of the antigenic epitope.

In contrast, the broad cross-reaction of fucosylated structures such as LDN-DF, explaining for example the binding of anti-schistosome antibodies to KLH (Dissous et al. 1986; Kantelhardt et al. 2002; Geyer et al. 2005) renders these unsuitable for diagnostic purposes. Further cross-reactions have been identified involving antibodies to truncated *N*-linked glycans (for example $Man_3GlcNAc_2$) which are present in helminths, plants, insects and vertebrates (van Remoortere et al. 2003a).

It was also found that *S. mansoni*-infected patients excrete egg-derived oligosaccharides into urine, offering a noninvasive diagnostic route to detect parasite glycans (Robijn et al. 2007b), most effectively accomplished with the antibody 114-4D12 which recognises a multiply fucosylated target (Robijn et al. 2007a).

7.5 Concluding Summary

Parasite glycans offer a rich and varied source of fascinating structures, some of which act directly on the host as immunomodulators (Harn et al. 2009) while others engage in forms of "glycan gimmickry" (van Die and Cummings 2010). This review has concentrated on the more prominent parasite systems, while also highlighting some of the important species for which little information has yet been garnered. Clearly, given the fascinating breadth and novelty thus far observed in parasite carbohydrate structures, this is an endeavour which should be greatly expanded.

The patterns of antibody recognition of parasite glycans, have established that many will serve as excellent targets for diagnostic purposes. Most interestingly, a number are now being identified as promising vaccine candidates for protective immunity (Nyame et al. 2004). Thus, these unusual and interactive structures are contributing in a very major way not only to our fundamental understanding of the host-parasite molecular dialogue, but also to new practical avenues of parasite detection, control, and ultimately eradication.

References

Aebischer T, Harbecke D, Ilg T (1999) Proteophosphoglycan, a major secreted product of intracellular *Leishmania mexicana* amastigotes, is a poor B-cell antigen and does not elicit a specific conventional CD4+ T-cell response. Infect Immun 67:5379–5385

Amer H, Hofinger A, Puchberger M, Kosma P (2001) Synthesis of O-methylated disaccharides related to excretory/secretory antigens of *Toxocara* larvae. J Carbohydr Chem 20:719–731

Atochina O, Da'dara AA, Walker M, Harn DA (2008) The immunomodulatory glycan LNFPIII initiates alternative activation of murine macrophages in vivo. Immunology 125:111–121

Bergwerff AA, van Dam GJ, Rotmans JP, Deelder AM, Kamerling JP, Vliegenthart JF (1994) The immunologically reactive part of immunopurified circulating anodic antigen from Schistosoma mansoni is a threonine-linked polysaccharide consisting of (→6)-(β-D-GlcpA-(1 → 3))-β-D-GalpNAc-(1 →)repeating units. J Biol Chem 269:31510–31517

Bickle Q, Helmby H (2007) Lack of galectin-3 involvement in murine intestinal nematode and schistosome infection. Parasite Immunol 29:93–100

Borst P, Rudenko G (1994) Antigenic variation in African trypanosomes. Science 264:1872–1873

Breuilh L, Vanhoutte F, Fontaine J, van Stijn CM, Tillie-Leblond I, Capron M, Faveeuw C, Jouault T, van Die I, Gosset P, Trottein F (2007) Galectin-3 modulates immune and inflammatory responses during helminthic infection: impact of galectin-3 deficiency on the functions of dendritic cells. Infect Immun 75:5148–5157

Bruschi F, Moretti A, Wassom D, Piergili Fioretti D (2001) The use of a synthetic antigen for the serological diagnosis of human trichinellosis. Parasite 8:S141–143

Campbell DH (1936) An antigenic polysaccharide fraction of *Ascaris lumbricoides* (from hog). J Infect Dis 59:266–280

Casaravilla C, Friere T, Malgor R, Medeiros A, Osinage E, Carmona C (2002) Mucin-type *O*-glycosylation in helminth parasites from major taxonomic groups: evidence for widespread distribution of the Tn antigens (GalNAc-Ser/Thr) and identification of UDP-GalNAc:polypeptide *N*-acetylgalactosamine transferase activity. J Parasitol 89:709–714

Collins JJ, King RS, Cogswell A, Williams DL, Newmark PA (2011) An atlas for *Schistosoma mansoni* organs and life-cycle stages using cell type-specific markers and confocal microscopy. PLoS Negl Trop Dis 5:e1009

Cummings RD, Nyame AK (1996) Glycobiology of schistosomiasis. FASEB J 10:838–848

Cummings RD, Nyame AK (1999) Schistosome glycoconjugates. Biochim Biophys Acta 1455:363–374

Dai WJ, Hemphill A, Waldvogel A, Ingold K, Deplazes P, Mossmann H, Gottstein B (2001) Major carbohydrate antigen of *Echinococcus multilocularis* induces an immunoglobulin G response independent of alphabeta + CD4+ T cells. Infect Immun 69:6074–6083

de Geus DC, van Roon AM, Thomassen EA, Hokke CH, Deelder AM, Abrahams JP (2009) Characterization of a diagnostic Fab fragment binding trimeric Lewis X. Proteins 76:439–447

Dell A, Haslam SM, Morris HR, Khoo K-H (1999) Immunogenic glycoconjugates implicated in parasitic nematode diseases. Biochim Biophys Acta 1455:353–362

Dematteis S, Pirotto F, Marqués J, Nieto A, Örn A, Baz A (2001) Modulation of the cellular immune response by a carbohydrate rich fraction from *Echinococcus granulosus* protoscoleces in infected or immunized Balb/c mice. Parasite Immunol 23:1–9

deSchoolmeester ML, Martinez-Pomares L, Gordon S, Else KJ (2009) The mannose receptor binds *Trichuris muris* excretory/secretory proteins but is not essential for protective immunity. Immunology 126:246–255

Descoteaux A, Turco SJ (1999) Glycoconjugates in *Leishmania* infectivity. Biochim Biophys Acta 1455:341–352

Díaz A, Fontana EC, Todeschini AR, Soulé S, González H, Casaravilla C, Portela M, Mohana-Borges R, Mendonça-Previato L, Previato JO, Ferreira F (2009) The major surface carbohydrates of the *Echinococcus granulosus* cyst: mucin-type *O*-glycans decorated by novel galactose-based structures. Biochemistry 48:11678–11691

Díaz A, Casaravilla C, Irigoín F, Lin G, Previato JO, Ferreira F (2011) Understanding the laminated layer of larval *Echinococcus* I: structure. Trends Parasitol 27:204–13

Dinglasan RR, Fields I, Shahabuddin M, Azad AF, Sacci JB Jr (2003) Monoclonal antibody MG96 completely blocks *Plasmodium yoelii* development in *Anopheles stephensi*. Infect Immun 71:6995–7001

Dissous C, Grzych JM, Capron A (1986) *Schistosoma mansoni* shares a protective oligosaccharide epitope with freshwater and marine snails. Nature 323:443–445

Dunne DW, Bickle QD, Butterworth AE, Richardson BA (1987) The blocking of human antibody-dependent, eosinophil-mediated killing of *Schistosoma mansoni* schistosomula by monoclonal antibodies which cross-react with a polysaccharide-containing egg antigen. Parasitology 94(Pt 2):269–280

Eberl M, Langermans JA, Vervenne RA, Nyame AK, Cummings RD, Thomas AW, Coulson PS, Wilson RA (2001) Antibodies to glycans dominate the host response to schistosome larvae and eggs: is their role protective or subversive? J Infect Dis 183:1238–1247

Ellis LA, Reason AJ, Morris HR, Dell A, Iglesias R, Ubeira FM, Appleton JA (1994) Glycans as targets for monoclonal antibodies that protect rats against *Trichinella spiralis*. Glycobiology 4:585–592

Ellis LA, McVay CS, Probert MA, Zhang J, Bundle DR, Appleton JA (1997) Terminal β-linked tyvelose creates unique epitopes in *Trichinella spiralis* glycan antigens. Glycobiology 7:383–390

Faveeuw C, Mallevaey T, Paschinger K, Wilson IBH, Fontaine J, Mollicone R, Oriol R, Altmann F, Lerouge P, Capron M, Trottein F (2003) Schistosome *N*-glycans containing core α3-fucose and core β2-xylose epitopes are strong inducers of Th2 responses in mice. Eur J Immunol 33:1271–1281

Fournet B, Leroy Y, Wieruszeski JM, Montreuil J, Poretz RD, Goldberg R (1987) Primary structure of an *N*-glycosidic carbohydrate unit derived from *Sophora japonica* lectin. Eur J Biochem 166:321–324

Geldhof P, Newlands GF, Nyame K, Cummings R, Smith WD, Knox DP (2005) Presence of the LDNF glycan on the host-protective H-gal-GP fraction from *Haemonchus contortus*. Parasite Immunol 27:55–60

Geyer H, Wuhrer M, Resemann A, Geyer R (2005) Identification and characterization of keyhole limpet hemocyanin *N*-glycans mediating cross-reactivity with *Schistosoma mansoni*. J Biol Chem 280:40731–40748

Glaser TA, Moody SF, Handman E, Bacic A, Spithill TW (1991) An antigenically distinct lipophosphoglycan on amastigotes of *Leishmania major*. Mol Biochem Parasitol 45:337–344

Gomez-Garcia L, Lopez-Marin LM, Saavedra R, Reyes JL, Rodriguez-Sosa M, Terrazas LI (2005) Intact glycans from cestode antigens are involved in innate activation of myeloid suppressor cells. Parasite Immunol 27:395–405

Grzych JM, Capron M, Bazin H, Capron A (1982) In vitro and in vivo effector function of rat IgG2a monoclonal anti-*S. mansoni* antibodies. J Immunol 129:2739–2743

Grzych J-M, Dissous C, Capron M, Torres S, Lambert PH, Capron A (1987) *Schistosoma mansoni* shares a protective epitope with keyhole limpet hemocyanin. J Exp Med 165:865–878

Guha-Niyogi A, Sullivan DR, Turco SJ (2001) Glycoconjugate structures of parasitic protozoa. Glycobiology 11:45R–59R

Handman E (2001) Leishmaniasis: current status of vaccine development. Clin Microbiol Rev 14:229–243

Harn DA, Mitsuyama M, David JR (1984) *Schistosoma mansoni*. Anti-egg monoclonal antibodies protect against cercarial challenge in vivo. J Exp Med 159:1371–1387

Harn DA, McDonald J, Atochina O, Da'dara AA (2009) Modulation of host immune responses by helminth glycans. Immunol Rev 230:247–257

Haslam SM, Coles GC, Munn EA, Smith TS, Smith HF, Morris HR, Dell A (1996) *Haemonchus contortus* glycoproteins contain *N*-linked oligosaccharides with novel highly fucosylated core structures. J Biol Chem 271:30561–30570

Haslam SM, Khoo K-H, Houston KM, Harnett W, Morris HR, Dell A (1997) Characterisation of the phosphorylcholine-containing *N*-linked oligosaccharides in the excretory–secretory 62 kDa glycoprotein of *Acanthocheilonema viteae*. Mol Biochem Parasitol 85:53–66

Haslam SM, Houston KM, Harnett W, Reason AJ, Morris HR, Dell A (1999) Structural studies of N-glycans of filarial parasites. Conservation of phosphorylcholine-substituted glycans among species and discovery of novel chito-oligomers. J Biol Chem 274:20953–20960

Hewitson JP, Harcus YM, Curwen RS, Dowle AA, Atmadja AK, Ashton PD, Wilson RA, Maizels RM (2008) The secretome of the filarial parasite, *Brugia malayi*: proteomic profile of adult excretory–secretory products. Mol Biochem Parasitol 160:8–21

Hewitson JP, Filbey KJ, Grainger JR, Dowle AA, Pearson M, Murray J, Harcus Y, Maizels RM (2011) *Heligmosomoides polygyrus* elicits a dominant nonprotective antibody response directed at restricted glycan and peptide epitopes. J Immunol in press

Hintz M, Kasper M, Stahl N, Geyer R, Kalinowski H-O, Karas M, Kühnhardt S, Schott H-H, Conraths FJ, Zahner H, Stirm S (1996) Dimethylaminoethanol is a major component of the *Litomosoides carinii* microfilarial sheath. Mol Biochem Parasitol 76:325–328

Hirzmann J, Hintz M, Kasper M, Shresta TR, Taubert A, Conraths FJ, Geyer R, Stirm S, Zahner H, Hobom G (2002) Cloning and expression analysis of two mucin-like genes encoding microfilarial sheath surface proteins of the parasitic nematodes *Brugia* and *Litomosoides*. J Biol Chem 27:27

Hokke CH, Deelder AM (2001) Schistosome glycoconjugates in host–parasite interplay. Glycoconj J 18:573–587

Hokke CH, Yazdanbakhsh M (2005) Schistosome glycans and innate immunity. Parasite Immunol 27:257–264

Hokke CH, Deelder AM, Hoffmann KF, Wuhrer M (2007) Glycomics-driven discoveries in schistosome research. Exp Parasitol 117:275–283

Ilg T, Harbecke D, Wiese M, Overath P (1993) Monoclonal antibodies directed against *Leishmania* secreted acid phosphatase and lipophosphoglycan. Partial characterization of private and public epitopes. Eur J Biochem 217:603–615

Ilg T (2000) Proteophosphoglycans of *Leishmania*. Parasitol Today 16:489–497

Jang-Lee J, Curwen RS, Ashton PD, Tissot B, Mathieson W, Panico M, Dell A, Wilson RA, Haslam SM (2007) Glycomics analysis of *Schistosoma mansoni* egg and cercarial secretions. Mol Cell Proteomics 6:1485–1499

Kang S, Cummings RD, McCall JW (1993) Characterization of the *N*-linked oligosaccharides in glycoproteins synthesized by microfilariae of *Dirofilaria immitis*. J Parasitol 79:815–828

Kantelhardt SR, Wuhrer M, Dennis RD, Doenhoff MJ, Bickle Q, Geyer R (2002) Fuc(α1 $\rightarrow$ 3) GalNAc-: the major antigenic motif of *Schistosoma mansoni* glycolipids implicated in infection sera and keyhole-limpet haemocyanin cross-reactivity. Biochem J 366:217–223

Kariuki TM, Farah IO, Wilson RA, Coulson PS (2008) Antibodies elicited by the secretions from schistosome cercariae and eggs are predominantly against glycan epitopes. Parasite Immunol 30:554–562

Khoo K-H, Maizels RM, Page AP, Taylor GW, Rendell N, Dell A (1991) Characterisation of nematode glycoproteins: the major *O*-glycans of *Toxocara* excretory secretory antigens are methylated trisaccharides. Glycobiology 1:163–171

Khoo K-H, Nieto A, Morris HR, Dell A (1997a) Structural characterization of the *N*-glycans from *Echinococcus granulosus* hydatid cyst membrane and protoscoleces. Mol Biochem Parasitol 86:237–248

Khoo KH, Chatterjee D, Caulfield JP, Morris HR, Dell A (1997b) Structural mapping of the glycans from the egg glycoproteins of *Schistosoma mansoni* and *Schistosoma japonicum*: identification of novel core structures and terminal sequences. Glycobiology 7:663–677

Khoo KH, Huang HH, Lee KM (2001) Characteristic structural features of schistosome cercarial N-glycans: expression of Lewis X and core xylosylation. Glycobiology 11:149–163

Kooyman FNJ, de Vries E, Ploeger HW, van Putten JPM (2007a) Antibodies elicited by the bovine lungworm, *Dictyocaulus viviparus*, cross-react with platelet-activating factor. Infect Immun 75:4456–4462

Kooyman FNJ, Ploeger HW, Hoglund J, Putten JPM (2007b) Differential *N*-glycan- and protein-directed immune responses in *Dictyocaulus viviparus*-infected and vaccinated calves. Parasitology 134:269–279

Kooyman FNJ, van Balkom BWM, de Vries E, van Putten JPM (2009) Identification of a thrombospondin-like immunodominant and phosphorylcholine-containing glycoprotein (GP300) in *Dictyocaulus viviparus* and related nematodes. Mol Biochem Parasitol 163:85–94

Lee JJ, Dissanayake S, Panico M, Morris HR, Dell A, Haslam SM (2005) Mass spectrometric characterisation of *Taenia crassiceps* metacestode *N*-glycans. Mol Biochem Parasitol 143:245–249

Loukas AC, Hintz M, Tetteh KKA, Mullin NP, Maizels RM (2000) A family of secreted mucins from the parasitic nematode *Toxocara canis* bear diverse mucin domains but share similar flanking six-cysteine (SXC) repeat motifs. J Biol Chem 275:39600–39607

Macedo CS, Schwarz RT, Todeschini AR, Previato JO, Mendonça-Previato L (2010) Overlooked post-translational modifications of proteins in *Plasmodium falciparum*: N- and O-glycosylation – a review. Mem Inst Oswaldo Cruz 105:949–956

Maizels RM, Kennedy MW, Meghji M, Robertson BD, Smith HV (1987) Shared carbohydrate epitopes on distinct surface and secreted antigens of the parasitic nematode *Toxocara canis*. J Immunol 139:207–214

Mangold BL, Dean DA (1992) The role of IgG antibodies from irradiated cercaria-immunized rabbits in the passive transfer of immunity to *Schistosoma mansoni*-infected mice. Am J Trop Med Hyg 47:821–829

Marinets A, Zhang T, Guillén N, Gounon P, Bohle B, Vollmann U, Scheiner O, Wiedermann G, Stanley SL, Duchêne M (1997) Protection against invasive amebiasis by a single monoclonal antibody directed against a lipophosphoglycan antigen localized on the surface of *Entamoeba histolytica*. J Exp Med 186:1557–1565

McConville MJ, Bacic A, Mitchell GF, Handman E (1987) Lipophosphoglycan of *Leishmania major* that vaccinates against cutaneous leishmaniasis contains an alkylglycerophosphoinositol lipid anchor. Proc Natl Acad Sci USA 84:8941–8945

McConville MJ, Bacic A (1989) A family of glycoinositol phospholipids from *Leishmania major*. Isolation, characterization, and antigenicity. J Biol Chem 264:757–766

McVay CS, Tsung A, Appleton J (1998) Participation of parasite surface glycoproteins in antibody-mediated protection of epithelial cells against *Trichinella spiralis*. Infect Immun 66:1941–1945

McVay CS, Bracken P, Gagliardo LF, Appleton J (2000) Antibodies to tyvelose exhibit multiple modes of interference with the epithelial niche of *Trichinella spiralis*. Infect Immun 68:1912–1918

Meevissen MHJ, Wuhrer M, Doenhoff MJ, Schramm G, Haas H, Deelder AM, Hokke CH (2010) Structural characterization of glycans on omega-1, a major *Schistosoma mansoni* egg glycoprotein that drives Th2 responses. J Proteome Res 9:2630–2642

Meevissen MHJ, Balog CI, Koeleman CAM, Doenhoff MJ, Schramm G, Haas H, Deelder AM, Wuhrer M, Hokke CH (2011) Targeted glycoproteomic analysis reveals that kappa-5 is a major, uniquely glycosylated component of *Schistosoma mansoni* egg antigens. Mol Cell Proteomics 10(5):M110.005710

Moody SF, Handman E, Bacic A (1991) Structure and antigenicity of the lipophosphoglycan from *Leishmania major* amastigotes. Glycobiology 1:419–424

Moody-Haupt S, Patterson JH, Mirelman D, McConville MJ (2000) The major surface antigens of *Entamoeba histolytica* trophozoites are GPI-anchored proteophosphoglycans. J Mol Biol 297:409–420

Naderer T, Vince JE, McConville MJ (2004) Surface determinants of *Leishmania* parasites and their role in infectivity in the mammalian host. Curr Mol Med 4:649–665

Naus CW, van Remoortere A, Ouma JH, Kimani G, Dunne DW, Kamerling JP, Deelder AM, Hokke CH (2003) Specific antibody responses to three schistosome-related carbohydrate structures in recently exposed immigrants and established residents in an area of *Schistosoma mansoni* endemicity. Infect Immun 71:5676–5681

Norden AP, Strand M (1985) Identification of antigenic *Schistosoma mansoni* glycoproteins during the course of infection in mice and humans. Am J Trop Med Hyg 34:495–507

Nyame AK, Debose-Boyd R, Long TD, Tsang VCW, Cummings RD (1998) Expression of Le^x antigen in *Schistosoma japonicum* and *S.haematobium* and immune responses to Le^x in infected animals: lack of Le^x expression in other trematodes and nematodes. Glycobiology 8:615–624

Nyame AK, Lewis FA, Doughty BL, Correa-Oliveira R, Cummings RD (2003) Immunity to schistosomiasis: glycans are potential antigenic targets for immune intervention. Exp Parasitol 104:1–13

Nyame AK, Kawar ZS, Cummings RD (2004) Antigenic glycans in parasitic infections: implications for vaccines and diagnostics. Arch Biochem Biophys 426:182–200

Omer Ali P, Smithers SR, Bickle Q, Phillips SM, Harn D, Simpson AJ (1988) Analysis of the anti-*Schistosoma mansoni* surface antibody response during murine infection and its potential contribution to protective immunity. J Immunol 140:3273–3279

Page AP, Hamilton AJ, Maizels RM (1992a) *Toxocara canis:* monoclonal antibodies to carbohydrate epitopes of secreted (TES) antigens localize to different secretion-related structures in infective larvae. Exp Parasitol 75:56–71

Page AP, Rudin W, Fluri E, Blaxter ML, Maizels RM (1992b) *Toxocara canis*: a labile antigenic coat overlying the epicuticle of infective larvae. Exp Parasitol 75:72–86

Pöltl G, Kerner D, Paschinger K, Wilson IB (2007) *N*-glycans of the porcine nematode parasite *Ascaris suum* are modified with phosphorylcholine and core fucose residues. FEBS J 274:714–726

Previato JO, Sola-Penna M, Agrellos OA, Jones C, Oeltmann T, Travassos LR, Mendonça-Previato L (1998) Biosynthesis of *O*-*N*-acetylglucosamine-linked glycans in *Trypanosoma cruzi*. Characterization of the novel uridine diphospho-*N*-acetylglucosamine:polypeptide N-acetylglucosaminyltransferase-catalyzing formation of *N*-acetylglucosamine $\alpha 1 \rightarrow$ *O*-threonine. J Biol Chem 273:14982–14988

Previato JO, Wait R, Jones C, DosReis GA, Todeschini AR, Heise N, Previato LM (2004) Glycoinositolphospholipid from *Trypanosoma cruzi*: structure, biosynthesis and immunobiology. Adv Parasitol 56:1–41

Reason AJ, Ellis LA, Appleton JA, Wisnewski N, Grieve RB, McNell M, Wassom DL, Morris HR, Dell A (1994) Novel tyvelose-containing tri- and tetra-antennary *N*-glycans in the immunodominant antigens of the intracellular parasite *Trichinella spiralis*. Glycobiology 4:593–603

Richter D, Incani RN, Harn DA (1996) Lacto-*N*-fucopentaose III ($Lewis^x$), a target of the antibody response in mice vaccinated with irradiated cercariae of *Schistosoma mansoni*. Infect Immun 64:1826–1831

Ritter M, Gross O, Kays S, Ruland J, Nimmerjahn F, Saijo S, Tschopp J, Layland LE, Prazeres da Costa C (2010) *Schistosoma mansoni* triggers Dectin-2, which activates the Nlrp3 inflammasome and alters adaptive immune responses. Proc Natl Acad Sci USA 107:20459–20464

Robijn ML, Koeleman CA, Wuhrer M, Royle L, Geyer R, Dwek RA, Rudd PM, Deelder AM, Hokke CH (2007a) Targeted identification of a unique glycan epitope of *Schistosoma mansoni* egg antigens using a diagnostic antibody. Mol Biochem Parasitol 151:148–161

Robijn MLM, Koeleman CAM, Hokke CH, Deelder AM (2007b) *Schistosoma mansoni* eggs excrete specific free oligosaccharides that are detectable in the urine of the human host. Mol Biochem Parasitol 151:162–172

Robinson MJ, Sancho D, Slack EC, LeibundGut-Landmann S, Reise SC (2006) Myeloid C-type lectins in innate immunity. Nat Immunol 7:1258–1265

Saunders SP, Walsh CM, Barlow JL, Mangan NE, Taylor PR, McKenzie AN, Smith P, Fallon PG (2009) The C-type lectin SIGNR1 binds *Schistosoma mansoni* antigens in vitro, but SIGNR1-deficient mice have normal responses during schistosome infection. Infect Immun 77:399–404

Schabussova I, Amer H, van Die I, Kosma P, Maizels RM (2007) *O*-Methylated glycans from *Toxocara* are specific targets for antibody binding in human and animal infections. Int J Parasitol 37:97–109

Schofield L, Hackett F (1993) Signal transduction in host cells by a glycosylphosphatidylinositol toxin of malaria parasites. J Exp Med 177:145–153

Schramm G, Hamilton JV, Balog CI, Wuhrer M, Gronow A, Beckmann S, Wippersteg V, Grevelding CG, Goldmann T, Weber E, Brattig NW, Deelder AM, Dunne DW, Hokke CH, Haas H, Doenhoff MJ (2009) Molecular characterisation of kappa-5, a major antigenic glycoprotein from *Schistosoma mansoni* eggs. Mol Biochem Parasitol 166:4–14

Todeschini AR, da Silveira EX, Jones C, Wait R, Previato JO, Mendonca-Previato L (2001) Structure of *O*-glycosidically linked oligosaccharides from glycoproteins of *Trypanosoma cruzi* CL-Brener strain: evidence for the presence of *O*-linked sialyl-oligosaccharides. Glycobiology 11:47–55

Todeschini AR, de Almeida EG, Agrellos OA, Jones C, Previato JO, Mendonca-Previato L (2009) α-N-acetylglucosamine-linked *O*-glycans of sialoglycoproteins (Tc-mucins) from *Trypanosoma cruzi* Colombiana strain. Mem Inst Oswaldo Cruz 104(Suppl 1):270–274

Tretter V, Altmann F, Kubelka V, März L, Becker WM (1993) Fucose alpha 1,3-linked to the core region of glycoprotein N-glycans creates an important epitope for IgE from honeybee venom allergic individuals. Int Arch Allergy Immunol 102:259–266

Ubillos L, Medeiros A, Cancela M, Casaravilla C, Saldana J, Dominguez L, Carmona C, Le Pendu J, Osinaga E (2007) Characterization of the carcinoma-associated Tk antigen in helminth parasites. Exp Parasitol 116:129–136

van Dam GJ, Bergwerff AA, Thomas-Oates JE, Rotmans JP, Kamerling JP, Vliegenthart JF, Deelder AM (1994) The immunologically reactive O-linked polysaccharide chains derived from circulating cathodic antigen isolated from the human blood fluke *Schistosoma mansoni* have Lewis x as repeating unit. Eur J Biochem 225:467–482

van de Vijver KK, Hokke CH, van Remoortere A, Jacobs W, Deelder AM, Van Marck EA (2004) Glycans of *Schistosoma mansoni* and keyhole limpet haemocyanin induce hepatic granulomas in vivo. Int J Parasitol 34:951–961

van de Vijver KK, Deelder AM, Jacobs W, Van Marck EA, Hokke CH (2006) LacdiNAc- and LacNAc-containing glycans induce granulomas in an in vivo model for schistosome egg-induced hepatic granuloma formation. Glycobiology 16:237–243

van den Berg TK, Honing H, Franke N, van Remoortere A, Schiphorst WECM, Liu F-T, Deelder AM, Cummings RD, Hokke CH, van Die I (2004) LacdiNAc-glycans constitute a parasite pattern for galectin-3-mediated immune recognition. J Immunol 173:1902–1907

van der Kleij D, van Remoortere A, Schuitemaker JH, Kapsenberg ML, Deelder AM, Tielens AG, Hokke CH, Yazdanbakhsh M (2002) Triggering of innate immune responses by schistosome egg glycolipids and their carbohydrate epitope GalNAcβ1-4(Fucα1-2Fucα1-3)GlcNAc. J Infect Dis 185:531–539

van Die I, Gomord V, Kooyman FNJ, van den Berg TK, Cummings RD, Vervelde L (1999) Core α1→-fucose is a common modification of N-glycans in parasitic helminths and constitutes an important epitope for IgE from *Haemonchus contortus* infected sheep. FEBS Lett 463:189–193

van Die I, van Vliet SJ, Kwame Nyame A, Cummings RD, Bank CM, Appelmelk B, Geijtenbeek TB, Van Kooyk Y (2003) The dendritic cell specific C-type lectin DC-SIGN is a receptor for *Schistosoma mansoni* egg antigens and recognizes the glycan antigen Lewis-x. Glycobiology 13:471–478

van Die I, Cummings RD (2010) Glycan gimmickry by parasitic helminths: a strategy for modulating the host immune response? Glycobiology 20:2–12

van Liempt E, van Vliet SJ, Engering A, García Vallejo JJ, Bank CMC, Sanchez-Hernandez M, van Kooyk Y, van Die I (2007) *Schistosoma mansoni* soluble egg antigens are internalized by human dendritic cells through multiple C-type lectins and suppress TLR-induced dendritic cell activation. Mol Immunol 44:2605–2615

van Remoortere A, Hokke CH, van Dam GJ, van Die I, Deelder AM, van den Eijnden DH (2000) Various stages of *Schistosoma* express Lewis^x, LacdiNAc, GalNAcβ1-4(Fucα1-3)GlcNAc and GalNAcβ1-4(Fucα1-2Fucα1-3)GlcNAc carbohydrate epitopes: detection with monoclonal antibodies that are characterized by enzymatically synthesized neoglycoproteins. Glycobiology 10:601–609

van Remoortere A, van Dam GJ, Hokke CH, van den Eijnden DH, van Die I, Deelder AM (2001) Profiles of immunoglobulin M (IgM) and IgG antibodies against defined carbohydrate epitopes in sera of *Schistosoma*-infected individuals determined by surface plasmon resonance. Infect Immun 69:2396–2401

van Remoortere A, Bank CMC, Nyame AK, Cummings RD, Deelder AM, van Die I (2003a) *Schistosoma mansoni*-infected mice produce antibodies that cross-react with plant, insect, and mammalian glycoproteins and recognize the truncated biantennary *N*-glycan $Man_3GlcNAc_2$-R. Glycobiology 13:217–225

van Remoortere A, Vermeer HJ, van Roon AM, van die I, van den Eijnden DH, Ágoston K, Kérèkgyarto J, Vliegenthart JFG, Kamerling JP, van dam GJ, Hokke CH, Deelder AM (2003b) Dominant antibody responses to Fucα1-3GalNAc and Fucα1-2Fucα1-3GlcNAc containing carbohydrate epitopes in *Pan troglodytes* vaccinated and infected with *Schistosoma mansoni*. Exp Parasitol 105:219–225

van Stijn CM, van den Broek M, Vervelde L, Alvarez RA, Cummings RD, Tefsen B, van Die I (2010) Vaccination-induced IgG response to Galα1-3GalNAc glycan epitopes in lambs protected against *Haemonchus contortus* challenge infection. Int J Parasitol 40:215–222

Vasta GR (2009) Roles of galectins in infection. Nat Rev Microbiol 7:424–438

Velupillai P, Harn DA (1994) Oligosaccharide-specific induction of interleukin 10 production by $B220^+$ cells from schistosome infected mice: a mechanism for regulation of $CD4^+$ T-cell subsets. Proc Natl Acad Sci USA 91:18–22

Velupillai P, Secor WE, Horauf AM, Harn DA (1997) B-1 cell ($CD5^+B220^+$) outgrowth in murine schistosomiasis is genetically restricted and is largely due to activation by polylactosamine sugars. J Immunol 158:338–344

Vervelde L, Bakker N, Kooyman FN, Cornelissen AW, Bank CM, Nyame AK, Cummings RD, van Die I (2003) Vaccination-induced protection of lambs against the parasitic nematode *Haemonchus contortus* correlates with high IgG antibody responses to the LDNF glycan antigen. Glycobiology 13:795–804

Wagner U, Hirzmann J, Hintz M, Beck E, Geyer R, Hobom G, Taubert A, Zahner H (2011) Characterization of the DMAE-modified juvenile excretory–secretory protein Juv-p120 of *Litomosoides sigmodontis*. Mol Biochem Parasitol 176:80–89

Wilson IB, Harthill JE, Mullin NP, Ashford DA, Altmann F (1998) Core α1,3-fucose is a key part of the epitope recognized by antibodies reacting against plant N-linked oligosaccharides and is present in a wide variety of plant extracts. Glycobiology 8:651–661

Wisnewski N, McNeil M, Grieve RB, Wassom DL (1993) Characterization of novel fucosyl- and tyvelosyl-containing glycoconjugates from *Trichinella spiralis* muscle stage larvae. Mol Biochem Parasitol 61:25–36

Wuhrer M, Dennis RD, Doenhoff MJ, Lochnit G, Geyer R (2000) *Schistosoma mansoni* cercarial glycolipids are dominated by Lewis X and pseudo-Lewis Y structures. Glycobiology 10:89–101

Wuhrer M, Balog CI, Catalina MI, Jones FM, Schramm G, Haas H, Doenhoff MJ, Dunne DW, Deelder AM, Hokke CH (2006a) IPSE/α-1, a major secretory glycoprotein antigen from schistosome eggs, expresses the Lewis X motif on core-difucosylated N-glycans. FEBS J 273:2276–2292

Wuhrer M, Koeleman CA, Fitzpatrick JM, Hoffmann KF, Deelder AM, Hokke CH (2006b) Gender-specific expression of complex-type N-glycans in schistosomes. Glycobiology 16:991–1006

Yamano K, Goto A, Nakamura-Uchiyama F, Nawa Y, Hada N, Takeda T (2009) Galβ1-6Gal, antigenic epitope which accounts for serological cross-reaction in diagnosis of *Echinococcus multilocularis* infection. Parasite Immunol 31:481–487

Zodda DM, Phillips SM (1982) Monoclonal antibody-mediated protection against *Schistosoma mansoni* infection in mice. J Immunol 129:2326–2328

Human IgE Antibodies Against Cross-Reactive Carbohydrate Determinants

8

Wolfgang Hemmer

8.1 Introduction

Immunoglobulin (Ig) E-mediated allergic diseases in humans are for the greatest part caused by protein allergens derived from various natural sources such as pollens, foods, animal dander and molds as well as mites and insect venoms. IgE responses to small non-protein molecules are far less common but do occur and may represent important clinical issues like in the case of drug allergy and occupation-related sensitization to isocyanates. However, it is well-documented in allergology now that IgE antibodies may be directed also against carbohydrates attached to carrier proteins. Scientific studies thus far have focused on asparagine-linked glycans (*N*-glycans) displaying core α(1→3)-linked fucose and/or β(1→2)-linked xylose, both representing common posttranslational modifications of plant, insect and some other invertebrate (mollusks, helminths) glycoproteins. These complex *N*-glycans have been denominated "cross-reactive carbohydrate determinants" (or CCDs) and are now recognized by allergists as the most important IgE-binding oligosaccharides. However, more recently also other protein-attached carbohydrates involved in IgE-mediated allergic reactions have been discovered, namely β-arabinose-containing *O*-linked glycans in mugwort pollen allergy, and α-galactose (αGal) in allergic reactions to meat and certain biologicals.

W. Hemmer (✉)
Floridsdorf Allergy Centre, Franz Jonas Platz 8/6, 1210 Vienna, Austria
e-mail: hemmer@faz.at

P. Kosma and S. Müller-Loennies (eds.), *Anticarbohydrate Antibodies*,
DOI 10.1007/978-3-7091-0870-3_8, © Springer-Verlag/Wien 2012

8.2 Cross-Reactive Carbohydrate Determinants (CCDs): *N*-Linked Oligosaccharides with Core α(1→3)-Fucose and/or β(1→2)-Xylose

The discovery of CCDs as relevant IgE binding structures dates back to 1981 when Aalberse et al. (1981) described a patient with an extraordinarily broad IgE reactivity profile towards a large number of pollens, plant foods as well as honeybee venom while clinical hypersensitivity to all these allergens was absent. The causative involvement of a common non-protein epitope in these antibody responses was apparent from inhibition studies showing equivalent reciprocal cross-inhibition between grass pollen, plant foods and honeybee venom which could not be reasonably explained by shared protein epitopes. Periodate treatment of extracts led to a complete loss of their IgE binding capacity suggesting that carbohydrate determinants were the cause of the observed IgE (cross-) reactivity. The molecular basis for this phenomenon became evident when plant-like *N*-glycans displaying core α(1→3)-fucose were demonstrated in honeybee venom phospholipase and hyaluronidase (Kubelka et al. 1993, 1995). Using small glycopeptides derived from pineapple bromelain no longer harboring protein epitopes, Tretter et al. (1993) were subsequently able to prove that human IgE may selectively bind to the carbohydrate moiety of glycoproteins and that such antibodies are not uncommon among venom-allergic subjects.

In addition to α(1→3)-fucosylation, core β(1→2)-xylose defines a distinct and independent IgE epitope of plant, snail and helminth (but not insect) *N*-glycans, however, according to current data IgE against xylose appears to be less common than IgE against α(1→3)-fucose.

8.2.1 Distribution and Structure of Allergenic N-Glycans

8.2.1.1 Cross-Reactive Carbohydrate Determinants of Plants

CCDs are produced by virtually all seed-bearing plants and probably also by non-*Spermatophyta* like horsetails and ferns (Altmann 2007). With special reference to allergy, it must be emphasized that CCDs are regularly found, though in different amounts, in all important plant allergen sources, i.e. pollens, foods (wheat, nuts, fruits, vegetables, etc.) as well as rubber latex.

The immunogenicity of plant *N*-glycans is based on the occurrence of core α(1→3)-linked fucose at the innermost GlcNAc and β(1→2) xylosylation of the core mannosyl residue, both substitutions being absent in human *N*-glycans (Fig. 8.1). Large Lewis[a] antennae, as known from some conifer pollen allergens and many plant foods (Alisi et al. 2001; Fötisch and Vieths 2001; Wilson et al. 2001) are currently considered not important in IgE binding (van Ree et al. 2000). The ubiquitous complex *N*-glycan of the MMXF[3] structure may be seen as the "prototype" allergenic *N*-glycan in plants. It is equally common in pollens, plant foods and rubber latex allergens, and is the major *N*-glycan in horseradish peroxidase (HRP), a non-allergenic model glycoprotein frequently employed for the study of carbohydrate-based IgE cross-reactivity. In contrast, pineapple bromelain, another commonly used research glycoprotein, predominantly contains truncated $MUXF^3$ glycans lacking the second, $\alpha(1\rightarrow3)$-linked mannose residue.

While all plants typically produce all types of *N*-glycans, substantial quantitative differences may exist with regard to particular glycan types (Wilson and Altmann 1998, 2001). For example, tree pollen *N*-glycans often bear terminal non-reducing GlcNAc residues which may diminish IgE binding (Wilson and Altmann 1998). Some well-characterized allergens are either very poor in $\alpha(1\rightarrow3)$ fucose (e.g., the major olive pollen allergen Ole e 1) or completely lack core fucosylation, as is the case in the vicilin-type 7 S globulins from hazelnut (Cor a 11) and peanut (Ara h 1) (van Ree et al. 2000; Kolarich and Altmann 2000). The glycoproteins from Bermuda grass pollen carry predominantly non-xylosylated glycans, mainly MMF^3, as typical for insect glycoproteins (Ohsuga et al. 1996).

8.2.1.2 Cross-Reactive Carbohydrate Determinants of Insects/Insect Venoms

Regularly found in honeybee, vespid and other *Hymenoptera* venoms is an $\alpha(1\rightarrow3)$ fucosylation of *N*-glycans. Hyaluronidase represents a major glycoallergen in these venoms (Kubelka et al. 1995; Kolarich et al. 2005) and is the primary cause for serologic cross-reactions between different *Hymenoptera* venoms (Hemmer et al. 2001, 2004; Kochuyt et al. 2005; Jappe et al. 2006; Jin et al. 2010). Honeybee venom contains also glycosylated phospholipase A2 and quite a number of high molecular weight glycoproteins most of which probably have limited relevance as protein allergens (Hemmer et al. 2004; Mahler et al. 2006; Hoffman 2006). Insect *N*-glycans are mainly of the MMF^3 or MUF^3 type and are often accompanied by a second core fucosylation in $\alpha(1\rightarrow6)$ position (MMF^3F^6, MUF^3F^6) (Fig. 8.1) (Staudacher et al. 1992; Kolarich et al. 2005). For allergy diagnosis it is important to consider that fucosylated *N*-glycans are not restricted to venoms but occur in other tissues as well (Koshte et al. 1989). CCDs are thus ubiquitous IgE epitopes in insect whole body extracts which are currently used in the diagnosis of hypersensitivity to bites from blood-feeding insects (e.g., mosquitoes, horseflies) and respiratory insect allergy (e.g., cockroach allergy).

Xylose does not occur in insects. Interestingly, despite the close phylogenetic proximity, the other arthropod groups *Arachnida* (including dust mites) and *Crustacea* appear to lack *N*-glycans with core $\alpha(1\rightarrow3)$-fucosylation (Wilson et al. 1998).

8.2.1.3 Cross-Reactive Carbohydrates of Other Invertebrates (Parasitic Helminths, Mollusks)

Parasitic helminths contain a broad repertoire of carbohydrate antigens which constitute a major target for the host immune system and which have been shown capable of modulating host immune responses by polarizing naïve T-cells into Th2 cells, initiating production of sugar-specific IgE antibodies, or induction of regulatory IL-10 producing T-cells (van Die and Cummings 2010). Complex *N*-glycans bearing core $\alpha(1\rightarrow3)$ fucose and/or xylose have been found in substantial amounts in several (but not all) helminths (Fig. 8.1), including trematodes (*Schistosoma*,

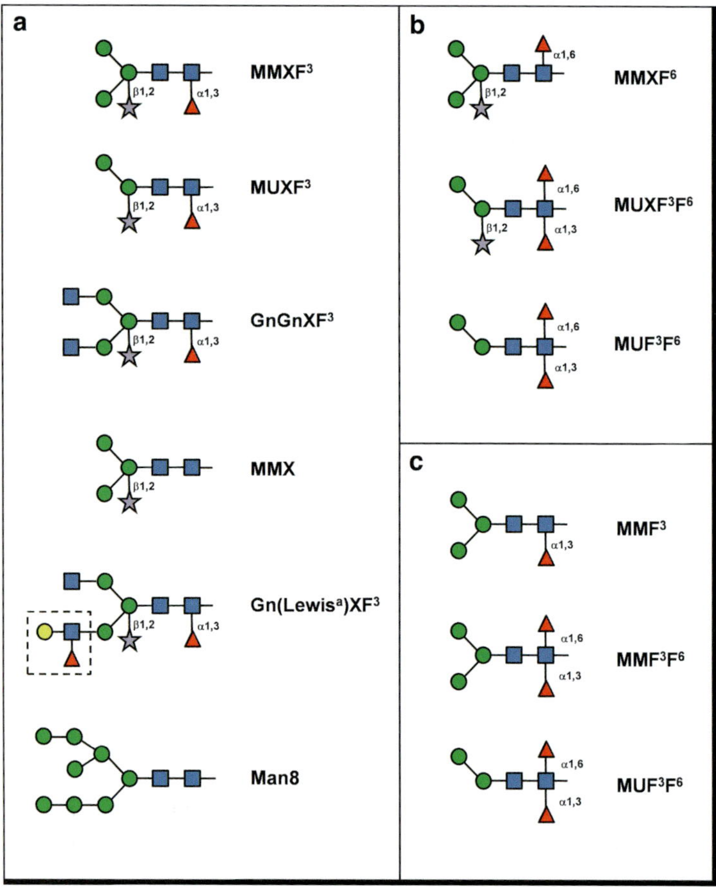

Fig. 8.1 Common allergenic and non-allergenic *N*-glycans from plants (**a**), parasitic helminths (**b**) and *Hymenoptera* venoms (**c**). *Blue squares*: GlcNAc, *green circles*: mannose, *red triangles*: fucose, *violet asterisks*: xylose, *yellow circles*: galactose

Trichobilharzia) as well as nematodes (*Haemonchus contortus*, *Dirofilaria immitis*) (Haslam et al. 1996; van Die et al. 1999). In *Schistosoma mansoni*-infected mice and *H. contortus*-infected sheep, both fucose and xylose are targets of the IgE immune response (van Die et al. 1999). While IgE antibodies against the parasite glycoconjugates appear to protect from further parasite infections, they have not yet been directly associated with allergic reactions. True allergy to helminth antigens is well-documented for the fish parasite *Anisakis simplex* causing pathogen-induced anaphylaxis when infected fish is ingested by sensitized humans. However, in this case clinically relevant IgE antibodies are directed against a panel of excreted/secreted and somatic proteins but not against helminth glycans (Lorenzo et al. 2000; Audicana and Kennedy 2008).

CCDs have been found also in glycoproteins of several snail species (Lommerse et al. 1997; Gutternigg et al. 2004). They contain xylose, whereas core α(1→3)-fucosylation appears to be largely absent despite the presence of α(1→3)-fucosyltransferase in the great pond snail *Lymnaea stagnalis* (van Tetering et al. 1999). Interestingly, small amounts of α(1→3) fucose, but no xylose, have been detected in the Eastern oyster (*Crassostrea virginica*) (Wilson, personal communication). Food allergic reactions to snails (and other mollusks) are mainly known from patients with house dust mite allergy due to cross-reactions between conserved muscle tropomyosins. There are no clear data supporting a role of carbohydrate antigens in such adverse reactions.

8.2.2 Specificity of Anti-CCD Antibodies

The relevant monosaccharides defining the antigenicity/allergenicity of *N*-glycans have been extensively studied using monoclonal or polyclonal rabbit, rat or goat antisera as well as human IgE. Early researchers identified xylose as the crucial element (Faye and Chrispeels 1988; Lauriere et al. 1988), whereas in later studies antibody-binding to xylose was not or less commonly observed (Wilson et al. 1998; Petersen et al. 1996; Bencurova et al. 2004). Within the context of allergy, IgE reactivity to α(1→3) fucose is nowadays considered more essential, although the prevalence may depend in part on patient selection criteria. The contribution of α(1→3) fucose was first demonstrated by Kurosaka et al. (1991) for polyclonal goat anti-HRP IgG, and shortly thereafter for human IgE in several studies of honeybee venom allergens (Kubelka et al. 1993; Tretter et al. 1993). Xylose and α(1→3) fucose are sterically apart, being attached to different sites of the glycan core, and thus represent distinct and independent epitopes (Lommerse et al. 1995). This is evident also from inhibition experiments using well-defined artificial glycoforms of human transferrin (Bencurova et al. 2004) and the possibility to separate by affinity chromatography polyclonal antisera into a xylose- and a α(1→3) fucose-specific fraction (Faye et al. 1993; van Die et al. 1999; van Ree et al. 2000).

Although the distal mannose of complex *N*-glycans is not antigenic in its own right, it may influence to some extent antibody binding. This may particularly apply to antibodies directed against xylose (Kurosaka et al. 1991; Bencurova et al. 2004). In accordance with this, bromelain has been found less sensitive for detecting CCD-positive sera than HRP and ascorbate oxidase in some studies (Malandain et al. 2007; Coutinho et al. 2008). *N*-Glycans lacking both terminal mannose residues have a drastically reduced binding capacity also for fucose-specific antibodies. Recent attempts to further dissect the specificity of anti-HRP antibodies using small CCD tri- and tetrasaccharides (containing either xylose or α(1→3) fucose) surprisingly revealed no or only weak binding to the CCD fragments (Collot et al. 2011) supporting a critical role of other sugar residues in antibody binding. Anti-CCD antibodies may thus be better referred to as fucose- or xylose-"dependent" rather than fucose- or xylose-"specific", as proposed by Altmann (2007).

Also substitution of the non-reducing glycan termini by GlcNAc (e.g., GnGnXF, Fig. 8.1) appears to reduce antibody binding, possibly by sterically hindering antibody access to the oligosaccharide core (Bencurova et al. 2004). In agreement with this, tree pollens, whose carbohydrate repertoire is dominated by $GnGnXF^3$ and high mannose-type *N*-glycans (Wilson and Altmann 1998), are less reactive with most CCD-positive sera than grass, rapeseed and ragweed pollen which contain large amounts of $MMXF^3$ and $MUXF^3$ glycans. Anyhow, GnGnX-specific antibodies could be induced in immunized rabbits (Jin et al. 2006).

8.2.3 Prevalence and Origin of Anti-CCD IgE Antibodies in Allergic Patients

The prevalence of anti CCD-IgE antibodies has been first studied in patients with venom allergy. Tretter et al. (1993), focusing on honeybee venom allergy, reported that among 47 sera positive for purified honeybee phospholipase A2, 74% had IgE antibodies reactive with the phospholipase glycans which could be effectively inhibited by MUXF bromelain glycopeptides conjugated to BSA. More recently, CCDs have been identified as a major cause for honeybee-vespid double-positivity which is seen in more than 50% of venom-allergic patients (Hemmer et al. 2001, 2004). Among such double-positive cases, 75% were found positive to oilseed rape pollen extracts used as a hypoallergenic glycoprotein source rich in CCDs, whereas this was quite unusual in honeybee or wasp single-positive sera (Hemmer et al. 2001). Importantly, in most patients anti-CCD IgE antibodies were the only cause for the observed double-positivity. Similar observations were made in a number of subsequent studies describing IgE-binding to bromelain in 52–74% of double-positive sera (Jappe et al. 2006; Müller et al. 2009; Mittermann et al. 2010). Summarizing these data, the prevalence of anti-CCD IgE antibodies among venom-allergic patients is as high as 25–40%. In a study by Kochuyt et al. (2005), at least 16% of unselected venom-allergic patients were found CCD-positive, although their true number may have been underestimated in this study. It appears likely that the high rate of latent venom sensitization found in the general population (up to 27%) (Schäfer and Przybilla 1996) is often due to CCD-specific IgE, although the exact percentage needs to be explored yet.

While glycosylation might not be essential for the allergenicity of venom allergens (Okano et al. 1999), it is quite obvious that insect stings themselves are potent inducers of an anti-carbohydrate IgE response. This can be concluded from the remarkably high prevalence of anti-CCD IgE antibodies in venom-allergic patients and the absence of other allergic diseases in the majority of them (Kochuyt et al. 2005).

The occurrence of anti-CCD IgE antibodies correlates also with atopy (i.e., the genetic predisposition to mount IgE responses to many different environmental allergens) and total IgE levels (Mari 2002; Linneberg et al. 2010). Among a large population of 1,831 patients with suspect respiratory allergy, Mari (2002) detected IgE to bromelain in 23% of atopic patients, but in only 5% of non-atopics.

Pollen allergy represents a special risk factor since the prevalence was 31% in pollen-sensitized patients (further increasing in subjects with multiple pollen sensitization) but only 10% in those sensitized to non-pollen allergens. Very similar results were published by other investigators reporting 17–24% CCD-positivity among patients with grass pollen allergy or multiple pollen sensitization (Bencurova et al. 2004; Ebo et al. 2004). Interestingly, monovalent birch pollen allergy was not associated with anti-CCD IgE in these studies. Extraordinarily high percentages of 65–80% were described from patients with olive and cypress pollen allergy (Batanero et al. 1999; Iacovacci et al. 2002). It may be concluded from these data that the development of anti-CCD IgE in atopic subjects is causally related to respiratory sensitization to certain pollens. Concerning gender and age, anti-CCD IgE antibodies are slightly more frequent in males whereas only marginal differences exist with regard to age (Mari 2002).

A high prevalence of CCD-positivity of up to 80% has been observed also among patients with allergy to foods, such as carrot, celery, orange, and banana (Ballmer-Weber et al. 2001; Luttkopf et al. 2000; Ahrazem et al. 2006; Palacin et al. 2011). Unless assuming a clinically relevant role of CCDs in these allergic reactions (see below), these high figures might rather mirror the strong atopic background of these patients, and may in part also be an overestimate due to a bias in patient selection in these studies.

Remarkably, a couple of recent papers identified alcohol intake as another independent risk factor for the development of anti-CCD IgE antibodies (Gonzalez-Quintela et al. 2008; Linneberg et al. 2010). These effects can be possibly ascribed to the ethanol metabolite acetaldehyde, since a linkage was found with certain class 1 alcohol dehydrogenase polymorphisms associated with rapid ethanol conversion (Linneberg et al. 2010). However, the measured serum anti-CCD IgE levels were throughout low and a significant rise in prevalence was only seen in non-atopic heavy drinkers. In atopics, prevalence was generally high without a significant difference between drinkers and abstainers, suggesting that the influence of alcohol consumption on IgE production is modest as compared to that of atopic predisposition.

It is worth mentioning that levels of anti-CCD IgE antibodies in CCD-positive sera are fairly low in most cases (<5 ng/ml = <2 kU/l) (van Ree et al. 2000; Mari 2002; Jappe et al. 2006; Bauermeister et al. 2009; Linneberg et al. 2010), although quite high values exceeding 20 kU/l may be seen in some (Mari et al. 1999, 2008; Mari 2002; Jappe et al. 2006). There is not much known about the time course of CCD-specific IgE. In venom-allergic subjects, venom-specific IgE is rather short-lived with a rapid conversion to negative serology within few years if patients are not re-stung (Mauriello et al. 1984) and this seems to apply also to the CCD-specific fraction (Hemmer, unpublished). Accordingly, everyday exposure to large amounts of inhaled or ingested CCDs through pollens and plant food does not maintain activation of CCD-specific B-cells in this population. The secretion of CCD-specific IgE might be more persistent in atopic patients (e.g., pollen allergic patients) (Mari et al. 1999), possibly linked to boosting of protein-specific immune responses during the pollen season, but this has to be dealt with in future studies.

8.2.4 Clinical Significance of Anti-CCD IgE

The clinical significance of anti-CCD IgE antibodies is still a matter of debate, but nowadays most allergists consider these antibodies to have no or very limited clinical relevance. Allergy diagnosis is basically limited by the fact that the mere presence of allergen-specific IgE neither predicts the emergence of clinical symptoms upon allergen exposure nor is the quantity of serum specific IgE closely correlated with disease severity (Ebo et al. 2004; Westritschnig et al. 2008; Blum et al. 2011). The progressing identification and molecular characterization of single protein allergens over the last years and the resulting insight into individual sensitization profiles made clear that the potency of different allergens to cause mediator release translating into clinical allergy differs considerably. Even if anti-CCD IgE antibodies are clinically relevant in rare cases, on a scale listing allergenic molecules according to their clinical "penetrance", CCDs are undoubtedly at the very end of this scale.

The assumption of lacking clinical relevance of anti-CCD IgE antibodies is based on several lines of evidence:

- CCD-positive patients always show broad IgE reactivity against pollens, plant food, latex and (commonly) insect venoms, but do not show clinical hypersensitivity to most of these allergens (Aalberse et al. 1981; van der Veen et al. 1997; Mari 2002; Ebo et al. 2004; Malandain 2004, 2005; Kochuyt et al. 2005; Malandain et al. 2007; Coutinho et al. 2008).
- Allergens recognized by patients' IgE merely via CCDs cause very weak skin test responses or no reactions at all, signifying low biologic activity of the carbohydrate-specific IgE (Mari et al. 1999; Mari 2002; Hemmer et al. 2001; Ebo et al. 2004; Kochuyt et al. 2005; Ahrazem et al. 2006; Gonzalez-Quintela et al. 2009; Mertens et al. 2010).
- In many allergic conditions, such as peanut, latex and venom allergy, patients' IgE is virtually always directed against protein epitopes of the respective allergens, while restricted reactivity to CCDs is extremely uncommon and may just be failure to detect the protein allergen (Astier et al. 2006; Ebo et al. 2004; Jappe et al. 2006; Jin et al. 2010).

Systematic studies on the (ir)relevance of anti-CCD IgE have mainly focused on conditions associated with life-threatening anaphylaxis, such as peanut, latex and venom allergy.

A classical study by van der Veen et al. (1997) described that CCD-positive grass pollen-allergic patients regularly react with peanut extracts *in vitro* but do not develop clinical symptoms despite peanut-specific IgE levels of up to 30 ng/ml. Basophils of grass pollen-allergic patients needed 100–10,000-fold higher amounts of peanut allergen for significant histamine release than true peanut-allergic subjects, indicating poor biologic activity of the carbohydrate-directed antibodies. Likewise, in a survey by Mari (2002) in 161 CCD-positive patients with discrepant test results to peanut (negative skin test/positive *in vitro* test), none had a history of peanut hypersensitivity. The very same was found in a couple of other papers (Guilloux et al. 2009; Vidal et al. 2009). In contrast, manifest peanut allergy is evidently associated with the regular presence of IgE against peptide epitopes (Astier et al. 2006).

Ebo et al. (2004) studied sensitization patterns in latex-positive patients with either clinically manifest latex allergy or asymptomatic sensitization. While patients with confirmed latex allergy did not react with CCDs, 81% of the asymptomatic subjects did, indicating that CCDs are a common cause of latent latex sensitization but do not represent clinically relevant epitopes. Subsequent studies in a large group of CCD-positive venom-allergic patients and heavy drinkers confirmed, that CCD-dependent reactivity with latex allergens is not associated with clinical hypersensitivity (Mahler et al. 2006; Coutinho et al. 2008). In latex-associated fruit allergy, clinical food allergy was found tightly associated with IgE to latex hevein (Hev b 6) and cross-reactivity with food class 1 chitinases harboring homologous hevein-like domains (Diaz-Perales et al. 1999). The presence of serum IgE against CCDs, however, was never associated with clinical food allergy despite strong antibody binding to immunoblotted food extracts.

Insect venom allergy is a field where the role of carbohydrates has been most intensely studied. Here, CCDs have been recognized as a major cause of double-positive *in vitro* results to honeybee and vespid venom (Hemmer et al. 2001, 2004; Kochuyt et al. 2005; Jappe et al. 2006; Mahler et al. 2006). While double-positivity is found in up to 60% of patients, the rarity of clinical hypersensitivity to both insects underlines the lacking relevance of anti-CCD antibodies. Further support comes from the observation that IgE against the culprit venom is virtually always directed against peptide epitopes, whereas CCDs are responsible for *in vitro* antibody binding to the (irrelevant) second venom (Hemmer et al. 2004; Jappe et al. 2006; Jin et al. 2010). Simultaneous *in vitro* reactivity of CCD-positive patients' sera with pollen and latex CCDs was found clinically irrelevant throughout (Kochuyt et al. 2005; Mahler et al. 2006). There is preliminary evidence from a prospective study confirming that sensitization to venom CCDs is a frequent cause of latent venom sensitization in the general population and not associated with positive sting challenge (Sturm, personal communication).

Finally, the irrelevance of anti-CCD IgE antibodies is illustrated by observations in occupational allergy to wood dusts showing that only reactivity with protein epitopes, but not CCDs, correlates with working place-related health problems (Kespohl et al. 2010). An interesting study was performed by Gonzalez-Quintela et al. (2011) reporting that heavy drinkers commonly develop IgE antibodies against CCDs which strongly bind in western blots to glycoproteins present in wine. Nevertheless, although wine glycoproteins were able to activate basophils *in vitro*, none of the patients ever experienced adverse reactions to wine consistent with allergy.

This body of evidence questioning the clinical relevance of anti-carbohydrate IgE in allergy is faced with a couple of contradicting papers claiming clinical relevance in at least certain conditions. Relevant studies have thus far focused on a limited number of pollens and (rare) food allergens such as tomato, celery, and zucchini (Fötisch et al. 2003, 1999; Bublin et al. 2003; Reindl et al. 2000). A major reasoning behind this is the ability of glycoproteins to activate basophils from allergic donors *in vitro* and the loss of this activity upon protein de-glycosylation.

Fötisch et al. (2003) observed that stimulation of basophils from tomato-allergic subjects with purified tomato fructofuranosidase (Lyc e 2) and HRP induces significant mediator release in four of ten sera (though at relatively high protein concentrations), while no release is obtained with recombinant non-glycosylated Lyc e 2 and de-glycosylated HRP. The same group also described basophil activation by a synthetic glycoprotein displaying bromelain glycans (MUXF-BSA) in two celery-allergic patients reacting in western blots selectively with celery CCDs, and the loss of reactivity upon protein de-glycosylation (Fötisch et al. 1999). Similar observations in a celery-allergic patient were made by Bublin et al. (2003) observing moderate basophil histamine release by purified glycosylated Api g 5 but not by the chemically de-glycosylated allergen. In a later survey of celery allergy, however, the releasing capacity of purified Api g 5 in CCD-positive patients was negligible as compared to recombinant celery Api g 1 and birch pollen Bet v 1 (Bauermeister et al. 2009).

A major functional role was alleged to carbohydrate epitopes in cypress pollen allergy where IgE-binding to the major cypress pollen allergen Cup c 1 is entirely due to CCDs in up to 80% of patients (Afferni et al. 1999; Iacovacci et al. 2002). A dose-dependent histamine release from patients' basophils could be obtained only with natural Cup c 1 (starting at a relatively high concentration of 0.5 μg/ml) but not with the *E. coli*-expressed non-glycosylated recombinant variant (Iacovacci et al. 2002). A similar role has been claimed for the *N*-glycans of the major olive pollen allergen Ole e 1 (Batanero et al. 1999), however, due to serious methodological shortcomings the findings of this study require verification by further investigators. Because native Ole e 1 (the major olive pollen allergen) and isolated *N*-glycans chemically removed from Ole e 1 by PNGase F treatment revealed equivalent histamine release from basophils, it was concluded that allergenicity essentially rests upon the carbohydrate moieties. Regardless of the circumstance that only xylosylated (but not $\alpha(1\rightarrow3)$-fucosylated) *N*-glycans can be removed by PNGase F from the protein core, these findings require verification by further investigators since efficient IgE receptor cross-linking by such monovalent oligosaccharides is hard to envisage.

The potency of CCDs to stimulate basophils has been examined very recently also by basophil activation test (BAT) using venom allergy as a model (Mertens et al. 2010). The authors provided convincing evidence that venom CCDs as well as HRP may up-regulate basophil CD203c expression in up to 67% of CCD-positive venom-double-positive patients, whereas activation is no longer achieved with periodate-treated proteins. While these data might taint in some way the reputation of BAT as a diagnostic method of superior specificity, it must be emphasized that, similar to most other papers reporting CCD-induced basophil activation, stimulation by CCDs was poor as compared to protein epitopes and only seen at 10–1,000-fold higher protein concentrations.

As a consequence of the aforementioned observations the indispensability of glycosylated allergens in allergy diagnosis has been emphasized by some authors, at least in the context of certain allergen sources or in certain patients (Fötisch and Vieths 2001; Fötisch et al. 2003; Iacovacci et al. 2002). However, up to now no data exist specifying and substantiating to which allergen sources this might apply and how patients with respectively relevant and irrelevant antibodies can be reliably distinguished. It remains to be explored why the same set of carbohydrate epitopes may exert dissimilar biological activity in the environment of different glycoproteins and why anti-CCD IgE antibodies may behave biologically diverse in different individuals. Furthermore, as pointed out previously by van Ree (2002) it is important to differentiate between biological activity (i.e., mediator release from effector cells) of anti-CCD IgE and clinical relevance, since mediator release does not necessarily translate into clinical allergy. Mari et al. (2008) showed in a limited number of grass pollen-allergic patients with high anti-CCD IgE production, that oral provocation with "plantified" recombinant human lactoferrin expressed in rice did not provoke any symptoms, although half of the patients exhibited significant basophil histamine release *in vitro* (though only with concentrations several orders of magnitude higher than necessary for the grass pollen allergen Phl p 5).

8.2.5 Reasons for the Clinical Insignificance of CCDs

Because mediator release from effector cells requires cross-linking of two occupied IgE receptors, only allergens displaying at least two epitopes may exert biologic activity. Monovalency of glycoproteins, i.e. presence of a single IgE-binding glycan, might thus reasonably explain the poor biologic activity of CCDs. In concordance with this, bromelain (carrying a single glycan) did not elicit positive skin prick test responses in a large group of CCD-positive patients, whereas at least 21% reacted positively to polyglycosylated HRP (although reactions were weak throughout and predominantly seen in patients with high anti-CCD IgE levels) (Mari et al. 1999; Mari 2002). Many well-characterized allergens have been shown to be monoglycosylated, e.g. orange Cit s 1, latex Hev b 2, hazelnut Cor a 11, peanut Ara h 1, grass pollen Phl p 1, honeybee Api m 1, and this monovalency may explain their poor allergenicity in skin testing or basophil activation in CCD-positive patients (Ahrazem et al. 2006; Pöltl et al. 2007; Lauer et al. 2004; Yagami et al. 2002; Wicklein et al. 2004). On the other hand, even though polyvalent glycoproteins such as HRP do prove biologically active in skin tests and basophil activation tests, positive responses are only seen in a subgroup of patients and are generally modest as compared to those elicited by protein allergens (Mari 2002; Mertens et al. 2010). Considering that among the high number of glycoproteins present in plant foods and pollens at least some are likely to be "polyvalent", monovalency alone does not sufficiently explain the low relevance of CCDs.

Other factors contributing to the low biological activity of anti-CCD IgE antibodies may be their mostly low serum concentrations and the positive correlation with total IgE levels (Mari 2002). This might favour IgE receptor saturation on effector cells and increasing scattering of IgE antibodies of the same specificity reducing the likelihood of successful IgE receptor cross-linking.

Low affinity of anti-CCD antibodies has been repeatedly proposed as an explanation for the low clinical relevance (van Ree and Aalberse 1999; van Ree 2002). However, recent studies using surface plasmon resonance revealed a surprisingly high affinity of purified rabbit IgG and human IgE antibodies against CCDs comparable to that of protein-specific antibodies (Jin et al. 2006, 2008) making low affinity an unlikely explanation.

Alternatively, protection may be ensured by high-affinity anti-CCD IgG/IgG4 antibodies functioning as "blocking" antibodies. Blocking antibodies are believed to play a crucial role in successful allergen immunotherapy by competing with IgE for binding to allergen epitopes and by mediating FcγRIIb-dependent inhibition of cell signalling in mast cells and basophils (Flicker and Valenta 2003; Strait et al. 2006). Concerning CCDs, such antibodies may arise from the everyday contact of the immune system with high amounts of CCDs derived from edible plants and inhaled pollens. Their induction has been understood as a kind of natural "glyco-immunotherapy" (Altmann 2007), possibly comparable to the generation of high levels of allergy-protective IgG4 antibodies in cat owners with strong exposure to cat allergens (Platts-Mills et al. 2001). Naturally occurring IgM and IgG1 (although not IgG4) against xylose or $\alpha(1\rightarrow3)$ fucose has been found in the sera of at least 50% of non-atopic blood donors (Bardor et al. 2003), but to date still little is known about the prevalence and quantity of IgG/IgG4 antibodies and the IgE/IgG ratio in allergic subjects.

8.2.6 Diagnostic Implications of Anti-CCD IgE Antibodies

Although the discovery of IgE antibodies against cross-reactive sugar determinants of plant and insect glycoproteins dates back to the early 1980s, this observation was ignored by most allergists for quite a long time. Once the dimension of anti-CCD antibody cross-reactivity and its implication for *in vitro* allergy diagnosis became more evident, much work has been dedicated to this issue more recently. The current shift in *in vitro* allergy diagnosis towards the increased usage of recombinant molecules has been strongly influenced by the growing awareness about the interference of anti-CCD IgE antibodies with correct allergy diagnosis. Notwithstanding the yet unsettled dispute about the clinical (ir)relevance of anti-CCD IgE antibodies, the increasing awareness of clinicians of the huge number of misleading "false-positive" *in vitro* results caused by CCDs has prompted different approaches to overcome the problem and to increase the specificity and predictive value of IgE determination.

Routine IgE screening by RAST or ELISA for bromelain, HRP, or other glycoprotein sources can be used as a simple measure to identify CCD-positive sera (Mari et al. 1999; Mari 2002; Hemmer et al. 2001; Kochuyt et al. 2005; Jappe et al. 2006; Müller et al. 2009). A positive result will caution doctors to over-interpret positive *in vitro* test results obtained with other plant or insect allergens, however, it needs to be emphasized that the simple proof of anti-CCD IgE antibodies in the serum does not reliably exclude "true" sensitization to a particular allergen, since protein- and carbohydrate-specific IgE may occur side by side (Hemmer et al. 2004; Jappe et al. 2006).

Destruction of carbohydrate epitopes by periodate treatment has been widely used in scientific research (Mari et al. 1999; Aalberse et al. 1981; Afferni et al. 1999; Hemmer et al. 2004; Mahler et al. 2006). Unfortunately, also protein conformation may be altered by this treatment (Hemmer et al. 2004; Léonard et al. 2005), leading to reduced sensitivity and false-negative test results. Therefore, periodate oxidation has never been implemented in commercial IgE assays.

A more reliable though simple method to get rid of CCD interference is serum inhibition, i.e. pre-incubation of samples with appropriate CCD inhibitors prior to specific IgE measurement (e.g., RAST inhibition). Serum inhibition has been a standard tool in scientific research, but has been put forward as a feasible measure in routine allergy diagnosis, too (Malandain et al. 2007). To obtain best results, a mixture of different glycoproteins, e.g. bromelain (mostly displaying $MUXF^3$) and HRP (mostly displaying $MMXF^3$), is probably necessary to cover all anti-CCD IgE specificities present in individual sera (Malandain et al. 2007; Altmann 2007). Alternatively, isolated glycopeptides obtained from these natural sources may be conjugated to inert carrier proteins such as BSA. A more sophisticated alternative to generate appropriate CCD inhibitors is the targeted modification of human glycoproteins (e.g., transferrin) by using appropriate glycosidases and recombinant glycosyltransferases which allows optimal standardization with regard to glycan repertoire and molarity (Bencurova et al. 2004; Jin et al. 2006). An even more elegant way than serum inhibition is to clear patients' sera from CCD-specific antibodies by micro-affinity chromatography using immobilized plant glycans (Jin et al. 2009). However, the disadvantage of all these procedures is their time need and the necessity of additional manual manipulation of blood samples which probably does not comply with the needs of today's routine labs.

A promising strategy to improve specificity of *in vitro* IgE determination is component-resolved diagnosis by (non-glycosylated) recombinant allergens. This technique not only eliminates the problem of CCDs but in addition provides valuable information about individual sensitization profiles improving accuracy of therapy and patient management (Valenta et al. 2007; De Knop et al. 2010). A substantial part of recent research has focused on insect venom allergy, where the diagnostic superiority of recombinant technology has been impressively demonstrated in a couple of papers (Müller et al. 2009; Mittermann et al. 2010; Seismann et al. 2010). Similarly, component-resolved diagnosis eliminating CCDs has been proven advantageous in the diagnosis of latex allergy (Raulf-Heimsoth et al. 2007; Ebo et al. 2010). CCD-free recombinant allergens may be obtained by protein expression in *E. coli* or yeasts, but correct folding of naturally glycosylated proteins can be a problem (Soldatova et al. 1998). The use of insect cell lines with low-level α1,3 fucosyltransferase activity, such as Sf9 cells, appears to guarantee allergen glycosylation with at worst just traces of unwanted CCDs along with proper protein folding (Seismann et al. 2010; Hancock et al. 2008).

8.3 Allergenic *O*-Glycans

A novel type of IgE-binding *O*-glycans has been identified on the major mugwort pollen allergen Art v 1 (Himly et al. 2003; Léonard et al. 2005). Art v 1 is a peculiar protein consisting of a globular cysteine-stabilized defensin-like domain and a proline-rich C-terminal tail with a prominent branched arabinogalactan polysaccharide and a number of single β-arabinosyl residues attached to hydroxylated proline residues. Results from de-glycosylation and inhibition experiments using rabbit antiserum against posttranslationally modified Art v 1 and sera from mugwort-allergic patients revealed that it is the β-arabinosylated hydroxyprolines (occurring as clusters of two or three) that represent IgE-binding determinants (Léonard et al. 2005). An approach to the identification of the minimal epitope has been recently undertaken by synthesis of dimers of the β-arabinosyl-hydroxyproline motif (Xie and Taylor 2010). Contradicting findings were obtained in another study reporting generation of monoclonal antibodies from a synthetic human recombinant antibody library by subtractive phage display specifically binding to the α-arabinosyl residues on the Art v 1 arabinogalactan polysaccharide (Gruber et al. 2009). In some mugwort-allergic patients, IgE antibodies against natural Art v 1 do not or less strongly bind to *E. coli*-expressed recombinant Art v 1, suggesting that the identified carbohydrate moieties represent important epitopes (Himly et al. 2003; Gruber et al. 2009). Support for a clinical relevance of the oligosaccharides comes from skin tests and nasal provocation tests showing stronger responses to native Art v 1 than to the recombinant molecule (Schmid-Grendelmeier et al. 2003).

There is thus far no evidence for an important role of mugwort glycans as cross-reactive epitopes to mind in allergy diagnosis. Rabbit antisera against Art v 1 β-arabinose glycans did not bind to the homologous ragweed pollen allergen Amb a 4, which contains two arabinogalactan polysaccharides similar to those of Art v 1 as well as single β-arabinosylated hydroxyprolines (Léonard et al. 2010). This lack of cross-reactivity may be due to the fact that hydroxyprolines in Amb a 4 do not occur pairwise like in Art v 1 (Léonard et al. 2010). There is also no cross-reactivity with arabinose-containing *O*-glycans from potato and tomato lectins (Léonard et al. 2005). In all, there is currently no evidence for an important role of *O*-glycan cross-reactivity in allergy diagnosis comparable to that of fucosylated/xylosylated *N*-glycans.

8.4 α-Gal, a Mammalian IgE-Binding Glycan

Galactose-α(1→3)-galactose (briefly termed αGal) is a common modification of glycoproteins and glycolipids from nearly all mammals, which remarkably is absent in old-world monkeys (including man) and other vertebrates (Macher and Galili 2008), cartilaginous fishes making an interesting exception (Harvey et al. 2009). αGal is highly immunogenic for humans, who regularly produce high levels of αGal-specific IgG antibodies representing the major cause for hyperacute tissue rejection following xenotransplantation (Macher and Galili 2008). αGal has been first recognized as a relevant allergen in patients with anaphylaxis to the humanized mouse monoclonal IgG1 antibody Cetuximab, caused by pre-existing anti-αGal IgE antibodies reacting with αGal in the murine part of Cetuximab (Chung et al. 2008), but shortly thereafter also an association with allergy to red meat became evident (Commins et al. 2009; Jacquenet et al. 2009; Commins and Platts-Mills 2009).

On *in vitro* testing, αGal-positive sera show comparable reactivity with different kinds of mammalian meats as well as with animal dander (e.g., cat, dog) and cow's milk indicating that all these allergen sources contain substantial amounts of αGal (Jacquenet et al. 2009; Commins and Platts-Mills 2009). The responsible αGal-expressing glycoproteins are not yet known in detail. αGal has been identified as a relevant epitope of cat salivary IgA (Grönlund et al. 2009), but also other Ig might represent relevant sources of αGal in view of the presence of galactosylated oligosaccharides sometimes bearing terminal αGal in the heavy chain variable regions of IgG and IgM (Endo et al. 1995; Harvey et al. 2009). Glycolipids are another potential source of αGal. The retarded gastrointestinal resorption of such glycolipids might explain the untypical delay in symptom onset observed in most αGal-positive meat-allergic patients (Commins et al. 2009; Commins and Platts-Mills 2009). Another remarkable finding of αGal-mediated meat allergy is the poor reactivity of patients in skin prick tests with meat extracts, reminding of the situation in α1,3-fucosylated/xylosylated *N*-glycans. Clearly positive skin test reaction are only obtained with intradermal testing (Commins et al. 2009).

Screening sera from different geographical regions for anti-αGal IgE revealed unexpected differences in prevalence leading to the hypothesis that primary sensitization to αGal has not occurred by meat itself. Tick bites have been suspected as a possible origin encouraged by the observation of cutaneous hypersensitivity reactions after tick bites in many patients (Commins et al. 2009; Commins and Platts-Mills 2009; van Nunen et al. 2009). However, αGal is thus far not known from ticks or mites or any other arthropods. Exposure to αGal during infection with helminth parasites might be another route of αGal sensitization (Commins et al. 2009). Although αGal does not seem ubiquitous in parasites, it has been proven in a few nematodes (Duffy et al. 2006; Khoo et al. 1997) and in the liver fluke *Fasciola hepatica* (Wuhrer et al. 2004). Anyhow, evidence for a causal relationship between worm infection and αGal sensitization in these patients is still lacking. The possibility of sensitization to αGal via drugs of bovine origin (e.g., thrombin, aprotinin) should not be completely disregarded.

8.5 Summary

N-Glycans displaying core α(1→3) fucose and/or xylose represent important cross-reactive carbohydrate determinants (CCDs) of plant and insect glycoproteins binding IgE from around 10–30% of allergic subjects. Based on a body of epidemiologic and experimental evidence, the clinical significance of IgE directed against CCDs appears to be extremely low, even if the reasons for this are not yet completely understood. Although clinical relevance in exceptional cases cannot be ruled out with absolute certainty, CCDs are now broadly acknowledged by clinicians as a major cause of "false-positive" results severely interfering with proper allergy diagnosis. Current strategies to overcome the problem include elimination of carbohydrate-directed IgE from samples by serum inhibition as well as component-based diagnosis using non-glycosylated recombinant allergens. Still little is known about the epitope structure and function of IgE-binding β-arabinosylated *O*-glycans recently discovered in mugwort pollen. While there exist some clues to a clinical relevance of these sugar antigens in allergic reactions, they unlikely play a prominent role as cross-reactive epitopes comparable to that of fucosylated/xylosylated *N*-glycans. The identification of galactose-α(1→3)-galactose (αGal) as an IgE-binding sugar epitope of mammalian origin has revived the interest in allergy to red meat and may be relevant also with respect to allergy to milk, animal danders and drugs of bovine origin. Major future tasks comprise confirmation of the relevance of these anti-αGal IgE antibodies in meat allergy by controlled oral provocation test and clarification of the alleged relationship with tick bites and helminth infection.

Acknowledgement I thank Friedrich Altmann, Vienna, for careful reading of the manuscript and his helpful suggestions.

References

Aalberse RC, Koshte V, Clemens JG (1981) Immunoglobulin E antibodies that crossreact with vegetable foods, pollen, and Hymenoptera venom. J Allergy Clin Immunol 68:356–364

Afferni C, Iacovacci P, Barletta B, Di Felice G, Tinghino R, Mari A, Pini C (1999) Role of carbohydrate moieties in IgE binding to allergenic components of *Cupressus arizonica* pollen extract. Clin Exp Allergy 29:1087–1094

Ahrazem O, Ibanez MD, Lopez-Torrejon G, Sanchez-Monge R, Sastre J, Lombardero M, Barber D, Salcedo G (2006) Orange germin-like glycoprotein Cit s 1: an equivocal allergen. Int Arch Allergy Immunol 139:96–103

Alisi C, Afferni C, Iacovacci P, Barletta B, Tinghino R, Butteroni C, Puggioni EM, Wilson IB, Federico R, Schininà ME, Ariano R, Di Felice G, Pini C (2001) Rapid isolation, characterization, and glycan analysis of Cup a 1, the major allergen of Arizona cypress (*Cupressus arizonica*) pollen. Allergy 56:978–984

Altmann F (2007) The role of protein glycosylation in allergy. Int Arch Allergy Immunol 142:99–115

Astier C, Morisset M, Roitel O, Codreanu F, Jacquenet S, Franck P, Ogier V, Petit N, Proust B, Moneret-Vautrin DA, Burks AW, Bihain B, Sampson HA, Kanny G (2006) Predictive value of skin prick tests using recombinant allergens for diagnosis of peanut allergy. J Allergy Clin Immunol 118:250–256

Audicana MT, Kennedy MW (2008) *Anisakis simplex*: from obscure infectious worm to inducer of immune hypersensitivity. Clin Microbiol Rev 21:360–379

Ballmer-Weber BK, Wüthrich B, Wangorsch A, Fötisch K, Altmann F, Vieths S (2001) Carrot allergy: double-blinded, placebo-controlled food challenge and identification of allergens. J Allergy Clin Immunol 108:301–307

Bardor M, Faveeuw C, Fitchette AC, Gilbert D, Galas L, Trottein F, Faye L, Lerouge P (2003) Immunoreactivity in mammals of two typical plant glyco-epitopes, core α(1,3)-fucose and core xylose. Glycobiology 13:427–434

Batanero E, Crespo JF, Monsalve RI, Martin-Esteban M, Villalba M, Rodriguez R (1999) IgE binding and histamine-release capabilities of the main carbohydrate component isolated from the major allergen of olive tree pollen, Ole e 1. J Allergy Clin Immunol 103:147–153

Bauermeister K, Ballmer-Weber BK, Bublin M, Fritsche P, Hanschmann KM, Hoffmann-Sommergruber K, Lidholm J, Oberhuber C, Randow S, Holzhauser T, Vieths S (2009) Assessment of component-resolved *in vitro* diagnosis of celeriac allergy. J Allergy Clin Immunol 124:1273–1281

Bencurova M, Hemmer W, Focke-Tejkl M, Wilson IB, Altmann F (2004) Specificity of IgG and IgE antibodies against plant and insect glycoprotein glycans determined with artificial glycoforms of human transferrin. Glycobiology 14:457–466

Blum S, Gunzinger A, Müller UR, Helbling A (2011) Influence of total and specific IgE, serum tryptase, and age on severity of allergic reactions to Hymenoptera stings. Allergy 66:222–228

Bublin M, Radauer C, Wilson IB, Kraft D, Scheiner O, Breiteneder H, Hoffmann-Sommergruber K (2003) Cross-reactive N-glycans of Api g 5, a high molecular weight glycoprotein allergen from celery, are required for immunoglobulin E binding and activation of effector cells from allergic patients. FASEB J 17:1697–1699

Chung CH, Mirakhur B, Chan E, Le QT, Berlin J, Morse M, Murphy BA, Satinover SM, Hosen J, Mauro D, Slebos RJ, Zhou Q, Gold D, Hatley T, Hicklin DJ, Platts-Mills TA (2008) Cetuximab-induced anaphylaxis and IgE specific for galactose-α-1,3-galactose. N Engl J Med 358:1109–1117

Collot M, Wilson IB, Bublin M, Hoffmann-Sommergruber K, Mallet JM (2011) Synthesis of cross-reactive carbohydrate determinants fragments as tools for *in vitro* allergy diagnosis. Bioorg Med Chem 19:1306–1320

Commins SP, Platts-Mills TA (2009) Anaphylaxis syndromes related to a new mammalian cross-reactive carbohydrate determinant. J Allergy Clin Immunol 124:652–657

Commins SP, Satinover SM, Hosen J, Mozena J, Borish L, Lewis BD, Woodfolk JA, Platts-Mills TA (2009) Delayed anaphylaxis, angioedema, or urticaria after consumption of red meat in patients with IgE antibodies specific for galactose-α-1,3-galactose. J Allergy Clin Immunol 123:426–433

Coutinho V, Vidal C, Garrido M, Gude F, Lojo S, Linneberg A, Gonzalez-Quintela A (2008) Interference of cross-reactive carbohydrates in the determination of specific IgE in alcohol drinkers and strategies to minimize it: the example of latex. Ann Allergy Asthma Immunol 101:394–401

De Knop KJ, Bridts CH, Verweij MM, Hagendorens MM, De Clerck LS, Stevens WJ, Ebo DG (2010) Component-resolved allergy diagnosis by microarray: potential, pitfalls, and prospects. Adv Clin Chem 50:87–101

Diaz-Perales A, Collada C, Blanco C, Sanchez-Monge R, Carrillo T, Aragoncillo C, Salcedo G (1999) Cross-reactions in the latex-fruit syndrome: a relevant role of chitinases but not of complex asparagine-linked glycans. J Allergy Clin Immunol 104:681–687

Duffy MS, Morris HR, Dell A, Appleton JA, Haslam SM (2006) Protein glycosylation in *Parelaphostrongylus tenuis* – first description of the Galα1-3Gal sequence in a nematode. Glycobiology 16:854–862

Ebo DG, Hagendorens MM, Bridts CH, De Clerck LS, Stevens WJ (2004) Sensitization to crossreactive carbohydrate determinants and the ubiquitous protein profilin: mimickers of allergy. Clin Exp Allergy 34:137–144

Ebo DG, Hagendorens MM, De Knop KJ, Verweij MM, Bridts CH, De Clerck LS, Stevens WJ (2010) Component-resolved diagnosis from latex allergy by microarray. Clin Exp Allergy 40:348–358

Endo T, Wright A, Morrison SL, Kobata A (1995) Glycosylation of the variable region of immunoglobulin G – site specific maturation of the sugar chains. Mol Immunol 32:931–940

Faye L, Chrispeels MJ (1988) Common antigenic determinants in the glycoproteins of plants, molluscs and insects. Glycoconj J 5:245–256

Faye L, Gomord V, Fitchette-Laine AC, Chrispeels MJ (1993) Affinity purification of antibodies specific for Asn-linked glycans containing α1→3 fucose or β1→2 xylose. Anal Biochem 209:104–108

Flicker S, Valenta R (2003) Renaissance of the blocking antibody concept in type I allergy. Int Arch Allergy Immunol 132:13–24

Fötisch K, Altmann F, Haustein D, Vieths S (1999) Involvement of carbohydrate epitopes in the IgE response of celery-allergic patients. Int Arch Allergy Immunol 120:30–42

Fötisch K, Vieths S (2001) *N*- and *O*-linked oligosaccharides of allergenic glycoproteins. Glycoconj J 18:373–390

Fötisch K, Westphal S, Lauer I, Retzek M, Altmann F, Kolarich D, Scheurer S, Vieths S (2003) Biological activity of IgE specific for cross-reactive carbohydrate determinants. J Allergy Clin Immunol 111:889–896

Gonzalez-Quintela A, Garrido M, Gude F, Campos J, Linneberg A, Lojo S, Vidal C (2008) Sensitization to cross-reactive carbohydrate determinants in relation to alcohol consumption. Clin Exp Allergy 38:152–160

Gonzalez-Quintela A, Garrido M, Gude F, Campos J (2009) Discordant positive results of multiallergen immunoglobulin E tests in relation to cross-reactive carbohydrate determinants and alcohol consumption. J Investig Allergol Clin Immunol 19:70–71

Gonzalez-Quintela A, Gomez-Rial J, Valcarcel C, Campos J, Sanz ML, Linneberg A, Gude F, Vidal C (2011) Immunoglobulin-E reactivity to wine glycoproteins in heavy drinkers. Alcohol 45:113–122

Grönlund H, Adédoyin J, Commins SP, Platts-Mills TA, van Hage M (2009) The carbohydrate galactose-α-1,3-galactose is a major IgE-binding epitope on cat IgA. J Allergy Clin Immunol 123:1189–1191

Gruber P, Gadermaier G, Bauer R, Weiss R, Wagner S, Leonard R, Breiteneder H, Ebner C, Ferreira F, Egger M (2009) Role of the polypeptide backbone and post-translational modifications in cross-reactivity of Art v 1, the major mugwort pollen allergen. Biol Chem 390:445–451

Guilloux L, Morisset M, Codreanu F, Parisot L, Moneret-Vautrin DA (2009) Peanut allergy diagnosis in the context of grass pollen sensitization for 125 patients: roles of peanut and cross-reactive carbohydrate determinants specific IgE. Int Arch Allergy Immunol 149:91–97

Gutternigg M, Ahrer K, Grabher-Meier H, Burgmayr S, Staudacher E (2004) Neutral N-glycans of the gastropod *Arion lusitanicus*. Eur J Biochem 271:1348–1356

Hancock K, Narang S, Pattabhi S, Yushak ML, Khan A, Lin S, Plemons R, Betenbaugh MJ, Tsang VCW (2008) False positive reactivity of recombinant, diagnostic, glycoproteins produced in High Five™ insect cells: Effect of glycosylation. J Immunol Methods 330:130–136

Harvey DJ, Crispin M, Moffatt BE, Smith SL, Sim RB, Rudd PM, Dwek RA (2009) Identification of high-mannose and multiantennary complex-type N-linked glycans containing α-galactose epitopes from Nurse shark IgM heavy chain. Glycoconj J 26:1055–1064

Haslam SM, Coles GC, Munn EA, Smith TS, Smith HF, Morris HR, Dell A (1996) *Haemonchus contortus* glycoproteins contain N-linked oligosaccharides with novel highly fucosylated core structures. J Biol Chem 271:30561–30570

Hemmer W, Focke M, Kolarich D, Wilson IB, Altmann F, Wöhrl S, Götz M, Jarisch R (2001) Antibody binding to venom carbohydrates is a frequent cause for double positivity to honeybee and yellow jacket venom in patients with stinging-insect allergy. J Allergy Clin Immunol 108:1045–1052

Hemmer W, Focke M, Kolarich D, Dalik I, Götz M, Jarisch R (2004) Identification by immunoblot of venom glycoproteins displaying immunoglobulin E-binding N-glycans as cross-reactive allergens in honeybee and yellow jacket venom. Clin Exp Allergy 34:460–469

Himly M, Jahn-Schmid B, Dedic A, Kelemen P, Wopfner N, Altmann F, van Ree R, Briza P, Richter K, Ebner C, Ferreira F (2003) Art v 1, the major allergen of mugwort pollen, is a modular glycoprotein with a defensin-like and a hydroxyproline-rich domain. FASEB J 17:106–108

Hoffman DR (2006) Hymenoptera venom allergens. Clin Rev Allergy Immunol 30:109–128

Iacovacci P, Afferni C, Butteroni C, Pironi L, Puggioni EM, Orlandi A, Barletta B, Tinghino R, Ariano R, Panzani RC, Di Felice G, Pini C (2002) Comparison between the native glycosylated and the recombinant Cup a1 allergen: role of carbohydrates in the histamine release from basophils. Clin Exp Allergy 32:1620–1627

Jacquenet S, Moneret-Vautrin DA, Bihain BE (2009) Mammalian meat-induced anaphylaxis: clinical relevance of anti-galactose-α-1,3-galactose IgE confirmed by means of skin tests to cetuximab. J Allergy Clin Immunol 124:603–605

Jappe U, Raulf-Heimsoth M, Hoffmann M, Burow G, Hübsch-Müller C, Enk A (2006) In vitro hymenoptera venom allergy diagnosis: improved by screening for cross-reactive carbohydrate determinants and reciprocal inhibition. Allergy 61:1220–1229

Jin C, Bencurova M, Borth N, Ferko B, Jensen-Jarolim E, Altmann F, Hantusch B (2006) Immunoglobulin G specifically binding plant N-glycans with high affinity could be generated in rabbits but not in mice. Glycobiology 16:349–357

Jin C, Hantusch B, Hemmer W, Stadlmann J, Altmann F (2008) Affinity of IgE and IgG against cross-reactive carbohydrate determinants on plant and insect glycoproteins. J Allergy Clin Immunol 121:185–190

Jin C, Nitsch S, Hemmer W, Altmann F (2009) Improving allergy diagnosis by removal of CCD-specific IgE from patients' sera. In: XVIII congress of the european academy of allergy and clinical immunology, Warsaw, 6–10 June 2009

Jin C, Focke M, Léonard R, Jarisch R, Altmann F, Hemmer W (2010) Reassessing the role of hyaluronidase in yellow jacket venom allergy. J Allergy Clin Immunol 125:184–190

Kespohl S, Schlünssen V, Jacobsen G, Schaumburg I, Maryska S, Meurer U, Brüning T, Sigsgaard T, Raulf-Heimsoth M (2010) Impact of cross-reactive carbohydrate determinants on wood dust sensitization. Clin Exp Allergy 40:1099–1106

Khoo KH, Nieto A, Morris HR, Dell A (1997) Structural characterization of the N-glycans from *Echinococcus granulosus* hydatid cyst membrane and protoscoleces. Mol Biochem Parasitol 86:237–248

Kochuyt AM, Van Hoeyveld EM, Stevens EA (2005) Prevalence and clinical relevance of specific immunoglobulin E to pollen caused by sting-induced specific immunoglobulin E to cross-reacting carbohydrate determinants in Hymenoptera venoms. Clin Exp Allergy 35: 441–447

Kolarich D, Altmann F (2000) N-Glycan analysis by matrix-assisted laser desorption/ionization mass spectrometry of electrophoretically separated nonmammalian proteins: application to peanut allergen Ara h 1 and olive pollen allergen Ole e 1. Anal Biochem 285:64–75

Kolarich D, Leonard R, Hemmer W, Altmann F (2005) The N-glycans of yellow jacket venom hyaluronidases and the protein sequence of its major isoform in *Vespula vulgaris*. FEBS J 272:5182–5190

Koshte VL, Kagen SL, Aalberse RC (1989) Cross-reactivity of IgE antibodies to caddis fly with arthropoda and mollusca. J Allergy Clin Immunol 84:174–183

Kubelka V, Altmann F, Staudacher E, Tretter V, März L, Hard K, Kamerling JP, Vliegenthart JF (1993) Primary structures of the N-linked carbohydrate chains from honeybee venom phospholipase A2. Eur J Biochem 213:1193–1204

Kubelka V, Altmann F, März L (1995) The asparagine-linked carbohydrate of honeybee venom hyaluronidase. Glycoconj J 12:77–83

Kurosaka A, Yano A, Itoh N, Kuroda Y, Nakagawa T, Kawasaki T (1991) The structure of a neural specific carbohydrate epitope of horseradish peroxidase recognized by antihorseradish peroxidase antiserum. J Biol Chem 266:4168–4172

Lauer I, Fötisch K, Kolarich D, Ballmer-Weber BK, Conti A, Altmann F, Vieths S, Scheurer S (2004) Hazelnut (*Corylus avellana*) vicilin Cor a 11: molecular characterization of a glycoprotein and its allergenic activity. Biochem J 383:327–334

Lauriere C, Lauriere M, Sturm A, Faye L, Chrispeels MJ (1988) Characterization of β-fructosidase, an extracellular glycoprotein of carrot cells. Biochimie 70:1483–1491

Léonard R, Petersen BO, Himly M, Kaar W, Wopfner N, Kolarich D, van Ree R, Ebner C, Duus JO, Ferreira F, Altmann F (2005) Two novel types of O-glycans on the mugwort pollen allergen Art v 1 and their role in antibody binding. J Biol Chem 280:7932–7940

Léonard R, Wopfner N, Pabst M, Stadlmann J, Petersen BO, Duus JO, Himly M, Radauer C, Gadermaier G, Razzazi-Fazeli E, Ferreira F, Altmann F (2010) A new allergen from ragweed (*Ambrosia artemisiifolia*) with homology to Art v 1 from mugwort. J Biol Chem 285:27192–27200

Linneberg A, Fenger RV, Husemoen LL, Vidal C, Vizcaino L, Gonzalez-Quintela A (2010) Immunoglobulin E sensitization to cross-reactive carbohydrate determinants: epidemiological study of clinical relevance and role of alcohol consumption. Int Arch Allergy Immunol 153:86–94

Lommerse JP, Kroon-Batenburg LM, Kamerling JP, Vliegenthart JF (1995) Conformational analysis of the xylose-containing N-glycan of pineapple stem bromelain as part of the intact glycoprotein. Biochemistry 34:8196–8206

Lommerse JP, Thomas-Oates JE, Gielens C, Preaux G, Kamerling JP, Vliegenthart JF (1997) Primary structure of 21 novel monoantennary and diantennary N-linked carbohydrate chains from αD-hemocyanin of *Helix pomatia*. Eur J Biochem 249:195–222

Lorenzo S, Romarís F, Iglesias R, Audícana MT, Alonso JM, Leiro J, Ubeira FM (2000) O-glycans as a source of cross-reactivity in determinations of human serum antibodies to *Anisakis simplex* antigens. Clin Exp Allergy 30:551–559

Luttkopf D, Ballmer-Weber BK, Wüthrich B, Vieths S (2000) Celery allergens in patients with positive double-blind placebo-controlled food challenge. J Allergy Clin Immunol 106: 390–399

Macher BA, Galili U (2008) The Galα1,3Galβ1,4GlcNAc-R (α-Gal) epitope: a carbohydrate of unique evolution and clinical relevance. Biochim Biophys Acta 1780:75–88

Mahler V, Gutgesell C, Valenta R, Fuchs T (2006) Natural rubber latex and hymenoptera venoms share immunoglobin E-epitopes accounting for cross-reactive carbohydrate determinants. Clin Exp Allergy 36:1446–1456

Malandain H (2004) Widening sensitization spectrum through carbohydrate panepitopes – a hypothesis. Allerg Immunol (Paris) 36:297–299

Malandain H (2005) IgE-reactive carbohydrate epitopes – classification, cross-reactivity, and clinical impact. Allerg Immunol (Paris) 37:122–128

Malandain H, Giroux F, Cano Y (2007) The influence of carbohydrate structures present in common allergen sources on specific IgE results. Eur Ann Allergy Clin Immunol 39:216–220

Mari A, Iacovacci P, Afferni C, Barletta B, Tinghino R, Di Felice G, Pini C (1999) Specific IgE to cross-reactive carbohydrate determinants strongly affect the *in vitro* diagnosis of allergic diseases. J Allergy Clin Immunol 103:1005–1011

Mari A (2002) IgE to cross-reactive carbohydrate determinants: analysis of the distribution and appraisal of the in vivo and *in vitro* reactivity. Int Arch Allergy Immunol 129:286–295

Mari A, Ooievaar-de Heer P, Scala E, Giani M, Pirrotta L, Zuidmeer L, Bethell D, van Ree R (2008) Evaluation by double-blind placebo-controlled oral challenge of the clinical relevance of IgE antibodies against plant glycans. Allergy 63:891–896

Mauriello PM, Barde SH, Georgitis JW, Reisman RE (1984) Natural history of large local reactions from stinging insects. J Allergy Clin Immunol 74:494–498

Mertens M, Amler S, Mörschbacher BM, Brehler R (2010) Cross-reactive carbohydrate determinants strongly affect the results of the basophil activation test in hymenoptera-venom allergy. Clin Exp Allergy 40:1333–1345

Mittermann I, Zidarn M, Silar M, Markovic-Housley Z, Aberer W, Korosec P, Kosnik M, Valenta R (2010) Recombinant allergen-based IgE testing to distinguish bee and wasp allergy. J Allergy Clin Immunol 125:1300–1307

Müller UR, Johansen N, Petersen AB, Fromberg-Nielsen J, Häberli G (2009) Hymenoptera venom allergy: analysis of double positivity to honey bee and Vespula venom by estimation of IgE antibodies to species-specific major allergens Api m1 and Ves v5. Allergy 64:543–548

Ohsuga H, Su SN, Takahashi N, Yang SY, Nakagawa H, Shimada I, Arata Y, Lee YC (1996) The carbohydrate moiety of the Bermuda grass antigen BG60. New oligosaccharides of plant origin. J Biol Chem 271:26653–26658

Okano M, Nishizaki K, Satoskar AR, Yoshino T, Masuda Y, Harn DA (1999) Involvement of carbohydrate on phospholipase A2, a bee-venom allergen, in *in vivo* antigen-specific IgE synthesis in mice. Allergy 54:811–818

Palacin A, Quirce S, Sanchez-Monge R, Bobolea I, Diaz-Perales A, Martin-Muñoz F, Pascual C, Salcedo G (2011) Sensitization profiles to purified plant food allergens among pediatric patients with allergy to banana. Pediatr Allergy Immunol 22:186–195

Petersen A, Vieths S, Aulepp H, Schlaak M, Becker WM (1996) Ubiquitous structures responsible for IgE cross-reactivity between tomato fruit and grass pollen allergens. J Allergy Clin Immunol 98:805–815

Platts-Mills T, Vaughan J, Squillace S, Woodfolk J, Sporik R (2001) Sensitisation, asthma, and a modified Th2 response in children exposed to cat allergen: a population-based cross-sectional study. Lancet 357:752–756

Pöltl G, Ahrazem O, Paschinger K, Ibañez MD, Salcedo G, Wilson IB (2007) Molecular and immunological characterization of the glycosylated orange allergen Cit s 1. Glycobiology 17:220–230

Raulf-Heimsoth M, Rihs HP, Rozynek P, Cremer R, Gaspar A, Pires G, Yeang HY, Arif SA, Hamilton RG, Sander I, Lundberg M, Brüning T (2007) Quantitative analysis of immunoglobulin E reactivity profiles in patients allergic or sensitized to natural rubber latex (*Hevea brasiliensis*). Clin Exp Allergy 37:1657–1667

Reindl J, Anliker MD, Karamloo F, Vieths S, Wüthrich B (2000) Allergy caused by ingestion of zucchini (*Cucurbita pepo*): characterization of allergens and cross-reactivity to pollen and other foods. J Allergy Clin Immunol 106:379–385

Schäfer T, Przybilla B (1996) IgE antibodies to hymenoptera venoms in the serum are common in the general population and are related to indication of atopy. Allergy 51:372–377

Schmid-Grendelmeier P, Holzmann D, Himly M, Weichel M, Tresch S, Ruckert B, Menz G, Ferreira F, Blaser K, Wüthrich B, Crameri R (2003) Native Art v 1 and recombinant Art v 1 are able to induce humoral and T cell-mediated *in vitro* and in vivo responses in mugwort allergy. J Allergy Clin Immunol 111:1328–1336

Seismann H, Blank S, Braren I, Greunke K, Cifuentes L, Grunwald T, Bredehorst R, Ollert M, Spillner E (2010) Dissecting cross-reactivity in hymenoptera venom allergy by circumvention of α-1,3-core fucosylation. Mol Immunol 47:799–808

Soldatova LN, Crameri R, Gmachl M, Kemeny DM, Schmidt M, Weber M, Müller UR (1998) Superior biologic activity of the recombinant bee venom allergen hyaluronidase expressed in baculovirus-infected insect cells as compared with *Escherichia coli*. J Allergy Clin Immunol 101:691–698

Staudacher E, Altmann F, März L, Hard K, Kamerling JP, Vliegenhart JF (1992) α1-6(α1-3)-Difucosylation of the asparagine-bound N-acetylglucosamine in honeybee venom phospholipase A2. Glycoconj J 9:82–85

Strait RT, Morris SC, Finkelman FD (2006) IgG-blocking antibodies inhibit IgE-mediated anaphylaxis in vivo through both antigen interception and FcγRIIb cross-linking. J Clin Invest 116:833–841

Tretter V, Altmann F, Kubelka V, März L, Becker WM (1993) Fucose α1,3-linked to the core region of glycoprotein N-glycans creates an important epitope for IgE from honeybee venom allergic individuals. Int Arch Allergy Immunol 102:259–266

Valenta R, Twaroch T, Swoboda I (2007) Component-resolved diagnosis to optimize allergen-specific immunotherapy in the Mediterranean area. J Investig Allergol Clin Immunol 17(Suppl 1):36–40

van der Veen MJ, van Ree R, Aalberse RC, Akkerdaas J, Koppelman SJ, Jansen HM, van der Zee JS (1997) Poor biologic activity of cross-reactive IgE directed to carbohydrate determinants of glycoproteins. J Allergy Clin Immunol 100:327–334 van Die I, Gomord V, Kooyman FN, van den Berg TK, Cummings RD, Vervelde L (1999) Core α1→3-fucose is a common modification of N-glycans in parasitic helminths and constitutes an important epitope for IgE from *Haemonchus contortus* infected sheep. FEBS Lett 463:189–193

van Die I, Cummings RD (2010) Glycan gimmickry by parasitic helminths: a strategy for modulating the host immune response? Glycobiology 20:2–12

van Nunen SA, O'Connor KS, Clarke LR, Boyle RX, Fernando SL (2009) An association between tick bite reactions and red meat allergy in humans. Med J Aust 190:510–511

van Ree R, Aalberse RC (1999) Specific IgE without clinical allergy (editorial). J Allergy Clin Immunol 103:1000–1001

van Ree R, Cabanes-Macheteau M, Akkerdaas J, Milazzo JP, Loutelier-Bourhis C, Rayon C, Villalba M, Koppelman S, Aalberse R, Rodriguez R, Faye L, Lerouge P (2000) β(1,2)-Xylose and α(1,3)-fucose residues have a strong contribution in IgE binding to plant glycoallergens. J Biol Chem 275:11451–11458

van Ree R (2002) Carbohydrate epitopes and their relevance for the diagnosis and treatment of allergic diseases. Int Arch Allergy Immunol 129:189–197

van Tetering A, Schiphorst WE, van den Eijnden DH, van Die I (1999) Characterization of a core α1→3-fucosyltransferase from the snail *Lymnaea stagnalis* that is involved in the synthesis of complex-type N-glycans. FEBS Lett 461:311–314

Vidal C, Vizcaino L, Díaz-Peromingo JA, Garrido M, Gomez-Rial J, Linneberg A, Gonzalez-Quintela A (2009) Immunoglobulin-E reactivity to a glycosylated food allergen (peanuts) due to interference with cross-reactive carbohydrate determinants in heavy drinkers. Alcohol Clin Exp Res 33:1322–1328

Westritschnig K, Horak F, Swoboda I, Balic N, Spitzauer S, Kundi M, Fiebig H, Suck R, Cromwell O, Valenta R (2008) Different allergenic activity of grass pollen allergens revealed by skin testing. Eur J Clin Invest 38:260–267

Wicklein D, Lindner B, Moll H, Kolarich D, Altmann F, Becker WM, Petersen A (2004) Carbohydrate moieties can induce mediator release: a detailed characterization of two major timothy grass pollen allergens. Biol Chem 385:397–407

Wilson IB, Altmann F (1998) Structural analysis of N-glycans from allergenic grass, ragweed and tree pollens: core α1,3-linked fucose and xylose present in all pollens examined. Glycoconj J 15:1055–1070

Wilson IB, Harthill JE, Mullin NP, Ashford DA, Altmann F (1998) Core α1,3-fucose is a key part of the epitope recognized by antibodies reacting against plant N-linked oligosaccharides and is present in a wide variety of plant extracts. Glycobiology 8:651–661

Wilson IB, Zeleny R, Kolarich D, Staudacher E, Stroop CJ, Kamerling JP, Altmann F (2001) Analysis of Asn-linked glycans from vegetable foodstuffs: widespread occurrence of Lewis a, core α1,3-linked fucose and xylose substitutions. Glycobiology 11:261–274

Wuhrer M, Grimm C, Dennis RD, Idris MA, Geyer R (2004) The parasitic trematode *Fasciola hepatica* exhibits mammalian-type glycolipids as well as Gal(α1-6)Gal-terminating glycolipids that account for cestode serological cross-reactivity. Glycobiology 14:115–126

Xie N, Taylor CM (2010) Synthesis of a dimer of β-(1,4)-L-arabinosyl-(2 S,4R)-4-hydroxyproline inspired by Art v 1, the major allergen of mugwort. Org Lett 12:4968–4971

Yagami T, Osuna H, Kouno M, Haishima Y, Nakamura A, Ikezawa Z (2002) Significance of carbohydrate epitopes in a latex allergen with β-1,3-glucanase activity. Int Arch Allergy Immunol 129:27–37

Structural Glycobiology of Antibody Recognition in Xenotransplantation and Cancer Immunotherapy

9

Mark Agostino, William Farrugia, Mauro S. Sandrin, Andrew M. Scott, Elizabeth Yuriev, and Paul A. Ramsland

9.1 Introduction

Carbohydrate antigens recognized by "natural" or preformed and elicited antibodies are central to transplantation/transfusion rejection across ABO blood group and species (xenotransplantation) barriers and are also promising candidates for cancer immunotherapy (Ramsland 2005). The key carbohydrate determinants (epitopes) recognized by antibodies are synthesized by a series of intracellular glycosyltransferases and are expressed on the surface of cells as glycolipids and glycoproteins. Often the minimal carbohydrate epitopes are located at the terminal end of more complex oligosaccharide chains, which result in these epitopes being displayed at a wide range of surface densities and contexts (e.g., glycolipids or glycoproteins). For example, many tumor-associated carbohydrate antigens are broadly expressed at very high densities on the cell surface of primary and

M. Agostino • E. Yuriev
Medicinal Chemistry and Drug Action, Monash Institute of Pharmaceutical Sciences, Monash University, Parkville, VIC 3052, Australia

W. Farrugia
Centre for Immunology, Burnet Institute Melbourne, VIC 3004, Australia

M.S. Sandrin
Department of Surgery Austin Health, University of Melbourne, Heidelberg, VIC 3084, Australia

A.M. Scott
Tumour Targeting Program, Ludwig Institute for Cancer Research Melbourne, VIC 3084, Australia

P.A. Ramsland (✉)
Centre for Immunology, Burnet Institute Melbourne, VIC 3004, Australia

Department of Surgery Austin Health, University of Melbourne, Heidelberg, VIC 3084, Australia

Department of Immunology, Monash University, Alfred Medical Research and Education Precinct, Melbourne, VIC 3004, Australia
e-mail: pramsland@burnet.edu.au

P. Kosma and S. Müller-Loennies (eds.), *Anticarbohydrate Antibodies*,
DOI 10.1007/978-3-7091-0870-3_9, © Springer-Verlag/Wien 2012

metastatic tumors, but the same carbohydrates occur at much lower levels and are typically restricted to a few cell types in healthy tissues (Scott and Renner 2001; Ezzelarab et al. 2005; Kobata and Amano 2005; Cazet et al. 2010). Thus, antibodies with similar specificities for individual carbohydrate epitopes can display different and often selective cell-binding profiles, based on the unique presentation of the carbohydrates on the target cells.

In this chapter, we discuss the structural glycobiology of the key antibody–carbohydrate interactions important in xenotransplantation and cancer immunotherapy. Progress in both fields is reliant on further mechanistic knowledge of the underlying complex biosynthetic pathways and the structural basis for antibody recognition of isolated and cellular forms of the target carbohydrates. Recent progress in bioinformatics, synthesis of complex carbohydrates and analysis of their interactions with proteins [reviewed in (Seeberger 2008; Taylor and Drickamer 2009; Frank and Schloissnig 2010)] is facilitating the experimental determination and interpretation of three-dimensional (3D) structures of antibody–carbohydrate complexes. Furthermore, advances in computational (*in silico*) methods [reviewed in (DeMarco and Woods 2008; Woods and Tessier 2010; Yuriev et al. 2011)] are revealing much needed complementary 3D information about antibody recognition of carbohydrates.

9.2 Antibody Recognition of Carbohydrate Xenoantigens

Two approaches have been used to overcome the critical worldwide shortage of human donor organs and tissues for transplantation. The first approach is to use ABO incompatible organs (Holgersson et al. 2005). This was not until recently possible, as grafting across an ABO incompatibility would result in immediate graft loss due to hyperacute rejection. This precipitous rejection is mediated by naturally occurring anti-ABO antibodies of the recipient binding to the incompatible ABO blood group carbohydrates on the surface of endothelium of the donor organ, resulting in complement-dependent organ destruction. Depletion or blocking of the anti-ABO antibodies or removal of antibody producing cells before the incompatible organ graft has, in many cases, led to stable transplants even after the reappearance of the anti-ABO antibodies, in a process termed graft accommodation (Crew and Ratner 2010; Dipchand et al. 2010). The second approach is to use organs from other species, or xenotransplantation. Similar to naturally occurring anti-ABO antibodies in humans lacking these antigens, all humans have high levels of natural antibodies recognizing carbohydrates containing terminal αGal(1→3)Gal epitopes (designated as αGal), present in most mammals except Old World monkeys, apes and humans (Galili et al. 1987; Good et al. 1992; Sandrin et al. 1993). While the barrier posed by αGal in xenotransplantation may have been successfully overcome by the genetic manipulation of donor animals (see Sect. 9.2.3), it is still of fundamental interest to understand how antibodies recognize αGal and related carbohydrates. Furthermore, it is critical to identify and characterize antibody recognition of non-αGal carbohydrate antigens that are likely to pose future obstacles to successful clinical xenotransplantation of pig organs in humans.

9.2.1 Structural Studies of Antibodies Against αGal Carbohydrate Xenoantigens

The nature of antibody–carbohydrate interactions and the method by which carbohydrate ligands fit into antibody binding sites are important in understanding the antibody–carbohydrate recognition process. However, detailed structural knowledge of this recognition is currently limited. Specifically, there are currently no experimentally determined (X-ray crystallography and NMR) antibody-αGal complexes, in contrast to several crystal structures of lectin-αGal complexes [reviewed in (Ramsland et al. 2003; Yuriev et al. 2009)]. *In silico* techniques offer attractive alternatives to experimental methods for the study of antibody–carbohydrate structures. In particular, homology modeling and molecular docking provide information about protein-ligand interactions in systems that are difficult to study with experimental techniques. Our group has previously generated homology models of mouse anti-αGal antibodies and used docking approaches to investigate their recognition of carbohydrates bearing αGal epitopes and cross-reactive peptides (Milland et al. 2007; Yuriev et al. 2008). Homology models of human αGal antibodies have also been generated and used in conjunction with site-directed mutagenesis data and docking to investigate xenoantigen recognition (Kearns-Jonker et al. 2007). An important general observation from these studies is that key amino acids within the binding sites of αGal-binding antibodies can be readily identified by homology modeling and docking.

Our *in silico* approach for exploring antibody–carbohydrate recognition and findings when applied to a panel of mouse αGal-binding monoclonal antibodies are outlined below. Despite recent developments in the docking field (Yuriev et al. 2011), it is important to test or validate a docking protocol against suitable test systems. Initially we assessed several popular docking programs for their ability to accurately dock carbohydrates to antibodies (Agostino et al. 2009a). Comparison of top ranking poses with high resolution crystal structures highlighted the strengths and weaknesses of these programs. Rigid docking, in which the protein conformation remains static, and flexible docking, where both the protein and ligand are treated as flexible, were compared. This study revealed that, in general, molecular docking of carbohydrates to antibodies was performed best by the Glide program (Friesner et al. 2004). Furthermore, the antibody binding site shape and carbohydrate flexibility were both observed to influence the capacity of docking programs to reproduce the experimentally determined carbohydrate binding poses.

The validated Glide-based docking protocol has been used to study carbohydrate recognition by a series of αGal-binding monoclonal antibodies (Agostino et al. 2009b). Considering that these antibodies display a range of binding site shapes, we developed a "site mapping" technique, which was validated against a series of high resolution antibody–carbohydrate crystal structures. Site mapping involves the use of molecular docking to generate a series of antibody–carbohydrate complexes, followed by analysis of the hydrogen bonding and van der Waals interactions occurring in each complex, which are tallied and then mapped (based on their relative contribution) onto the antibody binding site surface. Thus, the contributions to binding of a variety of potential carbohydrate binding modes are taken into consideration to compensate for differences in antibody binding site shapes and flexibility of the carbohydrates. When applied to αGal carbohydrate-antibody interactions, site mapping indicated that there was a significant overlap of the antibody regions engaging the xenoantigens across the panel of six monoclonal antibodies examined. The consensus recognition site for αGal carbohydrates was comprised of nine amino acid positions in five out of the six antibody complementarity determining regions (CDR) of the light (L) and heavy (H) chain variable (V) domains. When an additional six amino acids were included (forming the extended consensus site), more than 80% of all potential αGal carbohydrate interactions were accounted for across the panel of monoclonal antibodies.

Recently, we expanded the *in silico* approach to identify positions within the carbohydrate ligands, which are most important for recognition (carbohydrate maps), and to take into account the conformational preferences in docked carbohydrate poses (Agostino et al. 2010). This protocol exploits the tendency of certain carbohydrate linkages to cluster at specific conformational minima, which can be used to "filter" carbohydrate poses generated by molecular docking. Interaction-based filters using the antibody site maps and the carbohydrate maps are then applied to select the carbohydrate poses exhibiting the most preferred binding characteristics. When applied to a series of αGal carbohydrates and the panel of mouse monoclonal antibodies, a notable feature was the apparent restricted conformation of βGal(1→4)Glc/GlcNAc linkages. The most populated conformational cluster of βGal(1→4)Glc/GlcNAc linkages corresponded well to experimental structures and this property was used as a filter to select preferred binding modes of αGal-terminating trisaccharide (or longer) carbohydrates. In contrast, the conformation of the terminal αGal(1→3)Gal linkage varies depending on the antibody binding site topography, although it is possible that some of the antibodies recognize more than one αGal(1→3)Gal conformation. Carbohydrate interaction maps revealed that, across the panel of antibodies, the predominant interactions occurred with the terminal αGal(1→3)Gal disaccharide, but potential interactions occur with the third saccharide unit, which was either GlcNAc or Glc in the different xenoantigens. The obtained binding modes indicate that each antibody uses distinct mechanisms in recognizing the target antigens.

The preferred binding modes that were identified for the αGal(1→3)βGal(1→4) GlcNAc trisaccharide illustrated the similarities and differences in the recognition displayed by different antibodies that bind this xenoantigen (Fig. 9.1). All carbohydrate ligands were located in the binding sites formed by the unique conformations of the CDRs. The carbohydrate ligands were generally extended in conformation and either bound relatively flatly in grooves (Fig. 9.1a, d) or were in a more upright position with a single monosaccharide unit entering the binding site first and anchoring in a cavity by a process of end-on insertion (Fig. 9.1b, c, e, f).

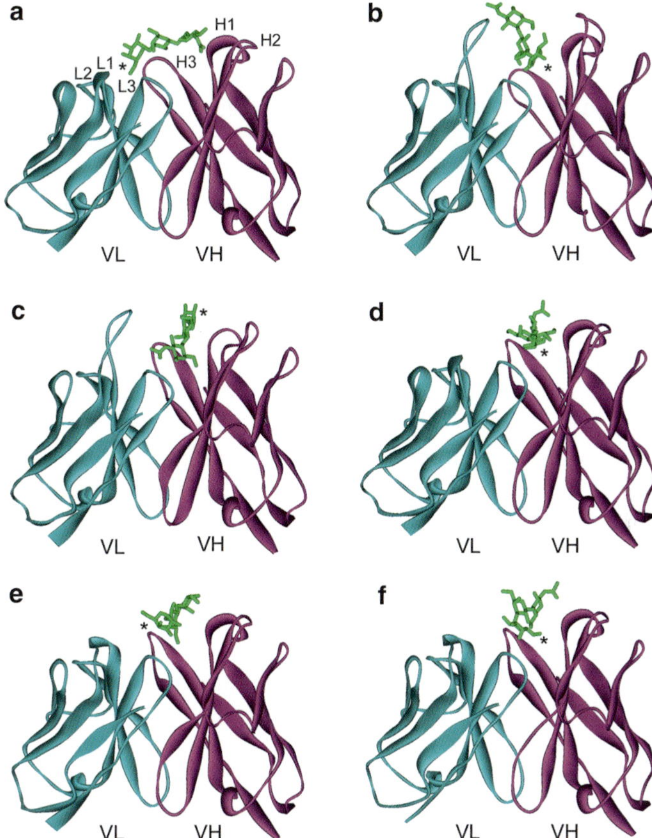

Fig. 9.1 *In silico* predictions of αGal carbohydrate recognition by antibodies. Preferred binding modes for αGal(1→3)βGal(1→4)GlcNAc trisaccharides are shown for a panel of monoclonal antibodies: (**a**) 6.13; (**b**) 22.121; (**c**) 24.7; (**d**) 12.15; (**e**) 15.101; (**f**) 8.17. The antibody variable domains (VL *cyan*, VH *magenta*) are shown as ribbons-style representations and carbohydrates as stick representations (*green*). The locations of CDR of the L (L1-3) and H (H1-3) chains are indicated only in panel (**a**). The position of the terminal αGal residue in each binding site is shown (*asterisk*). The preferred αGal carbohydrate binding modes were determined as previously described (Agostino et al. 2010)

In general, the terminal αGal residue entered the binding site first and was surrounded by residues of the antibody binding site. One exception was the 24.7 antibody (Fig. 9.1c) where the trisaccharide was reversed in orientation and the terminal αGal was pinned in place at the top of the binding site mainly by interactions with a residue (Asn 109 H) in VH CDR3, which was not found in the other antibody sequences. Collectively, αGal carbohydrate recognition by antibodies (Agostino et al. 2009b, 2010) is similar to lectins, where both end-on insertion and groove-type binding are involved in recognition αGal carbohydrate xenoantigens (Ramsland et al. 2003; Yuriev et al. 2009).

9.2.2 Potential Non-αGal Carbohydrate Xenoantigens

The high levels of αGal antibodies in human sera have until recently complicated the identification of non-αGal carbohydrate antigens. The availability of animals with minimal or no αGal has led to renewed efforts in characterizing non-αGal xenoantigens (Rood et al. 2005, 2007; Tseng et al. 2006; Harnden et al. 2010; Lin et al. 2010). We will outline two categories of potential carbohydrate xenoantigens, which are possible barriers to xenotransplantation.

Removal of αGal in genetically modified animals has revealed new antigenic determinants by exposing terminal βGal residues, which are normally masked. It has been proposed that the exposed LacNAc [βGal(1→4)GlcNAc] could be a target for natural or elicited antibodies (Lucq et al. 2000; Milland et al. 2005). Indeed most humans produce natural antibodies against LacNAc (I blood group) and these antibodies are better known as cold agglutinins (Cairns et al. 1996). However, it remains to be shown in a pig-to-primate model (or in humans) if naturally occurring or elicited antibodies against LacNAc are involved in graft rejection. Exposure of terminal βGal residues may also promote recognition by the various carbohydrate-binding receptors of innate immunity resulting in antibody independent xenograft rejection (Christiansen et al. 2006; Yuriev et al. 2009).

Perhaps the most likely non-αGal carbohydrate to act as xenoantigen in pig-to-human xenotransplant rejection is a sialic acid, *N*-glycolylneuraminic acid (Neu5Gc). This is one of the two abundant sialic acids in mammals, *N*-acetylneuraminic acid (Neu5Ac) being the other and only naturally occurring sialic acid in humans. Humans lack the functional enzyme that synthesizes endogenous Neu5Gc by hydroxylation of the Neu5Ac substrate (Chou et al. 1998). Even chimpanzees (our closest primate relative) express the enzyme for production of Neu5Gc, which results in an abundant surface expression of carbohydrates terminating in Neu5Gc in all mammals other than humans, and most human sera contain natural antibodies to Neu5Gc (Zhu and Hurst 2002; Tangvoranuntakul et al. 2003; Miwa et al. 2004). Furthermore, repeated intravenous exposure of humans to animal blood or blood products can cause "serum sickness" mediated by agglutinating antibodies specific for Neu5Gc or the Hanganutziu-Deicher (HD) antigen (Higashi et al. 1977). The potential for anti-Neu5Gc human natural antibodies to contribute to complement-dependent cytotoxicity (CDC) has recently been demonstrated by comparing CDC of human sera against thymocytes from wild-type, αGal knockout and Neu5Gc knockout mice. While most of the CDC against wild-type could be decreased with the removal of αGal, it was reduced further by the removal of Neu5Gc in double-knockout animals. Interestingly, unlike αGal specificity, where a large proportion of natural human antibodies are IgM, the anti-Neu5Gc antibodies are predominantly IgG, suggesting that antibody-dependent killing mechanisms other than CDC (e.g., Fc receptor mediated) may be important for xenograft rejection. However, this remains to be examined (Basnet et al. 2010). In another study of the pig enzyme for production of Neu5Gc, it appeared that most of the natural human antibodies against Neu5Gc were IgM, which were confirmed to cause CDC of cells transfected with the pig enzyme (Song et al. 2010). While the discrepancy in data on natural human antibody classes specific for Neu5Gc may need further examination, it is clear that preformed or elicited antibodies with Neu5Gc or HD specificity have the potential to cause delayed (or acute) antibody-mediated rejection of xenografts in human recipients. The presence of Neu5Gc in nonhuman primate tissues will complicate the preclinical analysis, but knocking out the enzyme that converts Neu5Ac into Neu5Gc in αGal knockout pigs would be a prudent consideration.

As mentioned above, the complications from the increased exposure of βGal and the presence of Neu5Gc are the two most likely sources of future carbohydrate xenoantigens after removal of αGal. However, there are other possibilities that await discovery, such as the recent suggestion by Byrne et al. (2011) that an Sd^a-like carbohydrate may represent a new carbohydrate antigen in xenotransplantation. Using presensitized baboon sera (cardiac heterotopic xenograft recipients), they identified β(1→4)GalNAc transferase 2 (B4GALNT2) after screening for IgG binding to cell surface expression libraries generated from CD46 transgenic and α(1→3)Gal transferase knockout pig aortic endothelial cells. The B4GALNT2 enzyme transfers GalNAc in β(1→4)-linkage to α(2→3)-sialylated Gal residues to generate the Sd^a or CAD antigen (Byrne et al. 2011). Although greater than 90% of humans express the Sd^a antigen, individuals that lack this antigen show a strong antibody response to the Sd^a (CAD) determinant (Donald et al. 1983). Along with other carbohydrates, the identification of this putative Sd^a-like xenoantigen suggests that before clinical xenotransplantation is common practice, the following question still needs to be answered: "*Just how human do we need to make the pig*?" (Ramsland 2005).

9.2.3 Progress Towards Clinical Xenotransplantation

The availability of genetically modified pigs with the gene for α(1→3)-galactosyltransferase knocked out (αGT-KO) has provided a source of αGal-deficient organs for xenotransplants, initially in nonhuman primates. Removal of the αGal epitopes, the target of most anti-pig natural antibodies, has largely eliminated hyperacute rejection and allowed organ grafts to function for several months. However, even in heavily immunosuppressed nonhuman primates, the xenografts are eventually rejected by antibody and cellular responses. Similar decreases in hyperacute and delayed xenograft rejection have occurred with pigs genetically engineered to express human complement regulatory genes (e.g., CD46, CD55 or CD59), which act on the effector complement mechanism for natural αGal antibodies [reviewed in (Ekser and Cooper 2010; Cooper and Ayares 2011)]. As discussed above for non-α Gal carbohydrate xenoantigens, the presence of foreign pig proteins and carbohydrates, in addition to αGal, are possible initiators of delayed xenograft rejection by adaptive and innate immune processes. Thus, the development of pigs with multiple modifications is required before clinical xenotransplantation will be a viable alternative to allotransplantation. Briefly, two of the genetic modifications that are being tested are: (1) the expression of human leukocyte antigens (HLA-E and HLA-G) on pig endothelial cells to inhibit the innate natural killer (NK) cellular response (Forte et al. 2001; Weiss et al. 2009), and (2) introduction of human coagulation regulators with the goal of overcoming an incompatibility between human and pig coagulation pathways (Cowan et al. 2009). With recent developments in approaches to rapidly introduce multiple genetic modifications onto the αGT-KO or complement-regulator pig backgrounds (Nottle et al. 2010), it is only a matter of time before donor pigs suitably compatible with human transplant recipients are developed. However, understanding the recognition of carbohydrates by antibodies and innate receptors will almost certainly impact on the future success of clinical xenotransplantation.

9.3 Antibody Targeting of Tumor-Associated Carbohydrate Antigens

Characterization of the composition and structure of blood group antigens was initially determined not from erythrocytes, but from benign cyst and stomach secretions. Monoclonal antibody technology was subsequently used to show that many blood group and related carbohydrate determinants are aberrantly or over-expressed in cancer, and that specific monoclonal antibodies could be generated that selectively recognize these tumor-associated carbohydrate antigens [see commentary and references therein by (Ramsland 2005)]. Among the numerous changes in glycosylation associated with cancer are the altered expression of A, B, H (O blood group) and Lewis carbohydrates (Le^a, Le^b, Le^x and Le^y and their sialylated forms) on the surfaces of many tumor cells (Sakamoto et al. 1986; Hakomori 1999; Kobata and Amano 2005). The altered expression of multiple glycosyltransferases in cancer has also led to markedly different expression of gangliosides (ceramide-based glycolipids containing one or more sialic acids) in many tumors compared to healthy tissues, making certain gangliosides (e.g., GD2 and GD3) promising candidates for cancer immunotherapy (Hakomori 2001). Another glycolipid over-expressed in many cancers is Globo H, which is widely expressed on many cancers of epithelial origin and has been identified on a population of breast cancer stem cells (Slovin et al. 2005; Chang et al. 2008). In addition to blood group related carbohydrates and glycolipids, neoepitopes are formed in many cancers by the underglycosylation of glycoproteins. Common examples are truncated *O*-linked carbohydrates including the Thomsen-Friedenreich (TF or T), the Thomsen-nouvelle (Tn) and their sialylated antigenic forms (sTF and sTn). These truncated *O*-linked carbohydrates occur at high densities in tumor-associated mucins such as MUC1 and MUC4, are found at lower densities on many other tumor proteins, and are expressed in a wide range of cancers (Slovin et al. 2005; Cazet et al. 2010; Reis et al. 2010). A summary of the key carbohydrate determinants associated with tumors that are recognized by antibodies is presented in Table 9.1.

Crystallographic 3D structures have been determined for several antibodies specific for tumor-associated carbohydrate antigens (Table 9.2). As previously

Table 9.1 Examples of carbohydrate tumor-associated antigens recognized by antibodies

Antigen name	Carbohydrate determinant[a]	Tumor types[b]
Lewis carbohydrates[c]		
Le^a	βGal(1→3)[αFuc(1→4)]GlcNAc–R	Colon, gastric, small cell lung cancer
Le^x	βGal(1→4)[αFuc(1→3)]GlcNAc–R	Epithelial cancers
Le^b	αFuc(1→2)βGal(1→3)[αFuc(1→4)]GlcNAc–R	Gastric cancer
Le^y	αFuc(1→2)βGal(1→4)[αFuc(1→3)]GlcNAc–R	Epithelial cancers and small cell lung cancer
Gangliosides/glycolipids		
GD3	αNeu5Ac(2→8)αNeu5Ac(2→3)βGal(1→4) Glc–Cer	Melanoma, neuroblastoma, glioblastoma
GD2	αNeu5Ac(2→8)αNeu5Ac(2→3)[βGalNAc (1→4)]βGal(1→4)Glc–Cer	Neuroblastoma, melanoma, sarcoma
GM3	αNeu5Ac(2→3)βGal(1→4)Glc–Cer	Meningioma, melanoma, neuroblastoma
GM2	αNeu5Ac(2→3)[βGalNAc(1→4)]βGal(1→4) Glc–Cer	Melanoma, neuroblastoma, glioblastoma
Globo H	αFuc(1→2)βGal(1→3)βGalNAc(1→3)αGal (1→4)βGal(1→4)Glc–Cer	Breast, colon, small cell lung cancer
Truncated O-glycans[c]		
T or TF	βGal(1→3)GalNAc–Ser/Thr	Breast, colon cancer
Tn	GalNAc–Ser/Thr	Colon, ovarian cancer

[a]R, a variety of short or long carbohydrate chains attached to glycolipids or glycoproteins; Cer, ceramide

[b]Some common examples of cancers known to express the tumor-associated carbohydrate antigens [reviewed in (Scott and Renner 2001; Slovin et al. 2005; Cazet et al. 2010)]

[c]In addition to the core determinants, sialylated forms of most of these antigens are frequently over-expressed in cancer

discussed, antibody recognition of carbohydrate epitopes resembles the binding of small molecules by antibodies generated against haptens (Ramsland et al. 2003). A predominant binding mode involves the end-on insertion of an anchoring group, which in the case of carbohydrates is often a monosaccharide unit within the carbohydrate determinant. In most cases, the anchoring group enters a pocket, varying in size and accessibility between antibodies, located between the CDR3 loops of both the light and heavy chains. In contrast to small molecules where the binding site normally lacks ordered solvent molecules, carbohydrates tend to bind in a more accessible site that can include a considerable number of solvent molecules. However, the anchoring saccharide units are often bound in a solvent-protected subsite. Depending on the size and branching patterns of the carbohydrate epitope, an antibody combining site recognizing a carbohydrate can vary from a pocket or cavity, to an extended groove, as well as a combination of the two (i.e., a groove leading into a deeper cavity).

Table 9.2 Crystal structures of antibodies against carbohydrate tumor-associated antigens

PDB	Resolution (Å)	Antibody	Specificity (C/U)[a]	Reference
1CLY	2.50	chBR96 Fab	Le^y (C)	Jeffrey et al. (1995)
1CLZ	2.80	muBR96 Fab	Le^y (C)	Jeffrey et al. (1995)
1UCB	2.50	chBR96 Fab	Le^y (U)	Sheriff et al. (1996)
1S3K	1.90	hu3S193 Fab	Le^y (C)	Ramsland et al. (2004)
3EYV	2.50	hu3S193 Fab	Le^y (C and U)	Farrugia et al. (2009)
1UZ6	2.05	291-2-G3-A Fab	Le^x (U)	van Roon et al. (2004)
1UZ8	1.80	291-2-G3-A Fab	Le^x (C)	van Roon et al. (2004)
1BZ7	2.50	R24 Fab	GD3 (U)	Kaminski et al. (1999b)
1R24	3.10	R24 Fab	GD3 (U)	Kaminski et al. (1999b)
1PSK	2.80	ME361 Fab	GD2 (U)	Pichla et al. (1997)
1RIH	2.50	14-F7 Fab	N-glycolyl GM3 (U)	Krengel et al. (2004)
3-IU4	1.75	chP3 Fab	N-glycolyl GM3 (U)	Talavera et al. (2009)
3IET	2.20	237mAb Fab	Tn, G[TNY[b]]KPPL (C)	Brooks et al. (2010)
3IF1	2.20	237mAb Fab	Tn, GalNAc (C)	Brooks et al. (2010)

[a]C = complexed with antigen and U = unliganded
[b]TNY = GalNAc modified threonine residue of the glycopeptide

A range of carbohydrate binding modes can be seen in the crystal structures of antibody complexes with tumor-associated carbohydrate antigens (Fig. 9.2). End-on insertion of a key monosaccharide is observed in most of the structures, with the possible exception of the Le^x binding antibody 291-2-G3-A, where two stacked saccharide units (Fuc and Gal) of the trisaccharide anchor into the binding pocket. For the two Le^y antibody complexes (chBR96 and hu3S193), a dominant feature of recognition is the tight binding of the $\alpha(1\rightarrow3)$-linked Fuc residue that enters deeply and is completely buried from bulk solvent (Ramsland et al. 2004). The glycopeptide-specific antibody, 237mAb, binds the Thr-linked GalNAc residue (Tn antigen) by end-on insertion and concomitantly recognizes the peptide in an elongated groove located higher up in the binding site (Fig. 9.2d, e) (Brooks et al. 2010). An overlay of all structures shows that the carbohydrate epitopes are located almost centrally (shifted slightly towards H chain) between the VL and VH domains, and all ligands penetrate the space between LCDR3 and HCDR3 to approximately equivalent depths (see Fig. 9.2f). Thus, binding of tumor-associated carbohydrates often (but not always) involves antibody residues in a deep pocket in a structurally equivalent location. In addition, the specificities for different epitopes depend on differences in shapes (topographies) and surface chemistries (constituent residues) across the antibody combining sites.

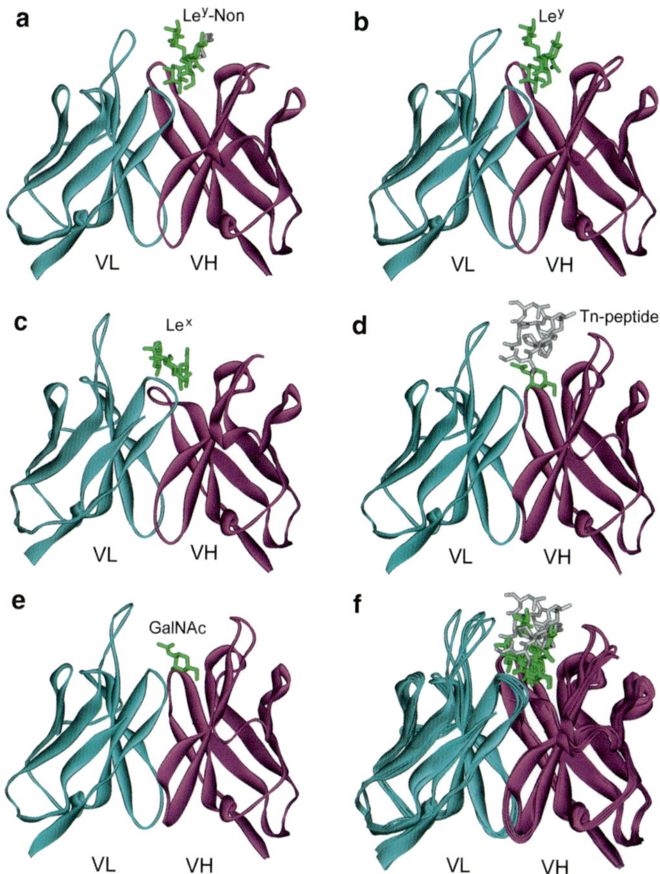

Fig. 9.2 Crystal structures of antibodies in complexes with their tumor-associated carbohydrate antigens. (**a**) Chimeric BR96 (PDB ID: 1CLY) with bound Le^y-nonoate (Non) ester; (**b**) hu3S193 (PDB ID: 1S3K) with the bound Le^y tetrasaccharide; (**c**) 291-2G3-A (PDB ID: 1UZ8) with bound Le^x trisaccharide; (**d**) 237mAb (PDB ID: 3IET) with a bound glycopeptide (carbohydrate epitope is Tn; GalNAc-α-*O*-Thr) from the protein podoplanin; (**e**) 237mAb (PDB ID: 3IF1) with bound GalNAc monosaccharide; (**f**) rigid-body overlay of variable regions of all complexes shown in panels **a**–**e**. The antibody variable domains (VL *cyan*, VH *magenta*) are shown as ribbons-style representations. Bound ligands are shown as stick representations with carbohydrate portions in *green* and non-carbohydrate portions in *grey*. Table 9.2 provides further information about the crystal structures depicted in this figure

9.3.1 Recognition of Blood Group Related Lewis Carbohydrates by Antibodies

Of the various Lewis carbohydrates that are over-expressed in cancer, crystal structures for antibody complexes have only been determined with Le^y and Le^x determinants (Table 9.2). The BR96 monoclonal antibody has been reported as complexes with a Le^y nonoate ester for both the murine and chimeric (murine-human) versions, and the chimeric version in its unliganded form (Jeffrey et al. 1995; Sheriff et al. 1996). We have determined the structures of a humanized monoclonal antibody (hu3S193) from two crystal forms in complex with the Le^y tetrasaccharide (Ramsland et al. 2004; Farrugia et al. 2009). Interestingly, the interactions with the Le^y carbohydrate were extremely similar when the BR96 and hu3S193 antibodies were compared (Ramsland et al. 2004). Contacts with the Le^x portion of the ligand were almost identical and involved a dominant contribution from aromatic binding site residues through hydrophobic and multiple hydrogen bonding interactions. The convergent recognition strategies of the BR96 and hu3S193 antibodies for Le^y have resulted in binding sites with equivalent shapes and surface chemistries, which are particularly apparent in regions surrounding the Le^x portion of the ligands (Ramsland et al. 2004; Yuriev et al. 2005). Differences between the two antibody interactions reside in the $\alpha(1\rightarrow2)$-linked Fuc moiety, the addition of which converts Le^x into Le^y. In hu3S193, this Le^y-specific Fuc is held in place by hydrogen bonding to an Asn residue in LCDR1, but due to subtle differences in the binding site topography, these contacts do not occur in the BR96 interaction with Le^y. The only other difference is due to the form of the Le^y ligands used for co-crystallization with the antibodies. Specifically, the nonoate ester group attached to the Le^y tetrasaccharide in BR96 is bound in a shallow groove between HCDR1 and HCDR3 that is not present in the hu3S193 binding site, which was crystallized with the free Le^y tetrasaccharide (Ramsland et al. 2004). Regardless of these minor differences, the overall similarity in recognition of Le^y by the BR96 and hu3S193 antibodies is shown in Fig. 9.2a, b.

Since the hu3S193 Fab complex with Le^y was determined at a resolution of 1.9 Å, we were able to examine the role of solvent in antibody recognition (Ramsland et al. 2004). Two of the key waters were also observed in an independent crystal form of the hu3S193 Fab in complex with Le^y, which was determined at a resolution of 2.5 Å (Farrugia et al. 2009). In the high resolution hu3S193 structure, a total of 13 ordered water molecules are involved directly and these greatly increase the complementarity between the hu3S193 binding site and the Le^y tetrasaccharide (Ramsland et al. 2004; Yuriev et al. 2005). The waters function as either bridges between carbohydrate and hu3S193 antibody residues or are believed, through hydrogen bonding directly to the carbohydrate, to influence the shape of the Le^y determinant. The role of water in maintaining the biologically active conformation of free Le^y and Le^x carbohydrates has been examined in detail using molecular dynamics (MD) simulations (Reynolds et al. 2008). Remarkably, the water molecule bridging events and solvent structure around free Le^y observed by MD closely corresponded to the hydrogen bonding network (water and binding site residues) involved in the hu3S193 interaction with Le^y (Ramsland et al. 2004; Reynolds et al. 2008).

The Le^x specific antibody 291-2-G3-A was not generated against tumor cells, but from mice infected with schistosomes, which express complex Le^x-containing saccharides on their surface. All three residues of the Le^x ligand are bound in a shallow pocket and contact residues are contributed by all six CDRs in the 291-2-G3-A binding site (van Roon et al. 2004). Consequently, the 291-2-G3-A binding site shape and the orientation of Le^x (Fig. 9.2c) bear no resemblance to the binding of

Le^y by the tumor-specific BR96 and hu3S193 antibodies (Yuriev et al. 2005). This dissimilarity could be due to how the 291-2-G3-A antibody was generated (i.e., against a non-tumor source of the Le^x antigen). However, the Le^x interaction with 291-2-G3-A does illustrate that an alternate binding mode may occur in tumor-specific antibodies generated against the various Lewis carbohydrates.

Although the antibody bound structures of Le^y and Le^x have shown the detailed basis for recognition of these carbohydrate determinants, the same epitopes are presented at high surface densities as both glycoproteins and glycolipids on tumor cells. The restricted tissue distributions and lower expression levels in most healthy adult tissues suggest that in vivo Le^y and Le^x are relatively inaccessible to antibodies. Comparisons of both free and bound conformations of Lewis determinants revealed an overall structural similarity and rigid nature of this family of histo-blood group and tumor-associated carbohydrate antigens (Yuriev et al. 2005). Combined with the studies of solvent structure (outlined above), it appears that the biologically active conformation of Lewis determinants is almost identical for the free and bound forms, which is presumably similar for tumors and healthy tissues. Therefore, for an antibody to selectively interact with Lewis-expressing tumors the probable mechanism is carbohydrate cluster recognition (i.e., high local densities of carbohydrates that promote multivalent antibody binding). We recently reported the crystal structure of hu3S193 Fab and Le^y derived from a crystal grown in the presence of divalent zinc ions, which promoted the formation hu3S193 Fab–Fab interactions in crystals and in solution (Farrugia et al. 2009). A similar metallic ion mediated association of hu3S193 *in vivo* is potentially involved in binding to the high densities of Le^y on tumor cells. Another mechanism for carbohydrate cluster recognition has been reported for a HIV-1 gp120 binding antibody, 2-G12, where domain swapped 2-G12 Fab homodimers were observed in crystals, resulting in tightly packed carbohydrate recognition sites (Calarese et al. 2003, see also Chap. 7). Furthermore, homophilic antibody binding and VH-VH β-pairing in crystals was reported for the GD3 binding R24 antibody (Kaminski et al. 1999b). These and other examples of antibody-antibody interactions may promote the close association of antibody binding sites to facilitate carbohydrate cluster recognition of tumor cells.

9.3.2 Antibody Recognition of Gangliosides

Structural studies with antibodies specific for tumor-associated gangliosides have been performed, but no crystal structures have so far been determined for antibody-ganglioside complexes (Table 9.2). Unliganded Fab structures have been determined for murine and chimeric R24 antibody that recognizes the disialoganglioside GD3. The binding site of R24 is proposed to be formed by the three CDRs from the heavy chain, which form a pocket lined by polar (Ser, Thr and His) and some Tyr residues. The proposed R24 binding pocket was suggested to accommodate the terminal sialic acid residue of GD3 (Kaminski et al. 1999b). The GD2 specific ME36.1 Fab has also been examined by crystallography at a resolution of 2.8 Å.

The ME36.1 binding site is formed by the six CDR loops that form a relatively large groove at the VL-VH interface, with approximate dimensions of 20 Å × 10 Å × 8 Å. In the absence of a co-crystal, the GD2 tetrasaccharide was manually fitted into the binding site to examine possible interactions with the ME36.1 antibody. The best fit placed the GD2 saccharide in the groove so that interactions were proposed between five of the six ME36.1 CDRs (Pichla et al. 1997). While this method of antibody-carbohydrate modeling could be reassessed using modern docking techniques, the groove-type binding site of the unliganded ME36.1 Fab was clearly of sufficient size to accommodate most of the tetrasaccharide headgroup of GD2.

The binding sites of two antibodies (14-F7 and chP3) specific for the *N*-glycolylneuraminic acid form of GM3 (*N*-glycolyl GM3) have been examined by crystallography (Krengel et al. 2004; Talavera et al. 2009). As discussed (Sect. 9.2.2), humans cannot produce endogenous Neu5Gc, but it has been shown that Neu5Gc can be present at low levels in some human tissues and at higher levels in certain cancers. The source of Neu5Gc in both cases is most likely dietary (Tangvoranuntakul et al. 2003). Using a combination of visual inspection, carbohydrate docking and mutagenesis approaches, *N*-glycolyl GM3 was proposed to bind in a site formed exclusively by the three HCDR loops. Binding modes for *N*-glycolyl GM3 were suggested to involve end-on insertion of the terminal Neu5Gc residue in a deep pocket, which may explain the specificity of 14-F7 and chP3 for *N*-glycolyl GM3 over the *N*-acetyl GM3 (i.e., Neu5Ac residues) that is the predominant form in healthy human tissues.

Previous attempts to determine the structures of ganglioside-antibody complexes have focused largely on the selection of a single pose obtained from molecular docking which is deemed to fit best with other experimental data (e.g., site-directed mutagenesis). Our site mapping technique, which considers multiple binding modes, may be used to augment or enhance the output of molecular docking (Agostino et al. 2009a, 2010). Thus, we applied site mapping to reassess ligand recognition by the four anti-ganglioside antibodies.

Site mapping predicts that antibodies 14-F7 and chP3, both of which recognize *N*-glycolyl GM3, employ a tightly arranged set of residues for hydrogen bonding to the target ligand (Fig. 9.3). The functionalities of the key hydrogen bonding residues are similar in each case, although their arrangement is somewhat "rotated" between 14-F7 and chP3. The similarity in ligand recognition between these two antibodies is surprising, given their dramatically different combining site organization; the binding site of 14-F7 consists of a small cavity made entirely of heavy chain residues, whereas the binding site of chP3 is a very large, open cavity consisting of residues from both the light chain and heavy chain. The binding site topographies, in conjunction with these site maps, may be useful in explaining the observed selectivity by these two antibodies for their *N*-glycolyl ganglioside antigens (Vázquez et al. 1995; Carr et al. 2000).

The antibodies R24 and ME36.1 recognize GD3 and GD2 respectively, both of which terminate in αNeu5Ac residues. Like the antibodies specific for *N*-glycolyl GM3, R24 and ME36.1 both employ a tightly arranged set of residues for hydrogen bonding to the ligand (Fig. 9.4). However, ME36.1 has a much larger, broader

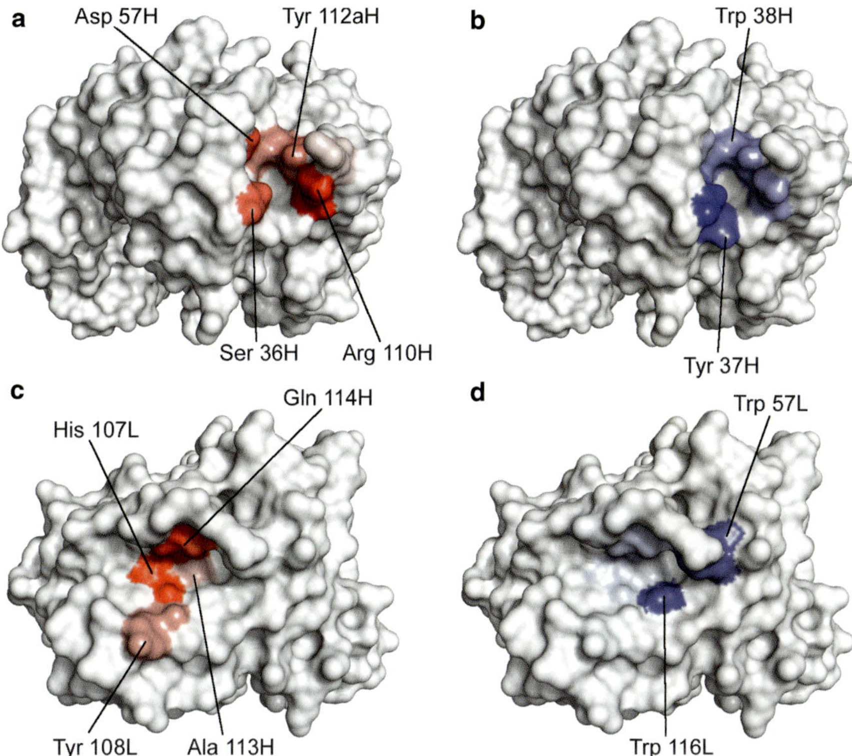

Fig. 9.3 Site maps of anti-*N*-glycolyl GM3 antibodies. (**a**) Hydrogen bond map of 14-F7 Fab. (**b**) van der Waals map of 14-F7. (**c**) Hydrogen bond map of chP3 Fab. (**d**) van der Waals map of chP3 Fab. (**a** and **b**) Generated using PDB ID: 1RIH (Krengel et al. 2004). (**c** and **d**) Generated using PDB ID: 3-IU4 (Talavera et al. 2009). Site maps were generated as previously described (Agostino et al. 2009b), but using GOLD (Jones et al. 1997) to carry out the initial docking. The missing portion of HCDR3 in PDB ID: 3-IU4 was modeled using Prime 2.2 (Schrödinger 2010a). Residues most important for interactions are indicated on the maps. Antibodies are numbered using the IMGT convention (Lefranc et al. 2003). Images generated using PyMOL (Schrödinger 2010b)

binding site compared to R24 and employs Tyr 55 of LCDR2 in ligand recognition, primarily via van der Waals interactions. It is possible that this tyrosine residue is involved in recognition of the GalNAc moiety of GD2 via a CH-π stacking interaction between the hydrophobic face of the GalNAc and the phenol portion of the tyrosine. This type of interaction has also been proposed for carbohydrate recognition by anti-αGal antibodies and, in that particular case, may be important in explaining the observed ligand selectivity (Agostino et al. 2010). Further *in silico* studies with the ganglioside and other sialic acid containing carbohydrates recognized by antibodies are currently underway and will be described in detail elsewhere (Agostino et al., unpublished data).

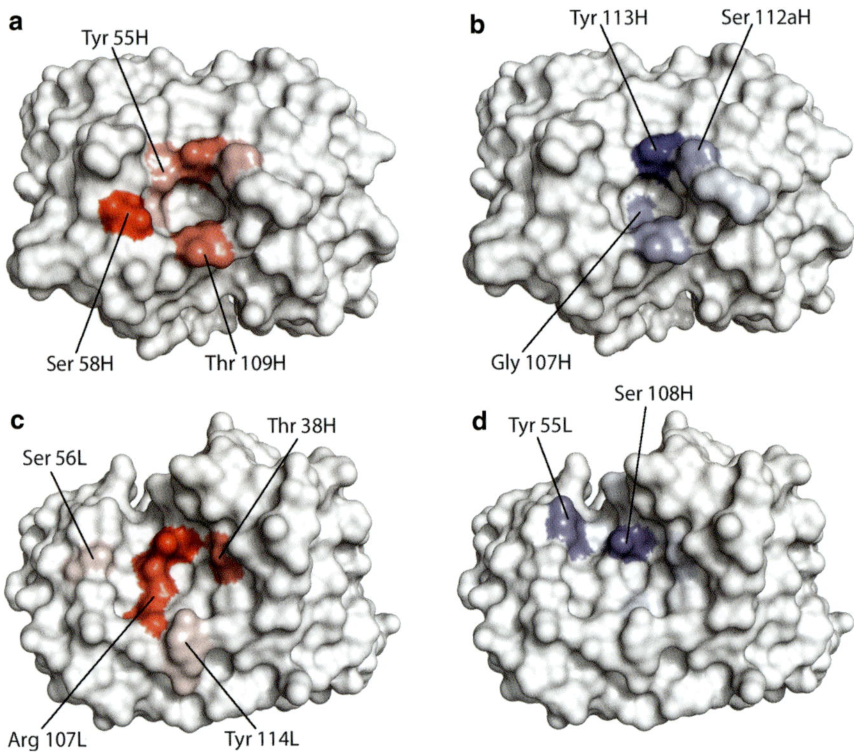

Fig. 9.4 Site maps of GD3 and GD2 binding antibodies. (**a**) Hydrogen bond map of R24 Fab. (**b**) van der Waals map of R24. (**c**) Hydrogen bond map of ME36.1 Fab. (**d**) van der Waals map of ME36.1 Fab. (**a** and **b**) Generated using PDB ID: 1BZ7 (Kaminski et al. 1999a). (**c** and **d**) Generated using PDB ID: 1PSK (Pichla et al. 1997). Site maps were generated as previously described (Agostino et al. 2009b), but using GOLD to carry out the initial docking. Residues most important for interactions are indicated. Antibodies are numbered using the IMGT convention (Lefranc et al. 2003). Images generated using PyMOL (Schrödinger 2010b)

9.3.3 Other Antigens Resulting from Modified Glycosylation in Tumors

Cryptic or neoepitopes can be unmasked in cancer as a result of loss of glycosyltransferases involved in *N*- and *O*-linked carbohydrate synthesis. The crystal structures of a tumor-specific antibody (237mAb) bound to its truncated *O*-linked glycopeptide (containing the Tn antigen) and the GalNAc monosaccharide were recently determined (Brooks et al. 2010). The GalNAc was recognized by 237mAb in a protected pocket that was formed by germline antibody residues, while the peptide is located in a groove near the entrance to the binding site (Fig. 9.2d). In the GalNAc complex with 237mAb, the free saccharide binds in the same binding pocket as for the Tn-glycopeptide (Fig. 9.2e) and is consequently an example of anchored or end-on recognition. In binding assays, only the Tn-glycopeptide (not the unglycosylated peptide or GalNAc) was shown to interact with 237mAb. Since the Tn-glycopeptide sequence was derived from a mouse tumor-associated protein (podoplanin), selectivity by 237mAb occurs by recognition of the Tn antigen only in the context of the underglycosylated podoplanin protein (Brooks et al. 2010). Antibodies with similar binding profiles against human tumor-associated glycoproteins bearing Tn and TF antigens may be promising candidates for cancer immunotherapy.

Another strategy for antibody recognition of tumor-associated glycoproteins is the direct binding to protein residues that are unmasked by the decrease in glycosylation. The SM3 antibody is an example of an antibody that binds to the MUC1 protein that is underglycosylated in many epithelial tumors such as breast cancer. The crystal structure for SM3 Fab in complex with a MUC1 peptide shows that the potential *O*-linked sites (Thr/Ser residues) are not directly involved in the interaction. It was suggested that conformational changes induced by the underglycosylation of MUC1 are responsible for the tumor specificity of SM3 (Dokurno et al. 1998). However, it is possible that this antibody only recognizes a cryptic MUC1 epitope that is unmasked in tumors, but is normally shielded by the extensive *O*-linked glycosylation of this mucin in healthy tissues.

9.3.4 Potential Clinical Application for Antibody Targeting of Carbohydrates in Cancer

Antibodies that specifically bind to tumor-associated carbohydrate antigens have enormous potential for the immunotherapy of cancer. Although several antibodies have been approved and are in general clinical use for treatment of certain cancers (Gura 2002; Glennie and van de Winkel 2003), so far, none of these antibodies bind directly to carbohydrate epitopes. However, a wide range of carbohydrate binding antibodies are currently being explored in preclinical and clinical trials. Herein, we summarize some studies of human in vivo antibody targeting of the Le^y, GD3 and GD2 antigens from two categories of tumor-associated carbohydrate antigens (Table 9.1).

The Le^y antigen is expressed in over 70% of epithelial cancers (e.g., breast, colon, ovary and lung) and is an attractive target for monoclonal antibody based therapy (Kitamura et al. 1994). Several clinical trials with Le^y binding antibodies have now been conducted. Early Phase I trials in patients with breast, colon and small cell lung cancers were conducted with murine anti-Le^y monoclonals (e.g., BR55-2 and ABL-364) and showed some minor indications of clinical efficacy. Side-effects were mostly low grade including nausea and vomiting, diarrhoea and hematuria. However, human anti-murine antibody responses (HAMA) prevented repeated treatment cycles (Schlimok et al. 1995). A chimeric (mouse-human) BR96-doxorubicin construct has been evaluated in a range of patients with advanced Le^y-positive cancers including metastatic breast and colon cancer. There was some indication of partial responses in a Phase I trial from the maximum tolerated dose (700 mg/m^2) of BR96-doxorubicin (Saleh et al. 2000). In Phase II trials, the clinical efficacy was limited to one partial response in 14 metastatic breast cancer patients (Tolcher et al. 1999) or no objective responses in 15 patients with advanced Le^y-positive gastric adenocarcinomas (Ajani et al. 2000). In these studies, nausea and vomiting (mostly controlled by premedication) due to upper gastro-intestinal tract toxicity was the most common side effect from BR96-doxorubicin treatment, but mild hematemesis due to hemorrhagic gastritis occurred in a proportion of patients, which may have been related to the doxorubicin component of the construct.

The murine Le^y binding monoclonal antibody 3-S193 was developed, and a detailed specificity, affinity and cytotoxicity analysis of 3-S193 showed it to be superior to BR55-2 and other anti-Le^y murine monoclonal antibodies (Kitamura et al. 1994). A CDR grafted humanized version of murine 3-S193 has been produced (hu3S193), and has undergone extensive preclinical testing (Clarke et al. 2000a,b; Scott et al. 2000). Hu3S193 has high affinity for the Le^y antigen, and has superior immune effector function (CDC $IC_{50} = 1.0$ μg/ml and antibody-dependent cellular-cytotoxicity (ADCC) $IC_{50} = 5.0$ μg/ml) compared to the mouse 3-S193 antibody. The mediation of potent immune effector function, combined with the humanization of this construct (reduced immunogenicity), indicates hu3S193 is an excellent candidate for immunotherapy of Le^y-expressing epithelial carcinomas such as breast cancer. The hu3S193 antibody has been evaluated in the clinic, and shown excellent targeting of Le^y-expressing tumors, a long half-life, retention of immune function *in vivo*, and no evidence of immunogenicity (Scott et al. 2007). Preclinical studies have shown efficacy of hu3S193 as an immunotherapeutic and as a carrier of payloads to tumor cells (e.g., isotopes) (Clarke et al. 2000b; Kelly et al. 2007, 2009). Phase I clinical trials in colorectal, lung, and ovarian cancer have shown promising early results (Krug et al. 2007; Scott et al. 2007), and Phase II trials are ongoing. Hu3S193 has also been evaluated as an immunotoxin, linked to calicheamicin (CMD-193), in a Phase I trial (Herbertson et al. 2009).

Gangliosides such as GM2, GD2, and GD3 are promising targets for immunotherapy of human cancers because of their dominant expression on the tumor cell surface, particularly for neuroectodermal cancers. A number of mouse or rat monoclonal antibodies were previously established against a series of gangliosides to study the nature of the molecules on the cell surface (Hanai et al. 2000). The most promising antibodies were converted to chimeric or humanized versions with the aim of developing these antibodies for immunotherapy of human cancer. It is desirable for antibodies to remain on the cell surface for a long time so that they can exert effector functions such as CDC and ADCC. We found that antibodies to GM2, GD2, and GD3 remained on the cell surface for longer than 60 min after binding, while antibodies to other types of carbohydrate such as sialyl-Le^a are quickly internalized (Lee et al. 2001). A chimeric monoclonal antibody to GD3, KM871, bound to a variety of tumor cell lines, especially melanoma cells, including some cell lines to which R24 failed to bind (Hanai et al. 2000). *In vitro*, the chimeric KM871 antibody was more effective than its mouse counterpart KM641 in CDC and ADCC killing of GD3-expressing melanoma cells (Shitara et al. 1993). In a preclinical study, intravenous injection of KM871 markedly suppressed tumor growth, and radiolabeled KM871 efficiently targeted the tumor site in a nude mouse model (Hanai et al. 2000). The KM871 chimeric monoclonal antibody has been evaluated in a Phase I clinical trial in melanoma patients (Scott et al. 2001, 2005). The long *in vivo* half-life and lack of immunogenicity of KM871 in patients suggests that this antibody is a promising candidate for immunotherapy of GD3-expressing tumors.

Targeting of GD2 in neuroblastoma patients with antibody/fusion constructs, and payloads (e.g., isotopes), has also been shown to have clinical therapeutic efficacy. The 3-F8 antibody, directed against GD2, has been evaluated as a murine and humanized version and with payload delivery (e.g., I^{131}) both systemically and via cerebrospinal fluid, in a number of clinical trials in neuroblastoma patients (Modak and Cheung 2010). The antibody 14.18 has also been developed for targeting GD2 in neuroblastoma. Chimeric 14.18 has been explored alone and in conjunction with cytokines in children with neuroblastoma, and therapeutic responses have been observed, with manageable toxicity of pain, and capillary leak syndrome. In a recent large randomized trial of 226 children with high risk neuroblastoma and a response to induction therapy and stem cell transplantation, the addition of chimeric 14.18 and cytokines (GM-CSF and IL-2) to standard therapy of isotretinoin had a superior event-free survival and overall survival compared to isotretinoin alone (Yu et al. 2010). The humanized 14.18 antibody linked to the cytokine IL-2 (i.e., an antibody-fusion protein) has also been recently shown to achieve over 20% complete responses in children with small volume relapsed or recurrent neuroblastoma (Shusterman et al. 2010). Thus, the targeting of GD2 in neuroblastoma patients has great promise, and further trials are ongoing.

Along with the examples discussed above, there are currently numerous antibodies directed against carbohydrates and glycoprotein targets that are associated with tumors. The next several years will undoubtedly bring further developments in the design and testing of carbohydrate binding antibodies, some of which are anticipated to be suitable for antibody-based cancer immunotherapy.

9.4 Concluding Remarks

Recognition of αGal xenoantigens appears to occur by the binding of the extended carbohydrates in a variety of binding site shapes. Using *in silico* methods, it has been shown that both groove and end-on insertion type of mechanisms can occur, with the majority of antibody recognition towards the terminal αGal(1→3)Gal disaccharide. Since the production of αGal deficient pigs, the preferred donor animals for human xenotransplantation, the search has been on to identify non-αGal antigens responsible for antibody-mediated xenograft rejection. Structural and functional studies of non-αGal carbohydrate recognition by antibodies will continue to facilitate progress in xenotransplantation.

The numerous genetic and epigenetic changes in cancer have resulted in changes to the antigenicity of tumor cells. Of particular importance are the multiple differences in glycosyltransferase expression in cancer, which results in several categories of tumor-associated carbohydrate antigens, including: (1) the over-expression of blood group and related carbohydrates; (2) the altered expression of gangliosides, and; (3) the production of cryptic epitopes by expression of truncated oligosaccharide chains on tumor glycoproteins. Antibody recognition of these carbohydrates occurs through extensive interactions that are dominated by the anchored end-on insertion of one or two monosaccharide units, normally in a deep cavity between the VL and VH domains. Solvent networks are involved in maintaining the structure of free and bound carbohydrate tumor antigens. Carbohydrate cluster recognition probably has a major influence on antibodies selectively binding to their carbohydrate targets, which are expressed at high densities on the surface of tumor cells, but are at lower densities and with restricted expression profiles in healthy tissues.

Combining experimental techniques with *in silico* approaches for studying 3D structures of carbohydrate-protein interactions has resulted in a wealth of knowledge of antibody recognition of key tissue and blood group carbohydrate antigens. In particular, these carbohydrate determinants are important targets for antibodies in xenotransplantation and cancer immunotherapy. With recent advances in all areas of glycobiology, the prospects and future are bright for understanding and manipulating the recognition of carbohydrates by antibodies, which is likely to be of significant importance in medicine.

Acknowledgements This work was funded in part by grants ID566722 and ID542512 from the National Health and Medical Research Council of Australia (NHMRC). M Agostino is a recipient of an Australian Postgraduate Award (APA). PA Ramsland was a recipient of an R Douglas Wright Career Development Award (ID365209) from the NHMRC. The authors gratefully acknowledge the contribution to this work of the Victorian Operational Infrastructure Support Program received by the Burnet Institute and the Ludwig Institute for Cancer Research.

References

Agostino M, Jene C, Boyle T, Ramsland PA, Yuriev E (2009a) Molecular docking of carbohydrate ligands to antibodies: structural validation against crystal structures. J Chem Inf Model 49:2749–2760

Agostino M, Sandrin MS, Thompson PE, Yuriev E, Ramsland PA (2009b) In silico analysis of antibody–carbohydrate interactions and its application to xenoreactive antibodies. Mol Immunol 47:233–246

Agostino M, Sandrin MS, Thompson PE, Yuriev E, Ramsland PA (2010) Identification of preferred carbohydrate binding modes in xenoreactive antibodies by combining conformational filters and binding site maps. Glycobiology 20:724–735

Ajani JA, Kelsen DP, Haller D, Hargraves K, Healey D (2000) A multi-institutional phase II study of BMS-182248-01 (BR96-doxorubicin conjugate) administered every 21 days in patients with advanced gastric adenocarcinoma. Cancer J 6:78–81

Basnet NB, Ide K, Tahara H, Tanaka Y, Ohdan H (2010) Deficiency of N-glycolylneuraminic acid and Galα1-3Galβ1-4GlcNAc epitopes in xenogeneic cells attenuates cytotoxicity of human natural antibodies. Xenotransplantation 17:440–448

Brooks CL, Schietinger A, Borisova SN, Kufer P, Okon M, Hirama T, MacKenzie CR, Wang LX, Schreiber H, Evans SV (2010) Antibody recognition of a unique tumor-specific glycopeptide antigen. Proc Natl Acad Sci USA 107:10056–10061

Byrne GW, Stalboerger PG, Du Z, Davis TR, McGregor CG (2011) Identification of new carbohydrate and membrane protein antigens in cardiac xenotransplantation. Transplantation. doi:10.1097/TP.0b013e318203c27d

Cairns T, Lee J, Goldberg LC, Hakim N, Cook T, Rydberg L, Samuelsson B, Taube D (1996) Thomsen–Friedenreich and PK antigens in pig-to-human xenotransplantation. Transplant Proc 28:795–796

Calarese DA, Scanlan CN, Zwick MB, Deechongkit S, Mimura Y, Kunert R, Zhu P, Wormald MR, Stanfield RL, Roux KH, Kelly JW, Rudd PM, Dwek RA, Katinger H, Burton DR, Wilson IA (2003) Antibody domain exchange is an immunological solution to carbohydrate cluster recognition. Science 300:2065–2071

Carr A, Mullet A, Mazorra Z, Vázquez AM, Alfonso M, Mesa C, Rengifo E, Pérez R, Fernández LE (2000) A mouse IgG_1 monoclonal antibody specific for *N*-glycolyl GM3 ganglioside recognized breast and melanoma tumors. Hybridoma 19:241–247

Cazet A, Julien S, Bobowski M, Burchell J, Delannoy P (2010) Tumour-associated carbohydrate antigens in breast cancer. Breast Cancer Res 12:204

Chang WW, Lee CH, Lee P, Lin J, Hsu CW, Hung JT, Lin JJ, Yu JC, Shao LE, Yu J, Wong CH, Yu AL (2008) Expression of Globo H and SSEA3 in breast cancer stem cells and the involvement of fucosyl transferases 1 and 2 in Globo H synthesis. Proc Natl Acad Sci USA 105:11667–11672

Chou HH, Takematsu H, Diaz S, Iber J, Nickerson E, Wright KL, Muchmore EA, Nelson DL, Warren ST, Varki A (1998) A mutation in human CMP-sialic acid hydroxylase occurred after the Homo-Pan divergence. Proc Natl Acad Sci USA 95:11751–11756

Christiansen D, Mouhtouris E, Milland J, Zingoni A, Santoni A, Sandrin MS (2006) Recognition of a carbohydrate xenoepitope by human NKRP1A (CD161). Xenotransplantation 13:440–446

Clarke K, Lee FT, Brechbiel MW, Smyth FE, Old LJ, Scott AM (2000a) In vivo biodistribution of a humanized anti-Lewis Y monoclonal antibody (hu3S193) in MCF-7 xenografted BALB/c nude mice. Cancer Res 60:4804–4811

Clarke K, Lee FT, Brechbiel MW, Smyth FE, Old LJ, Scott AM (2000b) Therapeutic efficacy of anti-Lewis(y) humanized 3S193 radioimmunotherapy in a breast cancer model: enhanced activity when combined with taxol chemotherapy. Clin Cancer Res 6:3621–3628

Cooper DK, Ayares D (2011) The immense potential of xenotransplantation in surgery. Int J Surg. doi:10.1016/j.ijsu.2010.11.002

Cowan PJ, Roussel JC, d'Apice AJ (2009) The vascular and coagulation issues in xenotransplantation. Curr Opin Organ Transplant 14:161–167

Crew RJ, Ratner LE (2010) ABO-incompatible kidney transplantation: current practice and the decade ahead. Curr Opin Organ Transplant 15:526–530

DeMarco ML, Woods RJ (2008) Structural glycobiology: a game of snakes and ladders. Glycobiology 18:426–440

Dipchand AI, Pollock BarZiv SM, Manlhiot C, West LJ, VanderVliet M, McCrindle BW (2010) Equivalent outcomes for pediatric heart transplantation recipients: ABO-blood group incompatible versus ABO-compatible. Am J Transplant 10:389–397

Dokurno P, Bates PA, Band HA, Stewart LM, Lally JM, Burchell JM, Taylor-Papadimitriou J, Snary D, Sternberg MJ, Freemont PS (1998) Crystal structure at 1.95 A resolution of the breast tumour-specific antibody SM3 complexed with its peptide epitope reveals novel hypervariable loop recognition. J Mol Biol 284:713–728

Donald AS, Yates AD, Soh CP, Morgan WT, Watkins WM (1983) A blood group Sda-active pentasaccharide isolated from Tamm-Horsfall urinary glycoprotein. Biochem Biophys Res Commun 115:625–631

Ekser B, Cooper DK (2010) Overcoming the barriers to xenotransplantation: prospects for the future. Expert Rev Clin Immunol 6:219–230

Ezzelarab M, Ayares D, Cooper DK (2005) Carbohydrates in xenotransplantation. Immunol Cell Biol 83:396–404

Farrugia W, Scott AM, Ramsland PA (2009) A possible role for metallic ions in the carbohydrate cluster recognition displayed by a Lewis Y specific antibody. PLoS One 4:e7777

Forte P, Pazmany L, Matter-Reissmann UB, Stussi G, Schneider MK, Seebach JD (2001) HLA-G inhibits rolling adhesion of activated human NK cells on porcine endothelial cells. J Immunol 167:6002–6008

Frank M, Schloissnig S (2010) Bioinformatics and molecular modeling in glycobiology. Cell Mol Life Sci 67:2749–2772

Friesner RA, Banks JL, Murphy RB, Halgren TA, Klicic JJ, Mainz DT, Repasky MP, Knoll EH, Shelley M, Perry JK, Shaw DE, Francis P, Shenkin PS (2004) Glide: a new approach for rapid, accurate docking and scoring. 1. Method and assessment of docking accuracy. J Med Chem 47:1739–1749

Galili U, Clark MR, Shohet SB, Buehler J, Macher BA (1987) Evolutionary relationship between the natural anti-Gal antibody and the Gal $\alpha(1\rightarrow3)$Gal epitope in primates. Proc Natl Acad Sci USA 84:1369–1373

Glennie MJ, van de Winkel JG (2003) Renaissance of cancer therapeutic antibodies. Drug Discov Today 8:503–510

Good AH, Cooper DK, Malcolm AJ, Ippolito RM, Koren E, Neethling FA, Ye Y, Zuhdi N, Lamontagne LR (1992) Identification of carbohydrate structures that bind human antiporcine antibodies: implications for discordant xenografting in humans. Transplant Proc 24:559–562

Gura T (2002) Therapeutic antibodies: magic bullets hit the target. Nature 417:584–586

Hakomori S (1999) Antigen structure and genetic basis of histo-blood groups A, B and O: their changes associated with human cancer. Biochim Biophys Acta 1473:247–266

Hakomori S (2001) Tumor-associated carbohydrate antigens defining tumor malignancy: basis for development of anti-cancer vaccines. Adv Exp Med Biol 491:369–402

Hanai N, Nakamura K, Shitara K (2000) Recombinant antibodies against ganglioside expressed on tumor cells. Cancer Chemother Pharmacol 46(Suppl):S13–S17

Harnden I, Kiernan K, Kearns-Jonker M (2010) The anti-nonGal xenoantibody response to α1,3-galactosyltransferase gene knockout pig xenografts. Curr Opin Organ Transplant 15:207–211

Herbertson RA, Tebbutt NC, Lee FT, MacFarlane DJ, Chappell B, Micallef N, Lee ST, Saunder T, Hopkins W, Smyth FE, Wyld DK, Bellen J, Sonnichsen DS, Brechbiel MW, Murone C, Scott AM (2009) Phase I biodistribution and pharmacokinetic study of Lewis Y-targeting immunoconjugate CMD-193 in patients with advanced epithelial cancers. Clin Cancer Res 15:6709–6715

Higashi H, Naiki M, Matuo S, Okouchi K (1977) Antigen of "serum sickness" type of heterophile antibodies in human sera: indentification as gangliosides with N-glycolylneuraminic acid. Biochem Biophys Res Commun 79:388–395

Holgersson J, Gustafsson A, Breimer ME (2005) Characteristics of protein–carbohydrate interactions as a basis for developing novel carbohydrate-based antirejection therapies. Immunol Cell Biol 83:694–708

Jeffrey PD, Bajorath J, Chang CY, Yelton D, Hellstrom I, Hellstrom KE, Sheriff S (1995) The X-ray structure of an anti-tumour antibody in complex with antigen. Nat Struct Biol 2:466–471

Jones G, Willett P, Glen RC, Leach AR, Taylor R (1997) Development and validation of a genetic algorithm for flexible docking. J Mol Biol 267:727–748

Kaminski MJ, MacKenzie CR, Mooibroek MJ, Dahms TE, Hirama T, Houghton AN, Chapman PB, Evans SV (1999a) The role of homophilic binding in anti-tumor antibody R24 recognition of molecular surfaces. Demonstration of an intermolecular β-sheet between interaction between VH domains. J Biol Chem 274:5597–5604

Kaminski MJ, MacKenzie CR, Mooibroek MJ, Dahms TE, Hirama T, Houghton AN, Chapman PB, Evans SV (1999b) The role of homophilic binding in anti-tumor antibody R24 recognition of molecular surfaces. Demonstration of an intermolecular beta-sheet interaction between VH domains. J Biol Chem 274:5597–5604

Kearns-Jonker M, Barteneva N, Mencel R, Hussain N, Shulkin I, Xu A, Yew M, Cramer DV (2007) Use of molecular modeling and site-directed mutagenesis to define the structural basis for the immune response to carbohydrate xenoantigens. BMC Immunol 8:3

Kelly MP, Lee FT, Tahtis K, Smyth FE, Brechbiel MW, Scott AM (2007) Radioimmunotherapy with alpha-particle emitting 213Bi-C-functionalized trans-cyclohexyl-diethylenetriaminepentaacetic acid-humanized 3S193 is enhanced by combination with paclitaxel chemotherapy. Clin Cancer Res 13:5604s–5612s

Kelly MP, Lee ST, Lee FT, Smyth FE, Davis ID, Brechbiel MW, Scott AM (2009) Therapeutic efficacy of 177Lu-CHX-A″-DTPA-hu3S193 radioimmunotherapy in prostate cancer is enhanced by EGFR inhibition or docetaxel chemotherapy. Prostate 69:92–104

Kitamura K, Stockert E, Garin-Chesa P, Welt S, Lloyd KO, Armour KL, Wallace TP, Harris WJ, Carr FJ, Old LJ (1994) Specificity analysis of blood group Lewis-y (Le(y)) antibodies generatedagainst synthetic and natural Le(y) determinants. Proc Natl Acad Sci USA 91: 12957–12961

Kobata A, Amano J (2005) Altered glycosylation of proteins produced by malignant cells, and application for the diagnosis and immunotherapy of tumours. Immunol Cell Biol 83:429–439

Krengel U, Olsson LL, Martinez C, Talavera A, Rojas G, Mier E, Angstrom J, Moreno E (2004) Structure and molecular interactions of a unique antitumor antibody specific for N-glycolyl GM3. J Biol Chem 279:5597–5603

Krug LM, Milton DT, Jungbluth AA, Chen LC, Quaia E, Pandit-Taskar N, Nagel A, Jones J, Kris MG, Finn R, Smith-Jones P, Scott AM, Old L, Divgi C (2007) Targeting Lewis Y (Le(y)) in small cell lung cancer with a humanized monoclonal antibody, hu3S193: a pilot trial testing two dose levels. J Thorac Oncol 2:947–952

Lee FT, Rigopoulos A, Hall C, Clarke K, Cody SH, Smyth FE, Liu Z, Brechbiel MW, Hanai N, Nice EC, Catimel B, Burgess AW, Welt S, Ritter G, Old LJ, Scott AM (2001) Specific localization, gamma camera imaging, and intracellular trafficking of radiolabelled chimeric anti-G(D3) ganglioside monoclonal antibody KM871 in SK-MEL-28 melanoma xenografts. Cancer Res 61:4474–4482

Lefranc M-P, Pommié C, Manuel R, Giudicelli V, Foulquier E, Truong L, Thouvenin-Contet V, Lefranc G (2003) IMGT unique numbering for immunoglobulin and T cell receptor variable domains and Ig superfamily V-like domains. Dev Comp Immunol 27:55–77

Lin CC, Ezzelarab M, Hara H, Long C, Lin CW, Dorling A, Cooper DK (2010) Atorvastatin or transgenic expression of TFPI inhibits coagulation initiated by anti-nonGal IgG binding to porcine aortic endothelial cells. J Thromb Haemost 8:2001–2010

Lucq J, Tixier D, Guinault AM, Greffard A, Loisance D, Pilatte Y (2000) The target antigens of naturally occurring human anti-β-galactose IgG are cryptic on porcine aortic endothelial cells. Xenotransplantation 7:3–13

Milland J, Christiansen D, Sandrin MS (2005) α1,3-Galactosyltransferase knockout pigs are available for xenotransplantation: are glycosyltransferases still relevant? Immunol Cell Biol 83:687–693

Milland J, Yuriev E, Xing PX, McKenzie IF, Ramsland PA, Sandrin MS (2007) Carbohydrate residues downstream of the terminal Galα(1,3)Gal epitope modulate the specificity of xenoreactive antibodies. Immunol Cell Biol 85:623–632

Miwa Y, Kobayashi T, Nagasaka T, Liu D, Yu M, Yokoyama I, Suzuki A, Nakao A (2004) Are N-glycolylneuraminic acid (Hanganutziu-Deicher) antigens important in pig-to-human xeno-transplantation? Xenotransplantation 11:247–253

Modak S, Cheung NK (2010) Neuroblastoma: therapeutic strategies for a clinical enigma. Cancer Treat Rev 36:307–317

Nottle MB, Vassiliev I, O'Connel PJ, d'Apice AJ, Cowan PJ (2010) On the need for porcine embryonic stem cells to produce Gal KO pigs expressing multiple transgenes to advance xenotransplantation research. Xenotransplantation 17:411–412

Pichla SL, Murali R, Burnett RM (1997) The crystal structure of a Fab fragment to the melanoma-associated GD2 ganglioside. J Struct Biol 119:6–16

Ramsland PA, Farrugia W, Yuriev E, Edmundson AB, Sandrin MS (2003) Evidence for structurally conserved recognition of the major carbohydrate xenoantigen by natural antibodies. Cell Mol Biol (Noisy-le-Grand) 49:307–317

Ramsland PA, Farrugia W, Bradford T, Hogarth PM, Scott AM (2004) Structural convergence of antibody binding of carbohydrate determinants in Lewis Y tumor antigens. J Mol Biol 340: 809–818

Ramsland P (2005) Blood brothers: carbohydrates in xenotransplantation and cancer immunotherapy. Immunol Cell Biol 83:315–317

Reis CA, Osorio H, Silva L, Gomes C, David L (2010) Alterations in glycosylation as biomarkers for cancer detection. J Clin Pathol 63:322–329

Reynolds M, Fuchs A, Lindhorst TK, Perez S (2008) The hydration features of carbohydrate determinants of Lewis antigens. Mol Simul 34:447–460

Rood PP, Hara H, Ezzelarab M, Busch J, Zhu X, Ibrahim Z, Ball S, Ayares D, Awwad M, Cooper DK (2005) Preformed antibodies to α1,3-galactosyltransferase gene-knockout (GT-KO) pig cells in humans, baboons, and monkeys: implications for xenotransplantation. Transplant Proc 37:3514–3515

Rood PP, Tai HC, Hara H, Long C, Ezzelarab M, Lin YJ, van der Windt DJ, Busch J, Ayares D, Ijzermans JN, Wolf RF, Manji R, Bailey L, Cooper DK (2007) Late onset of development of natural anti-nonGal antibodies in infant humans and baboons: implications for xenotransplantation in infants. Transpl Int 20:1050–1058

Sakamoto J, Furukawa K, Cordon-Cardo C, Yin BW, Rettig WJ, Oettgen HF, Old LJ, Lloyd KO (1986) Expression of Lewis^{a}, Lewis^{b}, X, and Y blood group antigens in human colonic tumors and normal tissue and in human tumor-derived cell lines. Cancer Res 46:1553–1561

Saleh MN, Sugarman S, Murray J, Ostroff JB, Healey D, Jones D, Daniel CR, LeBherz D, Brewer H, Onetto N, LoBuglio AF (2000) Phase I trial of the anti-Lewis Y drug immunoconjugate BR96-doxorubicin in patients with Lewis Y-expressing epithelial tumors. J Clin Oncol 18:2282–2292

Sandrin MS, Vaughan HA, Dabkowski PL, McKenzie IF (1993) Anti-pig IgM antibodies in human serum react predominantly with Gal(α1–3)Gal epitopes. Proc Natl Acad Sci USA 90:11391–11395

Schlimok G, Pantel K, Loibner H, Fackler-Schwalbe I, Riethmuller G (1995) Reduction of metastatic carcinoma cells in bone marrow by intravenously administered monoclonal antibody: towards a novel surrogate test to monitor adjuvant therapies of solid tumours. Eur J Cancer 31A:1799–1803

Schrödinger LLC (2010a) Prime, version 2.2. New York

Schrödinger LLC (2010b) The PyMOL molecular graphics system, Version 1.3r1, New York

Scott AM, Renner C (2001) Tumour antigens recognized by antibodies. In: Encyclopedia of life sciences. Wiley. doi:10.1038/npg.els.0001433, Chichester, UK

Scott AM, Geleick D, Rubira M, Clarke K, Nice EC, Smyth FE, Stockert E, Richards EC, Carr FJ, Harris WJ, Armour KL, Rood J, Kypridis A, Kronina V, Murphy R, Lee FT, Liu Z, Kitamura K, Ritter G, Laughton K, Hoffman E, Burgess AW, Old LJ (2000) Construction, production, and characterization of humanized anti-Lewis Y monoclonal antibody 3S193 for targeted immunotherapy of solid tumors. Cancer Res 60:3254–3261

Scott AM, Lee FT, Hopkins W, Cebon JS, Wheatley JM, Liu Z, Smyth FE, Murone C, Sturrock S, MacGregor D, Hanai N, Inoue K, Yamasaki M, Brechbiel MW, Davis ID, Murphy R, Hannah A, Lim-Joon M, Chan T, Chong G, Ritter G, Hoffman EW, Burgess AW, Old LJ (2001) Specific targeting, biodistribution, and lack of immunogenicity of chimeric anti-GD3 monoclonal antibody KM871 in patients with metastatic melanoma: results of a phase I trial. J Clin Oncol 19:3976–3987

Scott AM, Liu Z, Murone C, Johns TG, MacGregor D, Smyth FE, Lee FT, Cebon J, Davis ID, Hopkins W, Mountain AJ, Rigopoulos A, Hanai N, Old LJ (2005) Immunological effects of chimeric anti-GD3 monoclonal antibody KM871 in patients with metastatic melanoma. Cancer Immun 5:3

Scott AM, Tebbutt N, Lee FT, Cavicchiolo T, Liu Z, Gill S, Poon AM, Hopkins W, Smyth FE, Murone C, MacGregor D, Papenfuss AT, Chappell B, Saunder TH, Brechbiel MW, Davis ID, Murphy R, Chong G, Hoffman EW, Old LJ (2007) A phase I biodistribution and pharmacokinetic trial of humanized monoclonal antibody Hu3s193 in patients with advanced epithelial cancers that express the Lewis-Y antigen. Clin Cancer Res 13:3286–3292

Seeberger PH (2008) Automated carbohydrate synthesis as platform to address fundamental aspects of glycobiology – current status and future challenges. Carbohydr Res 343:1889–1896

Sheriff S, Chang CY, Jeffrey PD, Bajorath J (1996) X-ray structure of the uncomplexed anti-tumor antibody BR96 and comparison with its antigen-bound form. J Mol Biol 259:938–946

Shitara K, Kuwana Y, Nakamura K, Tokutake Y, Ohta S, Miyaji H, Hasegawa M, Hanai N (1993) A mouse/human chimeric anti-(ganglioside GD3) antibody with enhanced antitumor activities. Cancer Immunol Immunother 36:373–380

Shusterman S, London WB, Gillies SD, Hank JA, Voss SD, Seeger RC, Reynolds CP, Kimball J, Albertini MR, Wagner B, Gan J, Eickhoff J, DeSantes KB, Cohn SL, Hecht T, Gadbaw B, Reisfeld RA, Maris JM, Sondel PM (2010) Antitumor activity of hu14.18-IL2 in patients with relapsed/refractory neuroblastoma: a Children's Oncology Group (COG) phase II study. J Clin Oncol 28:4969–4975

Slovin SF, Keding SJ, Ragupathi G (2005) Carbohydrate vaccines as immunotherapy for cancer. Immunol Cell Biol 83:418–428

Song KH, Kang YJ, Jin UH, Park YI, Kim SM, Seong HH, Hwang S, Yang BS, Im GS, Min KS, Kim JH, Chang YC, Kim NH, Lee YC, Kim CH (2010) Cloning and functional characterization of pig CMP-*N*-acetylneuraminic acid hydroxylase for the synthesis of *N*-glycolylneuraminic acid as the xenoantigenic determinant in pig–human xenotransplantation. Biochem J 427:179–188

Talavera A, Eriksson A, Okvist M, Lopez-Requena A, Fernandez-Marrero Y, Perez R, Moreno E, Krengel U (2009) Crystal structure of an anti-ganglioside antibody, and modelling of the functional mimicry of its NeuGc-GM3 antigen by an anti-idiotypic antibody. Mol Immunol 46:3466–3475

Tangvoranuntakul P, Gagneux P, Diaz S, Bardor M, Varki N, Varki A, Muchmore E (2003) Human uptake and incorporation of an immunogenic nonhuman dietary sialic acid. Proc Natl Acad Sci USA 100:12045–12050

Taylor ME, Drickamer K (2009) Structural insights into what glycan arrays tell us about how glycan-binding proteins interact with their ligands. Glycobiology 19:1155–1162

Tolcher AW, Sugarman S, Gelmon KA, Cohen R, Saleh M, Isaacs C, Young L, Healey D, Onetto N, Slichenmyer W (1999) Randomized phase II study of BR96-doxorubicin conjugate in patients with metastatic breast cancer. J Clin Oncol 17:478–484

Tseng YL, Moran K, Dor FJ, Sanderson TM, Li W, Lancos CJ, Schuurman HJ, Sachs DH, Cooper DK (2006) Elicited antibodies in baboons exposed to tissues from α1,3-galactosyltransferase gene-knockout pigs. Transplantation 81:1058–1062

van Roon AM, Pannu NS, de Vrind JP, van der Marel GA, van Boom JH, Hokke CH, Deelder AM, Abrahams JP (2004) Structure of an anti-Lewis X Fab fragment in complex with its Lewis X antigen. Structure 12:1227–1236

Vázquez AM, Alfonso M, Lanne B, Karlsson K-A, Carr A, Barroso O, Fernández LE, Rengifo E, Lanio ME, Alvarez C, Zeuthen J, Pérez R (1995) Generation of a murine monoclonal antibody specific for *N*-glycolylneuraminic acid-containing gangliosides that also recognizes sulfated glycolipids. Hybridoma 14:551–556

Weiss EH, Lilienfeld BG, Muller S, Muller E, Herbach N, Kessler B, Wanke R, Schwinzer R, Seebach JD, Wolf E, Brem G (2009) HLA-E/human β2-microglobulin transgenic pigs: protection against xenogeneic human anti-pig natural killer cell cytotoxicity. Transplantation 87:35–43

Woods RJ, Tessier MB (2010) Computational glycoscience: characterizing the spatial and temporal properties of glycans and glycan–protein complexes. Curr Opin Struct Biol 20: 575–583

Yu AL, Gilman AL, Ozkaynak MF, London WB, Kreissman SG, Chen HX, Smith M, Anderson B, Villablanca JG, Matthay KK, Shimada H, Grupp SA, Seeger R, Reynolds CP, Buxton A,

Reisfeld RA, Gillies SD, Cohn SL, Maris JM, Sondel PM (2010) Anti-GD2 antibody with GM-CSF, interleukin-2, and isotretinoin for neuroblastoma. N Engl J Med 363:1324–1334

Yuriev E, Farrugia W, Scott AM, Ramsland PA (2005) Three-dimensional structures of carbohydrate determinants of Lewis system antigens: implications for effective antibody targeting of cancer. Immunol Cell Biol 83:709–717

Yuriev E, Sandrin MS, Ramsland PA (2008) Antibody-ligand docking: insights into peptide-carbohydrate mimicry. Mol Simul 34:461–468

Yuriev E, Agostino M, Farrugia W, Christiansen D, Sandrin MS, Ramsland PA (2009) Structural biology of carbohydrate xenoantigens. Expert Opin Biol Ther 9:1017–1029

Yuriev E, Agostino M, Ramsland PA (2011) Challenges and advances in computational docking: 2009 in review. J Mol Recognit 24:149–164

Zhu A, Hurst R (2002) Anti-N-glycolylneuraminic acid antibodies identified in healthy human serum. Xenotransplantation 9:376–381

Carbohydrate Mimetic Peptide Vaccines 10

Somdutta Saha, Anastas Pashov, Behjatolah Monzavi-Karbassi, Ann Marie Kieber-Emmons, Akashi Otaki, Ramachandran Murali, and Thomas Kieber-Emmons

10.1 Introduction

Post-translational modifications of lipids and proteins are important determinants in defining function in both normal- and disease-state biology (Apweiler et al. 1999; Bertozzi and Kiessling 2001; Shental-Bechor and Levy 2009; Varki 1993). In particular, the addition of glycan residues synthesized by the repertoire of glycosyltransferases and glycosidases provide the mammalian glycome a large array of glycan structures that add to the diversity already created by the proteome (Cattaruzza and Perris 2006). At the same time, many glycan structures are ubiquitous in nature (van Die and Cummings 2009). Pathogen glycans can mimic host mammalian glycosphingolipids, lending to their pathophysiology. This mimicry provides insight into the processes contributing to their pathophysiology, including elements of recognition, signaling, and evasion of the immune system by glycan processing (Tsai 2001).

Notable among the glycans expressed on pathogens are the lacto-, globo-, and ganglioside series (Apicella et al. 1994; Appelmelk et al. 1996, 1997; Mandrell and Apicella 1993; Moran et al. 1996), which are also often expressed on cancer cells, and are identified as tumor-associated carbohydrate antigens (TACAs) (Hakomori 2002). Changes in glycosylation are often a hallmark of the transition from normal to inflamed or neoplastic tissue (Magnani 1984; Meezan et al. 1969; Singhal and Hakomori 1990). This transition affects a myriad of processes that correlate with a poor prognosis of cancer, affecting cell signaling and communication, cell motility and adhesion, angiogenesis, and organ tropism (Hakomori 2001; Ono and Hakomori

S. Saha • A. Pashov • B. Monzavi-Karbassi • A.M. Kieber-Emmons • T. Kieber-Emmons (✉)
Department of Pathology, Winthrop P. Rockefeller Cancer Institute, University of Arkansas for Medical Sciences Little Rock, Little Rock, AR, USA
e-mail: TKE@uams.edu

A. Otaki • R. Murali
Department of Biomedical Sciences, Cedars Sinai Medical Center, Los Angeles, CA, USA

P. Kosma and S. Müller-Loennies (eds.), *Anticarbohydrate Antibodies*,
DOI 10.1007/978-3-7091-0870-3_10, © Springer-Verlag/Wien 2012

2004). Subsequently, the pathophysiological processes of infection and neoplasia are profoundly affected by similar, or the same, carbohydrate forms.

Multivalent glycans are danger signals for the immune system, often playing a role in immune recognition, but not necessarily the immune response. Many host cell types, including endothelial and epithelial cells, neutrophils, monocytes, natural killer cells, dendritic cells, and macrophages, play a role in host immune defense through the Toll-like receptors' glycan signature recognition (Medvedev et al. 2006). Antibodies can also be glycan signature-decoding agents, functioning not only as the first line of defense against pathogen infections but also targeting TACA-expressing cancer cells (Pashov et al. 2010; Vollmers and Brandlein 2009).

Glycans also initiate cellular responses leading to tissue rejection in organ transplantation. Natural antibodies targeting the xenogeneic galactosyl (Gal) carbohydrate antigen αGal(1→3)βGal(1→4)GlcNAc (αGal) mediate hyperacute rejection of xenotransplants (Galili 2005). The expression of αGal(1→3)Gal and the amount of αGal(1→3)Gal available for the binding of natural antibodies is generally determined by analyzing the binding of the *Griffonia simplicifolia* type I lectin (GS-I), which recognizes galactosyl moieties much like natural antibodies (Lin et al. 1998). Thus, lectins and antibodies that recognize common antigens are useful reagents for aiding in glycan identification, although some antibodies still cannot distinguish their presentation on *O*-glycans, *N*-glycans, or glycolipids. Nevertheless, these studies exemplify the critical need for understanding the role of glycans in a variety of cellular and immunological processes.

It is now evident that one antibody does not necessarily bind to a single antigen, but it may recognize antigens of similar structures. These findings draw attention to the molecular basis for cross-reactivity between structurally diverse molecules. Analysis of a larger repertoire of ligands reactive with an antibody-combining site might establish structure–function relationships not evident from binding to monoreactive antibodies. Functional antigen recognition is based on molecular interfaces rather than on backbone conformations. Heterologous binding by chemically unrelated moieties exposing homologous molecular surfaces may be a common phenomenon in antigen–antibody interactions. This is especially evidenced by antibody binding mimics aimed at translating the knowledge acquired from broadly reactive antibodies to the design of better immunogens for the induction of antitumor immune responses.

In this review, we focus on some of the structural features of carbohydrate–antibody complexes that allow development of antibody-based immune reagents and are important in developing vaccine-design strategies. Continued progress in immunotherapy depends on the identification of target molecules aberrantly expressed on cancer cells and more efficient approaches for enhancing the immunogenicity of weak antigens. TACAs are attractive targets for immunotherapy strategies because the majority of cell-surface proteins and lipids are glycosylated, and the glycosyl moiety is fundamental to the biological functions of these molecules in cancer cells (Hakomori 2001, 2004). A unique advantage in targeting TACAs is that multiple proteins and lipids on cancer cells can simultaneously be modified with the same carbohydrate structure. Thus, targeting TACAs broadens the spectrum of antigens recognized by the immune system. This multiple antigen targeting is crucial for thwarting tumor escape (Pashov et al. 2009).

10.2 Nature of Carbohydrate-Binding Antibodies

One of the key functions for natural immunoglobulin M (IgM) in limiting the severity of infection is its immediate interaction with invading pathogens. Being preformed, natural IgM functionality depends heavily on polyspecific binding, which enables it to recognize phylogenetically conserved structures, such as nucleic acids, phospholipids, and carbohydrates. In this context, induction of IgM-reactive antibodies to TACA-expressing tumor cells is akin to the role played by circulating natural IgM antibodies as a first-line immune surveillance for eradicating blood-borne pathogens. Interestingly, multivalency, avidity, and polyspecificity are more important factors in the biological function of IgM antibodies than affinity per se. However, even though carbohydrate-reactive IgM antibodies possess these features, they are not considered useful for therapeutics due to their transient nature.

10.2.1 IgM Antibodies at the Forefront

IgM can exhibit antitumor activity by a variety of mechanisms and can be used as a biomarker to assess prognosis. Takahashi et al. (1999) suggested that carbohydrate-reactive IgM antibodies might play an important antitumor role, as antiganglioside IgM antibody levels correlated positively with improved survival in melanoma patients. Stimulation of TACA-reactive IgM may signify an early endogenous immune response to eliminate a "danger signal" from the tumor microenvironment and circulation (Ravindranath et al. 2005). The functions of IgM glycan-binding antibodies depend not only on the nature but also on the density of the target. Thus, specific targeting of tumor cells is due in part to overexpression of the carbohydrate antigen on tumor cells, which compensates for the low affinity of the carbohydrate cross-reactive antibodies (Zuckier et al. 2000).

Mechanisms by which antibodies can induce tumor cell clearance may also depend on whether the glycan is presented on glycolipids or glycoproteins (Ragupathi et al. 2005). To a large extent, IgM-facilitated tumor cell death depends on complement and complement receptors (Ragupathi et al. 2005; van Montfoort et al. 2007). While bound to a multivalent antigen, IgM antibodies change their conformations, which in turn facilitate complement fixation and thus render complement-mediated lysis more efficient. However, carbohydrate antibodies perform other functions as well, including the mediation of apoptosis (Brandlein et al. 2003; Monzavi-Karbassi et al. 2005; Vollmers and Brandlein 2005a, b; Vollmers and Brandlein 2009) and immune regulation (Ravindranath et al. 2005). Interestingly, the ratio of IgG to IgM may play a role in antitumor behavior (Ravindranath et al. 1998). TACA-directed approaches not only enforce a natural antitumor antibody response but also conform with a novel view of immunotherapy as being the control of complex immune processes more related to the interventions in autoimmunity, as opposed to a purely vaccinological view of tumor vaccines. A better understanding of the immunoregulatory aspect of anti-TACA responses, for example, will help us understand the link between TACA immunization, innate immunity, and cellular immunity.

10.2.2 Affinity Maturation and Structural Consequences

Affinity maturation provides important insights into the polyspecific and cross-reactive nature of antibodies. The repertoire of germline antibodies is sufficiently diverse to bind to any antigen. In fact, its completeness is ensured as much by its diversity as by the polyspecificity of each clone. Isotype switch from IgM to IgG roughly parallels but is not dependent on affinity maturation. For carbohydrate-reactive antibodies, there are consequences in this transition. Generally, the evolution of the antigen-driven maturation process involves somatic hypermutations that accumulate in the primary antibody repertoire, resulting in antibodies with improved recognition of cognate antigens. The driving force of this selection is increased affinity, which is argued to emerge from decreased flexibility and adjustment of the complementary surface features in the antibody–antigen interface. Epitope discrimination depends on fine-tuning of favorable interactions involving hydrogen bonds and electrostatic and van der Waals interactions, which also define antibody pliability.

Structural studies reveal that substitution mutations leading to antibody diversity occur more often in the loop regions of the complementarity-determining regions (CDRs) than in the framework regions, which predominantly have silent mutations. The question that arises is whether somatic hypermutation modifies contact residues, that is, those that are responsible for antigen binding during the primary immune response. This has a direct impact on antigen recognition by the humoral branch of adaptive immunity. The optimization of the binding by somatic mutations fixes the particular binding conformation, the flexible variable region of the precursor antibody attained upon antigen binding. In the context of evolution, the concept of convergence is usually reserved for the finding of different ways in which recognition occurs, or of antibodies originating from differing germline sequences that undergo mutations converging onto the recognition of a particular determinant. The possibility that some germline sequences have evolved to be adapted for carbohydrate binding in particular remains, but is not essential, as somatic mutations are observed within IgM antibodies.

Structural comparisons between antibody–antigen complexes of precursor or germline antibodies and the respective mature antibodies demonstrate improved short- and long-range interactions at the binding pocket. It might be expected that the network of intermolecular hydrogen bonds that antibodies employ to bind to an antigen increase upon antibody maturation, or that perhaps when compared against a germline antibody, the total electrostatic interaction energy in antigen binding might show enhancement. The immune system is able to solve the task of generating high-affinity receptors for the same ligand in multiple ways. Although reduced in the process of structural adaptation, the polyspecificity of the antigen-binding site does not have to disappear altogether. The different antibodies, evolved for binding the same carbohydrate epitope, then can display different spectra of cross-reactivity with additional structures.

10.2.3 A Case in Point

In early studies, we examined the recognition properties of the anti-Lewis Y (LeY) monoclonal antibody BR55-2 conferring LeY specificity compared to other LeY-reactive antibodies and GS-I (Blaszczyk-Thurin et al. 1996). The LeY determinant αFuc(1→2)βGal(1→4)[αFuc(1→3)]GlcNAc is a neolacto-structure (type 2), which is closely related to the lacto-series (type 1) of blood groups (Le^a and Le^b). LeY is long recognized as a potential target for anticancer immunotherapy because it is expressed in 70–90% of tumors of epithelial origin (breast, gastrointestinal, lung, prostate, and ovary) (Steplewski et al. 1990). The conformational properties of LeY and Le^b indicate that the core tetrasaccharide is very rigid (Blaszczyk-Thurin et al. 1996). Analysis of the binding profiles of lacto-series isomeric structures by BR55-2 suggested that the binding epitope includes the hydroxyls (OH-4, and OH-3 groups) of the β-D-galactose unit, the methyl (6-CH_3) groups of the two fucose units, and the *N*-acetyl group of the subterminal β-D-*N*-acetyl-glucosamine (β-D-GlcNAc) (Blaszczyk-Thurin et al. 1996). We observed that a major source of specificity for the LeY structure by anti-LeY antibodies emanates from interaction with the β-D-GlcNAc residue in addition to the nature of the structures that extend at the reducing site of the fucosylated lactosamine. The Gal(1→4)[Fuc(1→3)]GlcNAc (LeX) portion contributes to about 90% of the surface area buried by the binding to the BR55-2 antibody, with specificity for LeY over Le^b being dependent on the orientation of the GlcNAc moiety, in contrast to reactivity of Le^b and LeY with GS-I (Blaszczyk-Thurin et al. 1996).

Residues from the H chain form a highly complementary surface into which the LeX trisaccharide is nestled. In contrast, the LeY-specific terminal αFuc(1→2)Gal linkage resides at the top of the binding site and is stabilized by hydrogen bonding to an Asn at L28 of the L chain, but also remains largely immersed in the bulk solvent, much like that observed in the crystal structure of a humanized anti-LeY antibody, hu3S193 (Ramsland et al. 2004). Both hu3S193, its murine counterpart mu3S193, and the BR55-2 antibody are analogous to many antibodies that bind small molecules primarily through end-on insertion and anchored binding strategies (Ramsland et al. 2003, see also Chap. 9). Shape complementarity is not as apparent with residues of the L chain that participate in only a relatively small contact surface between CDR L1 and one face of the LeY-specific Fuc residue. The lack of contacts involving the L chain has effectively resulted in sizeable portions of a potential binding cavity remaining unoccupied by ligand.

Analysis of germline sequences for LeY-reactive antibodies suggests that the germline VH7183.a13.20/VH50.1 encodes the majority of LeY-reactive antibodies reported in the literature, with the light chain encoded by the *Vkcr1* germline gene

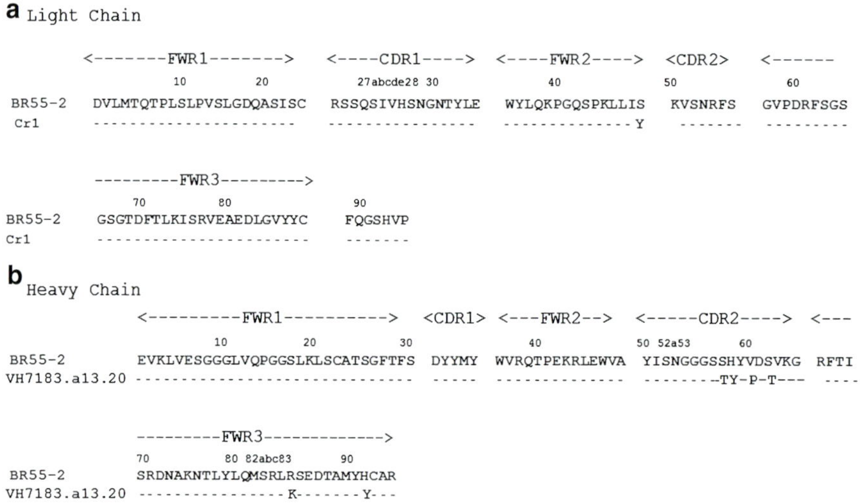

Fig. 10.1 Amino acid alignment of germline genes with BR55-2. Amino acid sequence alignment of the variable domains of (**a**) the light chain and (**b**) the heavy chains of BR55-2 and respective germline precursors. *Dashes* indicate identities with respect to BR55-2. Numbering corresponds to the Kabat numbering scheme

(Fig. 10.1). The single VH and VL gene segments used to encode LeY antibodies stands in contrast to the multiple VH and VL segments used by antibodies against other carbohydrate antigens. The use of a single VH segment from VH7183.a13.20/VH50.1 gene family by antibodies against at least three different ligand determinants (our unpublished data) is noteworthy. These structures provide insight into how inherited germline genes code for immunoglobulins of limited flexibility that are capable of binding a range of determinants from which affinity-matured antibodies are generated. Molecular dynamics calculations of antibody–LeY complexes, devoid of solvent effects, suggest that for the LeY-reactive antibodies BR55-2, B3, 1S3K, and mu3S193, major hydrogen bonding contacts are associated with residues found in the germline sequence (Table 10.1 and Fig. 10.1), yet each antibody can recognize different epitopes on the LeY determinant (our unpublished data). Only for BR96 have residue substitutions been identified that interact with LeY (i.e., H:GLN 52A).

It is generally accepted that normal follicular B cells undergo selection for mutations that lead to greater antigen-binding affinity. This selective pressure causes an enrichment of replacement mutations in the CDRs of the B-cell receptor (BCR), which have the most interaction with antigen, while they are limited in the framework regions. In normal germinal-center B cells, somatic hypermutation of the immunoglobulin genes occurs following stimulation of the BCR by antigen. Somatic hypermutation results in the substitution of nucleotides in the VDJ sequence of the immunoglobulin genes that can lead to either replacement or silent mutations. These changes lead to greater B-cell diversity by altering the binding

Table 10.1 Major LeY–antibody contact sites among anti-LeY antibodies

Antibody–LeY complex	Antibody contacting residues[a]
BR55-2	H:TYR50
	L:ASN28
	L:ASN28
	H:SER56
	H:SER56
B3	H:TYR35
	H:TYR35
	H:TYR35
	H:TYR50
	L:HIS27D
	L:ASN28
	L:HIS93
1S3K	L:HIS27D
	L:ASN28
	H:TYR33
	L:HIS93
	L:SER27E
BR96	H:TYR33
	H:GLN52A
mu3S193	H:TYR33
	L:SER27E
	H:TYR50
	L:HIS93

[a]Suggested contact residues are from molecular dynamics calculations of LeY–antibody complexes without solvent factors included in the calculations. Antibody residue numbering corresponds to that of Fig. 10.1

affinity of the BCR for the antigen. This pattern of replacement mutations indicates selection for immunoglobulins that have increased affinity for antigen yet have maintained their proper structure.

Because the maturation process is aimed at the development of antibodies with specificities for each antigenic determinant, amino acid residues forming the binding cavity should ideally undergo some sort of improvement in their binding capacity with maturation. However, the other side of this process is that distant mutations rigidify the best conformation out of those several that a flexible germline is capable of attaining. A glimpse of these processes is observed in analysis of a subset of murine anti-LeY antibodies and their germline precursor, which indicates that the contacting amino acid residues in the mature antibodies happen to be conserved even in the germline precursor. Selection rather acts on VDJ joining of CDR H3 and dictates the fine specificity of epitopes for the LeY determinate. This suggests that diversifying the repertoire of LeY reactivity does not confer any obvious advantages in terms of antigen-binding capacities as compared to the germline precursor.

We conclude that the repertoire for LeY reactivity did not confer any obvious advantages in terms of antigen-binding capacities from the germline precursor and is probably not an affinity-driven mechanism leading to convergence in binding of LeY-reactive antibodies. This further suggests that despite convergence in the antibody repertoire for an antigen, there is diversity in recognition of epitopes that define the antigen due to the fact that there are differences in the amino acid sequences, predominantly in the heavy-chain hypervariable (CDR H3) regions of the murine antibodies. Consequently, LeY-reactive antibodies might reflect the polyspecificities of natural antibodies with the use of a germline sequence that defines most of their interactions with the antigen, while VDJ diversity is used to reflect epitope specificity.

10.3 Molecular Mimicry Approach to Augment Anticarbohydrate Responses

10.3.1 Understanding Molecular Mimicry

Natural antibodies are inherently degenerate or polyspecific and thus cross-react with other structurally similar antigens with affinity in the micromolar range. The substitution of one antigen by another for antibody binding can be referred to as antigenic mimicry. There are numerous examples of antigenic mimicry of carbohydrate antigens in the context of replacing the carbohydrate binding to an antibody with a different ligand. Such surrogate antigens can also be immunogenic, inducing immune responses to the original, nominal antigen. Early studies suggested that anti-idiotypic (anti-Id) antibodies directed the triggering of pathogen-associated, antigen-specific immune responses to the polysaccharide capsules of *Escherichia coli* K13 (Stein and Soderstrom 1984), *E. coli* O111 (Klaerner et al. 1997), *Neisseria meningitidis* group C (Westerink et al. 1988), *Streptococcus pneumoniae* (McNamara et al. 1984), *N. gonorrhoeae* LOS (Gulati et al. 1996), and chlamydial exoglycolipid antigen (An et al. 1997); and to the lipopolysaccharide of *Pseudomonas aeruginosa* (Schreiber et al. 1991a, b) and the mucoid exopolysaccharide of *P. aeruginosa* (Schreiber et al. 1991a, b). Anti-Id antibodies that mimic tumor-associated carbohydrate antigens were described for αFuc(1→3)Gal (Diakun and Matta 1989), sialyl SSEA-1 (sialyl-LeX) (Tsuyuoka et al. 1996), sialyl-Le^{a} (Furuya et al. 1992), carbohydrates associated with tumor-associated glycoprotein TAG-72 (Schmolling et al. 1995), the Globo H saccharide epitope (Viale et al. 1987), the disialogangliosides GD2 (Sen et al. 1998) and GD3 (Chapman 2003), and the gangliosides GM2 (Chapman et al. 2000) and GM3 (Kanda et al. 1994), just to mention a few.

The structural basis for mimicry by such anti-Id antibodies is still not entirely clear. In one instance, it was found that both VH and VL regions contributed to the antigenicity of an anti-Id antibody that mimics the melanoma-associated ganglioside GM3 (Kanda et al. 1994). Crystallographic analysis of an anti-Id carbohydrate surrogate indicated that the anti-idiotope was found to be unable to carry an "internal image" of the antigen and therefore would not induce polysaccharide-specific "anti-anti-idiotopes" because the polysaccharide-binding cleft on the isolating antibody was too narrow and too deep to allow comprehensive contact with the binding site of the anti-Id antibody (Evans et al. 1994). Some structural mimicry has been observed in the complexes of several mimetic proteins. Examples include the complex of a camel heavy-chain antibody against lysozyme, where parts of some residues of the antibody mimic parts of the sugar substrate of lysozyme (Transue et al. 1998), and also the complex of porcine pancreatic-amylase with the proteinaceous inhibitor, where several specific hydrogen-bonding and hydrophobic interactions with the carbohydrate substrate are mimicked by the inhibitor (Bompard-Gilles et al. 1996).

In the case of the camel single-domain antibody, it was shown that a single variable domain fragment derived from a lysozyme-specific camel antibody naturally lacking light chains mimicked the oligosaccharide substrate functionally (inhibition constant for lysozyme, 50 nM) and structurally (lysozyme buried surface areas, hydrogen bond partners, and hydrophobic contacts similar to those seen in sugar-complex structures) (Transue et al. 1998). Most striking was the mimicry by the antibody's CDR 3 loop (which is longer than in murine or human antibodies), especially Ala104, which mimics the subsite C sugar 2-acetamido group. This group was previously identified as a key feature in binding lysozyme. Of particular note was the observation of the potential for the backbone of the CDR 3 loop to parallel the three-dimensional position of the linkages of the carbohydrate substrate within the binding site.

Insight also comes from an earlier analysis of amylase inhibitors (Mirkov et al. 1995; Murai et al. 1985). Seeds of the common bean contain three homologous proteins: phytohemagglutinin (PHA)-E, PHA-L, and the lectin-like protein α-amylase inhibitor. Structural studies suggest that the active site of α-amylase inhibitor consists of the tri-amino acid contacts Trp188, Arg74, and Tyr190, which define an analogous Trp-Arg-Tyr motif of loop 1 of tendamistat. In addition, the processing of the polypeptide at Asn77 may be necessary to bring these residues in close proximity. In tendamistat, loop 1 has the lowest B factors and is the major contributor to α-amylase binding. Most of the side chains composing this loop point in the same direction and are exposed to solvent. One of the two disulfide bonds in tendamistat connects the bases of the antiparallel β-strands flanking loop 1. This conformation is similar to that found for CDR 3 loops of antibodies. In this context, we found that the CDR H3 of the heavy chain of an anti-Id antibody that mimicked the C polysaccharide of *N. meningitidis* contained the residue tract YYRYD that contributed to the mimicry of the nominal antigen (Westerink et al. 1995). This peptide proved able to elicit a protective immune response against bacterial challenge (Westerink et al. 1995).

Just like anti-Id antibodies and natural proteins, peptides can substitute for carbohydrate compounds to target pathways involving either protein–carbohydrate interactions or carbohydrate-specific immunological reactions (Buchwald et al. 2005; Maitta et al. 2004; Melzer et al. 2003; Monzavi-Karbassi et al. 2002; Park et al. 2004; Prinz et al. 2004). Early on, it was observed that π–π (i.e., aromatic–aromatic) interactions appear to play a role as mimics for a variety of carbohydrate subunit interactions (Hoess et al. 1993; Murai et al. 1985; Oldenburg et al. 1992; Scott et al. 1992; Shikhman and Cunningham 1994; Shikhman et al. 1994; Valadon et al. 1996; Westerink et al. 1995). It is likely that the overall mechanism of a peptide binding to an antibody can differ from that of carbohydrate (Vyas et al. 2003), much like that observed for multiple peptides reacting with the same antibody (Keitel et al. 1997). Nevertheless, similar groups on lectins or antibodies can bind peptide mimetics as they do carbohydrate antigens (Luo et al. 2000). Structural similarity has been noted for a WYPY motif peptide, reactive with concanavalin A (ConA), that emulates an extended conformation observed in *Sesbania* mosaic virus coat protein. This extended conformation overlaps conformationally with the pentasaccharide within the ConA-binding site (Cunto-Amesty et al. 2001), much like that observed for the CDR 3 loop of camel heavy chains (Transue et al. 1998).

10.3.2 Carbohydrate Mimetic Peptides

With the use of chemical (peptide libraries) and immunological information, novel peptide immunogens have been defined that function as mimotopes generating immune responses to carbohydrate antigens. We previously reviewed the structural concepts and approaches used in vaccine design that illustrate the value and limitations of mimotopes targeting TACAs (Pashov et al. 2005) and the human immunodeficiency virus (Pashov et al. 2007). In this context, we showed early on that concepts associated with pharmacophore design could be used to define carbohydrate mimetic peptides (CMPs) applied to vaccine design (Cunto-Amesty et al. 2001; Luo et al. 2000). We demonstrated that a structure-assisted vaccine design approach, whereby small molecules, defined in crystallographic databases, could be used to theoretically define peptide mimetics emulating the three-dimensional interaction scheme of a native carbohydrate antigen (Luo et al. 2000). More important, it was shown that virtual screening led to experimental observation of motifs (Luo et al. 2000). We also showed that by use of this approach, an immunogenic peptide could be designed *de novo* (Cunto-Amesty et al. 2001).

The fine specificity of antibodies and lectins for glycan ligands can be used to guide the development of CMPs. Figure 10.2 outlines the general development of CMPs in vaccine design. However, the identification of patterns of amino acids common for antibody- and lectin-selected peptides is challenging because many of the carbohydrate binding antibodies and lectins are polyreactive and bind with varying affinities. Polyreactive natural antibodies were previously described to select diverse peptides that had either no obvious motif (Manivel et al. 2002) or a general amino acid bias toward proline (Tchernychev et al. 1997). However, there may be biasing in the type of amino acids that are found in peptides that bind to carbohydrate-binding proteins. Aromatic residues and hydrophobic and hydrogen-bonding amino acids seem favored. Such biased sequences do not necessarily converge on a canonical set of patterns, although some motifs stand out.

Fig. 10.2 Lectin-based vaccine design. CMPs can be defined in a four-step process. (1) Lectins that trigger apoptosis of tumor cells are defined. (2) Biopanning against a random peptide display library identifies potential CMPs, which are confirmed by carbohydrate-peptide inhibition assays. (3) The potential of the CMPs to induce TACA-reactive antibodies is evaluated, as is (4) the ability of CMP-induced antibodies to mediate apoptosis of tumor cells

Analysis of peptide selection by antibody–lectin templates suggests possibilities that can have an impact on design strategies. (1) Selected peptides can be considered as probes of the different conformations that the binding site can accommodate. Such is the situation observed for multiple peptides that react with the same antibody (Keitel et al. 1997). (2) Templates can bind to many peptides with different sets of molecular interactions. With few exceptions, most peptides display a significant number of interactions with the heavy chain of antibodies (Nair et al. 2000). It has been suggested that the judicious choice of peptides for testing should be based on the peptide interaction with both the heavy and light chain in order to induce antibodies with similar antigen-specific properties (Luo et al. 2000), as the combination of heavy and light chains will influence specificity (Kabat and Wu 1991). (3) If several carbohydrate-specific templates select the same peptide motif, the peptide might be considered a mimic of multiple carbohydrate antigens. Such a peptide either mimics a common epitope between diverse antigens (as we have described as a basis for antibody cross-reactivity with the C polysaccharide of *N. meningitidis* and the LeY antigen (Agadjanyan et al. 1997)) or is capable of adopting different conformations. (4) To further assess the value of the motifs identified and the amino acid–composition bias found, the structural features of the motifs must be evaluated by molecular modeling, nuclear magnetic resonance (NMR) spectroscopy, or crystallography.

Although structural analysis may raise confidence that the isolated peptide will have functional value, the induction of cross-reactive immune responses remains the ultimate proof of mimicry. In this context, we have shown that CMPs reactive with lectins can induce antibodies with the same functionality (Monzavi-Karbassi et al. 2005). To generate sustained immunity to TACAs, we developed CMPs as immunogens with overlapping B and T cell epitopes to link TACA reactive humoral responses with anti-tumor cellular responses. We observed that CMP immunization led to significant tumor growth inhibition in therapeutic and prophylactic mouse models, even when only the low-titer anti-TACA antibodies were elicited (Kieber-Emmons et al. 1999; Monzavi-Karbassi et al. 2002, 2005, 2007). CMPs can induce antitumor cellular responses, including CMP- and TACA-reactive T-helper 1 (Th1) $CD4^+$ cells and tumor-specific $CD8^+$ cells, which may compensate for low-titer humoral responses (Cunto-Amesty et al. 2001; Monzavi-Karbassi et al. 2005). Most of all, unlike TACAs, CMPs can prime for memory responses to TACAs (Monzavi-Karbassi et al. 2003), suggesting that CMPs facilitate cognate interactions between B cells and T cells that TACAs do not facilitate.

10.4 Making Use of Overlapping Recognition Sites That Define Epitopes on Determinant

Despite our success in using CMPs to induce cross-reactive immune responses to TACAs, surprisingly, we observed that the mimotopes induce low titers of serum antibodies that cross-reacted with TACAs. It is desirable to increase the TACA-reactive titers upon CMP immunization. Our working hypothesis is that this weak TACA-cross-reactive humoral immune response does not reflect the low immunogenicity of CMPs but rather their poor mimicry of TACAs. In support of this proposition is the fact that structural analysis of anti-Id antibody–antibody complexes or peptide surrogates of antigens in complex with monoclonal antibody (mAb) typically indicates that these molecules only approximate the topology of interactions and are therefore not exact structural mimics of the original antigen. The question of whether CMPs that elicit carbohydrate-binding antibodies are structural mimics of carbohydrates, or merely functional mimics that may interact with the antibody-combining site in a different manner from TACAs, is fundamental to our understanding of the immunological response parameters associated with mimotope immunization.

10.4.1 Improving Mimicry by Rational Design

One common theme in glycomimetic studies is that peptides selected on template biopanning do not necessarily mimic the structure of the nominal antigen; in addition, they bind to their cognate partner with micromolar affinity. This raises interesting questions: how is the weaker binding peptide able to mimic function and how important is structural mimicry? One possible explanation for lower affinity is that the carbohydrate–protein interactions involve solvents or metal ion at the binding site. In the ConA-peptide structures, no such feature is observed (Jain et al. 2000). It is possible that exclusion of solvents/ions by peptide might be responsible for the weaker affinity without sacrificing functionality, and a true structural mimic might require fidelity of chirality. These possibilities raise the question of how one can enhance the ability of TACA-mimetic peptides to induce TACA-specific antibodies with higher titers and association constants. We are testing the hypothesis that improving the hydrogen bond pattern through amino acid substitutions in a CMP, to be coincident with that for the carbohydrate ligand, will enhance the ability of CMPs to elicit anti-TACA antibodies with high titers and association constants.

Hydrogen bonds, which are highly directional, represent an important set of interactions to establish a basis for mimicry because they mainly confer the specificity in binding of the peptide and the carbohydrate antigen. We previously suggested that peptides could interact with similar amino acids on BR55-2 to those on LeY and GD2 interacting with an anti-GD2 antibody. Among peptides reactive with BR55-2 are those that contain a centralized WRY motif. We previously showed that WRY-containing peptides, such as P106, could bind to BR55-2 and that immunization with these CMPs could induce responses targeting LeY-expressing cell lines. Using the recognition properties of BR55-2 as a model system, we established a molecular perspective of peptide mimicry for LeY by comparing the three-dimensional-binding basis of BR55-2 to LeY with the binding of the same antibody to CMPs (Luo et al. 2000). In this case, computer-aided structural design was shown to agree with motifs identified from biopanning with BR55-2 against a random peptide library. Conformational studies indicate that the (W/Y)(R/L)Y and (W/Y)PY motifs can adopt extended turn-like structures, suggesting that a particular peptide structure is required for polysaccharide mimicry (Luo et al. 2000). The peptide mimics compete with LeY, as demonstrated by enzyme-linked immunosorbent assay (ELISA) and surface plasmon resonance (Biacore Life Sciences) analysis (Luo et al. 2000). The computer program LUDI (Accelrys, Corp., San Diego, CA) was used to map epitopes of the antibody-combining site, correlating peptide reactivity patterns. This approach identified amino acids interacting with the same BR55-2 functional residue groups that recognize the αFuc(1→3) moiety of LeY. Molecular modeling indicates that the peptides adopt an extended turn conformation within the BR55-2 combining site that serves to overlap the peptides with the LeY spatial position. Peptide binding is associated with only minor changes in BR55-2 relative to the BR55-2–LeY complex. Antipeptide serum distinguishes the αFuc(1→3) from the αFuc(1→4) linkage, therefore differentiating difucosylated neolacto-series antigens (Luo et al. 1998). These results indicate that peptides and carbohydrates can bind to the same antibody-binding site and that peptides can structurally and functionally mimic salient features of carbohydrate epitopes.

A WRY motif-containing CMP with the sequence GVVWRYTAPVHLGDG, referred to as P10, was also identified as a GD2 mimic by panning of a peptide library on the GD2-binding mAb ME36.1 (Qiu et al. 1999). P10 induces an antitumor immune response either as simply a multiple-antigen peptide (MAP) or after conjugation to KLH (Wondimu et al. 2008). The disialoganglioside βGalNAc (1→4)[αNeuAc(2→8)αNeuAc(2→3)]βGal(1→4)βGlc(1→1)Cer (GD2) is a cell-surface component that appears on the surface of metastatic melanoma cells and is a marker for disease progression. Determination of the crystal structure of the Fab fragment of ME36.1 shows that its CDR forms a groove-shaped binding site (Pichla et al. 1997). Molecular modeling has placed a four-residue sugar, representative of GD2, in the antigen-binding site that not only shows much of the interaction with GD2 contributed by heavy-chain interactions (predominated by His at position 35 of the heavy chain) but also displays strong interactions with Arg90 of the light chain (Pichla et al. 1997). On the basis of hydrogen-bonding schemes with the GD2 antigen, ME36.1 has the potential to interact with the GalNAc moiety of GD2 by ME36.1 residues Thr H33, Asn H59, and Asp H50; the Gal moiety of GD2 by ME36.1 residues Thr H33, His35, and Ser 100 H; αNeuAc(2→3) residue by Ser 100 H; and αNeuAc(2→8) residue by Tyr L93. This primary interaction scheme suggests that ME36.1 could react with GD2, possibly GD3, and perhaps with GM2, GM3, GD1b, and GD1a. Such broad specificity for these important tumor-associated TACAs in fact has been argued for by using ME36.1 in the clinic, and emphasizes the importance of inducing multiple specificity toward tumor antigens (i.e., binding of an antibody to two or more TACAs). Consequently, defining CMPs reactive with ME36.1 might in turn induce antibodies with a broader spectrum of ganglioside reactivity.

To understand how the CMP P10 might functionally mimic GD2 in binding to ME36.1, we used conformational and energy analysis (Pashov et al. 2005) to define potential binding modes of this peptide in the crystallographically defined ME36.1-binding pocket (Monzavi-Karbassi et al. 2007). However, modeling of GD2 showed that the sugar formed extensive interactions, including hydrogen bonds with CDR residues. The estimated free energy (ΔG_{GD2}) was about –10.6 kcal/mol. Comparison of the binding modes of P10 and GD2 showed a similar binding energetic ($\Delta G_{P10} = -17$ kcal/mol); the interaction pattern, however, is quite different. Whereas GD2 made at least two contacts each with CDR H1, H2, and H3, the peptide made only two contacts, with CDR H3 and H1; much of its binding energy derived from the hydrophobic contacts (Monzavi-Karbassi et al. 2007).

To relate the potential binding-mode conformation with solution structures, we performed NMR spectroscopy on the P10 peptide. Preliminary ^{13}C NMR spectroscopy analysis of P10 defined 199 possible solution conformations based on nuclear Overhauser effect distance constraints. Among these is a population of structures similar to the calculated binding-mode structure of P10 (a root-mean-square deviation of 2.2 Å). We calculated the transition energy (–2.8 kcal/mol) required to go from the average solution structure to the binding-mode structure, based on our previous approach to calculating transition energies. These data suggest that our modeling is sufficiently robust to define binding-mode structures that reflect solution structures.

10.4.2 Redesigning P10 and Defining the Structure for Mimicry

The P10 peptide inhibited the binding of ME36.1 to GD2 and induced antitumor immune responses (Wondimu et al. 2008). On the basis of hydrogen-bonding schemes with the GD2 antigen, we wanted to determine whether we could modify

P10 to increase the level of GD2 antigenic mimicry. From conformational studies, we surmised that removing the first three residues of P10 would result in a binding mode with ME36.1 with an increased number of hydrogen bonds in common with the way the GD2 antigen binds to ME36.1 (Monzavi-Karbassi et al. 2007). To reflect its shorter sequence (WRYTAPVHLGD), we refer to this peptide as P10 short (P10s). The redesigned CMP (P10s) shares five hydrogen bonds with GD2 in binding to ME36.1 (Monzavi-Karbassi et al. 2007). Molecular docking calculations indicated that the topographical binding mode of P10s overlaps that of GD2 in the ME36.1-combining site.

Because P10 was selected against ME36.1, it was of interest to determine whether P10s could also bind to another anti-GD2 mAb and compete with GD2 for binding to this second mAb. If cross-reactivity occurred with the second antibody, one could conclude that P10s reflected the most salient feature of GD2 underlying the recognition by anti-GD2 antibodies. The mAb 14G2a is an anti-GD2 antibody that has been tested clinically. As expected, P10s competed with GD2 for 14G2a binding (Fig. 10.3). In this assay, GD2 was incorporated into a lipid monolayer; incorporation was facilitated by coating onto a Biacore HPA sensor chip. This immobilization to the chip is likely to represent GD2‘s anchoring into cell membranes, better emulating the natural presentation of the antigen than in ELISAs.

Lectins, such as *Arachis hypogea* agglutinin/peanut lectin, *Amaranthus caudatus* lectin, or *Artocarpus integrifolia*/jacalin, have been extensively used to detect TACAs on cell surfaces. CMPs have previously been defined by biopanning with lectins. Binding of P10s to lectins would provide yet another perspective on the mimicry properties of P10s. The lectins used included wheat germ agglutinin (WGA), which is reactive with GlcNAc and sialic acid (αNeuAc) moieties; GS-I, which is reactive with the αGal and αGalNAc moieties; and *Vicia villosa*, which is reactive with αGalNAc moieties. Interestingly, GS-I and WGA showed the highest reactivity with P10s (Fig. 10.4), suggesting that P10s might be a mimic for Gal and GlcNAc/αNeuAc, which are sugar moieties found in ganglioside structures such as GD2 (βGalNAc(1→4)[αNeuAc(2→8)αNeuAc(2→3)]βGal(1→4)Glc (1→1)Cer) and the type 2 core structures [Gal(1→4)GlcNAc] of LeY αFuc (1→2)βGal(1→4)[αFuc(1→3)]βGlcNAc(1→3)-R and LeX βGal(1→4)[αFuc (1→3)]βGlcNAc(1→3)-R, respectively. P10 and P10s also contain a WRY motif. Therefore, we tested P10 and P10s for binding to the anti-LeY antibody BR55-2 by surface plasmon resonance analysis (Fig. 10.5), confirming the observation that BR55-2 can bind to WRY-containing peptides.

Our modeling studies indicated that the P10s peptide represented a more faithful mimic of ganglioside binding of the mAb ME36.1 than its P10 homologue, based on hydrogen bonding of ME36.1 to GD2. The loss of three residues in the *N*-terminus of P10s relative to the P10 peptide appeared to affect the P10s antibody binding-mode conformation, more faithfully contacting antibody side chains in a similar fashion to GD2 in its ME36.1-binding mode. P10s was observed to bind with higher affinity to the mAb and to induce more robust immune responses to the GD2 antigen without losing its ability to bind to LeY-binding antibodies.

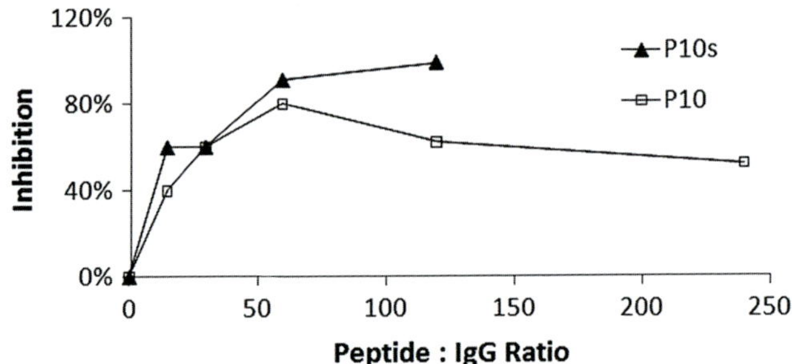

Fig. 10.3 Inhibition of binding of the anti-GD2 mAb 14G2a to GD2 with P10s. Inhibition of the binding of 14G2a antibody to GD2 by P10-MAP and P10s-MAP was measured by surface plasmon resonance. Hydrophobic surface chips (HPA, Biacore) were coated with phosphatidyl choline liposomes, and GD2 was incorporated into the lipid layer. The antibodies were passed over this surface at 1 μg/mL with or without the respective (P10 or P10s) CMP-MAP. The maximum binding and concentration of the ligand were optimized with BIAevaluation software (Biacore). The derived effective concentration of antibodies in the presence of inhibitor was used to calculate inhibition

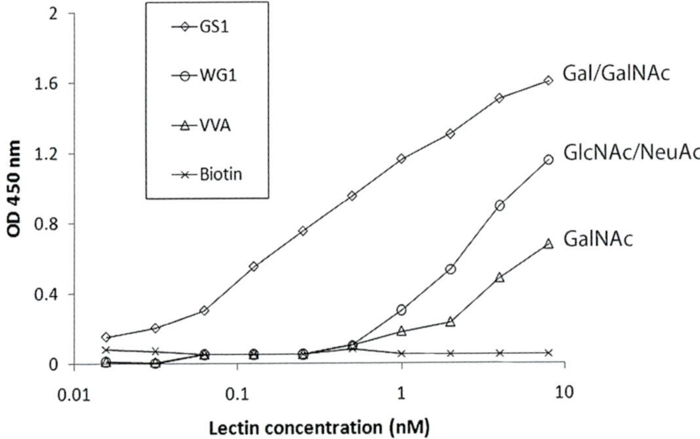

Fig. 10.4 Lectin binding to P10s peptide. Plates were coated with 20 μg/mL of P10s-MAP and incubated with serial concentrations of biotinylated lectins. Lectin binding was detected by streptavidin-peroxidase (1:10,000 dilution, 100 μL/well). Absorbance at 450 nm as read after 30 min of color development. Assays were performed in duplicate, and the average values are shown

Consequently, P10s displayed both increased antigenicity and humoral immunogenicity over the P10 peptide. This observation extended previous studies demonstrating that it was the topological or conformational similarity of the antigenic surfaces rather than sequence homology that dictated cross-reactivity and molecular mimicry. Such results confirmed that conformationally peptides and carbohydrates could bind to the same antibody-binding site and that peptides

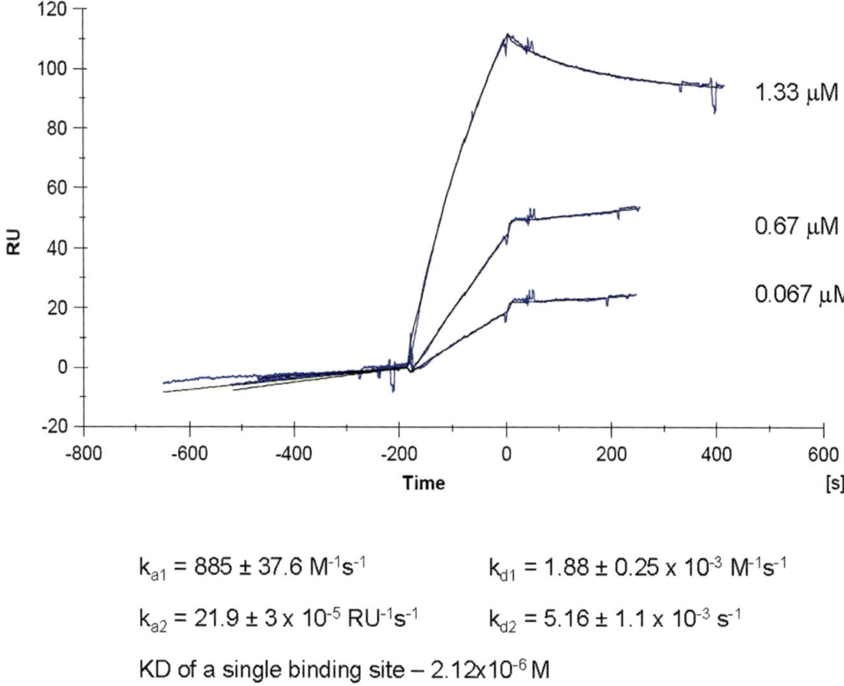

Fig. 10.5 BR55-2 binding to P10s. P10s was immobilized on a C1 chip to reduce interference with the dextran matrix. BR55-2 was run over the chip surface at 20 μL/min at 0.67 μM (*lower curve*) and 1.33 μM (*upper curve*) concentrations. The sensograms represent the difference between the positive and the control channels. The data were fitted by using the Langmuir binding model. The dissociation constant (K_d) for binding was calculated to be 1.2 × 10^{-7} M

could structurally mimic salient features of carbohydrate epitopes. Tuning the immune response by controlling the structural features of a designable immunogen can be achieved. The potential remains to further identify CMPs that are immunogenic to amplify functional carbohydrate-directed immune responses against circulating or disseminated tumor cells to have an impact on cancer survival.

10.4.3 P10s Binding to Human Antibodies

The broad carbohydrate cross-reactivity of P10s was mapped on the human preimmune IgG repertoire (intravenous immunoglobulin [IVIg]) with glycan arrays. The set of cross-reactive glycans included several tumor-associated antigens and short-chain gangliosides, but not the nominal antigen for the template antibody, ME36.1. Some non-self-reactivities, such as the anti-αGal epitope or the anti-globo-H epitope, were very high in the starting mixture, as these reactivities are normally highly represented in the IgG repertoire; although they are not highly enriched, they are very strong among the cross-reactivities of anti-P10s IgG. Other reactivities were very weak in the normal IgG repertoire (e.g., anti-GD3), as was expected because most of these antigens are well tolerated self-antigens. A high reactivity to these antigens in the P10s fraction led to very high enrichment ratios. As in the case of serum titers, these reactivities could not be attributed solely to affinity or concentration per se but were instead likely to represent the biologically relevant cross-reactivity of P10s.

Immunization of humans with CMPs will either induce new antibodies within the repertoire or perhaps stimulate B cells with carbohydrate specificities. The carbohydrate cross-reactivity of CMPs warrants searching for the respective specificities in the human repertoire of preimmune or natural antibodies. A large proportion of CMP-binding antibodies also bind to diverse carbohydrate epitopes in a polyspecific manner. Indeed we were able to precipitate, from a human IgG preparation for intravenous use (IVIg), IgG antibodies that bound to CMP as MAPs. Their broad specificity prompted investigation into the level of their specificity for different CMPs to rule out nonspecific stickiness. Immune complexes of IgG binding to the CMPs were precipitated from IVIg. The precipitated antibodies were predominantly of IgG2 isotype, which is in line with our hypothesis that these CMPs are recognized predominantly by carbohydrate-reactive antibodies (Fig. 10.6).

Because P10s is reactive with GS-I, we used a glycan array to compare the binding of the enriched P10s human IVIg fraction with the reactivity of GS-I. The polyspecificity of GS-I- and P10s-binding fractions of normal human IgG (Gammagard S/D) were compared for glycan-binding patterns (Fig. 10.7). Both reagents showed a degree of polyspecificity with a group of clearly negatively charged glycans. Correlation of the binding patterns suggested a weak cross-reactivity of the P10s-enriched serum antibodies with blood group A and B antigens, LeY, disulphated-Lewis X trisaccharide, and α-D-Gal, with a high binding affinity to βGalNAc (Tnβ) antigen. This observation paralleled earlier studies suggesting that the human anti-Tn antibodies that are able to bind to tumor tissue are more prone to bind to the beta form than to the alpha form of the synthetic antigen. Anti-Tnβ IgG titers have been found to correlate with the grade of gastrointestinal tumors (Smorodin et al. 2007). Possibly, this is the same reactivity as that we found in natural antibodies.

An essential feature of antibodies is the isotype distribution, which affects the involvement of different Fc and complement receptors and the subsequent functional effects. Among these effects that are of special interest in tumor immunotherapy is antigen cross-presentation. The isotype composition reactive with P10s and other CMPs verifies that CMPs are mimics of carbohydrates in that the predominant reactive isotype within the human repertoire is IgG2. In humans, IgG1 and IgG3 show higher affinity than IgG2 for most Fc receptors, which might translate into diminished functional activity for such antibodies. However, a portion of antibodies with the IgG1 isotype is reactive with P10s and other TACA forms. The cross-reactivity between natural antibodies and tumor-associated antigens and TACA, reflected, for example, by the high-molecular-weight mucin MUC-1, would suggest that it might be difficult to ascertain the contribution of a *de novo* antibody immune response to MUC-1 compared with a response by anti-TACA memory B

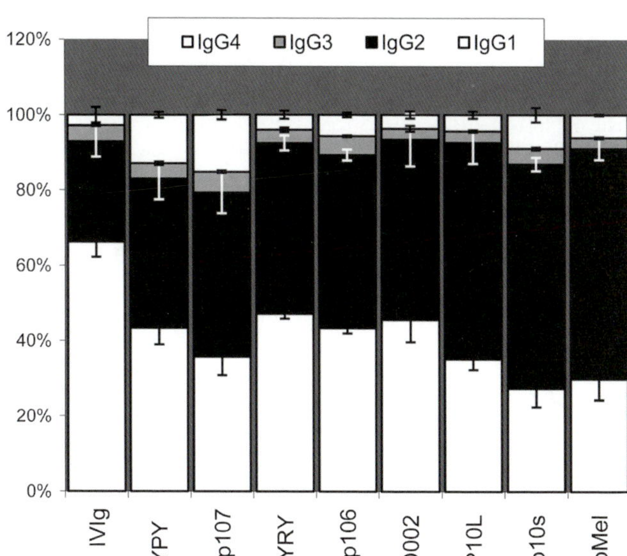

Fig. 10.6 Isotype composition of human preimmune IgG isolated from IgG by polyethylene glycol precipitation of immune complexes on different CMPs. Enrichment in IgG2 was generally observed. It is known that IgG2 antibodies (IgG3 in mice) can be produced in T cell-independent type 2 (TI-2) responses to carbohydrates. One-half of CMPs are also recognized by IgG4 antibodies, which share with IgG2 a lack of complement-activating activity but not a TI-2 origin. IgG4 antibodies represent some carbohydrate specificities and function, mostly as inhibitory and anti-inflammatory antibodies due to arm exchange. Apart from p106, P10, and P10s, the CMPs used included p107 (GGIYYRYDIYYRYDIYYRYD), PYPY (RGGLCYCPYPYCVCVGR), YPYRY (RGGLCYCY-PYRYCVCVGR), D002 (RGGLCYCRYRYCVCVGR), and pMel (VLYRYGSFSV), gp100 (476-485), or G10 (476)

cells stimulated in a thymus-independent manner. The presence of natural TACA-reactive antibodies that are polyreactive would lead to the formation of immune complexes taken up by macrophages and dendritic cells if the isotype of the complex lends itself to efficient uptake. In this context, uptake would facilitate cellular responses, providing new interventions for enhancing antitumor immunotherapy by facilitating epitope spreading.

10.5 Summary

As clinical correlates have highlighted carbohydrate-reactive IgM responses to cancer cells in humans, attention to antibody subsets is warranted to further understand and develop strategies to augment these responses, which might have a further impact on tumor-reactive cellular responses. Natural polyreactive antibodies that bind to tumor cells have been studied on several occasions. They are germline-encoded antibodies mostly from CD5^{+} B cells (the B1 genotype), and

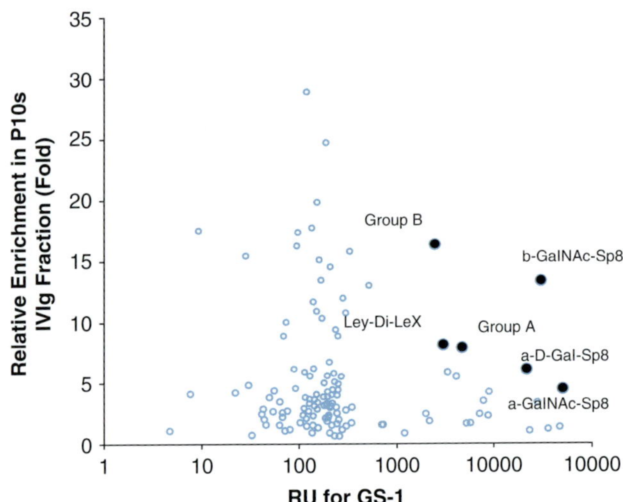

Fig. 10.7 Correlation between the polyspecificity of GS-I and anti-P10s antibody binding. The fraction of normal human IgG (IVIg, Gammagard S/D, Baxter/Hyland, Deerfield, IL) enriched on a P10s column was tested on glycan arrays (in collaboration with the Consortium for Functional Glycomics). The reactivity of GS-I is expressed in relative units after subtraction of the background, while that of the IVIg anti-P10s fraction is expressed as enrichment relative to the reactivity of the nonfractionated IVIg or the ratio of the response units (RU) of the P10s binding fraction and IVIg. The six reactivities that were strongest for both reagents are labeled. Note the overall orthogonal profile of the polyspecificity, with the common recognition of βGalNAc as the only true high binder for both P10s and GS-1

they bind to various tumor antigens, induce apoptosis of tumor cells, and detect not only malignant cells but also the precursor cellular stages. Natural polyreactive IgM autoantibodies, encoded by unmutated germline Ig V genes, represent a major fraction of the normal circulating IgM repertoire. Such antibodies fulfill the definition of autoantibodies, as they are self-reactive but have broad reactivity and bind mostly to altered antigens. Even in mouse models, nonimmunized mice of widely differing genetic backgrounds have detectable IgM antibodies to tumor cell-surface carbohydrates, their natural resistance to the tumor being related to their serum IgM levels. Analysis of functional antipathogen and antitumor immune responses involving glycan recognition suggests that multivalency, avidity, and polyreactivity are more important factors in the biological function of the antibodies than affinity per se. This provides insight into immune-surveillance paradigms to devise vaccine strategies.

Such analyses suggest that we pay more attention to the role of the major B-cell subpopulations and that carbohydrate-reactive IgM antibodies in particular may help bridge cellular responses. Expansion of the pool of memory B and T cells by CMP vaccination or activation of residual TACA memory B and T cells might be of benefit for the course of immunization. Multivalent CMPs target B1 cells and are hypothesized to facilitate the Th1 responses observed with CMPs. Understanding how to manipulate carbohydrate-reactive natural antibodies suggests that targeting the "natural memory" B-cell repertoire might provide novel mechanisms to prevent recurrence of disease mediated through $CD4^+$ T-cell responses. Unlike carbohydrate antigens and carbohydrate-conjugate vaccines, CMPs prime B and T cells for subsequent memory of carbohydrate antigens, facilitating long-term surveillance through recall of carbohydrate immune responses. This effect may minimize the need for constant boosting. In addition, CMPs can functionally emulate conserved structures of TACA, inducing antibodies that recognize multiple TACAs and therefore function like a TACA-multivalent vaccine. Therefore, we hypothesize that the immunotherapeutic potential of CMPs is related to their capacity to stimulate B-cell compartments that bridge innate and adaptive immunity.

References

Agadjanyan M, Luo P, Westerink MA, Carey LA, Hutchins W, Steplewski Z, Weiner DB, Kieber-Emmons T (1997) Peptide mimicry of carbohydrate epitopes on human immunodeficiency virus. Nat Biotechnol 15:547–551

An LL, Hudson AP, Prendergast RA, O'Brien TP, Stuart ES, Whittum HJ, MacDonald AB (1997) Biochemical and functional antigenic mimicry by a polyclonal anti-idiotypic antibody for chlamydial exoglycolipid antigen. Pathobiology 65:229–240

Apicella MA, Griffiss JM, Schneider H (1994) Isolation and characterization of lipopolysaccharides, lipooligosaccharides, and lipid A. [Review] [34 refs]. Methods Enzymol 235: 242–252

Appelmelk BJ, Simoons SI, Negrini R, Moran AP, Aspinall GO, Forte JG, De VT, Quan H, Verboom T, Maaskant JJ, Ghiara P, Kuipers EJ, Bloemena E, Tadema TM, Townsend RR, Tyagarajan K, Crothers JJ, Monteiro MA, Savio A, De GJ (1996) Potential role of molecular mimicry between *Helicobacter pylori* lipopolysaccharide and host Lewis blood group antigens in autoimmunity. Infect Immun 64:2031–2040

Appelmelk BJ, Negrini R, Moran AP, Kuipers EJ (1997) Molecular mimicry between *Helicobacter pylori* and the host. [Review] [31 refs]. Trends Microbiol 5:70–73

Apweiler R, Hermjakob H, Sharon N (1999) On the frequency of protein glycosylation, as deduced from analysis of the SWISS-PROT database. Biochim Biophys Acta 1473:4–8

Bertozzi CR, Kiessling LL (2001) Chemical glycobiology. Science 291:2357–2364

Blaszczyk-Thurin M, Murali R, Westerink MA, Steplewski Z, Co MS, Kieber-Emmons T (1996) Molecular recognition of the Lewis Y antigen by monoclonal antibodies. Protein Eng 9:447–459

Bompard-Gilles C, Rousseau P, Rouge P, Payan F (1996) Substrate mimicry in the active center of a mammalian alpha-amylase: structural analysis of an enzyme–inhibitor complex. Structure 4:1441–1452

Brandlein S, Pohle T, Ruoff N, Wozniak E, Muller-Hermelink HK, Vollmers HP (2003) Natural IgM antibodies and immunosurveillance mechanisms against epithelial cancer cells in humans. Cancer Res 63:7995–8005

Buchwald UK, Lees A, Steinitz M, Pirofski LA (2005) A peptide mimotope of type 8 pneumococcal capsular polysaccharide induces a protective immune response in mice. Infect Immun 73: 325–333

Cattaruzza S, Perris R (2006) Approaching the proteoglycome: molecular interactions of proteoglycans and their functional output. Macromol Biosci 6:667–680

Chapman PB, Morrissey DM, Panageas KS, Hamilton WB, Zhan C, Destro AN, Williams L, Israel RJ, Livingston PO (2000) Induction of antibodies against GM2 ganglioside by immunizing melanoma

patients using GM2-keyhole limpet hemocyanin + QS21 vaccine: a dose-response study. Clin Cancer Res 6:874–879
Chapman PB (2003) Vaccinating against GD3 ganglioside using BEC2 anti-idiotypic monoclonal antibody. Curr Opin Investig Drugs 4:710–715
Cunto-Amesty G, Dam TK, Luo P, Monzavi-Karbassi B, Brewer CF, Van Cott TC, Kieber-Emmons T (2001) Directing the immune response to carbohydrate antigens. J Biol Chem 276:30490–30498
Diakun KR, Matta KL (1989) Synthetic antigens as immunogens: Part III. Specificity analysis of an anti-anti-idiotypic antibody to a carbohydrate tumor-associated antigen. J Immunol 142:2037–2040
Evans SV, Rose DR, To R, Young NM, Bundle DR (1994) Exploring the mimicry of polysaccharide antigens by anti-idiotypic antibodies. The crystallization, molecular replacement, and refinement to 2.8 A resolution of an idiotope-anti-idiotope Fab complex and of the unliganded anti-idiotope Fab. J Mol Biol 241:691–705
Furuya A, Yoshida H, Hanai N (1992) Development of anti-idiotype monoclonal antibodies for Sialyl Le(a) antigen. Anticancer Res 12:27–31
Galili U (2005) The α-gal epitope and the anti-Gal antibody in xenotransplantation and in cancer immunotherapy. Immunol Cell Biol 83:674–686
Gulati S, McQuillen DP, Sharon J, Rice PA (1996) Experimental immunization with a monoclonal anti-idiotope antibody that mimics the *Neisseria gonorrhoeae* lipooligosaccharide epitope 2C7. J Infect Dis 174:1238–1248
Hakomori S (2001) Tumor-associated carbohydrate antigens defining tumor malignancy: basis for development of anti-cancer vaccines. Adv Exp Med Biol 491:369–402
Hakomori S (2002) Glycosylation defining cancer malignancy: new wine in an old bottle. Proc Natl Acad Sci USA 99:10231–10233
Hakomori S (2004) Carbohydrate-to-carbohydrate interaction, through glycosynapse, as a basis of cell recognition and membrane organization. Glycoconj J 21:125–137
Hoess R, Brinkmann U, Handel T, Pastan I (1993) Identification of a peptide which binds to the carbohydrate-specific monoclonal antibody B3. Gene 128:43–49
Jain D, Kaur K, Sundaravadivel B, Salunke DM (2000) Structural and functional consequences of peptide-carbohydrate mimicry. Crystal structure of a carbohydrate-mimicking peptide bound to concanavalin A. J Biol Chem 275:16098–16102
Kabat EA, Wu TT (1991) Identical V region amino acid sequences and segments of sequences in antibodies of different specificities. Relative contributions of VH and VL genes, minigenes, and complementarity-determining regions to binding of antibody-combining sites. J Immunol 147:1709–1719
Kanda S, Takeyama H, Kikumoto Y, Morrison SL, Morton DL, Irie RF (1994) Both VH and VL regions contribute to the antigenicity of anti-idiotypic antibody that mimics melanoma associated ganglioside GM3. Cell Biophys 25:65–74
Keitel T, Kramer A, Wessner H, Scholz C, Schneider-Mergener J, Hohne W (1997) Crystallographic analysis of anti-p24 (HIV-1) monoclonal antibody cross-reactivity and polyspecificity. Cell 91:811–820
Kieber-Emmons T, Luo P, Qiu J, Chang TY, Insug O, Blaszczyk-Thurin M, Steplewski Z (1999) Vaccination with carbohydrate peptide mimotopes promotes anti-tumor responses. Nat Biotechnol 17:660–665
Klaerner HG, Dahlberg PS, Acton RD, Battafarano RJ, Uknis ME, Johnston JW, Dunn DL (1997) Immunization with antibodies that mimic LPS protects against gram negative bacterial sepsis. J Surg Res 69:249–254
Lin SS, Parker W, Everett ML, Platt JL (1998) Differential recognition by proteins of α-galactosyl residues on endothelial cell surfaces. Glycobiology 8:433–443
Luo P, Agadjanyan M, Qiu J, Westerink MA, Steplewski Z, Kieber-Emmons T (1998) Antigenic and immunological mimicry of peptide mimotopes of Lewis carbohydrate antigens. Mol Immunol 35:865–879

Luo P, Canziani G, Cunto-Amesty G, Kieber-Emmons T (2000) A molecular basis for functional peptide mimicry of a carbohydrate antigen. J Biol Chem 275:16146–16154

Magnani JL (1984) Carbohydrate differentiation and cancer-associated antigens detected by monoclonal antibodies. Biochem Soc Trans 12:543–545

Maitta RW, Datta K, Pirofski LA (2004) Efficacy of immune sera from human immunoglobulin transgenic mice immunized with a peptide mimotope of *Cryptococcus neoformans* glucuronoxylomannan. Vaccine 22:4062–4068

Mandrell RE, Apicella MA (1993) Lipo-oligosaccharides (LOS) of mucosal pathogens: molecular mimicry and host-modification of LOS. [Review]. Immunobiology 187:382–402

Manivel V, Bayiroglu F, Siddiqui Z, Salunke DM, Rao KVS (2002) The primary antibody repertoire represents a linked network of degenerate antigen specificities. J Immunol 169:888–897

McNamara MK, Ward RE, Kohler H (1984) Monoclonal idiotope vaccine against *Streptococcus pneumoniae* infection. Science 226:1325–1326

Medvedev AE, Sabroe I, Hasday JD, Vogel SN (2006) Tolerance to microbial TLR ligands: molecular mechanisms and relevance to disease. J Endotoxin Res 12:133–150

Meezan E, Wu HC, Black PH, Robbins PW (1969) Comparative studies on the carbohydrate-containing membrane components of normal and virus-transformed mouse fibroblasts. II. Separation of glycoproteins and glycopeptides by sephadex chromatography. Biochemistry 8:2518–2524

Melzer H, Baier K, Felici F, von Specht BU, Wiedermann G, Kollaritsch H, Wiedermann U, Duchene M (2003) Humoral immune response against proteophosphoglycan surface antigens of *Entamoeba histolytica* elicited by immunization with synthetic mimotope peptides. FEMS Immunol Med Microbiol 37:179–183

Mirkov TE, Evans SV, Wahlstrom J, Gomez L, Young NM, Chrispeels MJ (1995) Location of the active site of the bean alpha-amylase inhibitor and involvement of a Trp, Arg, Tyr triad. Glycobiology 5:45–50

Monzavi-Karbassi B, Cunto-Amesty G, Luo P, Kieber-Emmons T (2002) Peptide mimotopes as surrogate antigens of carbohydrates in vaccine discovery. Trends Biotechnol 20:207–214

Monzavi-Karbassi B, Shamloo S, Kieber-Emmons M, Jousheghany F, Luo P, Lin KY, Cunto-Amesty G, Weiner DB, Kieber-Emmons T (2003) Priming characteristics of peptide mimotopes of carbohydrate antigens. Vaccine 21:753–760

Monzavi-Karbassi B, Artaud C, Jousheghany F, Hennings L, Carcel-Trullols J, Shaaf S, Korourian S, Kieber-Emmons T (2005) Reduction of spontaneous metastases through induction of carbohydrate cross-reactive apoptotic antibodies. J Immunol 174:7057–7065

Monzavi-Karbassi B, Hennings LJ, Artaud C, Liu T, Jousheghany F, Pashov A, Murali R, Hutchins LF, Kieber-Emmons T (2007) Preclinical studies of carbohydrate mimetic peptide vaccines for breast cancer and melanoma. Vaccine 25:3022–3031

Moran AP, Prendergast MM, Appelmelk BJ (1996) Molecular mimicry of host structures by bacterial lipopolysaccharides and its contribution to disease. [Review] [94 refs]. FEMS Immunol Med Microbiol 16:105–115

Murai H, Hara S, Ikenaka T, Goto A, Arai M, Murao S (1985) Amino acid sequence of protein alpha-amylase inhibitor from *Streptomyces griseosporeus* YM-25. J Biochem 97:1129–1133

Nair DT, Singh K, Sahu N, Rao KV, Salunke DM (2000) Crystal structure of an antibody bound to an immunodominant peptide epitope: novel features in peptide-antibody recognition. J Immunol 165:6949–6955

Oldenburg KR, Loganathan D, Goldstein IJ, Schultz PG, Gallop MA (1992) Peptide ligands for a sugar-binding protein isolated from a random peptide library. Proc Natl Acad Sci USA 89:5393–5397

Ono M, Hakomori S (2004) Glycosylation defining cancer cell motility and invasiveness. Glycoconj J 20:71–78

Park I, Choi IH, Kim SJ, Shin JS (2004) Peptide mimotopes of *Neisseria meningitidis* group B capsular polysaccharide. Yonsei Med J 45:755–758

Pashov A, Perry M, Dyar M, Chow M, Kieber-Emmons T (2005) Carbohydrate mimotopes in the rational design of cancer vaccines. Curr Top Med Chem 5:1171–1185

Pashov A, Perry M, Dyar M, Chow M, Kieber-Emmons T (2007) Defining carbohydrate antigens as HIV vaccine candidates. Curr Pharm Des 13:185–201

Pashov A, Monzavi-Karbassi B, Kieber-Emmons T (2009) Immune surveillance and immunotherapy: lessons from carbohydrate mimotopes. Vaccine 27:3405–3415

Pashov A, Monzavi-Karbassi B, Raghava GP, Kieber-Emmons T (2010) Bridging innate and adaptive antitumor immunity targeting glycans. J Biomed Biotechnol 2010:354068

Pichla SL, Murali R, Burnett RM (1997) The crystal structure of a Fab fragment to the melanoma-associated GD2 ganglioside. J Struct Biol 119:6–16

Prinz DM, Smithson SL, Westerink MA (2004) Two different methods result in the selection of peptides that induce a protective antibody response to *Neisseria meningitidis* serogroup C. J Immunol Methods 285:1–14

Qiu J, Luo P, Wasmund K, Steplewski Z, Kieber-Emmons T (1999) Towards the development of peptide mimotopes of carbohydrate antigens as cancer vaccines. Hybridoma 18:103–112

Ragupathi G, Liu NX, Musselli C, Powell S, Lloyd K, Livingston PO (2005) Antibodies against tumor cell glycolipids and proteins, but not mucins, mediate complement-dependent cytotoxicity. J Immunol 174:5706–5712

Ramsland PA, Farrugia W, Yuriev E, Edmundson AB, Sandrin MS (2003) Evidence for structurally conserved recognition of the major carbohydrate xenoantigen by natural antibodies. Cell Mol Biol (Noisy-le-Grand) 49:307–317

Ramsland PA, Farrugia W, Bradford TM, Mark Hogarth P, Scott AM (2004) Structural convergence of antibody binding of carbohydrate determinants in Lewis Y tumor antigens. J Mol Biol 340:809–818

Ravindranath MH, Kelley MC, Jones RC, Amiri AA, Bauer PM, Morton DL (1998) Ratio of IgG: IgM antibodies to sialyl Lewis(x) and GM3 correlates with tumor growth after immunization with melanoma-cell vaccine with different adjuvants in mice. Int J Cancer 75:117–124

Ravindranath MH, Muthugounder S, Presser N, Ye X, Brosman S, Morton DL (2005) Endogenous immune response to gangliosides in patients with confined prostate cancer. Int J Cancer 116:368–377

Schmolling J, Reinsberg J, Wagner U, Krebs D (1995) Antiidiotypic antibodies in ovarian cancer patients treated with the monoclonal antibody B72.3. Hybridoma 14:183–186

Schreiber JR, Nixon KL, Tosi MF, Pier GB, Patawaran MB (1991a) Anti-idiotype-induced, lipopolysaccharide-specific antibody response to *Pseudomonas aeruginosa*. II. Isotype and functional activity of the anti-idiotype-induced antibodies. J Immunol 146:188–193

Schreiber JR, Pier GB, Grout M, Nixon K, Patawaran M (1991b) Induction of opsonic antibodies to *Pseudomonas aeruginosa* mucoid exopolysaccharide by an anti-idiotypic monoclonal antibody. J Infect Dis 164:507–514

Scott JK, Loganathan D, Easley RB, Gong X, Goldstein IJ (1992) A family of concanavalin A-binding peptides from a hexapeptide epitope library. Proc Natl Acad Sci USA 89: 5398–5402

Sen G, Chakraborty M, Foon KA, Reisfeld RA, Bhattacharya CM (1998) Induction of IgG antibodies by an anti-idiotype antibody mimicking disialoganglioside GD2. J Immunother 21:75–83

Shental-Bechor D, Levy Y (2009) Folding of glycoproteins: toward understanding the biophysics of the glycosylation code. Curr Opin Struct Biol 19:524–533

Shikhman AR, Cunningham MW (1994) Immunological mimicry between *N*-acetyl-β-D-glucosamine and cytokeratin peptides. Evidence for a microbially driven anti-keratin antibody response. J Immunol 152:4375–4387

Shikhman AR, Greenspan NS, Cunningham MW (1994) Cytokeratin peptide SFGSGFGGGY mimics *N*-acetyl-β-D-glucosamine in reaction with antibodies and lectins, and induces in vivo anti-carbohydrate antibody response. J Immunol 153:5593–5606

Singhal A, Hakomori S (1990) Molecular changes in carbohydrate antigens associated with cancer. Bioessays 12:223–230

Smorodin EP, Kurtenkov OA, Sergeyev BL, Chuzmarov VI, Afanasyev VP (2007) The relation of serum anti-(GalNAc β) and -para-Forssman disaccharide IgG levels to the progression and histological grading of gastrointestinal cancer. Exp Oncol 29:61–66

Stein KE, Soderstrom T (1984) Neonatal administration of idiotype or antiidiotype primes for protection against *Escherichia coli* K13 infection in mice. J Exp Med 160:1001–1011

Steplewski Z, Blaszczyk-Thurin M, Lubeck M, Loibner H, Scholz D, Koprowski H (1990) Oligosaccharide Y specific monoclonal antibody and its isotype switch variants. Hybridoma 9:201–210

Takahashi T, Johnson TD, Nishinaka Y, Morton DL, Irie RF (1999) IgM anti-ganglioside antibodies induced by melanoma cell vaccine correlate with survival of melanoma patients. J Invest Dermatol 112:205–209

Tchernychev B, Cabilly S, Wilchek M (1997) The epitopes for natural polyreactive antibodies are rich in proline. Proc Natl Acad Sci USA 94:6335–6339

Transue TR, De Genst E, Ghahroudi MA, Wyns L, Muyldermans S (1998) Camel single-domain antibody inhibits enzyme by mimicking carbohydrate substrate. Proteins 32:515–522

Tsai CM (2001) Molecular mimicry of host structures by lipooligosaccharides of *Neisseria meningitidis*: characterization of sialylated and nonsialylated lacto-N-neotetraose (Galβ1-4GlcNAcβ1-3Galβ1-4Glc) structures in lipooligosaccharides using monoclonal antibodies and specific lectins. Adv Exp Med Biol 491:525–542

Tsuyuoka K, Yago K, Hirashima K, Ando S, Hanai N, Saito H, Yamasaki KM, Takahashi K, Fukuda Y, Nakao K, Kannagi R (1996) Characterization of a T cell line specific to an anti-Id antibody related to the carbohydrate antigen, sialyl SSEA-1, and the immundominant T cell antigenic site of the antibody. J Immunol 157:661–669

Valadon P, Nussbaum G, Boyd LF, Margulies DH, Scharff MD (1996) Peptide libraries define the fine specificity of anti-polysaccharide antibodies to *Cryptococcus neoformans*. J Mol Biol 261:11–22

van Die I, Cummings RD (2009) Glycan gimmickry by parasitic helminths: a strategy for modulating the host immune response? Glycobiology 20:2–12

van Montfoort N, de Jong JM, Schuurhuis DH, van der Voort EI, Camps MG, Huizinga TW, van Kooten C, Daha MR, Verbeek JS, Ossendorp F, Toes RE (2007) A novel role of complement factor C1q in augmenting the presentation of antigen captured in immune complexes to CD8+ T lymphocytes. J Immunol 178:7581–7586

Varki A (1993) Biological roles of oligosaccharides: all of the theories are correct. Glycobiology 3:97–130

Viale G, Grassi F, Pelagi M, Alzani R, Menard S, Miotti S, Buffa R, Gini A, Siccardi AG (1987) Anti-human tumor antibodies induced in mice and rabbits by "internal image" anti-idiotypic monoclonal immunoglobulins. J Immunol 139:4250–4255

Vollmers HP, Brandlein S (2005a) The "early birds": natural IgM antibodies and immune surveillance. Histol Histopathol 20:927–937

Vollmers HP, Brandlein S (2005b) Death by stress: natural IgM-induced apoptosis. Methods Find Exp Clin Pharmacol 27:185–191

Vollmers HP, Brandlein S (2009) Natural antibodies and cancer. Nat Biotechnol 25:294–298

Vyas NK, Vyas MN, Chervenak MC, Bundle DR, Pinto BM, Quiocho FA (2003) Structural basis of peptide-carbohydrate mimicry in an antibody-combining site. Proc Natl Acad Sci USA 100:15023–15028

Westerink MA, Campagnari AA, Wirth MA, Apicella MA (1988) Development and characterization of an anti-idiotype antibody to the capsular polysaccharide of *Neisseria meningitidis* serogroup C. Infect Immun 56:1120–1127

Westerink MA, Giardina PC, Apicella MA, Kieber-Emmons T (1995) Peptide mimicry of the meningococcal group C capsular polysaccharide. Proc Natl Acad Sci USA 92:4021–4025

Wondimu A, Zhang T, Kieber-Emmons T, Gimotty P, Sproesser K, Somasundaram R, Ferrone S, Tsao CY, Herlyn D (2008) Peptides mimicking GD2 ganglioside elicit cellular, humoral and tumor-protective immune responses in mice. Cancer Immunol Immunother 57:1079–1089

Zuckier LS, Berkowitz EZ, Sattenberg RJ, Zhao QH, Deng HF, Scharff MD (2000) Influence of affinity and antigen density on antibody localization in a modifiable tumor targeting model. Cancer Res 60:7008–7013

Antitumor Vaccines Based on Synthetic Mucin Glycopeptides 11

Ulrika Westerlind and Horst Kunz

11.1 Introduction

The interest in tumor-associated glycoconjugate antigens was particularly initiated by Springer, who published in 1984 that glycoproteins on the outer cell-membrane of epithelial tumor cells have an altered glycosylation consisting of the Thomsen-Friedenreich (T-) antigen and its precursor the T_N-antigen structure (Springer 1984). He and his coworkers also had found that monoclonal antibodies induced with glycoproteins from tumor cell membranes showed cross-reactivity to desialylated glycophorin A. It was concluded from these observations that the T-and T_N-glycoproteins on the epithelial tumor cells must be structurally related to asialoglycophorin A (Springer et al. 1983) (Fig. 11.1a). Glycophorin A is the major sialoglycoprotein on erythrocytes. In the *N*-terminal domain it contains cryptic T-antigen structures which are covered by sialylation in the 3′- and 6-position. The glycophorin exists in two blood group specificities M and N, which have identical glycoforms, but differ in two of the total 131 amino acids. One of those differences concerns the *N*-terminal amino acid which is a serine in blood group M, but a leucine in blood group N specificity (Tomita and Marchesi 1975). Stimulated by these results glycopeptide vaccines representing the *N*-terminal region of asialoglycophorin A were synthesized (Kunz and Birnbach 1986) (Fig. 11.1b). Antibodies induced in mice with such synthetic glycopeptide vaccine based on the blood group M *N*-terminal region of asialoglycophorin A specifically recognized the T-antigen glycan structure linked to the *N*-terminal M blood group

U. Westerlind
Gesellschaft zur Förderung der Analytischen Wissenschaften e.V, ISAS – Leibniz Institute for Analytical Sciences, Otto-Hahn-Str. 6b, D-44227 Dortmund, Germany

H. Kunz (✉)
Johannes Gutenberg-Universität Mainz, Institut für Organische Chemie, Duesbergweg 10-14, D-55128 Mainz, Germany
e-mail: hokunz@uni-mainz.de

P. Kosma and S. Müller-Loennies (eds.), *Anticarbohydrate Antibodies*,
DOI 10.1007/978-3-7091-0870-3_11,

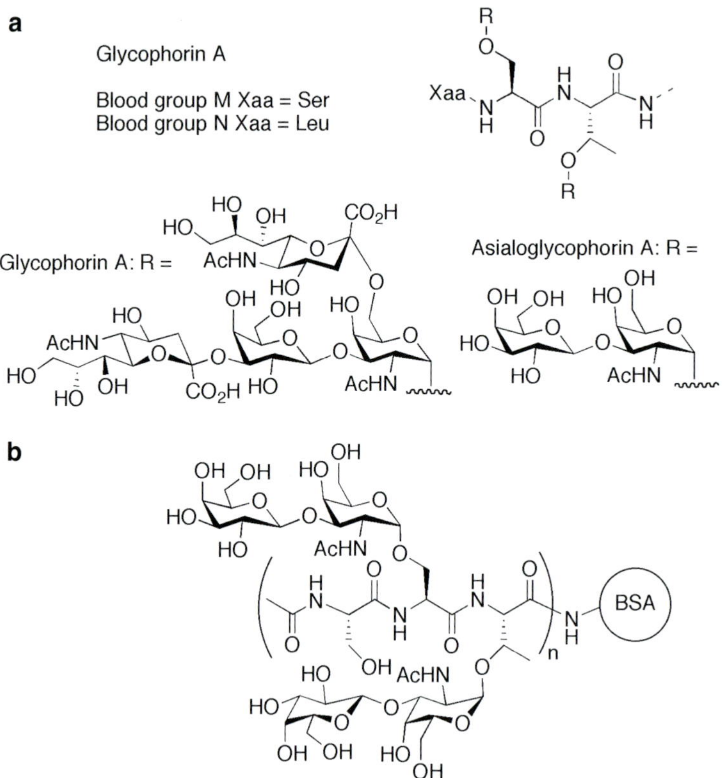

Fig. 11.1 (**a**) Glycophorin A and asialoglycophorin A with M and N blood group specificities and (**b**) immunogenic glycopeptide BSA conjugate consisting of clustered T-antigens

peptide backbone structure and differentiated between blood group M and N asialoglycophorin, showing that both the glycan and peptide backbone structure are relevant for the antibody binding specificity. These generated antibodies showed affinity to epithelial tumor tissues, but also bound to normal epithelial tissue. It was, concluded from these findings, that the synthetic T-antigen glycopeptide structure is tumor-associated, but not sufficiently tumor selective. In addition, the differentiation between the glycophorin blood group specificities observed with the induced antibodies suggested that in a potential antitumor vaccine a tumor-associated saccharide antigen should be combined with a tumor-selective peptide structure. In this context, more recent investigations of the tumor-associated epithelial mucin MUC1, expressed on almost all types of epithelial cells, had been of particular interest (Gendler et al. 1990).

Mucins are a class of extensively glycosylated proteins expressed on the surface of epithelial cells or secreted to function in mucus. They normally carry large *O*-linked carbohydrate structures that obscure the protein core. Among the mucins the membrane bound MUC1 is the most intensively studied glycoprotein with regard to cancer immunotherapy (Taylor-Papadimitriou et al. 1999; Hanisch 2001). Its large extracellular *N*-terminal region shares a structural feature common to all mucins, which consists of a (variable) number of peptide tandem repeats (VNTR). These repeats have identical or very similar amino acid sequences, which are rich in proline, serine and threonine residues. In MUC1, variable numbers (20–125) of tandem repeats consisting of 20 amino acids of the sequence HGV*TS*APD*T*R-PAPG*ST*APPA (Swallow et al. 1987), which includes five potential *O*-glycosylation sites (italized), have been found. On epithelial tumor cells, MUC1 is extensively overexpressed and its extracellular glycosylation pattern was found to be characteristically altered. Concomitant down-regulation of glycosyl transferases, in particular the core 2 β-1,6-*N*-acetylglucosaminyltransferase, and up-regulation of sialyltransferases results in short saccharides often with premature sialylation on the extracellular surface (Brockhausen et al. 1995; Brockhausen 1999; Burchell et al. 2001; Lloyd et al. 1996). As a consequence, T_N-, T-, sialyl-T_N-, (2,3)-sialyl-T- and (2,6)-sialyl-T-antigen structures constitute important examples of such tumor-associated saccharide antigens (Fig. 11.2). Furthermore, the underglycosylation of the mucin extracellular domain also results in the exposure of its peptide backbone. Tumor-associated epitopes consisting of both the saccharide and the peptide structures are exposed for interaction with components of the immune system.

By inducing sufficiently strong immune reactions specific to MUC1 tumor-associated antigens, it should be possible to break the natural tolerance of the immune system against these structures. In order to produce such a strong humoral immune response a naïve B cell needs to differentiate into an antibody-secreting plasma cell and to proliferate. To this end, additional stimulation by activated $CD4^+$ T helper cells is required. The naïve T-helper (T_H−) cells are activated when their T-cell receptor (TCR) binds to the peptide epitope presented by the major histocompatibility complex II (MHC II) on the surface of a antigen-presenting cell (APC). The peptide epitope presented by the APCs is to be generated by proteolytic fragmentation of the extracellular antigen that had been internalized via the B-cell receptor. The peptide fragments formed by proteolytic cleavage can then bind to the MHC class II complex resulting in T helper cell activation (Germain 1994).

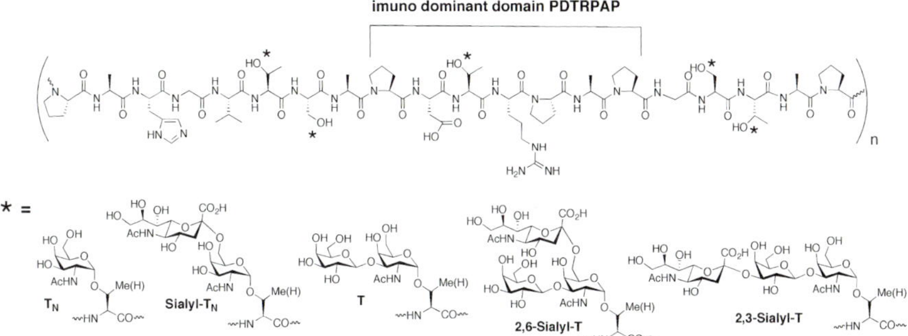

Fig. 11.2 Tumor-associated glycosylation on MUC1 tandem repeat peptides

A number of efforts have been made to synthesize MUC1 tandem repeat glycopeptides that represent the aberrant glycoforms of cell surface glycoprotein. These glycopeptides are the crucial antigens for the development of synthetic vaccines which should elicit antibodies useful for immunotherapy or as diagnostic tools. However, the tumor-associated MUC1 glycopeptides are only moderately immunogenic, and additional stimulation is necessary to generate a strong humoral immune response. Therefore, a foreign protein carrier, as for example keyhole limpet hemocyanine (KLH) or bovine serum albumin (BSA), or an immunostimulating T_H-cell peptide epitope, e.g. a peptide epitope from ovalbumin, needs to be linked to the MUC1 glycopeptides (Becker et al. 2006; Liakatos and Kunz 2007; Wilkinson et al. 2011). During immunization it is also necessary to support the innate immune system by adding an adjuvant to the vaccine, for example Freund's adjuvant or by using an adjuvant built into the vaccine, for example Pam_3Cys lipopeptide ligands of the Toll-like receptors 2 (Ingale et al. 2007; Wilkinson et al. 2011). Examples of synthetic vaccines based on tumor-associated MUC1 glycopeptides conjugated to various immunostimmulants will here be given.

11.2 Synthesis of T_N-, T-, Sialyl T_N-, Sialyl-T-Glycosyl Amino Acid Building Blocks

MUC1 tandem repeat glycopeptides are synthesized on solid-phase according to the Fmoc strategy using glycosylated amino acid building blocks. The chemical synthesis of glycosylated Fmoc-serine and threonine building blocks for solid phase peptide synthesis is a demanding task. The tumor-associated glycosyl amino acid structures are accessible from the T_N-antigen intermediate **12** by a unifying biomimetic strategy (Fig. 11.3). Exploiting the relatively high reactivity of the 6- and 3-hydroxyl groups of galactose towards electrophilic attack in combination with a proper protecting group strategy, regioselective glycosylations were achieved affording the 2,6-sialyl T_{N}-, 2,6-sialyl-T- and 2,3-sialyl-T-Fmoc-amino acid building blocks, respectively (Fig. 11.3).

The T_N-antigen threonine and serine conjugates are synthesized from acetobromogalactose (Lemieux 1963) **1** via the corresponding galactal (Shafizadeh 1963) **2** by azidonitration (Lemieux and Ratcliffe 1979) yielding an anomeric mixture of azido nitrate **3**, which is subsequently converted to the corresponding α-glycosyl bromide **4** by treatment with LiBr in acetonitrile (Lemieux and Ratcliffe 1979). Fmoc-threonine *t*-Bu-ester (Kunz 1997), or its serine counterpart (not shown) is then glycosylated with **4** under modified Koenigs–Knorr conditions (Koenigs and Knorr 1901; Paulsen and Hoelck 1982; Liebe and Kunz 1997a) providing **5**. The azido function is then converted to the corresponding acetamide **6**, for example by thioacetic acid (Rosen et al. 1988; Meinjohanns et al. 1996), and the *t*-Bu-ester is cleaved by TFA in presence of anisole as a scavenger, providing the fully protected T_N-antigen building block **7** which can be applied to solid phase peptide synthesis (SPPS) (Scheme 11.1).

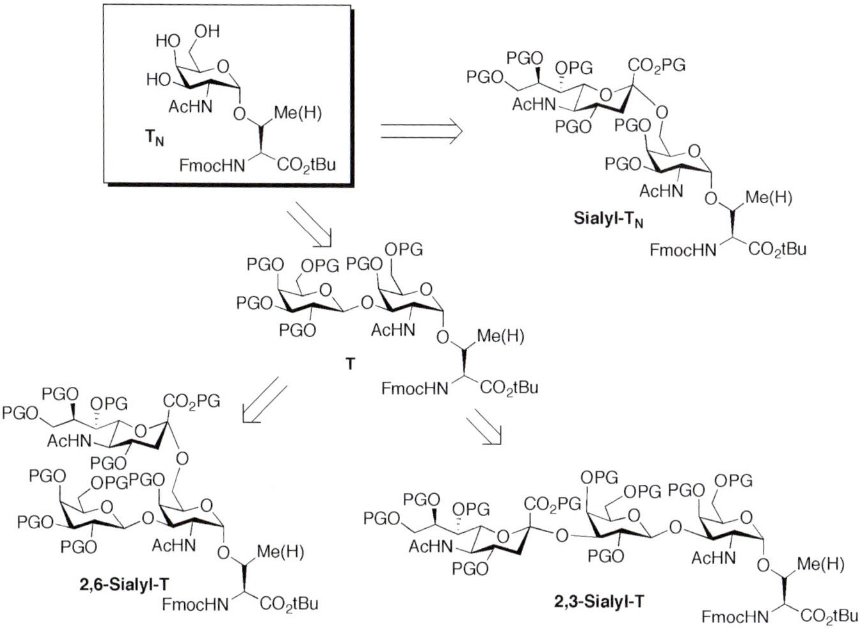

Fig. 11.3 Synthetic strategy for glycosylated amino acid building blocks

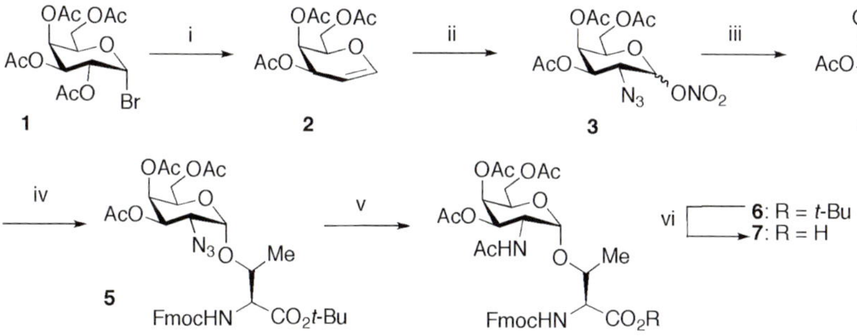

Scheme 11.1 Reagents and conditions: (i) Zn-dust, $CuSO_4$, H_2O, HOAc, 85%; (ii) Azidonitration, CAN, NaN_3, MeCN, 45%; (iii) LiBr, MeCN 92%; (iv) Fmoc-Thr-O*t*-Bu, Ag_2CO_3, $AgClO_4$ 80%; (v) AcSH, 75%; and (vi) TFA, anisole, 90%

The construction of 2,6-sialyl-T_N-antigen (Liebe and Kunz 1997a) requires the preparation of a sialyl donor **11**. It has been proven that glycosylation reactions with xanthate **11** activated through a thiophilic activator are superior to other sialic acid donors (Marra and Sinay 1989). Peracetylation of sialic acid **8** gives the fully acetylated intermediate **9**, which is deprotonated with cesium carbonate and benzylated to give **10** as an anomeric mixture (Furuhata et al. 1991). Treatment of **10** with acetyl chloride followed by in situ reaction with KS(CS)OEt affords xanthate **11** under thermodynamically controlled conditions as a single anomer.

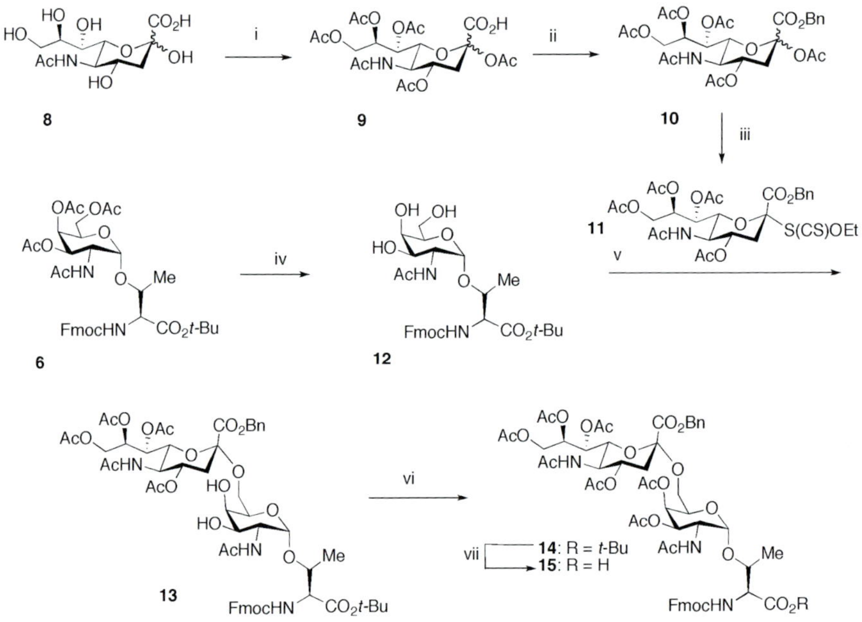

Scheme 11.2 Reagents and conditions: (i) Ac_2O, pyridine, quantitative; (ii) Cs_2CO_3, BnBr, 77%; (iii) 1. AcCl, H_2O; 2. KS(CS)OEt, 64%; (iv) NaOMe, MeOH; (v) MeSOTf, MeCN, CH_2Cl_2 59%; (vi) Ac_2O, Pyridine, 90%; and (vii) TFA, anisole, 94%

After careful deacetylation of T_N-antigen-Fmoc-threonine (Liebe and Kunz 1994, 1997b; Zemplen and Kuntz 1923) **6**, the resulting product **12** is sialylated regio- and stereoselectively in the 6-position using of xanthate **11** activated by MeSOTf (Dasgupta and Garegg 1988) in an acetonitrile containing solvent. At low temperature (−65°C), only the kinetically favored equatorial product is formed due to assistance of the nitrile solvent (Braccini et al. 1993; Loenn and Stenvall 1992; Schmidt et al. 1990). Further transformations include peracetylation of **13** and cleavage of the *t*-Bu-ester **14** to give the Fmoc-SPPS-building block **15** (Liebe and Kunz 1997a) (Scheme 11.2).

T_N-intermediate **12** can also be converted into the T-antigen building block **19** by a simple procedure. Treatment of **12** with benzaldehyde dimethyl acetal under controlled acid catalysis gives the corresponding 4,6-benzylidene acetal **16**, which is subjected to a subsequent Helferich glycosylation (Helferich and Wedemeyer 1949) with acetobromogalactose **1**, to form the disaccharide conjugate **17**. The benzylidene acetal can be hydrolyzed under mild acidic conditions (Smith et al. 1962) providing **18**. Peracetylation of **18** with acetic anhydride and pyridine followed by removal of the *t*-Bu-ester affords the fully protected T-antigen Fmoc-SPPS-building block **19** (Scheme 11.3).

The 2,3-sialyl-T-antigen is accessible from intermediate **16**, which is glycosylated with 6-*O*-benzyl-acetobromogalactose (Lergenmüller et al. 1998) **20.** The obtained product **21** is subsequently carefully deacetylated in order to prevent β-elimination.

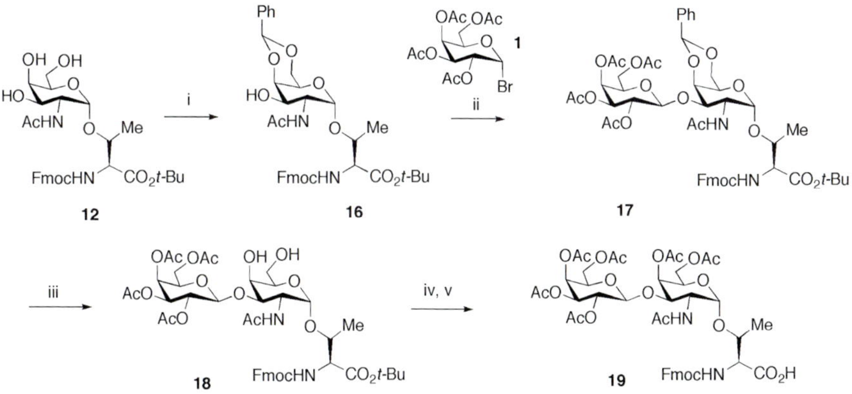

Scheme 11.3 Reagents and conditions: (i) $PhCH(OMe)_2$, TsOH, 75%; (ii) $Hg(CN)_2$, 68%; (iii) 80% aq. HOAc, 87%; (iv) Ac_2O, Pyridine, 92%; and (v) TFA, Anisole, 95%

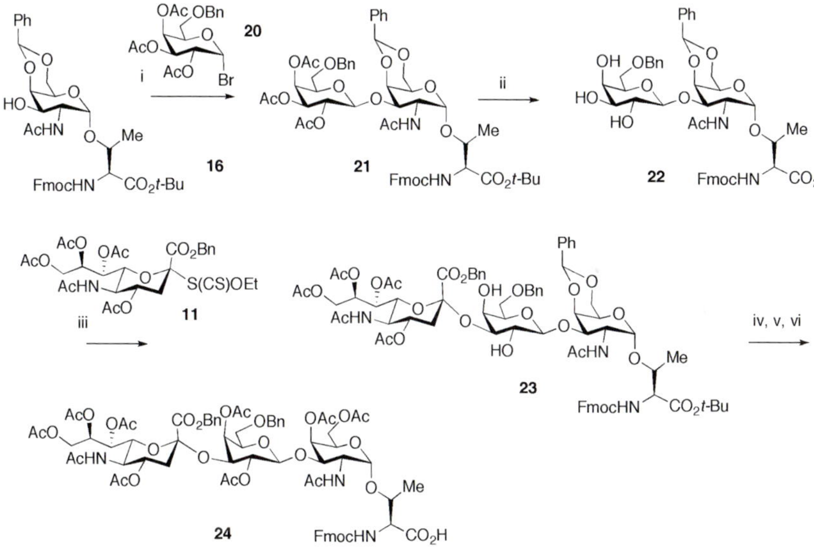

Scheme 11.4 Reagents and conditions: (i) $Hg(CN)_2$, 93%; (ii) cat NaOMe, pH 8.5, 34%; (iii) MeSOTf, 58%; (iv) 80% aq. HOAc; (v) Ac_2O, pyridine, cat. DMAP, 80% over two steps; and (vi) TFA, anisole, quantitative

Sialylation of the more reactive equatorial 3′-position using the sialic xanthate **11** under the conditions already described proceeds smoothly, thus providing **23**. The benzylidene acetal of **23** is removed under mild acidic (Smith et al. 1962) conditions. After acetylation the *t*-Bu-ester is removed providing the Fmoc-2,3-sialyl-T-building block **24** in good overall yield (Scheme 11.4).

The T-antigen intermediate **21** can also be transformed to the 2,6-sialyl-T-antigen by selective sialylation in the 6-position of **25**. Solvolytic removal of the

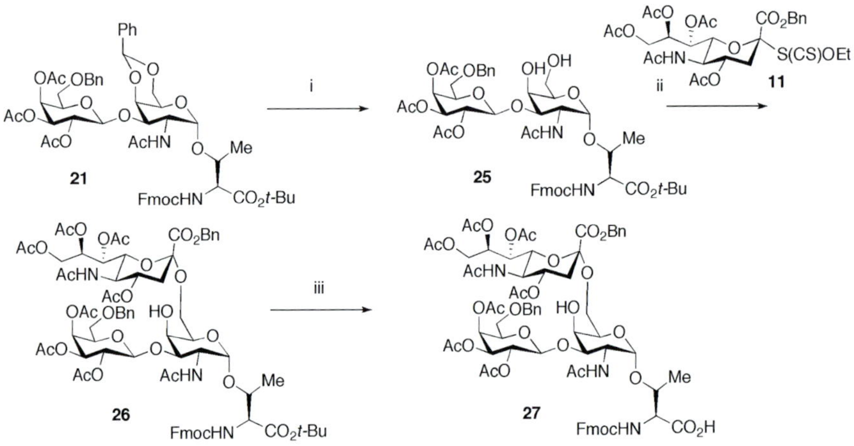

Scheme 11.5 Reagents and conditions: (i) 80% aq. HOAc; (ii) MeSOTf; and (iii) TFA, anisole, 98%

benzylidene acetal in **21** yields the acceptor **25** with free OH groups in the 4- and the 6-position. Due to the intrinsic low reactivity of the axial 4-OH of galactose, a highly selective sialylation reaction takes place, again employing xanthate **11** as the donor, providing **26**. Removal of the *t*-Bu ester gives the Fmoc-2,6-sialyl-T-antigen building block **27**. Note that the 4-OH group was left unprotected. Due to the steric hindrance by the sialic acid moiety, it is not necessary to protect this OH group (Scheme 11.5).

11.3 Synthesis of T_N-, T-, Sialyl-T_N-, Sialyl-T-Glycopeptides and Vaccines

The synthesis of glycopeptides can be realized by different strategies. Glycopeptides can be prepared by attachment of saccharides to the already completed target peptide (convergent synthesis), or by the use of glycosylated amino acid building blocks incorporated into the stepwise peptide assembly. The use of the convergent approach is limited since it is suffering from low yields of glycosylations due to reactivity problems. Problems with α and β selectivity are more pronounced when larger glycan structures should be coupled to serine/threonine residues within a peptide. Synthesis of *O*-glycopeptides by Fmoc solid phase peptide synthesis (SPPS) employing glycosylated amino acids is, therefore, the favorable approach (Kunz 1987; Meldal 1994; Kihlberg and Elofsson 1997; Herzner et al. 2000). During peptide backbone assembly, the glycosylated amino acid building blocks are commonly protected. This is because of the lability of the *O*-glycosidic bond to strong acid treatment. In addition, by treatment with a strong base *O*-glycopeptides can undergo β-elimination of the *O*-linked glycans or epimerization at the amino acid stereogenic centers (Sjölin et al. 1996). After cleavage of the synthesized glycopeptide from resin, the glycan protecting groups need to be removed under mild conditions. *O*-Acetyl protecting groups are commonly used for the saccharide portion which can be removed under mild conditions, e.g. using dilute sodium methoxide in methanol (Peters et al. 1992; Jansson et al. 1992) or hydrazine hydrate in methanol (Kunz et al. 1990; Bardaji et al. 1991). Glycopeptides can also be prepared employing an enzymatic approach (Schuster et al. 1994).

MUC1 tandem repeat glycopeptides are normally synthesized by solid-phase Fmoc peptide synthesis in a stepwise fashion starting with a suitable resin preloaded with the *C*-terminal amino acid. The choice of the linker and the resin depends on whether the peptide should later on be released with concomitant amino acid side chain deprotection or under milder conditions not affecting these amino acid side chain protective groups. For mild cleavage conditions preventing side chain deprotection the trityl linker resin (Frechet and Haque 1975) can be used. This linker is cleavable by 0.1% TFA. An alternative resin contains the PTMSEL linker (Wagner et al. 2003) from which the peptide is released by treatment with tetrabutylammonium fluoride (TBAF) in dichloromethane. Another linker is the allylic HYCRON linker (Seitz and Kunz 1997), which is cleavable by palladium (0)-catalyzed allyl transfer. If the side chain protective groups should be simultaneously removed from the peptide during cleavage, Wang resin (Wang 1973) is most commonly used and cleaved with a 95% TFA mixture. The choice of linker and resin is also dependent on the *C*-terminal peptide sequence and the question whether it is prone to diketopiperazine formation, such as proline and alanine containing sequences. In such a case, a bulky linker is required, such as the trityl or the fluoride-sensitive 2-phenyl-2-trimethylsilyl-ethylester linker (PTMSEL). The valuable glycosylated amino acid building blocks are often coupled manually using 1.5–2 equivalents activated with the more reactive coupling reagents *N*-[(dimethylamino)-1*H*-1,2,3-triazolo[4,5-*b*]pyridin-1-ylmethylene]-*N*-methylmethanaminium (HATU)/1-hydroxy-7-azabenzotriazole (HOAt) (Carpino 1993), while the other Fmoc amino acids normally are coupled automatically in a peptide synthesizer using 5–20 equivalents and activated with *N*-[(1*H*-benzotriazol-1-yl)(dimethylamino) methylene]-*N*-methylmethanaminium hexafluorophosphate *N*-oxide (HBTU)/1-hydroxybenzotriazole (HOBt) (Dourtoglou et al. 1984). After detachment from resin and purification by HPLC, the glycopeptides are either conjugated to the immune stimulating component, or the glycopeptides are deprotected in the glycan portions and then conjugated to the immunestimulant. Deprotection of the glycans are performed by hydrogenolytic removal of the sialic acid benzyl ester followed by removal of the *O*-acetyl protective groups by transesterification in methanol with catalytic amounts of NaOMe at pH 9–9.5.

11.3.1 Synthesis of MUC1 Glycopeptides Conjugated to a Peptide T-cell Epitope

Recently, sialyl-T_N- and T_N-mono-, di- and triglycosylated 38 amino acid MUC1 tandem repeat peptides connected to an $OVA_{323–339}$ T-cell peptide epitope via a non-immunogenic spacer (**28–30**), were synthesized (Westerlind et al 2008). The solid-phase synthesis was carried out according to above outlined strategy starting with Wang resin preloaded with Fmoc arginine. The glycosylated sialyl-T_N- (**15**) and T_N-amino acid (**7**) building blocks were used in two-fold excess and coupled with HATU/HOAt. The other amino acids were coupled according to the standard protocol (20 eq amino acid and HBTU/HOBt) in a peptide synthesizer. After cleavage from resin and purification by preparative reversed phase HPLC, the removal of the protective groups of the glycans was performed by hydrogenolysis of the sialic acid benzyl ester and subsequent removal of the *O*-acetyl protective groups by treatment with catalytic amounts of NaOMe in methanol at pH 9–9.5. After completing the global deprotection, the glycopeptide–OVA–vaccine constructs were purified again by preparative reversed phase HPLC and isolated in overall yields (calculated from resin) of 36% (**28**) 17% (**29**) and 32% (**30**) (Scheme 11.6). These fully synthetic vaccines were used in combination with complete Freund's adjuvant (CFA) for immunization of transgenic mice (DO11.10) whose T-cells express an OVA-specific CD4 receptor. High antibody titers specific to the corresponding MUC1-antigens were induced in one of three mice immunized with vaccine **28** and in two of three mice immunized with vaccine **29**. None of ten mice immunized with the triglycosylated vaccine **30**, containing additional glycosylation in the immunodominant PDTR domain, did generate an immune response. The antibodies generated from vaccines **28** and **29** were further investigated by ELISA and microarray binding specificity studies (Westerlind et al. 2009). The antibodies displayed a very similar binding specificity. It turned out that the antibodies were highly specific for glycosylation with sialyl-T_N in the HGVT position of the tandem repeat. If the glycan was removed or moved to another position within the tandem repeat sequence the binding was totally lost. Glycopeptides with the required sialyl-T_N-glycosylation in the HGVT region, but additional glycosylation with T_N or sialyl-T_N in the PDTR or GSTA region were accepted, and also glycopeptides consisting of more than one tandem repeat are recognized. In addition, it was found that the GSTA part was not important for binding recognition of these antibodies, while removal of the immunodominant PDTR region resulted in a complete loss of binding of the antibodies induced by **28** and **29** (Scheme 11.6).

11.3.2 Synthesis of MUC1-Glycopeptides Conjugated to Protein Carriers

Vaccines consisting of carrier protein conjugates such as conjugates to BSA or KLH, are well-established in immunology. A few examples of such vaccines obtained by different conjugation methods and employing different carrier proteins will here be outlined. MUC1-glycopeptides conjugated through coupling with diethyl squarate, or using an alkene-thiol reaction, a maleimide-thiol addition or glutaraldehyde coupling will be described. Common to all these reactions is that the MUC1-glycopeptide must be deprotected on the peptide side chains and glycans prior to the conjugation to the carrier protein.

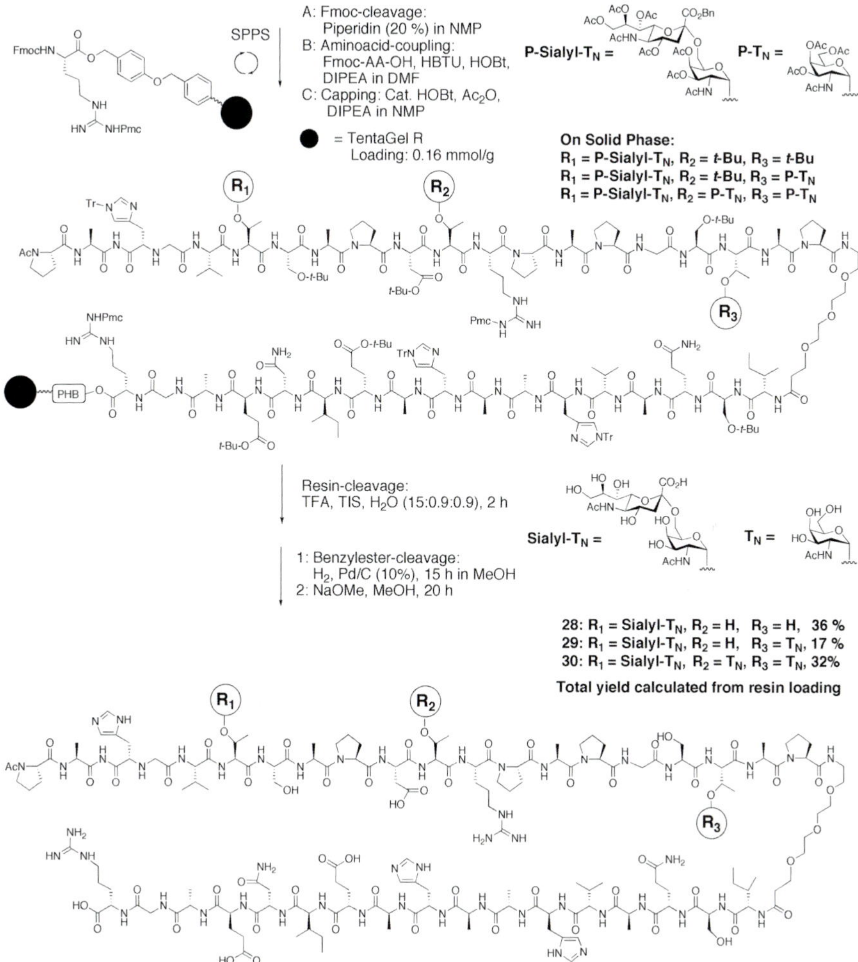

Scheme 11.6 Synthesis of sialyl-T_N MUC1-OVA$^{323-339}$ glycopeptide vaccines

Immunizations with MUC1-glycopeptides coupled through diethyl squarate to Tetanus Toxoid as an immune carrier have shown promising results (Kaiser et al. 2009; Hoffman-Röder et al. 2010). Tetanus Toxoid conjugates have already been applied to humans in several vaccines towards bacterial and viral targets. Therefore, this carrier protein is considered attractive for a MUC1 glycopeptide vaccine. MUC1 glycopeptides containing a sialyl-T_N- **31**, a T-antigen **32** or a di-fluoro-T-antigen **33** MUC1-glycopeptide equipped with an oligoethylene glycol spacer amino acid were conjugated to Tetanus Toxoid protein employing diethyl squarate (3,4-diethoxy-3-cyclobutene-1,2-dione) as the coupling reagent (Kaiser et al. 2009; Hoffman-Röder et al. 2010; Tietze et al. 1991) (Scheme 11.7). The MUC1-glycopeptides containing ST_N-, T- or di-fluoro-T-antigen and a triethylene glycol

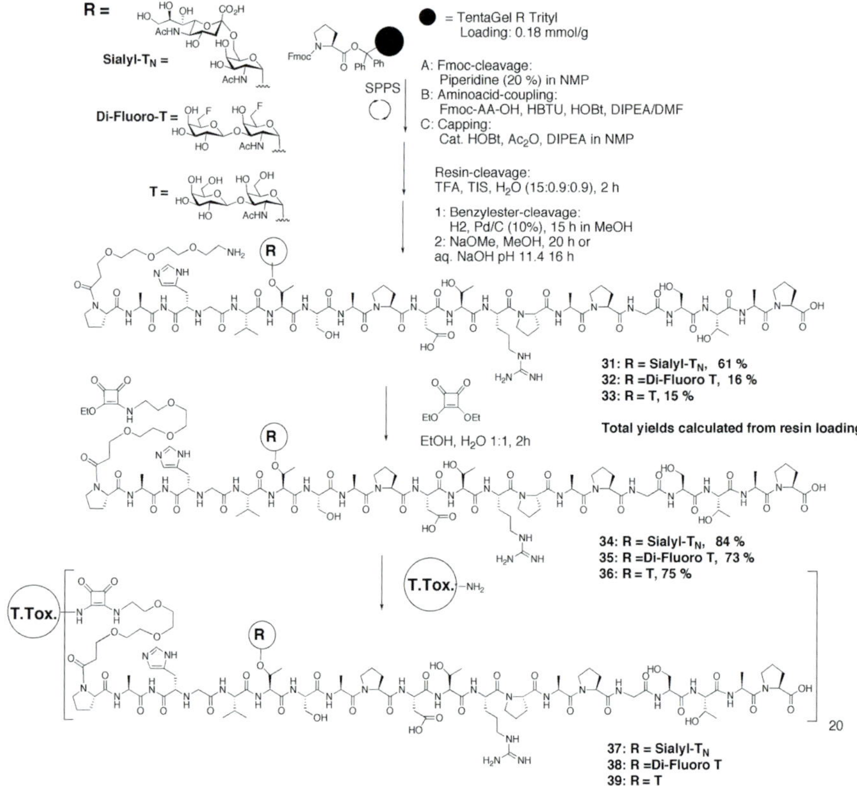

Scheme 11.7 Synthesis of sialyl-T_N-, T-, and di-fluoro-T MUC1-Tetanus Toxoid protein vaccines

spacer with a free amine at the *N*-terminus **(31–33)** were prepared by solid-phase synthesis according to Fmoc strategy in a similar fashion as described for the OVA-vaccines. In this case, a trityl resin was used in order to avoid diketopiperazine formation as the peptide sequence starts with Pro-Ala (Scheme 11.7). Employing TFA the fully assembled peptides were cleaved from the resin with simultaneous removal of the peptide side chain protective groups. The ST_N-disaccharide was then deprotected by hydrogenation using palladium on charcoal and subsequent deacetylation using NaOMe in methanol to yield the sialyl-T_N-MUC1-glycopeptide **(31)** in an overall yield of 61%. The T- and di-fluoro-T-glycopeptides are directly treated with base to give the deacetylated compounds **32** and **33**. The deprotected MUC1-glycopeptides reacted with diethyl squarate by stirring in a mixture of ethanol and water at pH 8 and yielded the activated constructs **34–36**. The squarate monoamide-glycopeptides were coupled to the Tetanus Toxoid in a sodium phosphate buffer at pH 9 and afforded vaccines **37–39** carrying on average more than 20 MUC1-glycopeptides conjugated to the protein. Immunological evaluation of these vaccines showed that very strong immune responses were induced in almost all of the immunized mice. The generated antibodies were further evaluated by ELISA and neutralization experiments as well as by glycopeptide microarrays. The results gave evidence that specific immune responses were elicited towards the MUC1 antigens present in the vaccines. Furthermore, the binding of antibodies induced by the T-antigen vaccines **38** and **39** to tumor cells were evaluated by FACS analysis. It was shown that the antibodies recognized MCF-7 and T47D breast cancer cells (Hoffman-Röder et al. 2010) (Scheme 11.7).

Sialyl-T and T MUC1 glycopeptide vaccines have also been prepared. In one example, these glycopeptides were connected to BSA as the carrier protein via a thioether linkage and a non-immunogenic spacer (Wittrock et al. 2007). The formation of thioethers via a radical-induced addition of thiols to alkenes appears favourable in comparison to the more common peptide-protein conjugation techniques employing squarates (Tietze et al. 1991) or maleimido (Shin et al. 2001; Keller and Rudinger 1975) linkers, which have immunogenic potential themselves. A 2,3-sialyl-T-MUC1 glycopeptide with a thiol amino acid spacer at the *N*-terminus was prepared starting from a trityl resin preloaded with proline. The peptide backbone assembly and cleavage from resin according to the procedure described above gave the partly protected glycopeptide **40** in 36% yield. Removal of the protective groups was performed to give the thiol glycopeptide **41**, which was coupled to olefin-modified BSA in water employing UV-radiation. After dialysis and lyophilization the pure antigen-BSA conjugate **42** was obtained (Scheme 11.8a). The reverse thioether linkage was also constructed by the synthesis of an allylamide-functionalized T-antigen MUC1 tandem repeat peptide **(43)** (39% overall yield) and its photochemical coupling to BSA carrying a thiol spacer to give **44** (Scheme 11.8b). These glycopeptides vaccines have so far not been employed in immunization experiments (Scheme 11.8).

Alternatively, enzymatic approaches have been used to prepare MUC1-glycopeptide vaccines. One example includes a 60-mer MUC1 tandem repeat peptide, which was enzymatically glycosylated with T_N- and sialyl-T_N-glycans and conjugated to KLH as carrier protein (Sorensen et al. 2006; Tarp et al. 2007). The MUC1 60-mer peptide consisting of three tandem repeats **(45)** was prepared through standard Fmoc solid-phase peptide synthesis. After cleavage and purification, the peptide was completely T_N glycosylated **(46)** *in vitro* through a concerted action of GalNAc-T2 and GalNAc-T4 glycosyltransferases. This reaction was performed by using UDP-GalNAc and *N*-acetylgalactosaminyl transferases (GalNAc T-2 and GalNAc T-4) in a sodium cacodylate, $MnCl_2$ and Triton X-100 buffer at pH 7.4, yielding peptide construct **46** fully glycosylated on all potential glycosylation sites. A part of the glycopeptide material was further sialylated with ST6GalNAc-I, a human α-*N*-acetylgalactosamine α-2,6-sialyltransferase, and generated a MUC1 60-mer with sialyl-T_N **(47)** at all 15 glycosylation sites. Sialylation was performed in a MES, EDTA and DTT buffer of pH 6.5 with CMP-NeuAc as donor. The sialyl-T_N- and T_N-MUC1 glycopeptides **46** and **47** were conjugated to KLH through reaction with glutaraldehyde resulting in a glycopeptide to conjugate ratio of 300:1 (Scheme 11.9). The resulting sialyl-T_N- and T_N-glycopeptide vaccines **48** and **49** were used for immunization of Balb/c mice and human MUC1 transgenic mice

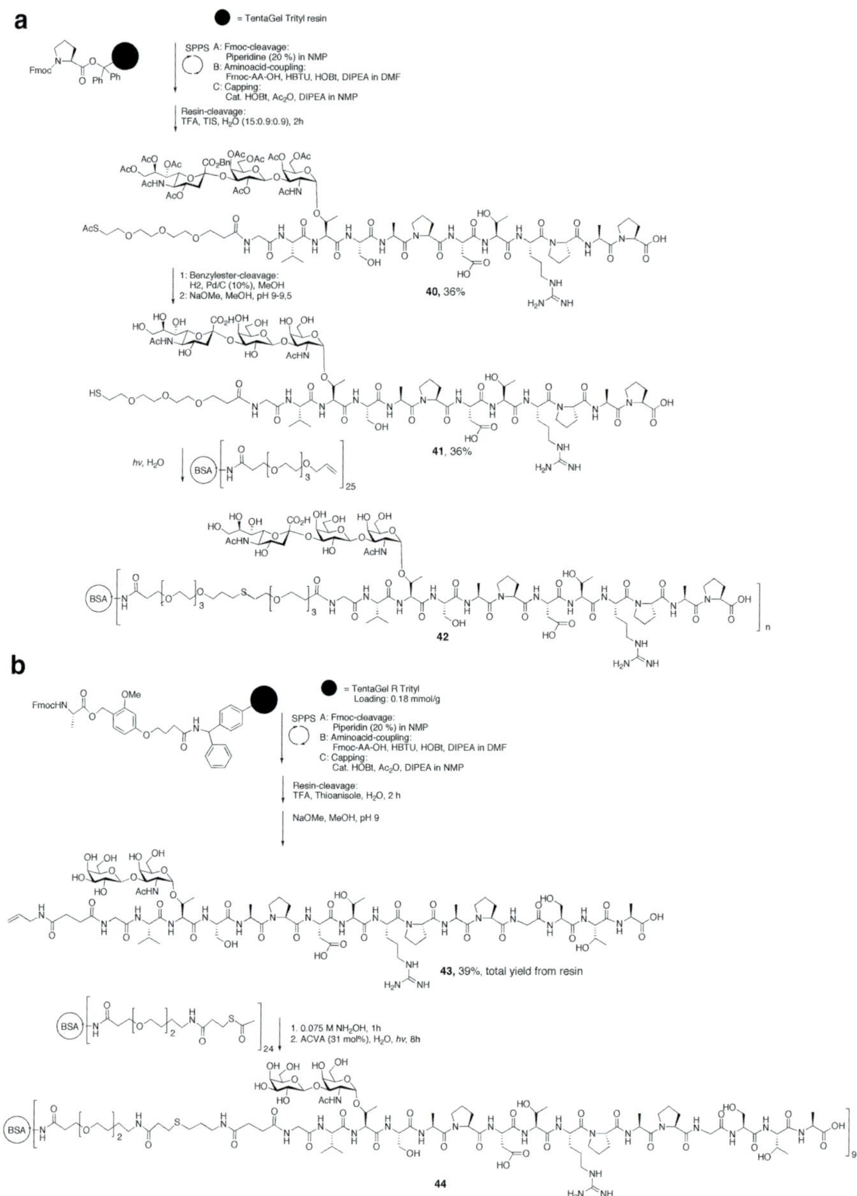

Scheme 11.8 Synthesis of (**a**) Sialyl-T-antigen BSA conjugate (**b**) T-antigen BSA conjugate through alkene-thiol reaction

(MUC1 Tg). Strong immune responses specific to the MUC1 60-mer 15 ST_N and T_N immunogen structures were elicited in both the Balb/c and MUC1 Tg mice. Serum generated from the T_N glycopeptide vaccine **48** reacted strongly with the

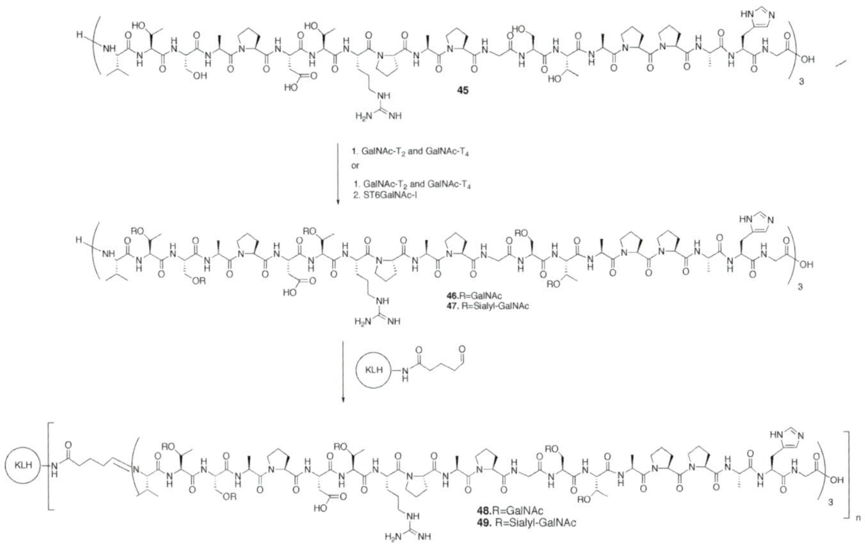

Scheme 11.9 Enzymatic Synthesis of Sialyl-T_N- and T_N-antigen KLH conjugate vaccine

human breast cancer cell line T47D, which mainly carries T_N- and some T- and sialyl-T-glycans, but weaker with the MCF7 breast cancer cell-line partially based on core 2 structures. The non-tumorigenic epithelial cell-line MTSV1-7, which expresses high levels of the core 2 β-1,6-GlcNAc transferase was not recognized by the sera. The sera generated from the sialyl-T_N-glycopeptide vaccine **49** stained primary breast cancer cells expressing MUC1 and ST_N and did not react with MCF7 breast cancer cells. Monoclonal antibodies (5E5) were also generated with the MUC1 60-mer 15 T_N-vaccine **48** as the immunogen. Antibody specificity studies showed that these antibodies were in particular specific to antigen structures glycosylated in the GSTA part of the MUC1 tandem repeat (Scheme 11.9).

Other examples of vaccines have been prepared consisting of glycan multi-epitope peptides conjugated to KLH as the carrier protein. It was considered attractive to prepare vaccines targeting more than one tumor-associated epitope during the immunization. This could be done by combining vaccines targeting different tumor associated glycosylation on the peptide backbone like T_N-, sialyl-T_N-, T-and sialyl-T-structures or by combining vaccines with variation of the position for glycosylation on the MUC1 tandem repeat. The problem with immunization using combined vaccines with different antigens separately conjugated to the immune carrier protein is that there is a risk that the increased level of the immune carrier, as for example KLH, can result in a decreased immunogenicity of the individual antigens. To avoid this problem, unimolecular multi-epitope vaccines were investigated (Zhu et al. 2009; Ragupathi et al. 2006; Lee and Danishefsky 2009). Hybrid glycopeptide KLH conjugate vaccines were prepared based on a mixture of tumor associated glycans linked through spacers to a peptide backbone. Both tumor associated glycolipid glycans, like Globo-H, GM2, and glycoprotein glycans like T_N, sialyl-T_N, and T were combined in this vaccine. These hybrid glycopeptides were prepared through stepwise coupling of the individual Fmoc protected glycosylated spacer amino acid building blocks employing EDCl, HOBt, Et_3N (scheme 11.11). The spacer glycosylated amino acid building blocks were prepared by different strategies. T_N-, sialyl-T_N- and T-glycosylated amino acids **50–53** with a four carbon spacer were obtained by coupling of glycosyl trichloroacetimidates with a *N*-Fmoc protected hydroxynorleucine benzyl ester in the presence of a Lewis acid, TMSOTf or $ZnCl_2$ (Scheme 11.10b). The GM2 and Globo-H amino acid building block **54** and **55** containing a six carbon spacer were prepared by coupling of the Globo-H pentenyl glycoside to protected allyl glycine through an olefin cross-methathesis in the presence of a ruthenium catalyst. Reduction of the alkene and concomitant removal of the benzyl ester protecting group generated the glycosylated amino acid building block (Scheme 11.10a).

After assembly of the peptide backbone, the Boc protecting group at the *C*-terminal diamine spacer was removed using TFA followed by introduction of a thiospacer and removal of acetates from the glycans and the spacer employing sodium hydroxide in methanol. The deprotected hybrid glycopeptide construct **56** was conjugated to KLH functionalized with a maleimide spacer by stirring at room temperature in a pH 6.5–7 phosphate buffer for 4 h. On average 505 hybrid glycopeptides consisting of Globo-H, GM2, T_N-, sialyl-T_N- and T-glycans had been linked per KLH molecule. The prepared vaccine construct **57** was used for immunization of mice. ELISA experiments with the obtained mice sera showed that both IgG and IgM antibodies were generated, which specifically recognized each individual carbohydrate antigen. Additional FACS analyses displayed that MCF-7 breast cancer cells were recognized by the sera. However, exclusively antibodies of short lived IgM type recognized the tumor cells (Scheme 11.11).

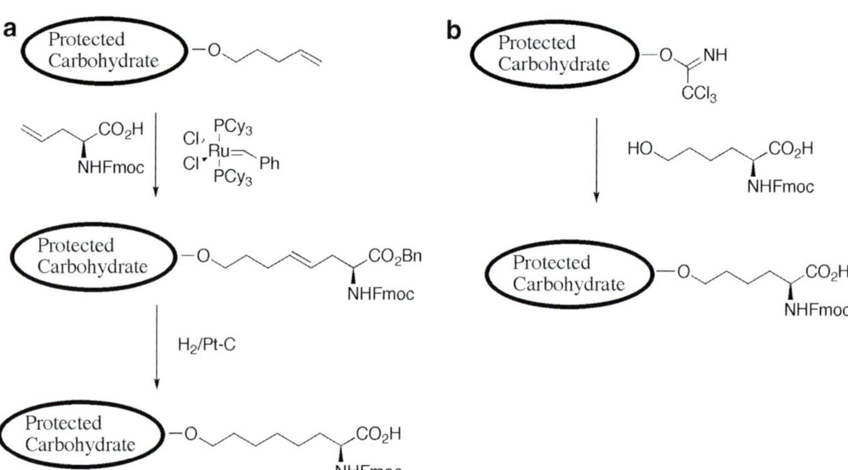

Scheme 11.10 Methods to prepare glycosylated amino acid mimics: (**a**) through olefin cross-metathesis and (**b**) through coupling with hydroxynorleucine to a trichloroacetimidate donor glycan in the presence of a Lewis acid

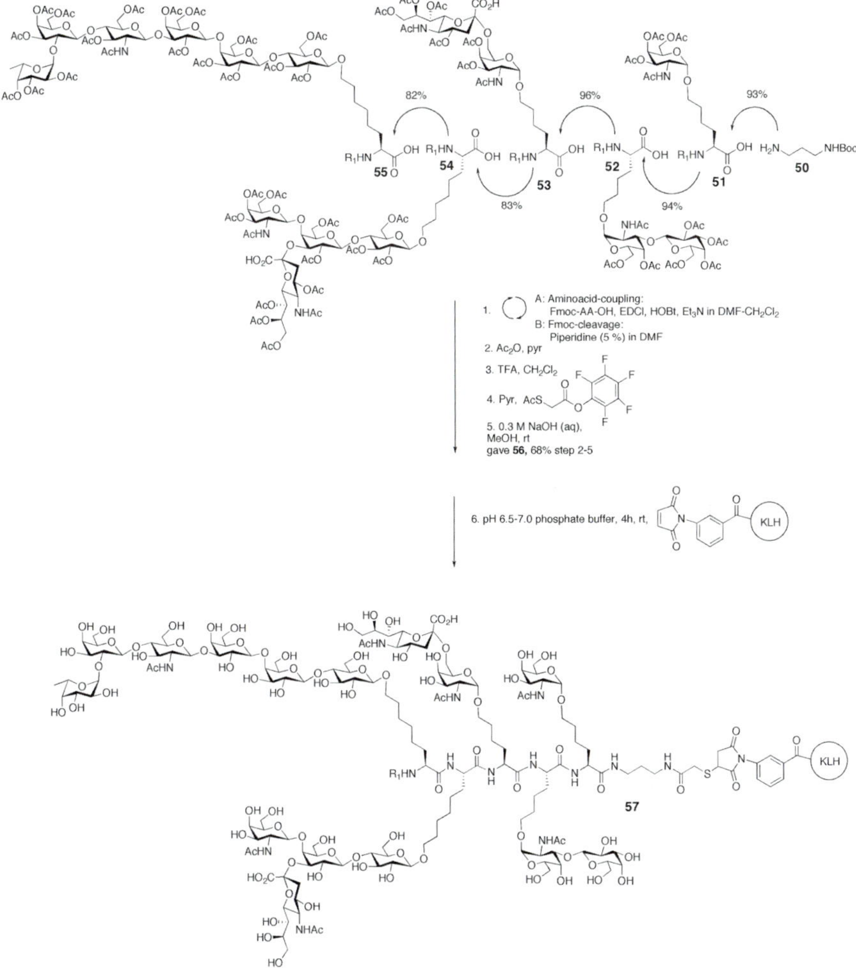

Scheme 11.11 Synthesis of a unimolecular pentavalent vaccine

11.3.3 Synthesis of MUC1-Glycopeptides Conjugated to a Built-in Immunostimulant and T-cell Epitope

Immunostimulants often have characteristic molecular patterns derived from pathogens to which the immune system is commonly pre-exposed. An example of a MUC1 glycopeptide vaccine conjugated to both an immunostimulant and a T-cell epitope will here be described (Ingale et al. 2009; Ingale et al. 2006, 2007) The used stimulant, *S*-[(*R*)-2,3-dipalmitoyloxy-propyl]-*N*-palmitoyl-(*R*)-cysteine (Pam_3Cys) (Bessler et al. 1998) is a ligand of the Toll-like receptor 2. Through interaction with the receptor, pro-inflammatory cytokines and chemokines are produced, which stimulates the APCs that can process and present the immunogenic epitopes contained in the vaccine to the T-cells. The lipopeptide Pam_3Cys also facilitates the formation of liposomes, which serves as efficient vaccine delivery vehicles. As a T_H-cell epitope, the peptide sequence 103-KLFAVWKITYKDT-115 derived from polio virus was included. The B-cell epitope consisted of a MUC1 decapeptide glycosylated with a GalNAc residue in the immunodominant domain.

The MUC1 glycopeptide was obtained by standard Fmoc solid-phase peptide synthesis, and the single glycosylation was introduced using a T_N-glycosylated Fmoc amino acid building block as previously described. A cysteine peptide was attached to the *N*-terminus prior to the release from the resin. The protective groups of the glycan were removed using aqueous hydrazine, and the peptide **58** containing the *N*-terminal cysteine was employed in a native chemical ligation (NCL) reaction with the T-cell epitope peptide. Applying a safety-catch sulfonamide resin (Backes et al. 1996) preloaded with a glycine, the T-cell epitope peptide **59** with an acetamidomethyl (Acm) protected cysteine at the *N*-terminus and a *S*-benzyl group at the *C*-terminus was obtained by general methods of peptide assembly. After alkylation of the *C*-terminal acyl sulfonamide linker, cleavage with benzyl mercaptan and sodium thiophenolate in THF yielded the peptide with protected side chains. After purification, this peptide was treated with a TFA cleavage cocktail, which removed the amino acid side chain protective groups and yielded **59**. The native chemical ligation was performed between the MUC1 peptide thiol **58** and the T-cell epitope thioester **59** in a phosphate buffer (pH 7.5) in the presence of tris-carboxyethyl phosphine and EDTA under ultrasonication. The ligation reaction was initiated by addition of 2-mercaptoethane sulphonate and was completed after 2 h. After removal of the acetamidomethyl protective group from the primary ligation product, peptide **60** was obtained in good yield. Subsequently, a second liposome-mediated NCL was performed with the synthesized Pam_3Cys peptide **61** having a *S*-benzyl group at the *C*-terminus, thus forming the three-component vaccine **62** (Scheme 11.12).

The T_N MUC1-polio$_{103\text{-}115}$ Pam_3Cys three-component vaccine **62** was incorporated into phospholipid based liposomes and used for immunization of mice. The antibody titers were detected by ELISA using microtiter plates coated with the 11-mer MUC1 glycopeptide conjugated to BSA. A strong IgG immune response was detected. These antibodies showed reactivity towards the MUC1 specific breast cancer tumor cell line (MCF-7) as was shown by FACS analysis.

Other examples of synthetic Pam_3Cys conjugate vaccines are two component vaccines containing the whole MUC1 tandem repeat peptide glycosylated with T_N-, T- or 2,6-sialyl-T-antigens (Kaiser et al. 2010). The unprotected MUC1-glycopeptides having a triethylene glycol spacer with a free amino group at the *N*-terminus (**63–65**) were prepared using Fmoc chemistry according to methods described above. Vaccines were generated by fragment condensation between the prepared Pam_3Cys lipopeptide **66** and the MUC1 peptides **63–65** employing HATU/HOAt activation in DMF to give construct **67–68**. The T-antigen vaccine **68** was used for immunization of mice resulting in the induction of glycopeptide-specific antibodies (Scheme 11.13).

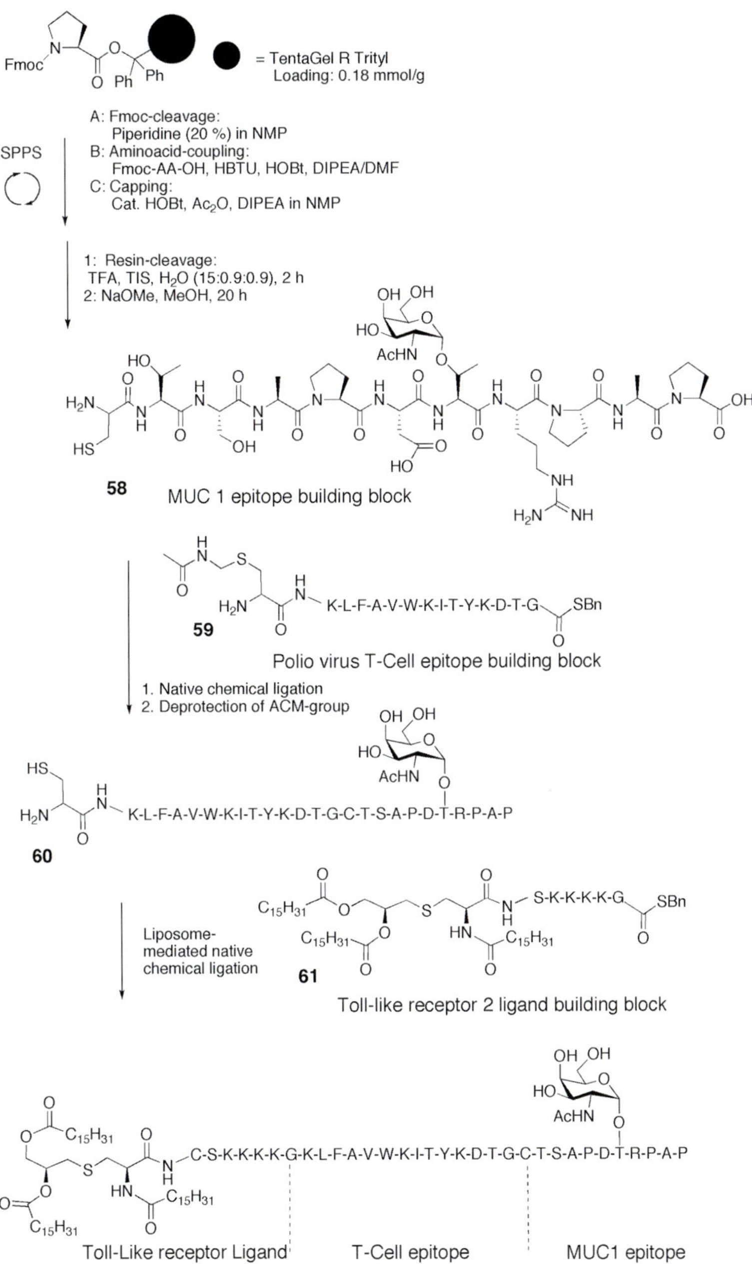

Scheme 11.12 Synthesis of Pam_3Cys polio T_N MUC1 three-component vaccine

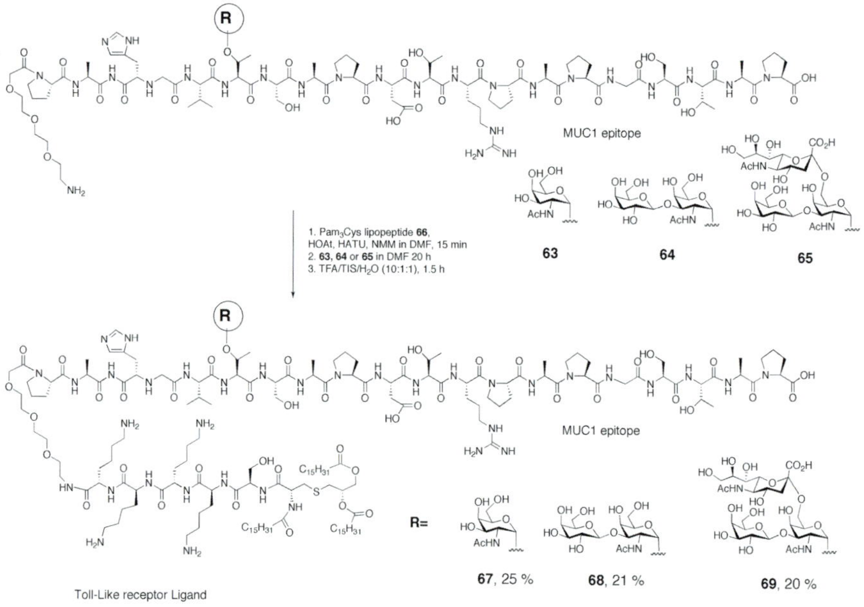

Scheme 11.13 T_N-, T- and Sialyl-T-MUC1 Pam_3Cys two-component vaccines

11.3.4 Synthesis of MUC1 Glycopeptide Dendrimer Vaccines

Employing multi-epitope presentation based on a dendrimer, as for example a oligo-lysine core (Tam 1988), carrier-induced immune suppression, often occurring during immunization with carrier protein vaccines, could be avoided. Vaccines based on multiple antigen presentation could also be favourable for the uptake and presentation of the antigen by antigen presenting cells. Synthesis of MUC1 and MUC4 T_N- and sialyl-T_N-glycopeptide dendrimer vaccines were recently reported (Becker et al. 2009; Keil et al. 2009). An example of a MUC1 sialyl-T_N-glycopeptide dendrimer vaccine based on a di-lysyl-lysine core will here be given. The vaccine was prepared either with or without an extra immunostimulating Tetanus Toxoid T-cell peptide epitope (Keil et al. 2001). In order to separate the B- and T-cell epitope and the di-lysyl-lysine core from each other a triethylene glycol spacer amino acid was incorporated in between them. The sialyl-T_N-MUC1-glycopeptide **70** and the Tetanus Toxoid T-cell epitope **71** with a triethylene glycol spacer at the *C*-terminal end were prepared by Fmoc-solid-phase peptide synthesis. Starting with aminomethyl-polystyrene resin (AMPS) functionalized with an allylic HYCRON linker (Seitz and Kunz 1997) and a triethylene glycol spacer, the loading with Fmoc-proline or Fmoc-valine amino acid and the assembly of the peptide backbone were performed according to standard procedures. The MUC1 *N*-terminal amine was then protected with an acetyl group, and the Tetanus Toxoid peptide amine was protected with a benzyloxycarbonyl group. Palladium(0)-catalyzed cleavage from allylic linker then gave the MUC1 glycopeptide **70** and the Tetanus Toxoid peptide **71** in overall yields of 36% and 42%, respectively (Keil et al. 2001) (Scheme 11.14).

The di-lysyl-lysine core for multiple antigen presentation was prepared starting with an amide coupling of di-benzyloxycarbonyl (Z) lysine to the lysine *tert*-butylester **72**. The formed Z-protected di-lysyl-lysine ester core **73** was hydrogenated over palladium on carbon to give the deprotected amine core **74** in 96% yield (Scheme 11.14a). For construction of the dendrimers, fragment condensation of sialyl-T_N-glycopeptide **70** (8 eq) to the di-lysyl lysine core **74**

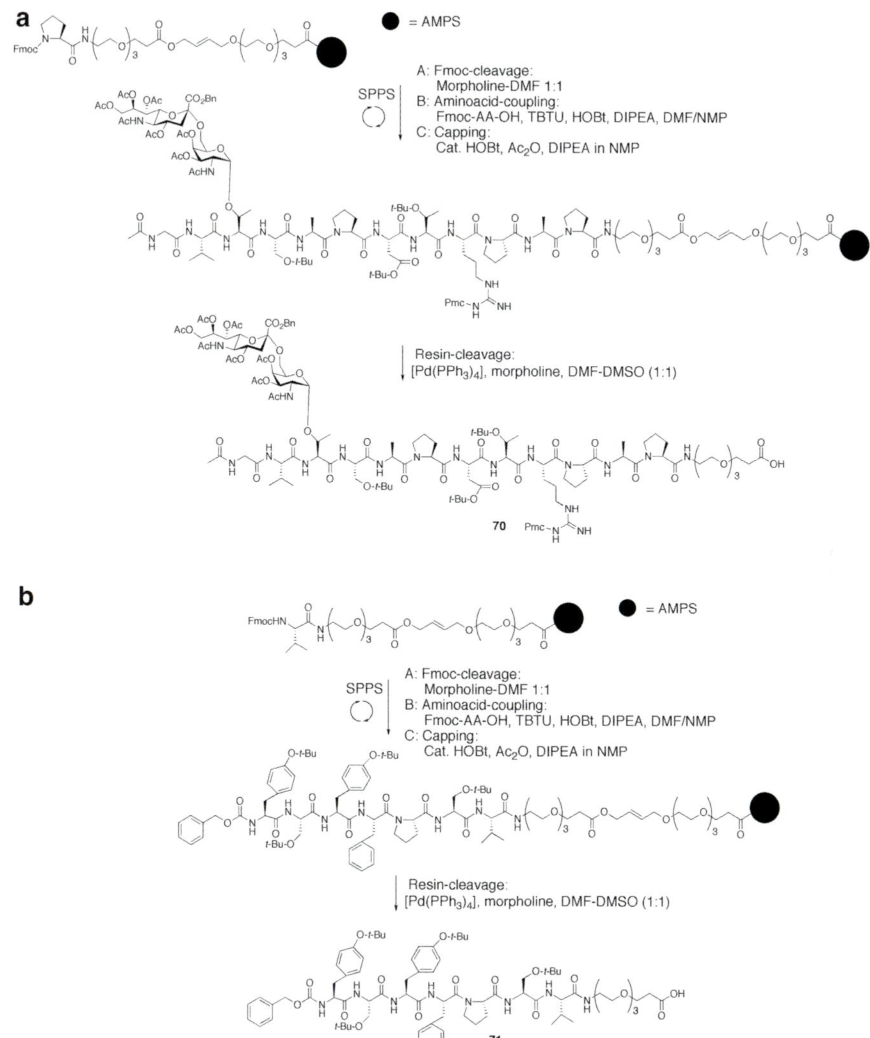

Scheme 11.14 Synthesis of (**a**) sialyl-T_N-MUC1-glycopeptide and (**b**) synthesis of Tetanus Toxoid peptide

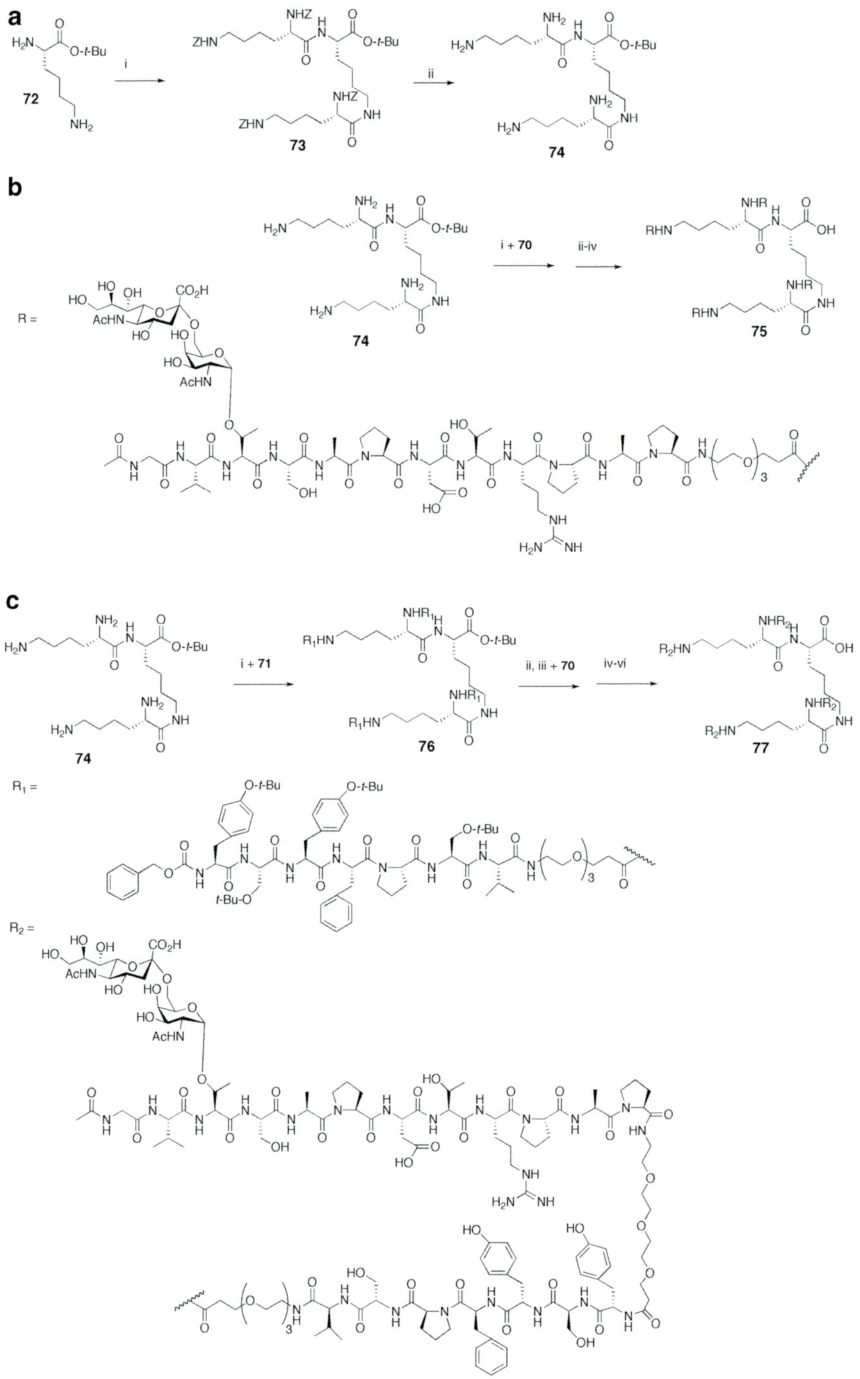

Scheme 11.15 Synthesis of (**a**) di-lysyl-lysine dendrimer core, (i) Z-Lys(Z)-OH, TBTU, HOBt, NMM, DMF, 20°C, 2 d, 36%; (ii) Pd/C (10%), H_2, MeOH, 20°C, 2 h, 93%. (**b**) sialyl-

was performed employing HATU/HOAt and *N*-methyl morpholine for activation and resulted in the MUC1-glycopeptide dendrimer. Acidolytic removal of the peptide side chain protecting groups and glycan deprotection by catalytic hydogenation of the benzyl ester and careful deacetylation using catalytic sodium methoxide in methanol generated the dendrimer vaccine **75** (Scheme 11.14b). In a similar fashion a glycopeptide dendrimer vaccine also including a Tetanus Toxoid T-cell epitope was prepared (Scheme 11.14c). Starting with a solid phase synthesis of the Tetanus Toxoid peptide (8 eq) followed by *N*-deprotection of the di-benzyloxycarbonyl group employing hydrogen over palladium on carbon, a fragment condensation to the solid-phase-linked **76** was carried out. Coupling of the carboxy-activated MUC1-glycopeptide (8 eq) and subsequent removal of the peptide and glycan protecting groups gave the dendrimer vaccine **77**. The prepared synthetic dendrimer vaccines are currently under investigation in immunization studies (Scheme 11.15).

Conclusions

During the recent years, a number of vaccines consisting of tumor-associated MUC1-glycopeptides containing the T_N-, T-, sialyl-T_N- and sialyl-T-saccharide antigens have been synthesized by their conjugation to various immunostimulants. Immunological evaluation of these vaccines has shown that antibodies were induced which are specific towards these tumor-associated glycopeptides and do recognize the membrane glycoproteins on cancer cells. A number of these synthetic vaccines showed promising effects, in particular the MUC1 Tetanus Toxoid vaccines. Tetanus Toxoid-based vaccines have already been applied in humans, and they generally induce very strong immune responses, which can override the natural tolerance of the immune system. Furthermore, the antibodies induced by the MUC1 Tetanus Toxoid vaccines are of the IgG type and specifically bind to epithelial tumor cells, such as the MCF-7 and T47D breast cancer cells. These properties make them promising candidates for the development of an active immunization against cancer diseases.

Scheme 11.15 (continued) T_N-MUC1-glycopeptide dendrimer, (i) HATU, HOAt, NMM, DMF, 20°C, 2 d, 65%; (ii) Pd/C (10%), H_2, MeOH, 20°C, 3 h; (iii) CH_2Cl_2/TFA/thioanisole/ethanthiol (10:10:1:1), 20°C, 4 h, 66%; (iii) NaOMe, MeOH, pH 8.5, 20°C, 18 h, prep. HPLC gave 30% pure **75** and 35% impure **75**. (**c**) sialyl-T_N-MUC1-T.Tox dendrimer vaccine, (i) HATU, HOAt, NMM, DMF, 20°C, 2 d, 49%; (ii) Pd/C (10%), H_2, MeOH, 20°C, 3 h; (iii) HATU, HOAt, NMM, DMF, 20°C, 2 d, 73%; (iv) Pd/C (10%), H_2, MeOH, 20°C, 4 h; CH_2Cl_2/TFA/thioanisole/ethanthiol (20:20:1:1), 20°C, 3 h, 23%, by-product 57%; (v) NaOMe, MeOH, pH 8.5, 20°C, 18 h, prep. HPLC gave **77**

References

Backes BJ, Virgilio AA, Ellman JA (1996) Activation method to prepare a highly reactive acylsulfonamide "Safety-Catch" linker for solid-phase synthesis. J Am Chem Soc 118:3055–3056

Bardaji E, Torres JL, Clapes P, Albericio F, Barany G, Rodriguez RE (1991) Synthesis and biological activity of O-glycosylated morphiceptin analogs. J Chem Soc Perkin Trans 1:1755

Becker T, Dziadek S, Wittrock S, Kunz H (2006) Synthetic glycopeptides from the mucin family as potential tools in cancer immunotherapy. Curr Cancer Drug Targets 6:491–517

Becker T, Kaiser A, Kunz H (2009) Synthesis of dendrimeric tumor-associated mucin-type glycopeptide antigens. 2009:1113–1122

Bessler WG, Heinewetter L, Wiesmueller KH, Jung G, Baier W, Huber M, Lorenz AR, van der Esche U, Mittenbuhler K, Hoffman P (1998) Bacterial cell wall components as immunomodulators. 1. Lipopeptides as adjuvants for parenteral and oral immunization. Int J Immunopharmacol 19:547–550

Braccini I, Derouet C, Esnault J, du Penhoat CH, Mallet JM, Michon V, Sinay P (1993) Conformational analysis of nitrilium intermediates in glycosylation reactions. Carbohydr Res 246:23–41

Brockhausen I, Yang JM, Bruchell J, Whitehouse C, Taylor-Papadimitriou J (1995) Mechanisms underlying aberrant glycosylation of MUC1 mucin in breast cancer cells. Eur J Biochem 233:607–17

Brockhausen I (1999) Pathways of O-glycan biosynthesis in cancer cells. Biochim Biophys Acta Gen Subj 1473:67–95

Burchell JM, Mungul A, Taylor-Papadimitriou J (2001) O-linked glycosylation in the mammary gland: changes that occur during malignancy. J Mammary Gland Biol Neoplasia 6:355–64

Carpino LA (1993) 1-Hydroxy-7-azabenzotriazole. An efficient peptide coupling additive. J Am Chem Soc 115:4397–8

Dasgupta F, Garegg PJ (1988) Use of sulfenyl halides in carbohydrate reactions. Part I. Alkyl sulfenyl triflate as activator in the thioglycoside-mediated formation of β-glycosidic linkages during oligosaccharide synthesis. Carbohydr Res 177:C13–C17

Dourtoglou V, Gross B, Lambropoulou V, Zioudrou C (1984) O-Benzotriazolyl-N,N,N′,N′-tetramethyluronium hexafluorophosphate as coupling reagent for the synthesis of peptides of biological interest. Synthesis 1984:572–4

Frechet JMJ, Haque KE (1975) Polymers as protecting groups in organic synthesis. II. Protection of primary alcohol functional groups. Tetrahedron Lett 16:3055–6

Furuhata K, Komiyama K, Ogura H, Hata T (1991) Studies on sialic acids. Part XXIII. Studies on glycosylation of the mitomycins. Syntheses of 7-N-(4-O-glycosylphenyl)-9a-methoxymitosanes. Chem Pharm Bull 39:255–9

Gendler S, Lancaster CA, Taylor-Papadimitriou J, Duhig T, Peal N, Bruchell J, Pemberton L, Lalani EN, Wilson P (1990) Molecular cloning and expression of human tumor-associated polymorphic epithelial mucin. J Biol Chem 265:15286–15293

Germain RN (1994) MHC-dependent antigen processing and peptide presentation: providing ligands for T lymphocyte activation. Cell 76:287–299

Hanisch F-G (2001) O-glycosylation of the mucin type. Biol Chem 382:143–149

Helferich B, Wedemeyer KF (1949) Preparation of glucosides from acetobromoglucose. Justus Liebigs Ann Chem 563:139–45

Herzner H, Reipen T, Schultz M, Kunz H (2000) Synthesis of glycopeptides containing carbohydrate and peptide recognition motifs. Chem Rev 100:4495–4537

Hoffman-Röder A, Kaiser A, Wagner S, Gaidzik N, Kowalczyk D, Westerlind U, Gerlitzki B, Schmitt E, Kunz H (2010) Synthetic antitumor vaccines from tetanus toxoid conjugates of MUC1 glycopeptides with the Thomsen-Friedenreich antigen and a fluorine-substituted analogue. Angew Chem Int Ed 4:8498–8503

Ingale S, Buskas T, Boons GJ (2006) Synthesis of glyco(lipo)peptides by liposome-mediated native chemical ligation. Org Lett 8:5785–5788

Ingale S, Wolfert MA, Gaekwad J, Buskas T, Boons GJ (2007) Robust immune responses elicited by a fully synthetic three-component vaccine. Nat Chem Biol 3:663–667

Ingale S, Wolfert MA, Buskas T, Boons GJ (2009) Increasing the antigenicity of synthetic tumor-associated carbohydrate antigens by targeting Toll-like receptors. Chembiochem 10:455–463

Jansson AM, Meldal M, Bock K (1992) Solid-phase synthesis and characterization of *O*-dimannosylated heptadecapeptide analogues of human insuline-like growth factor 1 (IGF-1). J Chem Soc Perkin Trans 1:1699–1707

Kaiser A, Gaidzik N, Westerlind U, Kowalczyk D, Hobel A, Schmitt E, Kunz H (2009) A synthetic vaccine consisting of a tumor-associated Sialyl-T_N-MUC1 tandem-repeat glycopeptide and tetanus toxoid: induction of a strong and highly selective immune response. Angew Chem Int Ed 48:7551–7555

Kaiser A, Gaidzik N, Becker T, Menge C, Groh K, Cai H, Li YM, Gerlitzki B, Schmitt E, Kunz H (2010) Fully synthetic vaccines consisting of tumor-associated MUC1 glycopeptides and a lipopeptide ligand of the toll-like receptor 2. Angew Chem Int Ed 49:3688

Keil S, Claus C, Dippold W, Kunz H (2001) Towards the development of antitumor vaccines: a synthetic conjugate of a tumor-associated MUC1 glycopeptide antigen and a tetanus toxin epitope. Angew Chem Int Ed 40:366–369

Keil S, Kaiser A, Syed F, Kunz H (2009) Dendrimers of vaccines consisting of tumor-associated glycopeptide antigens and T cell epitope peptides. Synthesis 2009:1355–1369

Keller O, Rudinger J (1975) Preparation and some properties of maleimido acids and maleoyl derivatives of peptides. Helv Chim Acta 58:531–541

Kihlberg J, Elofsson M (1997) Solid-phase synthesis of glycopeptides: immunological studies with T cell stimulating glycopeptides. Curr Med Chem 4:85–116

Koenigs W, Knorr E (1901) Derivatives of grape sugar and galactose. Ber Dtsch Chem Ges 34:957–981

Kunz H, Birnbach S (1986) Synthesis of tumor associated T_N- and T-antigen type O-glycopeptides and their conjugation to bovine serum albumin. Angew Chem Int Ed 25:360–362

Kunz H (1987) Synthesis of glycopeptides, partial structures of biological recognition components. Angew Chem Int Ed 26:294–308

Kunz H, Birnbach S, Wernig P (1990) Synthesis of glycopeptides with the T_N and T antigen structures, and their coupling to bovine serum albumin. Carbohydr Res 202:207–23

Kunz H (1997) O- and N-glycopeptides: synthesis of selectively deprotected building blocks. In: Hanessian S (ed) Preparative carbohydrate chemistry. Marcel Dekker, New York, pp 265–281

Lee D, Danishefsky SJ (2009) 'Biologic' level structures through chemistry: a total synthesis of a unimolecular pentavalent MUCI glycopeptide construct. Tetrahedron Lett 50:2167–2170

Lemieux RU (1963) Tetra-O-acetyl-D-glucopyranosyl bromide. In: Whistler RL, Wolfrom ML (eds) Methods in carbohydrate chemistry, vol 2. Academic, New York, pp 221–223

Lemieux RU, Ratcliffe RM (1979) The azidonitration of tri-O-acetyl-D-galactal. Can J Chem 57:1244–51

Lergenmüller M, Ito Y, Ogawa T (1998) Use of dichlorophthaloyl (DCPhth) group as an amino protecting group in oligosaccharide synthesis. Tetrahedron 54:1381–1394

Liakatos A, Kunz H (2007) Synthetic glycopeptides for the development of cancer vaccines. Curr Opin Mol Ther 9:35–44

Liebe B, Kunz H (1994) Synthesis of Sialyl-Tn antigen. Regioselective sialylation of a galactosamine threonine conjugate unblocked in the carbohydrate portion. Tetrahedron Lett 35:8777–8

Liebe B, Kunz H (1997a) Solid-phase synthesis of a tumor-associated sialyl-T_N antigen glycopeptide with a partial sequence of the "tandem repeat" of the MUC-1 mucin. Angew Chem Int Ed 36:618–621

Liebe B, Kunz H (1997b) Solid-phase synthesis of a sialyl-Tn-glycoundecapeptide of the MUC1 repeating unit. Helv Chim Acta 80:1473–1482

Lloyd KO, Burchell J, Kudryashov V, Yin BWT, Taylor-Papadimitriou J (1996) Comparison of O-linked carbohydrate chains in MUC-1 mucin from normal breast epithelial cell lines and breast carcinoma cell lines. Demonstration of simpler and fewer glycan chains in tumor cells. J Biol Chem 271:33325–33334

Loenn H, Stenvall K (1992) Exceptionally high yield in glycosylation with sialic acid. Synthesis of a GM3 glycoside. Tetrahedron Lett 33:115–16

Marra A, Sinay P (1989) Stereoselective synthesis of 2-thioglycosides of N-acetylneuraminic acid. Carbohydr Res 187:35–42

Meinjohanns E, Meldal M, Schleyer A, Paulsen H, Bock K (1996) Efficient syntheses of core 1, core 2, core 3 and core 4 building blocks for SPS of mucin O-glycopeptides based on the N-Dts-method. J Chem Soc Perkin Trans 1:985–993

Meldal M (1994) Glycopeptide synthesis. Neoglycoconjugates: Prep Appl 1994:145–98

Paulsen H, Hoelck JP (1982) Building blocks of oligosaccharides. Part XV. Synthesis of O-β-D-galactopyranosyl-(1→3)-O-(α-D-2-acetamido-2-deoxy-α-D-galactopyranosyl)-(1→3)-L-serine and -L-threonine glycopeptides. Carbohydr Res 109:89–107

Peters S, Bielfeldt T, Meldal M, Bock K, Paulsen H (1992) Multiple-column solid-phase glycopeptide synthesis. J Chem Soc Perkin Trans 1:1163–1171

Ragupathi G, Koide F, Livingstone PO, Cho YS, Endo A, Wan Q, Spassova M, Keding S, Allen J, Ouerfelli O, Wilson RM, Danishefsky SJ (2006) Preparation and evaluation of unimolecular pentavalent and hexavalent antigenic constructs targeting prostate and breast cancer: a synthetic route to anticancer vaccine candidates. J Am Chem Soc 128:2715–2725

Rosen T, Lico IM, Chu DTW (1988) A convenient and highly chemoselective method for the reductive acetylation of azides. J Org Chem 53:1580–2

Schmidt RR, Behrendt M, Toepfer A (1990) Glycosyl imidates. 48. Nitriles as solvents in glycosylation reactions: highly selective β-glycoside synthesis. Synlett 1990:694–6

Schuster M, Wang P, Paulson JC, Wong CH (1994) Solid-phase chemical-enzymic synthesis of glycopeptides and oligosaccharides. J Am Chem Soc 116:1135–1136

Seitz O, Kunz H (1997) HYCRON, an allylic anchor for high-efficiency solid phase synthesis of protected peptides and glycopeptides. J Org Chem 62:813–826

Shafizadeh F (1963) Galactal. In: Whistler RL, Wolfrom ML (eds) Methods in carbohydrate chemistry, vol 2. Academic, New York, pp 409–410

Shin I, Jung HJ, Lee MR (2001) Chemoselective ligation of maleimidosugars to peptides/protein for the preparation of neoglycopeptides/neoglycoprotein. Tetrahedron Lett 42:1325–1328

Sjölin P, Elofsson M, Khilberg J (1996) Removal of acyl protecting groups from glycopeptides: base does not epimerize peptide stereocenters, and β-elimination is slow. J Org Chem 61:560–565

Smith M, Rammler DH, Goldberg IH, Khorana HG (1962) Polynucleotides. XIV. Specific synthesis of the C3′-C5′ internucleotide linkage. Synthesis of uridylyl(3′→5′)-uridine and uridylyl-(3′→5′)-adenosine. J Am Chem Soc 84:430–40

Sorensen AL, Reis CA, Tarp MA, Mandel U, Ramachandran K, Sankaranarayanan V, Schwientek T, Graham J, Taylor-Papadimitriou J, Hollingsworth MA, Burchell J, Clausen H (2006) Chemoenzymatically synthesized multimeric Tn/STn MUC1 glycopeptides elicit cancer-specific anti-MUC1 antibody responses and override tolerance. Glycobiology 16:96–107

Springer GF, Desai RR, Fry WA, Goodale RL, Shearen JG, Scanlon EF (1983) T antigen, a tumor marker against which breast, lung and pancreas carcinoma patients mount immune responses. Cancer Detect Prev 6:111–118

Springer GF (1984) T and Tn, general carcinoma autoantigens. Science 224:1198–206

Swallow DM, Gendler S, Griffiths B, Corney G, Taylor-Papadimitriou J, Bramwell ME (1987) The human tumor-associated epithelial mucins are coded by an expressed hypervariable gene locus PUM. Nature 328:82–4

Tam JP (1988) Methionine ligation strategy in the biomimetic synthesis of parathyroid hormones. Proc Natl Acad Sci USA 85:5409–13

Tarp MA, Sorensen AL, Mandel U, Paulsen H, Burchell J, Taylor-Papadimitriou J, Clausen H (2007) Identification of a novel cancer-specific immunodominant glycopeptide epitope in the MUC1 tandem repeat. Glycobiology 17:197–209

Taylor-Papadimitriou J, Burchell J, Miles DW, Dalziel M (1999) MUC1 and cancer. Biochim Biophys Act, Mol Basis Dis 1455:301–313

Tietze LF, Arlt M, Beller M, Gluesenkamp KH, Jaehde E, Rajewsky MF (1991) Conjugation of p-aminophenyl glycosides with squaric acid diester to a carrier protein and the use of the neoglycoprotein in the histochemical detection of lectins. Chem Ber 124:1215–21

Tomita M, Marchesi VF (1975) Amino acid sequence and oligosaccharide attachment sites of human erythrocyte glycophorin. Proc Natl Acad Sci USA 72:2964–2968

Wagner M, Dziadek S, Kunz H (2003) The (2-phenyl-2-trimethylsilyl)ethyl-(PTMSEL)-linker in the synthesis of glycopeptide partial structures of complex cell surface glycoproteins. Chem Eur J 9:6018–6030

Wang SS (1973) p-Alkoxybenzyl alcohol resin and p-alkoxybenzyloxycarbonylhydrazide resin for solid phase synthesis of protected peptide fragments. J Am Chem Soc 95:1328–33

Westerlind U, Hobel A, Gaidzik N, Schmitt E, Kunz H (2008) Synthetic vaccines consisting of tumor-associated MUC1 glycopeptide antigens and a T-cell epitope for the induction of a highly specific humoral immune response. Angew Chem Int Ed 47:7551–7556

Westerlind U, Schröder H, Hobel A, Gaidzik N, Kaiser A, Niemeyer CM, Schmitt E, Waldmann H, Kunz H (2009) Tumor-associated MUC1 tandem-repeat glycopeptide microarrays to evaluate serum- and monoclonal-antibody specificity. Angew Chem Int Ed 48:8263–8267

Wilkinson BL, Day S, Malins LR, Apostolopoulos V, Payne RJ (2011) Self-adjuvanting multi-component cancer vaccine candidates combining per-glycosylated MUC1 glycopeptides and the toll-like receptor 2 agonist Pam_3CysSer. Angew Chem Int Ed 50:1635–1639

Wittrock S, Becker T, Kunz H (2007) Synthetic vaccines of tumor-associated glycopeptide antigens by immune-compatible thioether linkage to bovine serum albumin. Angew Chem Int Ed 46:5226–5230

Zemplén G, Kuntz A (1923) The sodium compounds of glucose and the saponification of the acylated sugars. Chem Ber 56B:1705–1710

Zhu J, Wan Q, Lee D, Yang G, Spassova M, Ouerfelli O, Ragupathi G, Damani P, Livingstone PO, Danishefsky SJ (2009) From synthesis to biologics: preclinical data on a chemistry derived anticancer vaccine. J Am Chem Soc 131:9298–9303

Glycan Microarray Analysis of Tumor-Associated Antibodies

12

Ola Blixt, Irene Boos, and Ulla Mandel

12.1 Introduction

A change in glycosylation is a common feature of tumor cells and may affect any type of glycoconjugate such as *N*-glycans and *O*-glycans on glycoproteins, and oligosaccharides on glycolipids and glycosaminoglycans (Altmann 2007; Hakomori 1985). These changes in glycan structures have marked influence on many diverse biological functions of complex carbohydrates and contribute to the malignant phenotype. Historically, changes in glycan structures on cancer cells have also served as the first biomarkers of cancer from early studies of histo-blood group antigens by immunohistochemistry (Hakomori 1984; Dabelsteen 1996; Kannagi et al. 2001) to more advanced techniques applied today involving mass spectrometry. Throughout the last 40+ years antibodies and, in particular, monoclonal antibodies (mAb) have served as a prominent tool for defining glycan changes in cancer, and a large number of antibodies to different carbohydrate structures have been developed and the fine specificities characterized by a number of different approaches (Heimburg-Molinaro and Rittenhouse-Olson 2009). In this chapter we review representative monoclonal antibodies with cancer-associated reactivity patterns and how their specificities can be analyzed by emerging microarray technologies.

Arguably the most widely studied tumor carbohydrate antigens are those produced by incomplete biosynthesis of mucin-type *O*-glycans (Springer 1984), and they constitute a good example for how cancer-associated glycans emerge through altered biosynthesis of glycosylation in cells (Fig. 12.1). At least the three tumor associated antigens (TACA), Tn, T and STn differ from other epitopes in that they are

O. Blixt (✉) • I. Boos • U. Mandel
Department of Cellular and Molecular Medicine, Copenhagen Center for Glycomics, University of Copenhagen, Blegdamsvej 3, DK-2200 Copenhagen, Denmark
e-mail: olablixt@sund.ku.dk

P. Kosma and S. Müller-Loennies (eds.), *Anticarbohydrate Antibodies*,
DOI 10.1007/978-3-7091-0870-3_12, © Springer-Verlag/Wien 2012

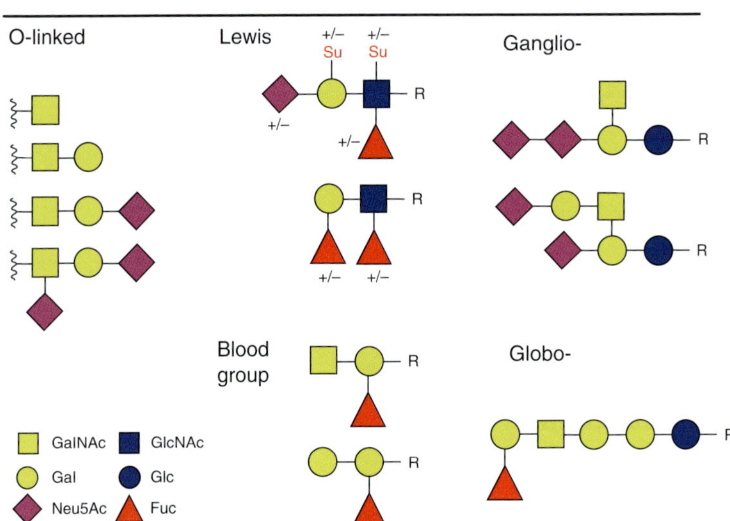

Fig. 12.1 Examples of tumor related carbohydrate epitopes. Abbreviations *Su* sulfate, *R* penultimate glycans or lipid

immunogenic in the host and every individual has an appreciable amount of natural antibodies to these epitopes (Kurtenkov et al. 2005)

Carbohydrates are immunogenic and many of the early studies of immunity to cancer cells in animals resulted in antibodies with cancer-associated reactivity that eventually were shown to be directed to distinct glycan epitopes. The first and most prominent example being an antibody specific for a colon carcinoma ganglio-oligosaccharide SLe[a] (Koprowski et al. 1981; Magnani et al. 1982) and many others followed this (for review see Kannagi and Hakomori 2001). Many antibodies to carbohydrate structures are more difficult to develop because of the T-cell-independent response to carbohydrates (Cunto-Amesty et al. 2001). This can result in the production of low affinity IgM antibodies and difficulties with screening technologies can cause selections of antibodies with low-affinity binding sites because of the net avidity enhancement. Unfortunately, the low-affinity binding site can also have a similar affinity for unwanted structures. However, several IgG antibodies do exist.

Production of antibodies using cellular extracts can result in antibodies that react with multiple related structures, and therefore the resultant bioassays have sensitivity or specificity problems. Protein conjugates of saccharides for the production of polyclonal and mAbs to carbohydrate structures can be used to solve these problems. The development of the hybridoma technique by Köhler and Milstein (1975) allowed the production of specific mAbs, which could help to identify specific proteins and glycoproteins for example in embryonic development, and cell differentiation as well as oncogenesis and several other diseases. The problem is that one need to isolate clones, grow them up and select them one by one but also are limited by responses in mice (and later rats, guinea pigs and man). A more recent technology is based on natural or random phage antibodies in phage display assays which allows for large screening and cloning of antibody domains (Nelson et al. 2010) which provides genes encoding recombinant antibodies against antigens of interest. This approach was recently applied towards production of anti-carbohydrate antibodies (Yuasa et al. 2010). It was also determined, that the use and production of IgY, a chicken immunoglobulin, has some advantage over mammalian IgG antibodies in immunodiagnostics. The IgY can be purified easy out of egg yolk, so that blood or cell collection is not necessary but additional research is required to make useful specific anti-carbohydrate-IgY comparable to hybridoma produced mAb (Kaltgrad et al. 2007).

Monoclonal antibody preparations can be used as either culture supernatant or ascites fluid. Further purification of immunoglobulins can be performed with affinity chromatography, and Protein A- or Protein G-Sepharose is applied based on the immunoglobulin binding ability of Protein A or Protein G respectively. Established methods for mAb characterization are dot- and western-blotting, agglutination tests, immunofluorescence as well as enzyme-linked immunosorbent assays (ELISA) (Geng et al. 2005). Monoclonal antibodies to oligosaccharides are particularly important in mapping the remarkably diverse cell-surface glycome but there is also considerable heterogeneity of the carbohydrate specificity of these antibodies to identify specific carbohydrate ligands involved in cell adhesion and various recognition events (Kannagi et al. 2001). Determination of the reactivity of the produced antibodies with related oligosaccharide structures is essential prior to utilization.

12.2 Methods for Characterization of Fine Specificities of Anti-Carbohydrate Antibodies

Characterization of anti-carbohydrate antibodies requires access to glycoconjugates with a single epitope as shown with glycolipids (Young et al. 1981) or later with neo-glycolipids produced from glycoproteins (Larkin et al. 1991). Initially libraries of glycolipids were used for fine specificity analysis but limited by availability and purity of carbohydrate antigens. Advances in the field of carbohydrate chemistry (Seeberger 2008) and chemoenzymatic synthesis (Blixt and Razi 2006) in combination with new technologies for high-throughput screening (Alvarez and Blixt 2006), have enabled further characterization of the fine specificities of these mAbs. Current methods for mAb binding to immobilized ligands are based on sandwich assays with fluorescently labeled mAbs or fluorescently labeled anti-mAb antibodies. Depending on methods used, significant differences in binding specificities can be obtained due to molecular presentation of the carbohydrate ligand (Rinaldi et al. 2009) as illustrated in Fig. 12.2. In addition, the glycan microarray approach mostly presents haptens and although this may be sufficient to map epitopes final confirmation with native glycoconjugates seems necessary.

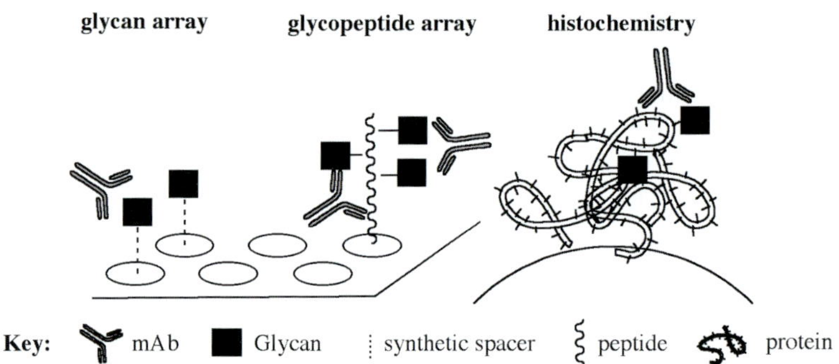

Fig. 12.2 Glycan-antibody interactions on surfaces

12.2.1 Printed Glycan Microarrays (PGA)

The glycan array technology offers a unique opportunity to display hundreds if not thousands of defined glycan structures in minute amounts at high density for probing fine specificities of mAbs or scarce serum antibodies in comparative analysis. Over the past decade several different platforms have been established containing respected numbers of glycan features (Rillahan and Paulson 2010). One of the most advanced glycan microarray with >600 unique glycans is offered from the Consortium for Functional Glycomics (CFG) and binding studies of animal and plant lectins, antibodies, toxins, and pathogens, including viruses and bacteria have been successfuly evaluated (Blixt et al. 2004). These printed glycan microarrays are sensitive, robust, and require very small quantities of glycans and glycan binding proteins (GBPs) which makes this technology also suitable for diagnostic developments. An inherent problem with carbohydrate-protein interactions is their often low affinity (mM–μM) due to fast-off rates resulting in reduced binding. However, this can be in many cases overcome by creating multimeric complexes to increase binding avidity (Blixt et al. 2004). Monoclonal antibodies have affinities that are generally stronger even for carbohydrate ligands and the glycan microarray performs relatively well in such binding studies as exemplified in sections below.

12.2.2 *O*-Glycopeptide Microarrays (O-GPM)

Much information on glycoprotein recognition has been derived by extrapolating data from glycan microarrays, which present the glycans in isolation. However, it does not fully account for the contributions from the larger glycoprotein environment that can have an important role in the specificity and recognition. The complexity and heterogeneity of non-template driven nature of *O*-glycan biosynthesis with the initiation step of the 20 distinct GalNAc transferases, together with the aberrant alteration of the *O*-glycosylation mechanism in disease, the formation of *O*-glycopeptide epitopes (O-PTMs) is large. In fact, development of

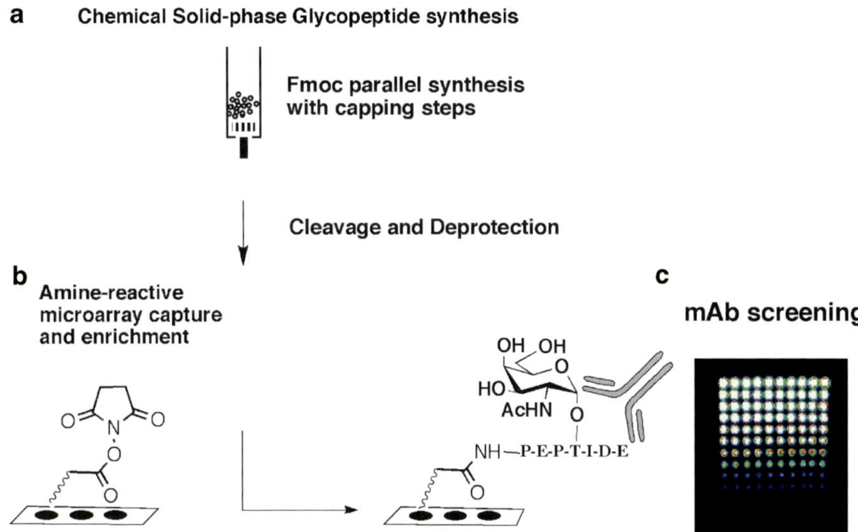

Fig. 12.3 Fabrication of *O*-glycopeptide microarrays. (**a**) Chemical synthesis with *N*-acetylation capping steps. (**b**) On-slide enrichment of crude product via amine-reactive *N*-hydroxysuccinimide microarray glass surface. (**c**) Microarray analysis with monoclonal antibodies followed by detection with fluorescent labeled secondary antibody

anti-carbohydrate mAbs occur in most cases through immunization protocols where the hapten is a conjugate of a non-natural protein or peptide carrier or attached to its native protein which complicates the identification of the target as the antigen can be found on numerous different peptide sequences and can be presented to the host as clusters or as individual small epitopes. Therefore it is imperative to also include libraries covering parts of the underlying peptide sequence that can have a profound effect on mAb recognition. We recently reported a strategy to assemble an *O*-glycopeptide microarray platform (Fig. 12.3) for screening and characterization of GBPs and anti-carbohydrate antibodies as well as serum antibodies (Blixt et al. 2010) and several examples are illustrated in the following sections.

12.3 Anti-Carbohydrate Tumor Antibody Specificities

One of the first anti-carbohydrate antibodies produced was the asialo-GM2 (Young et al. 1979). Since then many additional mAbs to other glycan determinants have been generated and their specificities are well established with different biochemical assays (Kannagi et al. 2001). Along with the new glycan microarray technology development in glycomics many of these mAbs are now being increasingly re-evaluated to confirm their specificities but also to gain new insights into potential cross-reactivities and/or fine subspecificities. In Table 12.1 we have

Table 12.1 Tumor associated carbohydrate antigens defined by monoclonal antibodies

Antibody clone name (isotype)	Tumor antigen (reference)	Immunogen	Reported cross-reactivity by array
HBTn/5 F4 (IgM)	Tn (Thurnher et al. 1993)	AOSM	Tn-cluster
1E3 (IgG2a)	Tn (Mandel et al. 1991)	AOSM	Tn-cluster
5E5 (IgG1)	Tn-MUC1 (Sorensen et al. 2006)	Tn-MUC1-peptide	Tn-peptide
2D9 (IgG1)	Tn- MUC1 (Tarp 2007)	Tn-MUC1-peptide	Tn-peptide
HBsTn/3F1 (IgG1)	STn (Clausen, unpublished)	OSM	STn-cluster
TKH2 (IgG1)	STn (Kjeldsen et al. 1988)	OSM	STn-cluster
B72.3 (TAG72) (IgG1)	STn (Nuti et al. 1982)	Breast cancer	STn-peptide
HH8 (IgM)	T (Clausen et al. 1988)	Galactosyl-A glycolipid	R-Tα-R
JAA-F11 (IgG3)	T- (Heimburg et al. 2006)	T-BSA	R-Tα-
3C9 (IgM)	T (Clausen et al. 1988)	Galactosyl-A glycolipid	Tα-
KL-6 (IgG)	ST- (Ohyabu et al. 2009)	MUC1	ST-MUC1 peptide
1B2 (IgM)	LacNAc (Young et al. 1981)	Glycolipid	Not tested
FH6 (IgM)	SLe^x (Fukushi et al. 1985)	Glycolipid	Specific
KM93 (IgM)	SLe^x (Shitara et al. 1987) CalBiochem	Lung cancer	Cross react Sialyl-lacNAc
Ab1 (IgM)	6-Su-SiaLe^x (Hirakawa et al. 2010)	CHO cells	Cross react with Le^c
NS-CA19-9 (IgG1)	SLe^a (Magnani et al. 1981) DAKO	Colon cancer	Specific
7E3 (IgM)	SLe^a (Sawada et al. 2011) MabVax Ther	SLe^a -KLH	Specific
2D3 (IgM)	SLe^a (Takada et al. 1991) Seikagaku	Pure lipid	Cross react
MC-480/SSEA-1 (IgM)	Le^x (Kannagi et al. 1982)	teratocarcinoma	Specific
SH1 (IgG3)	Le^x (Singhal, Cancer Res, 1990)	Purified glycolipid	Specific
7LE (IgG1)	Le^a (Rouger et al. 1987)	Ovarian cyst mucin	Cross react
2.25LE (IgG1)	Le^b (Rouger et al. 1987)	Ovarian cyst mucin	Le^a
AH6 (IgM)	Le^Y (Abe et al. 1983)	MKN74 carcinoma cell line	Cross react
9A (IgG3)	Blood group A (AbCam)	A431 carcinoma cells	Non-type specific
HH6 (IgG3)	PanA Blood group A (Clausen, unpublished)	Blood group A glycolipids	Non-type specific

(continued)

Table 12.1 (continued)

Antibody clone name (isotype)	Tumor antigen (reference)	Immunogen	Reported cross-reactivity by array
NaM87-1 F6 (IgG3)	Blood group A (Commercial various)		Non-type specific
CLCP-19B (IgM)	Blood group B (Commercial various)	ASPC-1 Pan Ca Cell Line	Unspec.
Z5H-2 (IgM)	Blood group B (Commercial various)	B human blood protein	Non-type specific
Bric231 (IgG1)	Blood group H (Commercial various)	HEL cell line	H-type-2 specific
17-206 (IgG3)	Blood group H (Commercial various)	SW-403 Col Ca Cell Line	H-type-1 specific
BE2 (IgM)	Blood group H (Young et al. 1981)	Glycolipid	H-type-2 specific
ME361	GD2 (Thurin et al. 1986)	Human melanoma	GD2 specific
GMR7	GD2 (Ozawa et al. 1992) Seikagaku	Glycolipid	GD2 specific

selected several commercially available anti-carbohydrate antibodies as well as other published mAbs where data are publically available on the CFG database. In the subsequent section we will highlight their reactivities while discussing the different methods used for their characterization.

12.3.1 Anti-Tn-, STn-, T- and -Antibodies

The GalNAc-(Tn-) antigen was initially described as carbohydrate antigen on erythrocytes (Dausset et al. 1959) or Tn-syndrome (Berger 1999). The extent to which the peptide backbone and pattern of Tn displayed (i.e. single versus clustered sites) has not been fully clarified for many anti Tn- and STn antibodies. One of the first describing the importance of this was Yamashina with mAb MLS 102 (Kurosaka et al. 1988). Since then it has been believed that GalNAc-Ser/Thr is involved in Tn-antigen but the exact epitope structure is unknown. It is well known that the Tn-antigen is a tumor-associated antigen (Springer 1989) and the fact that it is expressed in a variety of malignant disorders have opened up a new interest for this antigen as a cancer-associated marker (Hakomori 1985). The Tn-antigen shows some structural similarity to the A antigen, and blood type A individuals have less antibody immune response against the Tn antigens (Hirohashi et al. 1985). Specific expression of Tn-antigen on a surface of malignant cells enabled to develop anti-cancer vaccine containing Tn (Springer 1997; Xu et al. 2004). Research on passive administration of antibodies directed against carbohydrate antigens could also have a potential effect in cancer therapy (Zhang et al. 1998).

Several anti-Tn mAbs have been developed with Tn-antigens on different carrier molecules as immunogens. Despite a clear and defined structure of the carbohydrate part of Tn-antigen, the real epitope structure was found to have a complex nature (Li et al. 2010) and Tn-specific mAbs can recognize the Tn-antigen differently. A few examples of anti Tn-antibodies with distinct specificity differences are illustrated with the printed glycan array (PGA) (Sect. 12.2.1) and the glycopeptide microarray (Sect. 12.2.2) above. Either of the tested Tn-mAbs HBTn/5 F4 (Thurnher et al. 1993), 1E3 (Mandel et al. 1991), were able to bind significantly to the PGA although binding to other glycans have been reported for 1E3 on an alternative platform where glycans were conjugated to BSA (Li et al. 2009). It has been noted that a certain density of the Tn-epitope is needed for some Tn-mAbs to bind, whereas for others, it does not, illustrating the widespread characterization problem of these Tn-specific mAbs. The O-GPM array analysis of HBTn/5F4 and 1E3 is a representative example on how both, density and peptide sequence, affect binding (Fig. 12.4). The immunogen for HBTn/5F4 was AOSM and the mAb is commercially available for histochemistry analysis (Dako Cytomation, Carpenteria, CA). As illustrated in Fig. 12.4, a selection of Tn-glycopeptides from the MUC1 20mer tandem repeat covering all possible combination of glycosylation sites (Blixt et al. 2010) revealed a rather complex reactivity pattern of the HBTn/5F4 mAb. The mAb binds to both mono- and clustered di-glycosylated Tn-epitopes, influenced by the underlying peptide sequence. Specifically the GSTAPP epitope of MUC1a (Fig. 12.4) is preferred over other glycosylation sites (compare compounds 1–5). Binding can either be increased with addition of other distant sites (compound 9) or decreased (compound 14) but strongly increased with clustered di-glycosylated sequences in the GSTAPP site (compounds 23, 46, 54–59). The monovalent reactivity can also be influenced by the penultimate amino acids as illustrated in Fig. 12.5 for mAb HBTn/5F4.

The other Tn-hapten mAb, 1E3 (BM8) derived from immunization with AOSM (Mandel et al. 1991) showed a more restricted preference for clustered Tn-glycopeptides. Only di-glycosylated sequences were tolerated at the GSTAPP sequence site on MUC1 (Fig. 12.4). Both the HBTn and 1E3 mAbs are also reactive towards other Tn-peptides (not listed here) have also shown similar reactivities towards clustered Tn-antigens (Nakada et al. 1993; Coltart et al. 2002; Kato et al. 2008). Recently two Tn-glycopeptide specific mAbs, 5E5 and 2D9, were identified to be specific towards MUC1 expressing tumors (Sorensen et al. 2006) with a distinct preference for mono- and bis-Tn-peptide specific sequences (Blixt et al. 2010; Kracun et al. 2010).

A structurally related tumor hapten is the sialylated Tn-hapten, αNeu5Ac (2→6)αGalNAc(STn-) where several mAbs have been raised and evaluated in clinical studies, *in vitro* diagnostics, *in vivo* diagnostics, and active immunotherapy (Nuti et al. 1982; Kjeldsen et al. 1988). Because of its association with cancer, it has been suggested that STn epitopes are actively involved in the cell adhesion and metastatic spread of tumor cells to endothelial cell surfaces (Reddish et al. 1997). The mAb TKH2 which was generated following immunization with ovine submaxillary mucin (OSM), a well characterized mucin that displays clusters of STn and Tn epitopes (Nuti et al. 1982; Kjeldsen et al. 1988) and the mAb, HBsTn/3F1, demonstrate specific STn-binding to the PGA (Fig. 12.6) but with a preference for clustered di-STn-glycosylated peptide sequences using STn-glycopeptides (Reddish et al. 1997) (data not shown).

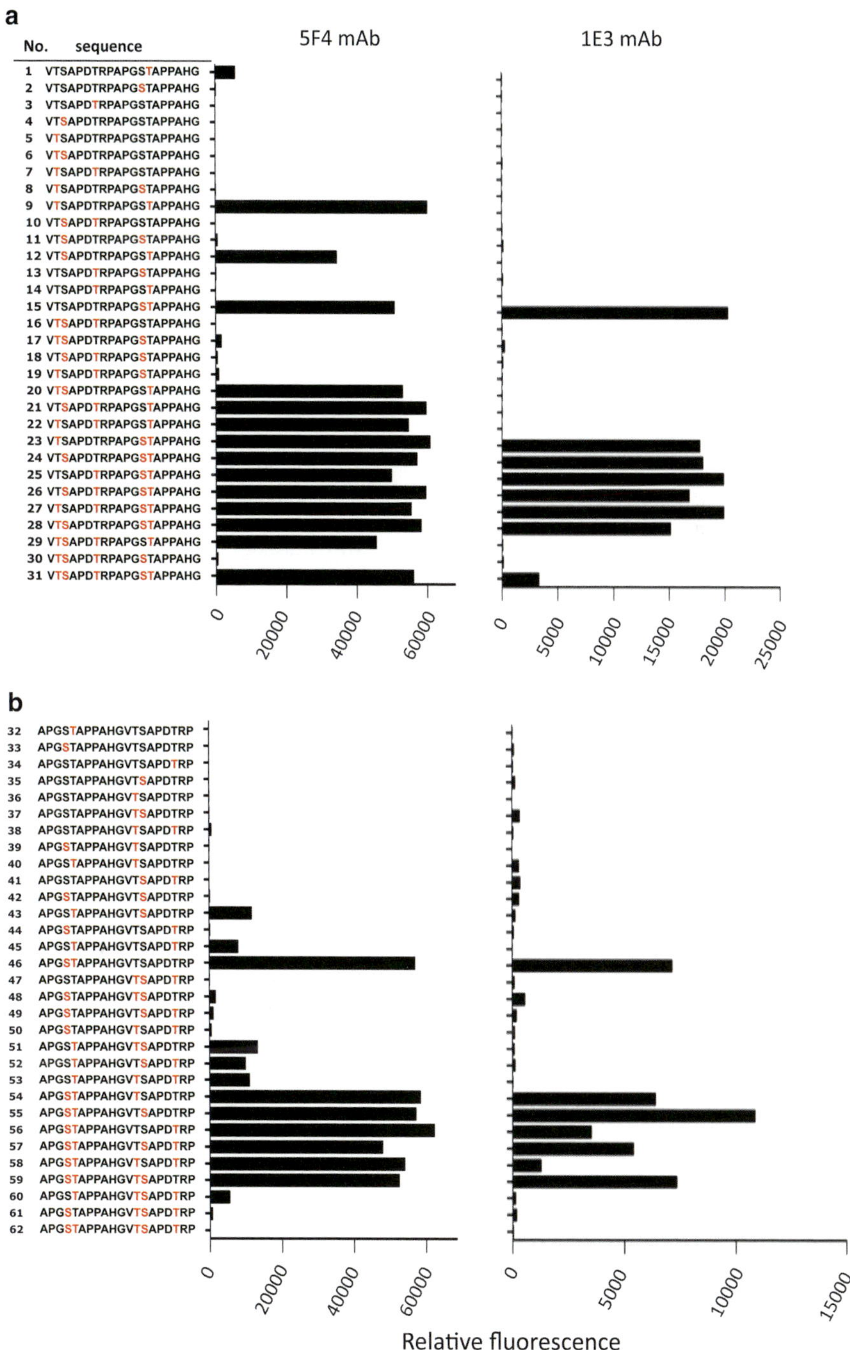

Fig. 12.4 Binding of HBTn/5F4 and 1E3 mAbs to a Tn-glycopeptide microarray (O-GPM array) detected with anti-mouse IgG-Cy3 labeled antibody. Glycopeptides (**a** 1–31, MUC1a-20mer of TR, **b** 32–62, MUC1b 10mer overlap of MUC1a TR) with marked amino acids in red are glycosylated with GalNAc

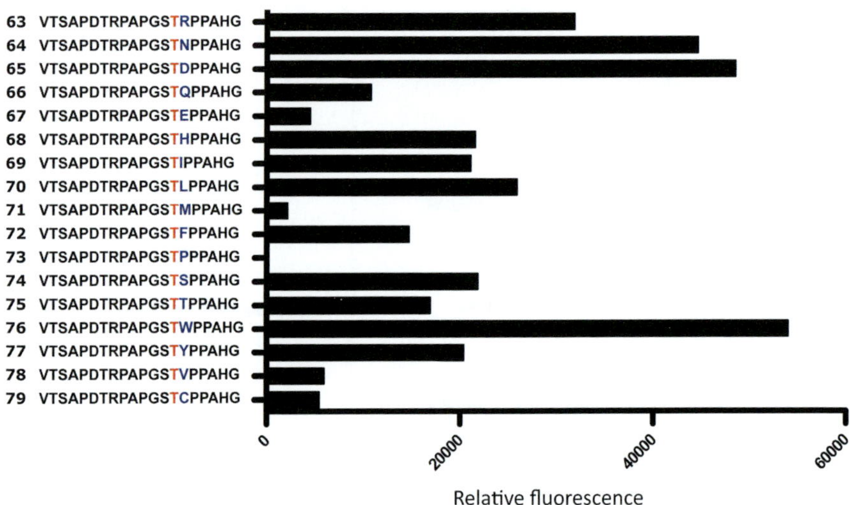

Fig. 12.5 Binding of HBTn/5F4 mAb to arrayed Tn-MUC1 analogs detected with anti-mouse IgG-Cy3 labeled antibody. Marked amino acids in *red* are glycosylated with GalNAc and amino acid marked in *blue* are mutations

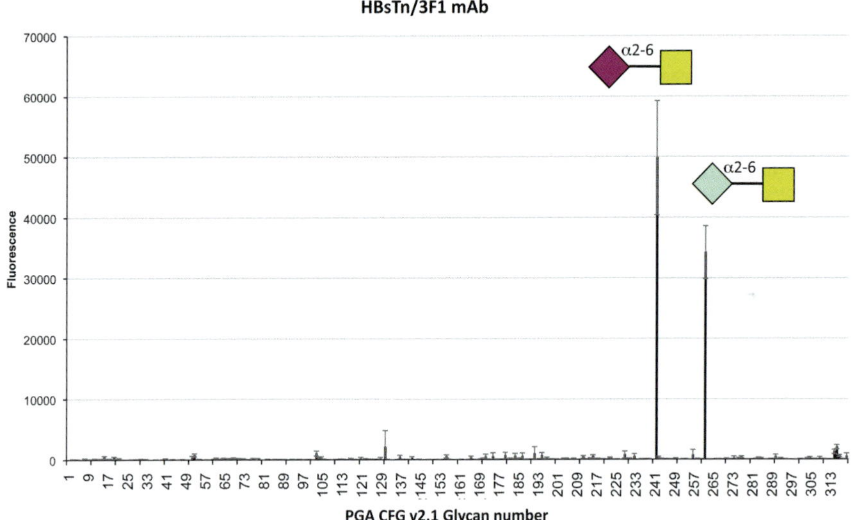

Fig. 12.6 Printed glycan microarray (PGA) analysis of HbsTn/3F1 mAb on the CFG v3.2 (www.functionalglycomics.org). Primary antibody was detected with anti-mouse-IgG-Cy3 labeled antibody. Symbols in figure: ◆ Neu5Ac; ◆ Neu5Gc; ■ GalNAc

The clustered reactivity might be due to the mucin glycoprotein specificity of these monoclonal reagents because mucins typically present multiple tandems of serine/threonine in the peptide core sequences. Interestingly, the related and commercially available B72.3 STn mAb (TAG72), raised against human, metastatic mammary carcinoma cells (Nuti et al. 1982), did show a more selective reactivity to the underlying peptide structure (Fig. 12.7a) as seen with the Tn-reactive mAbs. Only clustered bis-STn-epitopes within the G**ST**APP sequence were able to bind to B72.3 mAb after on-chip glycosylation with hST6GalNAc transferase (Blixt et al 2010) whereas mono-glycosylation either at serine or threonine within the same site were inactive. In addition, altered or extended glycoforms of the G**ST**APP site such as Core-1 and Core-3 structures were negative (Fig. 12.7b) (Blixt et al. 2011).

Thomsen-Friedenreich antigen (TF- or T-antigen), or more precisely, the epitope βGal(l→3)αGalNAc-attached to proteins by an *O*-serine or *O*-threonine linkage, is expressed in many carcinomas, including those of the breast, colon, bladder, and prostate. The T-antigen is important in adhesion and metastasis and therefore a potential immunotherapy target. Several mAbs to the T-antigen have been developed but many of these show cross-reactivities towards extended glycoforms (Heimburg-Molinaro and Rittenhouse-Olson 2009) as well as specificity for both anomeric forms of this disaccharide (TFα and TFβ, including related structures on glycolipids) (Dessureault et al. 1997; Karsten et al. 1995). Only a few anti T-antigen mAbs have been evaluated on the PGA, the JAA-F11 (Heimburg et al. 2006), HH8 (Clausen et al. 1988) and 3C9 (Bohm et al. 1997). All three mAbs showed specific binding to α-linked βGal(l→3)GalNAc-antigen and their extended glycoforms except for 3C9 that also bound β-linked T-antigen and the Core-2 branched glycoforms (Table 12.2). Both HH8 and 3C9 were derived from the same immunogen, a galactosyl-A glycolipid antigen having the terminal structure, βGal(l→3)α GalNAc(1→3)[αFuc(1→2)]βGal(l→R), which is the precursor for type 3 chain A (repetitive A) and type 3 chain H (A-associated H). On the PGA only HH8 did bind extended A oligosaccharides (Table 12.2, entries 13, 14) in agreement with a previous report with de-sialylated erythrocytes of O- and B-type (Clausen et al. 1988). The 3C9 mAb did not show any binding to blood group related antigens.

Another tumor related mAb, KL-6, used for determination of sialylated MUC1 is strongly expressed on various carcinomas (Inagaki et al. 2009). Recently the epitope was defined by a glycopeptide ELISA assay (Ohyabu et al. 2009) and confirmed by the O-GPM array to be a αNeuAc(2→3)T-PDTR-epitope on MUC1 (Blixt et al. 2011). Reactivity to the same epitope was previously described by the mAb MY.1E12 (Takeuchi et al. 2002).

12.3.2 Anti-Lewis Antibodies

Cancer-associated glycans, SLe^a and SLe^x are well established tumor markers and they were recently shown to appear after epigenetic silencing of some glycan genes during early carcinogenesis (Kannagi et al. 2001). Detection and appearance of tumor related Lewis antigens have been greatly facilitated with panels of anti-Lewis mAbs many that are now commercially available and frequently used in histology.

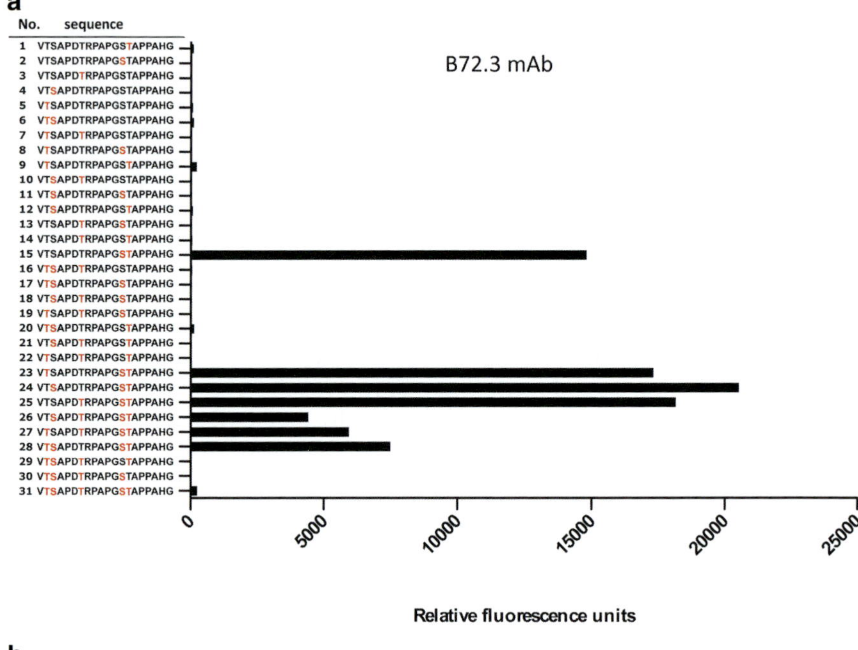

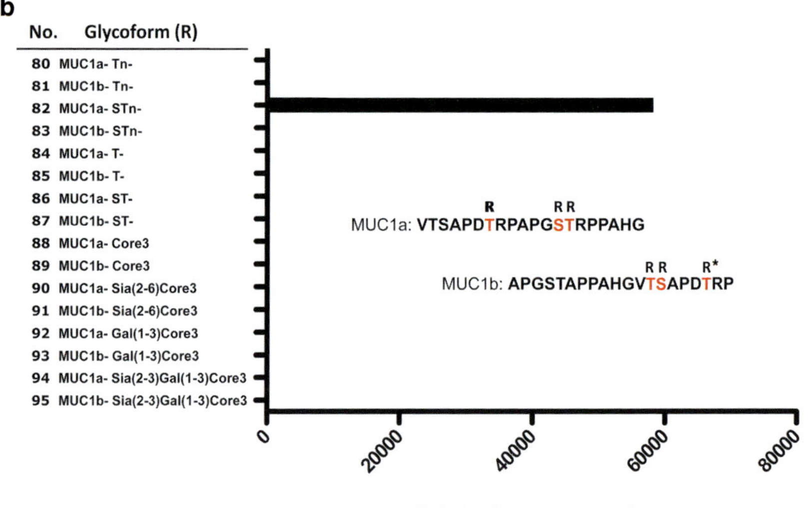

Fig. 12.7 Binding of B72.3 (TAG72) mAb to an *O*-glycosylated MUC1-20mer microarrays (Blixt et al. 2011). Primary antibody was detected with anti-mouse-IgG-Cy3 labeled antibody. (**a**) Analysis to STn-MUC1a glycoforms. Glycopeptides (1–31, MUC1a-20mer with marked amino acids in *red* are glycosylated with Neu5Ac(2-6)GalNAc. (**b**) Analysis to extended glycoforms of MUC1a and MUC1b. * = R not included for Core3 glycoforms

Table 12.2 Binding of anti-T-antigen mAbs to selected *O*-glycans. The mAbs JAA-F11 and HH8 were analyzed as described (www.functionalglycomics.org) and mAbs 3 C9 was applied as cell culture supernatant (1:4 dilution) and detected with anti-mouse-IgM-Cy3 labeled antibody. # Data for 3 C9 is unpublished and not available at CFG database

List no.	Glycan no. CFG v3.2	Selected glycan structures for T-antigen specific mAbs	mAb reactivity (+binding)		
			JAA	HH8	3C9#
1	124	Galβ1–3GalNAcα–Sp8	+	+	+
2	275	Galβ1–3GalNAc–Sp14			
3	125	Galβ1–3GalNAcβ–Sp8			+
4	160	GlcNAcβ1–3GalNAcα–Sp8			
5	121	Galβ1–3(Neu5Acα2–6)GalNAcα–Sp8	+	+	
6	122	Galβ1–3(Neu5Acβ2–6)GalNAcα–Sp8	+	+	
7	58	Fucα1–2Galβ1–3GalNAcα-Sp8			
8	120	Galβ1–3(GlcNAcβ1–6)GalNAcα–Sp8	+	+	+
9	119	Galβ1–3(Galβ1–4GlcNAcβ1–6) GalNAcα–Sp8	+	+	+
10	174	GlcNAcβ1–6GalNAcα–Sp8			
11	201	Neu5Acα2–3Galβ1–3GalNAcα–Sp8			
12	212	Neu5Acα2–3(Neu5Acα2–6)GalNAcα–Sp8			
13	376	Galβ1–3GalNAcα1–3(Fucα1–2) Galβ1–4GlcNAc–Sp14		+	not tested
14	387	Fucα1–2Galβ1–3GalNAcα1–3(Fucα1–2) Galβ1–4GlcNAcβ–Sp0			not tested

Two anti-sialyl Lewis X (SLe^{x}) mAbs, FH6 (Fukushi et al. 1985) and KM93 (Shitara et al. 1987), have been analyzed for their ability to bind to 16 human colon carcinoma cells by flow cytometry. The binding profiles of these two anti-SLe^{x} mAbs were different suggesting that they recognize different subtypes of SLe^{x} carbohydrate epitopes (Nemoto et al. 1998). Detailed PGA analysis of these mAbs showed different binding profiles (Table 12.3) where mAb KM93 demonstrated broader reactivities towards non-fucosylated and sulfated SLe^{x} ligands whereas mAb FH6 had a much stricter specificity towards the terminal SLe^{x} ligands. Another anti-sulfo-SLe^{x} mAb, Ab1 (Hirakawa et al. 2010), showed specific reactivity with sulfated Lewis structures, both fucosylated and non-fucosylated.

The isomeric sLe^{a} structure was discovered in patients with colon cancer and pancreatic cancer more than 30 years ago. Several SLe-specific mAbs have been used extensively for histochemistry and to aid in diagnosis of cancer. For example the commercially available mAb NS-19-9 (Magnani et al. 1982) and 7E3 mAb (MabVaxTher) are both directed to the SLe^{a} epitope and have been extensively utilized for diagnosis of colon and pancreatic cancers (Sawada et al. 2011). Analysis on the PGA showed strict specificities to the terminal SLe^{a} epitope present on linear oligosaccharide chains (Table 12.3). Another related mAb, 2D3 (Takada

Table 12.3 Binding of anti-Lewis-antigen mAbs to selected Lewis-structures. The mAbs were analyzed as described (www.functionalglycomics.org)

No.	Glycan no.CFG v3.2	Selected Lewis structures	Anti-Lewis antibody with reported specificity										
			FH6	KM93	Abl	CA19-9	7-E9	2D3	SSEA1	SHI	7LE	2.25LE	AH6
			SLe^x	SLe^x	suSLe^x	SLe^a	SLe^a	SLe^a	Le^x	Le^x	Le^a	Le^a	Le^y
1	132	Galβ1–3GlcNAcβ–SpO											
2	151	Galβ1–4GlcNAcβ–SpO											
3	31	[3OSO3]Galβ1–3GlcNAcβ–Sp8											
4	34	[3OSO3]Galβ1–4GlcNAcβ–Sp0	X										
5	33	[3OSO3]Galβ1–4[6OSO3]GlcNAcβ–Sp8											
6	35	[3OSO3]Galβ1–4GlcNAcβ–Sp8											
7	29	[3OSO3]Galβ1–3(Fucα1–4)GlcNAcβ–Sp8											
8	32	[3OSO3]Galβ–4(Fucα1–3)GlcNAcβ–Sp8											
9	63	Fucα1–2Galβ1–3GlcNAcβ–SpO									X		
10	71	Fucα1–2Galβ1–4GlcNAcβ–Sp0											
11	116	Galβ1–3(Fucα1–4)GlcNAcβ–SpO									X	X	
12	134	Galβ1–4(Fucα1–3)GlcNAcβ–Sp0							X	X			X
13	224	Neu5Acα2–3Galβ1–3GlcNAcβ–SpO						X					
14	235	Neu5Acα2–3Galβ–4GlcNAcβ–SpO		X									
15	226	Neu5Acα2–3Galβ1–4[6OSO3]GlcNAcβ–Sp8			X								
16	216	Neu5Acα2–3Galβ1–3(Fucα1–4)GlcNAcβ–Sp8				X	X	X				X	
17	229	Neu5Acα2–3Galβ1–4(Fucα1–3)GlcNAcβ–SpO	X	X									
18	207	Neu5Acα2–3(6–O–Su)Galβ1–4(Fucα1–3) GlcNAcβ–Sp8		X									
19	227	Neu5Acα2–3Galβ1–4(Fucα1–3)[6OSO3] GlcNAcβ–Sp8			X			X				X	
20	57	Fucα1–2Galβ1–3(Fucα1–4)GlcNAcβ–SpO											
21	67	Fucα1–2Galβ1–4(Fucα1–3)GlcNAcβ–SpO							X				X

et al. 1991) (Seikagaku), binds to the SLe^a but cross-reacts to sulfated and non-fucosylated analogs.

Monoclonal antibodies to the corresponding non-sialylated Lewis structures Le^x (Takada et al. 1991) and Le^a are also available and have been evaluated on the PGA (Rouger et al. 1987). Several mAbs have been raised to the stage-specific embryonic antigen SSEA-1 (Le^x) such as the anti-SSEA1 (480) (Kannagi et al. 1982) and SH1 mAb (Fukushi et al. 1984). Both mAbs react with Le^x, but SSEA-1 also showed additional binding to Le^y structure (Table 12.3). The Le^y antigen is also frequently observed in gastric cancers and to some extent in normal tissues. The mAb, AH6 developed by immunization with human gastric cancer cell line MKN74 (Abe et al. 1983), did react selectively to Le^y antigens on the PGA. Some cross-reactivity was seen to Le^x structures.

12.3.3 Anti-Blood Group Antibodies

Cell-surface glycoconjugates often carry carbohydrate structures related to the histo-blood-group (ABO) antigens, which are expressed in both normal and cancerous tissues. Aberrant expression of the ABO-antigens in tumor development is not clear but loss of antigen expression has been reported in carcinomas (Le Pendu et al. 2001; Mandel et al. 1992; Hakomori 1978) as well as incompatible expression (Breimer et al. 1987). A blood group A antibody 9A (AbCam) prepared by immunizing with human vulval squamous carcinoma cell line A431, had on the PGA terminal αGalNAc(1→3)Gal-antigen and type specific blood group A type-2 reactivity but not to type-1 or lactose chains (Table 12.4). A second general A-specific mAb, HH6 (H. Clausen unpublished), recognizes terminal A-tetrasaccharide epitopes (Table 12.4, entries 13–15) in a non-type specific manner (Abe et al. 1984). Blood group B antibodies such as CLCP and Z5H2 (Table 12.1) showed a similar un-restricted group B reactivity (Table 12.4, entries 6–10). In contrast, evaluated H-type specific mAbs, BRIC231, 17–206 and BE2 showed much better type-specificities. BRIC231 accepted αFuc(1→2)type-2 and αFuc(1→2)lactose structures whereas 17–206 and BE2 showed only αFuc(1→2) type-1 and type-2 restricted reactivity respectively (Young et al. 1981).

12.3.4 Anti-Ganglio- and Globo-Oligosaccharide Antibodies

Anti-carbohydrate mAbs directed to ganglio-oligosaccharides are the best-studied antibodies since methods for preparation, characterization and detection were established earlier than for other glycoconjugates. A few of these mAbs have been studied on the PGA. The GD2 ganglioside is an excellent target for active specific immunotherapy due to its restricted distribution in normal tissues and its high expression on tumors of neuroectodermal origin (Wondimu et al. 2008). The mAbs ME36.1 (Thurin et al. 1986) and GMR7 (Ozawa et al. 1992) showed

Table 12.4 Binding of anti-Lewis-antigen mAbs to selected Lewis-structures. The mAbs were analyzed as described (www.functionalglycomics.org)

No.	Glycan no. CFG v3.2	Selected histo blood group structures	Anti-blood group antibody with reported specificity							
			9A	HH6 Pan A	NaM87 – 1 F6	CLCP	Z5H2	Bric231	17–206	BE2
			A	A	A	B	B	H	H	H
1	74	Fucα1–2Galβ–Sp8								
2	73	Fucα1–2Galβ1–4Glcβ–Sp0						X		
3	63	Fucα1–2Galβ1–3GlcNAcβ–Sp0							X	
4	71	Fucα1–2Galβ–4GlcNAcβ–Sp0						X		X
5	319	Fucαl–2Galβ1–3GalNAcα–Spl4								
6	106	Galα1–3Galβ–Sp8				X				
7	98	Gaα–3(Fucαl–2)Galβ–Sp8				X	X			
8	97	Galα1–3(Fucαl–2) Galβ1–4Glcβ–Sp0				X	X			
9	94	Galα1–3(Fucαl–2) Galβ1–3GlcNAcβ–Sp0				X	X			
10	96	Galα1–3(Fucαl–2) Galβ1–4GlcNAcβ–Sp0				X	X			
11	85	GalNAcαl–3Galβ–Sp8	X							
12	83	GalNAcα1–3(Fucα1–2)Galβ–Sp8			X					
13	82	GalNAcα1–3(Fucα1–2) Gaβl–4Glcβ–SpO		X	X					
14	78	GalNAca1–3(Fucαl–2) Galβ1–3GlcNAcβ–Sp0		X	X					
15	80	GalNAcαl–3(Fucαl–2) Galβ–4GlcNAcβ–Sp0	X	X	X					
		Other non-blood group reactivities	X			X				

specific reactivity with the printed GD2 oligosacharide on the PGA (www.functionalglycomics.org).

The Blood group –H glycolipid oligosaccharide Globo H is a hexasaccharide, which is a member of a family of antigenic carbohydrates that are highly expressed on various types of cancers and is also targeted by the mAb MBr1 in immunohistochemistry studies (Canevari et al. 1983). Printed glycan microarray data showed that the minimal binding epitope of globo-H was the terminal trisaccharide epitope αFuc(1→2)βGal(1→3)α/βGalNAc- (Wang et al. 2008; Kaltgrad et al. 2007) in agreement with Clausen et al. (1986). Attempts to produce anti-carbohydrate IgY antibodies from chicken have proven to be an alternative path to obtain relative specific polyclonal reactivities. A unique feature of IgY antibodies is that they have a broader antigen-binding host range, due to the great evolutionary distance between chickens and mammals. The IgY production process is also non-invasive and accumulative from collecting eggs. One PGA example is the anti-globo-H-IgY antibody that also showed reactivities to the terminal trisaccharide structure as MBr1 (Kaltgrad et al. 2007) (Fig. 12.8).

12.3.5 Anti-Tumor Serum Antibodies

Very few reports in the literature describe human serum anti-glycan antibodies for diagnostic purposes, despite of the fact that the occurrence of tumor-associated carbohydrate antigens is reflected by altered glycosylation. A few anti-glycan antibodies directed towards tumor-associated cell-surface carbohydrates have been identified by glycan array technology (Huang et al. 2006; Lawrie et al. 2006). The anti-carbohydrate antibody repertoire in human sera is complex (Blixt et al. 2004, 2009; von Gunten et al. 2009) and makes identification of a specific response with biological significance problematic (Jacob et al. 2011).

Immune responses to peptides are more specific and *via* high-throughput screening methods, auto-antibodies to several tumor associated peptides have been identified (Tan et al. 2009). Recently, auto-antibodies to glyco-peptides (Fig. 12.9) were found elevated in various cancer patients compared to healthy controls (Blixt et al. 2011; Wandall et al. 2010). Altered *O*-glycosylation of proteins is a hallmark in cancer but immunity to their combined glyco-peptide sequences constitutes a relatively undiscovered set of biomarkers and further studies are warranted.

12.4 Perspectives

The microarray platform offers a major advance in detailed analysis of fine specificities of antibodies to glycans and glycoconjugates. A limiting factor is access to compound libraries, but combined use of chemical and enzymatic synthesis have in recent years allowed production of increasingly complex structures and international consortia such as CFG and EuroGlycoArray greatly facilitate access to libraries and glycan arrays. It is clearly necessary to validate identified binding

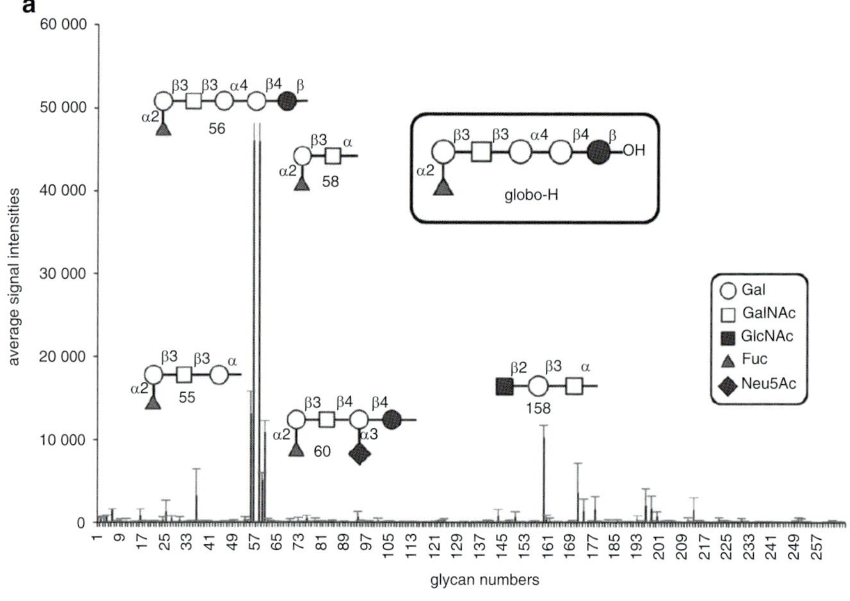

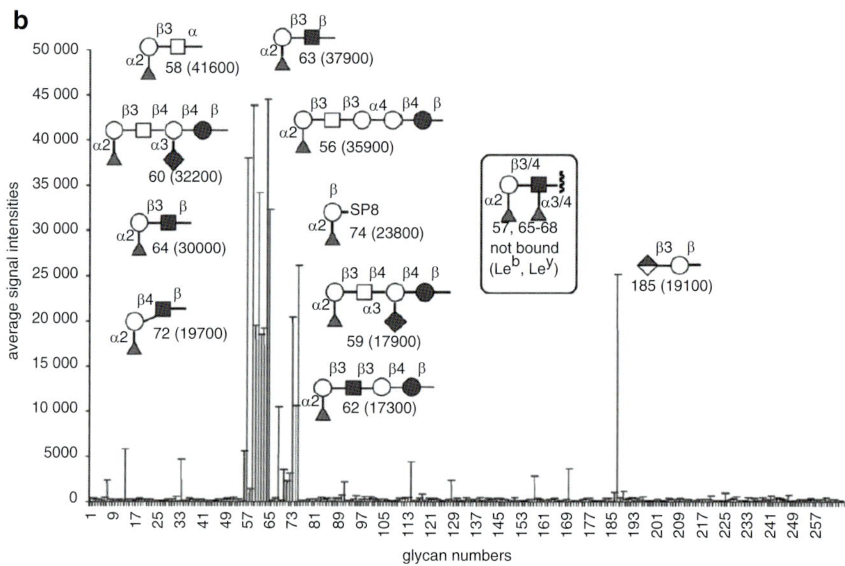

Fig. 12.8 Binding of MBr1 mAb (**a**) and anti-globo-H-IgY pAb (**b**) to PGA v2.0 (Diagram extracted and modified from Kaltgrad et al. (2007)

specificities with array analysis in more complex biological assays such as serum. It is also important to include libraries covering parts of the underlying peptide sequence that can have a profound effect on mAb recognition. We are now using

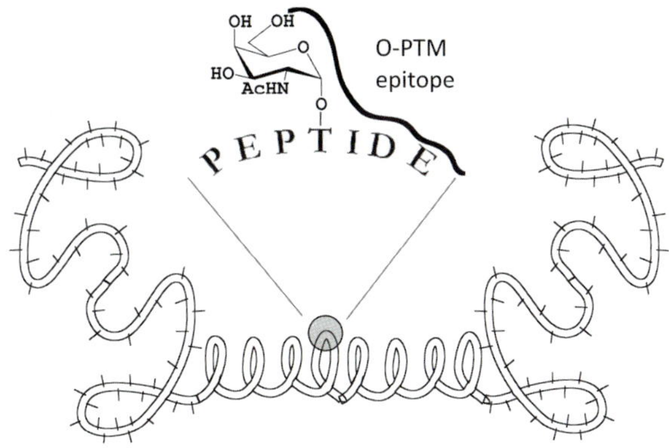

Fig. 12.9 *O*-glycopeptide epitopes (O-PTMs) as potential serum antibody biomarkers

glycopeptide arrays to further identify different binding specificities in polyclonal sera of immunized mice prior to development of screening strategies for isolation of valuable hybridoma mAbs. We foresee an increasing use of both the glycan and glycopeptide microarray array technologies to determine fine-specificities of GBPs and antibodies as well as for identification of new biomarker epitopes.

Acknowledgements This work was supported by National Institute of General Medical Sciences Grant GM62116 to the Consortium for Functional Glycomics, The Carlsberg Foundation, The Benzon Foundation, The Velux Foundation, The Danish Research Council, The Danish Agency for Science, Technology and Innovation (FTP), NIH PO1 CA052477 NIH (1U01CA128437-01), EU FP7-HEALTH-2007-A 201381, and University of Copenhagen Programme of Excellence.

References

Abe K, McKibbin JM, Hakomori S (1983) The monoclonal antibody directed to difucosylated type 2 chain (Fucα1→2Galβ1→4[Fucα1→3]GlcNAc; Y determinant). J Biol Chem 258(19):11793–11797

Abe K, Levery SB, Hakomori S (1984) The antibody specific to type 1 chain blood group A determinant. J Immunol 132(4):1951–1954

Altmann F (2007) The role of protein glycosylation in allergy. Int Arch Allergy Immunol 142(2):99–115

Alvarez RA, Blixt O (2006) Identification of ligand specificities for glycan-binding proteins using glycan arrays. Methods Enzymol 415:292–310

Berger EG (1999) Tn-syndrome. Biochim Biophys Acta 1455(2–3):255–268

Blixt O, Razi N (2006) Chemoenzymatic synthesis of glycan libraries. Methods Enzymol 415:137–153

Blixt O, Head S, Mondala T, Scanlan C, Huflejt ME, Alvarez R, Bryan MC, Fazio F, Calarese D, Stevens J, Razi N, Stevens DJ, Skehel JJ, van Die I, Burton DR, Wilson IA, Cummings R, Bovin N, Wong CH, Paulson JC (2004) Printed covalent glycan array for ligand profiling of diverse glycan binding proteins. Proc Natl Acad Sci USA 101(49):17033–17038

Blixt O, Kumagai-Braesch M, Tibell A, Groth CG, Holgersson J (2009) Anticarbohydrate antibody repertoires in patients transplanted with fetal pig Islets revealed by glycan arrays. Am J Transplant 9(1):83–90

Blixt O, Clo E, Nudelman AS, Sorensen KK, Clausen T, Wandall HH, Livingston PO, Clausen H, Jensen KJ (2010) A high-throughput O-glycopeptide discovery platform for seromic profiling. J Proteome Res 9(10):5250–5261

Blixt O, Bueti D, Burford B, Allen D, Julien S, Hollingsworth M, Gammerman A, Fentiman I, Taylor-Papadimitriou J, Burchell JM (2011) Autoantibodies to aberrantly glycosylated MUC1 in early stage breast cancer are associated with a better prognosis. Breast Cancer Res 13(2):R25

Bohm CM, Mulder MC, Zennadi R, Notter M, Schmitt-Graff A, Finn OJ, Taylor-Papadimitriou J, Stein H, Clausen H, Riecken EO, Hanski C (1997) Carbohydrate recognition on MUC1-expressing targets enhances cytotoxicity of a T cell subpopulation. Scand J Immunol 46(1):27–34

Breimer ME, Brynger H, Le Pendu J, Oriol R, Rydberg L, Samuelsson BE, Vinas J (1987) Blood group ABO-incompatible kidney transplantation biochemical and immunochemical studies of blood group A glycolipid antigens in human kidney and characterization of the antibody response (antigen specificity and antibody class) in O recipients receiving A2 grafts. Transplant Proc 19(1 Pt 1):226–230

Canevari S, Fossati G, Balsari A, Sonnino S, Colnaghi MI (1983) Immunochemical analysis of the determinant recognized by a monoclonal antibody (MBr1) which specifically binds to human mammary epithelial cells. Cancer Res 43(3):1301–1305

Clausen H, Holmes E, Hakomori S (1986) Novel blood group H glycolipid antigens exclusively expressed in blood group A and AB erythrocytes (type 3 chain H). II. Differential conversion of different H substrates by A1 and A2 enzymes, and type 3 chain H expression in relation to secretor status. J Biol Chem 261(3):1388–1392

Clausen H, Stroud M, Parker J, Springer G, Hakomori S (1988) Monoclonal antibodies directed to the blood group A associated structure, galactosyl-A: specificity and relation to the Thomsen-Friedenreich antigen. Mol Immunol 25(2):199–204

Coltart DM, Royyuru AK, Williams LJ, Glunz PW, Sames D, Kuduk SD, Schwarz JB, Chen XT, Danishefsky SJ, Live DH (2002) Principles of mucin architecture: structural studies on synthetic glycopeptides bearing clustered mono-, di-, tri-, and hexasaccharide glycodomains. J Am Chem Soc 124(33):9833–9844

Cunto-Amesty G, Luo P, Monzavi-Karbassi B, Lees A, Kieber-Emmons T (2001) Exploiting molecular mimicry to broaden the immune response to carbohydrate antigens for vaccine development. Vaccine 19(17–19):2361–2368

Dabelsteen E (1996) Cell surface carbohydrates as prognostic markers in human carcinomas. J Pathol 179(4):358–369

Dausset J, Moullec J, Bernard J (1959) Acquired hemolytic anemia with polyagglutinability of red blood cells due to a new factor present in normal human serum (Anti-Tn). Blood 14:1079–1093

Dessureault S, Koven I, Reilly RM, Couture J, Schmocker B, Damani M, Kirsh J, Ichise M, Sidlofsky S, McEwan AJ, Boniface G, Stern H, Gallinger S (1997) Pre-operative assessment of axillary lymph node status in patients with breast adenocarcinoma using intravenous 99mtechnetium mAb-170 H.82 (Tru-Scint AD). Breast Cancer Res Treat 45(1):29–37

Fukushi Y, Hakomori S, Nudelman E, Cochran N (1984) Novel fucolipids accumulating in human adenocarcinoma. II. Selective isolation of hybridoma antibodies that differentially recognize mono-, di-, and trifucosylated type 2 chain. J Biol Chem 259(7):4681–4685

Fukushi Y, Kannagi R, Hakomori S, Shepard T, Kulander BG, Singer JW (1985) Location and distribution of difucoganglioside (sialyl dimeric Le^x) in normal and tumor tissues defined by its monoclonal antibody FH6. Cancer Res 45(8):3711–3717

Geng D, Shankar G, Schantz A, Rajadhyaksha M, Davis H, Wagner C (2005) Validation of immunoassays used to assess immunogenicity to therapeutic monoclonal antibodies. J Pharm Biomed Anal 39(3–4):364–375

Hakomori SI (1978) Isolation of blood group ABH-active glycolipids from human erythrocyte membranes. Methods Enzymol 50:207–211

Hakomori S (1984) Tumor-associated carbohydrate antigens. Annu Rev Immunol 2:103–126

Hakomori S (1985) Aberrant glycosylation in cancer cell membranes as focused on glycolipids: overview and perspectives. Cancer Res 45(6):2405–2414

Heimburg J, Yan J, Morey S, Glinskii OV, Huxley VH, Wild L, Klick R, Roy R, Glinsky VV, Rittenhouse-Olson K (2006) Inhibition of spontaneous breast cancer metastasis by anti-Thomsen-Friedenreich antigen monoclonal antibody JAA-F11. Neoplasia 8(11):939–948

Heimburg-Molinaro J, Rittenhouse-Olson K (2009) Development and characterization of antibodies to carbohydrate antigens. Methods Mol Biol 534:341–357

Hirakawa J, Tsuboi K, Sato K, Kobayashi M, Watanabe S, Takakura A, Imai Y, Ito Y, Fukuda M, Kawashima H (2010) Novel anti-carbohydrate antibodies reveal the cooperative function of sulfated N- and O-glycans in lymphocyte homing. J Biol Chem 285(52):40864–40878

Hirohashi S, Clausen H, Yamada T, Shimosato Y, Hakomori S (1985) Blood group A cross-reacting epitope defined by monoclonal antibodies NCC-LU-35 and −81 expressed in cancer of blood group O or B individuals: its identification as Tn antigen. Proc Natl Acad Sci USA 82(20):7039–7043

Huang CY, Thayer DA, Chang AY, Best MD, Hoffmann J, Head S, Wong CH (2006) Carbohydrate microarray for profiling the antibodies interacting with Globo H tumor antigen. Proc Natl Acad Sci USA 103(1):15–20

Inagaki Y, Xu H, Nakata M, Seyama Y, Hasegawa K, Sugawara Y, Tang W, Kokudo N (2009) Clinicopathology of sialomucin: MUC1, particularly KL-6 mucin, in gastrointestinal, hepatic and pancreatic cancers. Biosci Trends 3(6):220–232

Jacob F, Goldstein DR, Bovin NV, Pochechueva T, Spengler M, Caduff R, Fink D, Vuskovic MI, Huflejt ME, Heinzelmann-Schwarz V (2011) Serum anti-glycan antibody detection of non-mucinous ovarian cancers by using a printed glycan array. Int J Cancer, in press

Kaltgrad E, Sen Gupta S, Punna S, Huang CY, Chang A, Wong CH, Finn MG, Blixt O (2007) Anti-carbohydrate antibodies elicited by polyvalent display on a viral scaffold. Chembiochem 8(12):1455–1462

Kannagi R, Hakomori S (2001) A guide to monoclonal antibodies directed to glycotopes. Adv Exp Med Biol 491:587–630

Kannagi R, Nudelman E, Levery SB, Hakomori S (1982) A series of human erythrocyte glycosphingolipids reacting to the monoclonal antibody directed to a developmentally regulated antigen SSEA-1. J Biol Chem 257(24):14865–14874

Karsten U, Butschak G, Cao Y, Goletz S, Hanisch FG (1995) A new monoclonal-antibody (A78-G/A7) to the Thomsen-Friedenreich pantumor antigen. Hybridoma 14(1):37–44

Kato K, Takeuchi H, Ohki T, Waki M, Usami K, Hassan H, Clausen H, Irimura T (2008) A lectin recognizes differential arrangements of O-glycans on mucin repeats. Biochem Biophys Res Commun 371(4):698–701

Kjeldsen T, Clausen H, Hirohashi S, Ogawa T, Iijima H, Hakomori S (1988) Preparation and characterization of monoclonal antibodies directed to the tumor-associated O-linked sialosyl-2 → 6α-N-acetylgalactosaminyl (sialosyl-Tn) epitope. Cancer Res 48(8):2214–2220

Köhler G, Milstein C (1975) Continuous cultures of fused cells secreting antibody of predefined specificity. Nature 256(5517):495–497

Koprowski H, Herlyn M, Steplewski Z, Sears HF (1981) Specific antigen in serum of patients with colon carcinoma. Science 212(4490):53–55

Kracun SK, Clo E, Clausen H, Levery SB, Jensen KJ, Blixt O (2010) Random glycopeptide bead libraries for seromic biomarker discovery. J Proteome Res 9(12):6705–6714

Kurosaka A, Kitagawa H, Fukui S, Numata Y, Nakada H, Funakoshi I, Kawasaki T, Ogawa T, Iijima H, Yamashina I (1988) A monoclonal antibody that recognizes a cluster of a disaccharide, NeuAc alpha(2–6)GalNAc, in mucin-type glycoproteins. J Biol Chem 263(18):8724–8726

Kurtenkov O, Klaamas K, Rittenhouse-Olson K, Vahter L, Sergejev B, Miljukhina L, Shljapnikova L (2005) IgG immune response to tumor-associated carbohydrate antigens (TF, Tn, αGal) in patients with breast cancer: impact of neoadjuvant chemotherapy and relation to the survival. Exp Oncol 27(2):136–140

Larkin M, Knapp W, Stoll MS, Mehmet H, Feizi T (1991) Monoclonal antibodies VIB-E3, IB5 and HB9 to the leucocyte/epithelial antigen CD24 resemble BA-1 in recognizing sialic acid-dependent epitope(s). Evidence that VIB-E3 recognizes NeuAcα2-6GalNAc and NeuAcα2-6Gal sequences. Clin Exp Immunol 85(3):536–541

Lawrie CH, Marafioti T, Hatton CS, Dirnhofer S, Roncador G, Went P, Tzankov A, Pileri SA, Pulford K, Banham AH (2006) Cancer-associated carbohydrate identification in Hodgkin's lymphoma by carbohydrate array profiling. Int J Cancer 118(12):3161–3166

Le Pendu J, Marionneau S, Cailleau-Thomas A, Rocher J, Le Moullac-Vaidye B, Clement M (2001) ABH and Lewis histo-blood group antigens in cancer. APMIS 109(1):9–31

Li Q, Anver MR, Butcher DO, Gildersleeve JC (2009) Resolving conflicting data on expression of the Tn antigen and implications for clinical trials with cancer vaccines. Mol Cancer Ther 8 (4):971–979

Li Q, Rodriguez LG, Farnsworth DF, Gildersleeve JC (2010) Effects of hapten density on the induced antibody repertoire. Chembiochem 11(12):1686–1691

Magnani JL, Brockhaus M, Smith DF, Ginsburg V, Blaszczyk M, Mitchell KF, Steplewski Z, Koprowski H (1981) A monosialoganglioside is a monoclonal antibody-defined antigen of colon carcinoma Science 212:55–6

Magnani JL, Nilsson B, Brockhaus M, Zopf D, Steplewski Z, Koprowski H, Ginsburg V (1982) A monoclonal antibody-defined antigen associated with gastrointestinal cancer is a ganglioside containing sialylated lacto-N-fucopentaose II. J Biol Chem 257(23):14365–14369

Mandel U, Petersen OW, Sorensen H, Vedtofte P, Hakomori S, Clausen H, Dabelsteen E (1991) Simple mucin-type carbohydrates in oral stratified squamous and salivary gland epithelia. J Invest Dermatol 97(4):713–721

Mandel U, Langkilde NC, Orntoft TF, Therkildsen MH, Karkov J, Reibel J, White T, Clausen H, Dabelsteen E (1992) Expression of histo-blood-group-A/B-gene-defined glycosyltransferases in normal and malignant epithelia: correlation with A/B-carbohydrate expression. Int J Cancer 52(1):7–12

Nakada H, Inoue M, Numata Y, Tanaka N, Funakoshi I, Fukui S, Mellors A, Yamashina I (1993) Epitopic structure of Tn glycophorin A for an anti-Tn antibody (MLS 128). Proc Natl Acad Sci USA 90(6):2495–2499

Nelson AL, Dhimolea E, Reichert JM (2010) Development trends for human monoclonal antibody therapeutics. Nat Rev Drug Discov 9(10):767–774

Nemoto Y, Izumi Y, Tezuka K, Tamatani T, Irimura T (1998) Comparison of 16 human colon carcinoma cell lines for their expression of sialyl LeX antigens and their E-selectin-dependent adhesion. Clin Exp Metastasis 16(6):569–576

Nuti M, Teramoto YA, Mariani-Costantini R, Hand PH, Colcher D, Schlom J (1982) A monoclonal antibody (B72.3) defines patterns of distribution of a novel tumor-associated antigen in human mammary carcinoma cell populations. Int J Cancer 29(5):539–545

Ohyabu N, Hinou H, Matsushita T, Izumi R, Shimizu H, Kawamoto K, Numata Y, Togame H, Takemoto H, Kondo H, Nishimura S (2009) An essential epitope of anti-MUC1 monoclonal antibody KL-6 revealed by focused glycopeptide library. J Am Chem Soc 131(47): 17102–17109

Ozawa H, Kotani M, Kawashima I, Tai T (1992) Generation of one set of monoclonal antibodies specific for b-pathway ganglio-series gangliosides. Biochim Biophys Acta 1123(2):184–190

Reddish MA, Jackson L, Koganty RR, Qiu D, Hong W, Longenecker BM (1997) Specificities of anti-sialyl-Tn and anti-Tn monoclonal antibodies generated using novel clustered synthetic glycopeptide epitopes. Glycoconj J 14(5):549–560

Rillahan CD, Paulson JC (2010) Glycan microarrays for decoding the glycome. Annu Rev Biochem 2011(80):797–823

Rinaldi S, Brennan KM, Goodyear CS, O'Leary C, Schiavo G, Crocker PR, Willison HJ (2009) Analysis of lectin binding to glycolipid complexes using combinatorial glycoarrays. Glycobiology 19(7):789–796

Rouger P, Tsikas G, Gane P, Oriol R, Salmon C (1987) Immunological approach of anti-H (9), anti-Lewis (6), anti-P (3) and anti-Pr (1) monoclonal antibodies. Rev Fr Transfus Immunohematol 30(5):663–669

Sawada R, Sun SM, Wu X, Hong F, Ragupathi G, Livingston PO, Scholz WW (2011) Human monoclonal antibodies to sialyl-LewisA (CA19.9) with potent CDC, ADCC, and antitumor activity. Clin Cancer Res 17(5):1024–1032

Seeberger PH (2008) Automated oligosaccharide synthesis. Chem Soc Rev 37(1):19–28

Shitara K, Hanai N, Yoshida H (1987) Distribution of lung adenocarcinoma-associated antigens in human tissues and sera defined by monoclonal antibodies KM-52 and KM-93. Cancer Res 47(5):1267–1272

Singhal AK, Orntoft TF, Nudelman E, Nance S, Schibig L, Stroud MR, Clausen H, Hakomori S (1990) Profiles of Lewis^{x}-containing glycoproteins and glycolipids in sera of patients with adenocarcinoma Cancer Res 50:1375–80

Sorensen AL, Reis CA, Tarp MA, Mandel U, Ramachandran K, Sankaranarayanan V, Schwientek T, Graham R, Taylor-Papadimitriou J, Hollingsworth MA, Burchell J, Clausen H (2006) Chemoenzymatically synthesized multimeric Tn/STn MUC1 glycopeptides elicit cancer-specific anti-MUC1 antibody responses and override tolerance. Glycobiology 16(2): 96–107

Springer GF (1984) T and Tn, general carcinoma autoantigens. Science 224(4654):1198–1206

Springer GF (1989) Tn epitope (N-acetyl-D-galactosamine α-O-serine/threonine) density in primary breast carcinoma: a functional predictor of aggressiveness. Mol Immunol 26(1):1–5

Springer GF (1997) Immunoreactive T and Tn epitopes in cancer diagnosis, prognosis, and immunotherapy. J Mol Med 75(8):594–602

Takada A, Ohmori K, Takahashi N, Tsuyuoka K, Yago A, Zenita K, Hasegawa A, Kannagi R (1991) Adhesion of human cancer cells to vascular endothelium mediated by a carbohydrate antigen, sialyl Lewis A. Biochem Biophys Res Commun 179(2):713–719

Takeuchi H, Kato K, Denda-Nagai K, Hanisch FG, Clausen H, Irimura T (2002) The epitope recognized by the unique anti-MUC1 monoclonal antibody MY.1E12 involves sialyl α 2-3galactosyl β1-3 *N*-acetylgalactosaminide linked to a distinct threonine residue in the MUC1 tandem repeat. J Immunol Methods 270(2):199–209

Tan HT, Low J, Lim SG, Chung MC (2009) Serum autoantibodies as biomarkers for early cancer detection. FEBS J 276(23):6880–6904

Thurin J, Thurin M, Herlyn M, Elder DE, Steplewski Z, Clark WH Jr, Koprowski H (1986) GD2 ganglioside biosynthesis is a distinct biochemical event in human melanoma tumor progression. FEBS Lett 208(1):17–22

Thurnher M, Clausen H, Sharon N, Berger EG (1993) Use of O-glycosylation-defective human lymphoid cell lines and flow cytometry to delineate the specificity of Moluccella laevis lectin and monoclonal antibody 5 F4 for the Tn antigen (GalNAc α1-O-Ser/Thr). Immunol Lett 36(3):239–243

Tarp MA, Sorensen AL, Mandel U, Paulsen H, Burchell J, Taylor-Papadimitriou J, Clausen H (2007) Identification of a novel cancer-specific immunodominant glycopeptide epitope in the MUC1 tandem repeat Glycobiology 17:197–209

von Gunten S, Smith DF, Cummings RD, Riedel S, Miescher S, Schaub A, Hamilton RG, Bochner BS (2009) Intravenous immunoglobulin contains a broad repertoire of anticarbohydrate antibodies that is not restricted to the IgG2 subclass. J Allergy Clin Immunol 123(6):1268–1276

Wandall HH, Blixt O, Tarp MA, Pedersen JW, Bennett EP, Mandel U, Ragupathi G, Livingston PO, Hollingsworth MA, Papadimitriou JT, Burchell J, Clausen H (2010) Autoantibody signatures to aberrant O-glycopeptide epitopes serve as undiscovered biomarkers of cancer. Cancer Res 70(4):1306–1313

Wang CC, Huang YL, Ren CT, Lin CW, Hung JT, Yu JC, Yu AL, Wu CY, Wong CH (2008) Glycan microarray of Globo H and related structures for quantitative analysis of breast cancer. Proc Natl Acad Sci USA 105(33):11661–11666

Wondimu A, Zhang T, Kieber-Emmons T, Gimotty P, Sproesser K, Somasundaram R, Ferrone S, Tsao CY, Herlyn D (2008) Peptides mimicking GD2 ganglioside elicit cellular, humoral and tumor-protective immune responses in mice. Cancer Immunol Immunother 57(7):1079–1089

Xu Y, Gendler SJ, Franco A (2004) Designer glycopeptides for cytotoxic T cell-based elimination of carcinomas. J Exp Med 199(5):707–716

Young WW Jr, MacDonald EM, Nowinski RC, Hakomori SI (1979) Production of monoclonal antibodies specific for two distinct steric portions of the glycolipid ganglio-N-triosylceramide (asialo GM2). J Exp Med 150(4):1008–1019

Young WW Jr, Portoukalian J, Hakomori S (1981) Two monoclonal anticarbohydrate antibodies directed to glycosphingolipids with a lacto-N-glycosyl type II chain. J Biol Chem 256(21): 10967–10972

Yuasa N, Zhang W, Goto T, Sakaue H, Matsumoto-Takasaki A, Kimura M, Ohshima H, Tsuchida Y, Koizumi T, Sakai K, Kojima T, Yamamoto K, Nakata M, Fujita-Yamaguchi Y (2010) Production of anti-carbohydrate antibodies by phage display technologies: potential impairment of cell growth as a result of endogenous expression. J Biol Chem 285(40): 30587–30597

Zhang S, Zhang HS, Reuter VE, Slovin SF, Scher HI, Livingston PO (1998) Expression of potential target antigens for immunotherapy on primary and metastatic prostate cancers. Clin Cancer Res 4(2):295–302

A Novel Mannose 6-phosphate Specific Antibody Fragment for Diagnosis of Mucolipidosis type II and III

13

Sandra Pohl, Thomas Braulke, and Sven Müller-Loennies

13.1 Introduction

Eukaryotic cells of animals have developed a specialized organelle for the degradation and recycling of macromolecules, called the lysosome (De Duve 1963). The breakdown of these macromolecules is carried out by more than 60 acid hydrolases such as proteases, nucleases, glycosidases, phosphatases, lipases etc. (Luzio et al. 2007). Newly synthesized lysosomal hydrolases are equipped with mannose 6-phosphate (Man6*P*) residues on high-mannose type *N*-glycans. This marker is generated in the Golgi apparatus in a two-step enzymatic process in which first a *N*-acetylglucosamine 1-phosphate (GlcNAc1*P*) residue is transferred to a terminal mannose (Man) residue. In a second step the enzymatic hydrolysis of the GlcNAc uncovers the Man6*P* residue. Man6*P* functions as recognition marker for specific receptors required for lysosomal targeting of acid hydrolases. Importantly, from a medical point of view, also extracellular Man6*P*-containing proteins can be internalized and transported to the lysosomes via Man6*P*-receptors which are located also at the plasma membrane (Kornfeld and Mellman 1989; Braulke and Bonifacino 2009). Whereas the majority of the over 50 known lysosomal storage disorders are caused by inherited defects of single lysosomal enzymes or lysosomal membrane proteins, the failure to generate Man6*P* leads to a deficiency of multiple enzymes resulting in mucolipidosis (ML) type II and type III (Futerman and van Meer 2004).

S. Pohl • T. Braulke
Department of Biochemistry, Children's Hospital, University Medical Center Hamburg-Eppendorf, Martinistr. 52; Bldg. N27, 20246 Hamburg, Germany

S. Müller-Loennies (✉)
Research Center Borstel, Leibniz-Center for Medicine and Biosciences, Parkallee 1-40, 23845 Borstel, Germany
e-mail: sml@fz-borstel.de

P. Kosma and S. Müller-Loennies (eds.), *Anticarbohydrate Antibodies*,
DOI 10.1007/978-3-7091-0870-3_13, © Springer-Verlag/Wien 2012

The diagnosis of MLII and III is only carried out in a few specialized laboratories throughout the world and is based on the biochemical and genetic analysis of biomaterial isolated from patients. Diagnosis of MLII and III would greatly benefit from the development of confirmatory assays easier to perform also in routine analytic laboratories on suspicious patients. For this purpose the specific detection of Man6*P* in glycoproteins by an antibody would be ideal.

This application in mind, we have immunized a rabbit with a neoglycoconjugate of a mixture of oligosaccharides from yeast containing Man6*P* residues and bovine serum albumin (BSA) known to induce a polyclonal anti-Man6*P* response (Braulke et al. 1987; Braulke et al. 1988). The antigen binding domain of an antibody can be expressed in *Escherichia coli* as a single-chain antibody fragment (scFv) in which the VH and VL domains of the antibody are joined by a flexible polypeptide linker (Bird et al. 1988; Huston et al. 1988) and genetically fused to surface proteins of, e.g., filamentous phage. The surface display then allows selection and amplification, a technique called "Phage Display" [for further information see (Barbas et al. 2001)]. Since the generation of monoclonal antibodies (mAb) from rabbits is far from being routine due to the lack of appropriate fusion cell lines, we have referred to phage display technology to generate a scFv specifically binding to Man6*P* (Müller-Loennies et al. 2010).

In this review we describe the genetic and biochemical background of mucolipidoses and the development of a novel antibody scFv (scFv M6P-1) for the

- Easy diagnosis of MLII and III by western blots.
- Selective purification of recombinant high-affinity uptake forms of lysosomal enzymes on an affinity matrix.
- Immunohistological staining of lysosomes.

Furthermore, scFv M6P-1 can be applied to the quantitation of Man6*P* in glycoproteins, the isolation of the Man6*P*-proteome of cells and organs and has aided in the investigation of alternative protein trafficking pathways to the lysosome.

13.1.1 Generation of the Man6*P* Recognition Marker

Soluble lysosomal enzymes and secretory proteins are synthesized in the endoplasmic reticulum (ER). The *N*-terminal signal sequence directs their translocation into the ER lumen and is subsequently cleaved off by the signal peptidase. For *N*-glycosylation a preformed oligosaccharide core composed of three glucoses (Glc), nine Man and two GlcNAc, ($Glc_3Man_9GlcNAc_2$) is transferred to selected asparagine residues on the nascent protein prior to protein folding [Fig. 13.1, (Rothman et al. 1978; Ruddock and Molinari 2006)]. The transferred core oligosaccharides are then subject to 'trimming' reactions initiated by glucosidase I in the ER before completion of translation (Kornfeld and Kornfeld 1985). The two other glucose residues are subsequently hydrolyzed by glucosidase II in the ER. The monoglucosylated core glycan intermediate is recognized by the lectins calnexin and calreticulin which function as molecular chaperones until the protein is properly folded

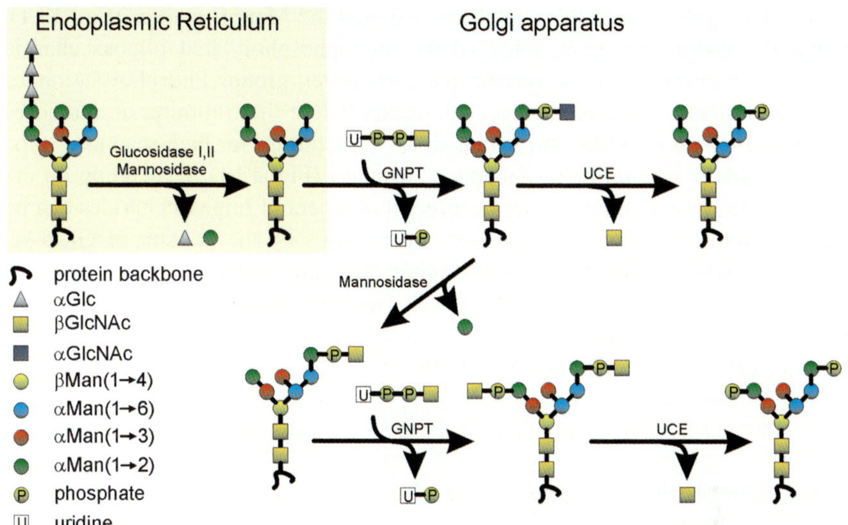

Fig. 13.1 Schematic drawing of the enzymatic formation of Man6*P* residues on *N*-glycans of lysosomal proteins. The generation of these residues is catalyzed in a two-step reaction initiated by the transfer of UDP-GlcNAc to selected C6 hydroxyl groups of mannoses in a *cis*-Golgi compartment by UDP-*N*-acetylglucosamine (UDP-GlcNAc):lysosomal enzyme *N*-acetylglucosamine-1-phosphotransferase (GNPT, GlcNAc-1-phosphotransferase; EC 2.7.8.17) followed by hydrolysis of the GlcNAc residue in the *trans*-Golgi apparatus by the *N*-acetylglucosamine-1-phosphodiester α-*N*-acetylglucosaminidase (UCE, 'uncovering enzyme'; EC 3.1.4.45). Some of the *N*-glycan chains are equipped with a second phosphodiester group. Phosphorylation of mannose residues in the α(1→6)-branch occurs before the trimming of mannoses in the α(1→3)-branch by α-mannosidase I. Therefore, phosphorylated glycans may contain 5–7 mannose residues. Depending on the lysosomal enzyme and the cell type, certain oligosaccharides are converted into hybrid or complex type sugar chains (not shown). Therefore, monophosphorylated oligosaccharides are also found in the α(1→6)-branch of hybrid-type oligosaccharides. The subcellular compartments in which the reactions take place are indicated as boxes

(Parodi 2000). The removal of the third glucose residue releases the folded glycoprotein from the chaperones and allows the attack of α-mannosidase I for further trimming reactions in the ER resulting in the formation of octamannosyl high-mannose type chains.

An important modification of *N*-glycans on lysosomal enzymes is the formation of Man6*P* residues distinguishing these glycoproteins from other classes of newly synthesized glycoproteins. Two enzymes catalyze the generation of Man6*P* residues: UDP-*N*-acetylglucosamine (UDP-GlcNAc):lysosomal enzyme *N*-acetylglucosamine-1-phosphotransferase (GlcNAc-1-phosphotransferase; EC 2.7.8.17) and the *N*-acetylglucosamine-1-phosphodiester α-*N*-acetylglucosaminidase ('uncovering enzyme', UCE; EC 3.1.4.45).

The initial transfer of GlcNAc1*P* from UDP-GlcNAc to selected C6 hydroxyl groups of mannoses occurs in a *cis*-Golgi compartment that results in a phosphodiester intermediate. The hydrolysis of the covering GlcNAc residue from the phosphodiester by the UCE in the *trans*-Golgi apparatus exposes the Man6*P* marker (Fig. 13.1). Within the Golgi apparatus, some of the monophosphorylated oligosaccharide chains are equipped with a second phosphodiester group. Phosphorylation of mannose residues in the $\alpha(1\rightarrow6)$-branch occurs before the trimming of mannoses in the $\alpha(1\rightarrow3)$-branch by α-mannosidase I, resulting in high-mannose type oligosaccharides containing 5–7 mannose residues (Fig. 13.1). Depending on the lysosomal enzyme and the cell type, different numbers of oligosaccharides can be converted into hybrid or complex type sugar chains by the transfer of GlcNAc, galactose (Gal), fucose (Fuc), or *N*-acetylneuraminic acid (Neu5Ac) residues. Therefore, monophosphorylated oligosaccharides are also found in the $\alpha(1\rightarrow6)$-branch of hybrid-type oligosaccharides (Varki and Kornfeld 1983; Goldberg and Kornfeld 1983; Lazzarino and Gabel 1989).

13.1.2 Mucolipidosis Type II and III

The GlcNAc-1-phosphotransferase complex is composed of three subunits ($\alpha_2\beta_2\gamma_2$) that are encoded by two genes, *GNPTAB* and *GNPTG* (Kollmann et al. 2010). The GlcNAc-1-phosphotransferase activity is lacking or reduced in two distinct autosomal recessive human diseases impairing lysosomal enzyme trafficking and lysosomal function, mucolipidosis (ML) II and MLIII, respectively. Although rare diseases, they have been the subject of extensive studies in the last 40 years since their first description. These studies were crucial for the discovery of the Man6*P*-dependent lysosomal enzyme trafficking pathway [reviewed in (Kornfeld and Sly 2001; Kollmann et al. 2010)].

Patients diagnosed with MLII alpha/beta or MLIII alpha/beta (formerly known as I-cell disease or MLII and MLIIIA, respectively) are either homozygotes or compound heterozygotes for mutations in the *GNPTAB* gene localized on chromosome 12q23.3 (Kudo et al. 2005; Tiede et al. 2005b). The MLIII gamma patients (formerly known as pseudo-Hurler polydystrophy or MLIIIC) are homozygotes or compound heterozygotes for mutations in the *GNPTG* gene localized on chromosome 16p13.3 (Raas-Rothschild et al. 2000). The revised nomenclature of mucolipidoses is based on the clinical phenotype and the disease-causing gene defect and is important for clinicians and patients, as *GNPTG* mutations cause a milder phenotype and have better prognosis than do *GNPTAB* mutations (Cathey et al. 2008). Until now approximately 100 mutations in the *GNPTAB* gene have been described whereas 20 different mutations were reported in the *GNPTG* gene of MLIII gamma patients (Kollmann et al. 2010).

Clinical symptoms of MLII patients are characterized by dwarfism, skeletal abnormalities, facial dysmorphism, stiff skin, delayed development, mental retardation and cardiomegaly leading to death between 5 and 8 years of age. In MLIII gamma patients a later onset of clinical symptoms and a more slowly progressive course is observed allowing survival into the 8th decade. Because of progressive stiffness of hands and shoulders and musculoskeletal changes, MLIII gamma is often misdiagnosed for a rheumatological disorder (Kelly et al. 1975; Spranger et al. 2002; Cathey et al. 2008).

13.1.3 Current Diagnostic Analysis of MLII and MLIII

The clinical diagnosis of MLII or III can be confirmed by biochemical analyses. The loss or reduced capability to generate Man6*P* leads to a massive secretion of the lysosomal enzymes into the extracellular milieu and the circulation, and an intracellular deficiency of multiple lysosomal enzymes (Kornfeld and Sly 2001). The intracellular deficiency of lysosomal enzymes causes subsequently an accumulation of undegraded material in lysosomes, which is visible by light microscopy as phase-dense inclusion bodies in fibroblasts of affected patients (Leroy and Demars 1967). The activity of several lysosomal enzymes (e. g. β-hexosaminidase, β-glucuronidase, β-galactosidase, α-mannosidase and arylsulfatase A) can be measured in serum, or media and cell extracts of cultured fibroblasts from clinically diagnosed MLII and MLIII patients. In comparison to cells of healthy individuals the activities of lysosomal enzymes are reduced in patient cells but increased in serum and conditioned cell media demonstrating the missorting of lysosomal enzymes (Kornfeld and Sly 2001). During the transport along the biosynthetic pathway in healthy cells many inactive lysosomal precursors undergo proteolytic processing steps leading to mature, active enzymes. The modifications of lysosomal enzymes are dependent on the pH and the intracellular compartment and can be used as an indicator for proper sorting processes (Hasilik and Neufeld 1980). Radioactive pulse-chase experiments in fibroblasts of diagnosed MLII or MLIII patients followed by immunoprecipitation of certain lysosomal enzymes is useful to demonstrate the missorting of lysosomal enzymes (Tiede et al. 2005a; Pohl et al. 2010b). The direct measurement of the GlcNAc-1-phosphotransferase activity in fibroblasts requires the synthesis and purification of metabolically labelled [^{32}P]UDP-GlcNAc (Reitman and Kornfeld 1981). Both methods are cumbersome and therefore cannot be routinely used for diagnosis.

Despite the major progress made during the last decade allowing the identification of the molecular defects in MLII and MLIII by direct sequencing of *GNPTAB* and *GNPTG*, these methods are laborious and expensive, and intronic mutations are not always detectable. Therefore, a rapid, convenient and sensitive method would greatly facilitate the diagnosis of MLII and MLIII.

13.2 Generation and Characterization of scFv M6P-1

13.2.1 Immunization and Selection

Upon mild hydrolysis of *Pichia (Hansenula) holstii* NRRLY-2448 yeast mannan oligosaccharides can be obtained which contain Man6*P*. The structural analysis revealed that the hydrolysate consists of a mixture of oligosaccharides (Fig. 13.2)

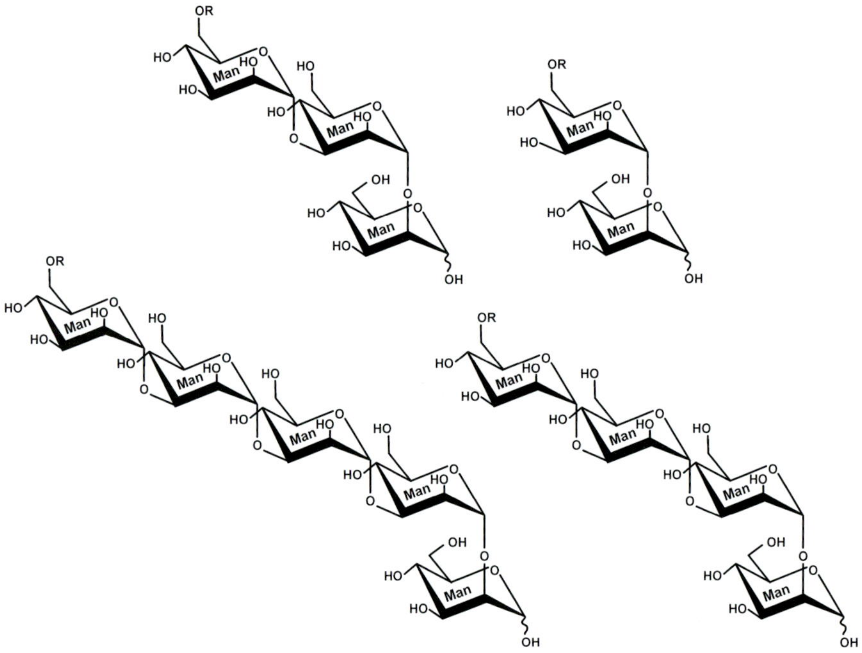

R=H, R = $PO(OH)_2$

Fig. 13.2 Chemical structures of Man6*P*-containing oligosaccharides from *Pichia (Hansenula) holstii* (Bretthauer et al. 1973; Parolis et al. 1998; Ferro et al. 2002)

and the majority are pentasaccharides (Bretthauer et al. 1973; Parolis et al. 1996; Parolis et al. 1998). Therefore, this preparation is referred to as pentamannose 6-phosphate (PMP). As opposed to *N*-glycans, in which the terminal phosphorylated mannose residues are connected αMan(1→2)αMan, the PMP contains terminal α(1→3)-linked mannoses in which only the reducing end is formed in an α(1→2)-linkage [Fig. 13.2, (Fischer et al. 1980; Parolis et al. 1996; Parolis et al. 1998)]. The conjugation of PMP to BSA and immunization with this conjugate induces a polyclonal antibody response in rabbits which binds Man6*P* also in glycoproteins [PMP-BSA, (Braulke et al. 1987)]. The basis for this observation is an apparent structural similarity of α(1→2)- and α(1→3)-linked Man_2 leading to a cross-reaction with antibodies.

For the generation of a Man6*P*-specific scFv from an immunized rabbit, a library of scFv was assembled by standard genetic procedures (Barbas et al. 2001). This was achieved by taking bone marrow from both legs and spleen, extraction of total RNA, reverse transcription into cDNA and PCR amplification of genes coding for the variable domains of antibody heavy (VH) and light (VL) chains. The amplified genes were then assembled into full length scFv by PCR overlap extension and ligated into the phagemid vector pComb3XSS (Barbas et al. 2001). Transformation of *E. coli* yielded 5.7×10^6 transformants and after induction of phage-production by superinfection with M13KO7 helper phage, 10^{12} phages were obtained for the selection. The selection and enrichment of phage bound scFv ("panning") specific for Man6*P* was performed on PMP-BSA immobilized on ELISA plates. The selection of carbohydrate antibodies by phage display is difficult to achieve due to often low avidities. Because the conditions to achieve optimum binding were unknown, we have varied the amounts of immobilized PMP-BSA (3–100 pmol/well) used for panning. The outcome of each panning round was analyzed by phage-ELISA and successful enrichment was only seen at 50 pmol immobilized antigen after five rounds of panning. Some binding was also seen after three rounds, which was, however, not specific for Man6*P*.

13.2.2 Expression and Biochemical Characterization

For purification by immobilized metal ion affinity chromatography (IMAC) and detection 5xHis-tag and a c-myc were attached to the *C*-terminus of the scFv M6P-1 protein sequence, respectively. Expression in *E. coli* following the protocol of MacKenzie and To (1998) yielded soluble protein, which was extracted from the periplasm by treatment of harvested cells with the polycationic membrane active peptide Polymyxin B (0.1 mg/ml final conc. in ice cold buffer). The soluble protein could be collected from the supernatants of three extractions by IMAC. Separation of monomers from oligomeric scFv was achieved by gel filtration (Fig. 13.3). The cDNA sequence analysis revealed an unpaired cysteine at the beginning of complementarity determining region (CDR) 2 VH (Fig. 13.4) which is also present in the germline sequence IGHV1S40*01 (Giudicelli et al. 2006). The substitution of this residue by serine (scFv M6P-1S) or alanine improved expression levels in *E. coli* three- to four-fold and increased the protein stability whereas the affinity towards Man6*P* was not affected (Fig. 13.5). After purification to homogeneity and lyophilization in phosphate buffered saline (PBS) pH 7.2 containing 1% PEG 8,000, 5 mM EDTA and 250 mM trehalose (Carpenter et al. 1993; Draber et al. 1995) the protein was stable for over a year without loss of activity.

13.2.3 Analysis of Binding by ELISA

To achieve comparable results in ELISA and ELISA inhibition studies using scFv, in general, freshly prepared solutions of purified mono- or dimer scFv should be used to avoid influences from avidity effects. Although scFv contain only a single antigen binding site, they are prone to form fully functional oligomers (Dolezal et al. 2000) and the ratio at equilibrium depends on the affinity between the VL and VH interfaces and the length of the linker (Glockshuber et al. 1990).

13.2.3.1 ELISA with Soluble scFv M6P-1

For ELISA, the outcome of the experiment largely depends on the amount of immobilized antigen and the concentration of the primary antibody. Due to the

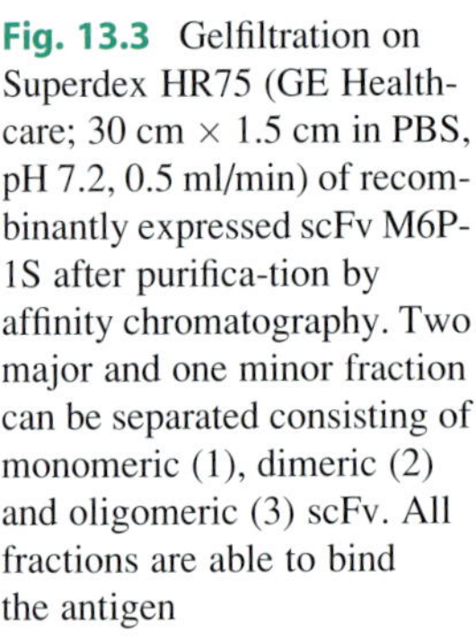

Fig. 13.3 Gelfiltration on Superdex HR75 (GE Healthcare; 30 cm × 1.5 cm in PBS, pH 7.2, 0.5 ml/min) of recombinantly expressed scFv M6P-1S after purifica-tion by affinity chromatography. Two major and one minor fraction can be separated consisting of monomeric (1), dimeric (2) and oligomeric (3) scFv. All fractions are able to bind the antigen

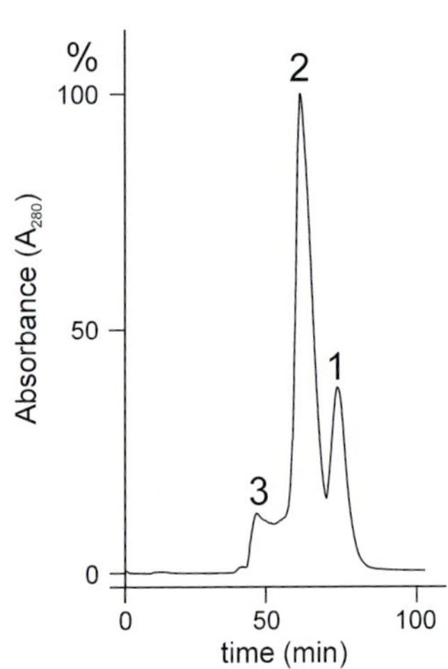

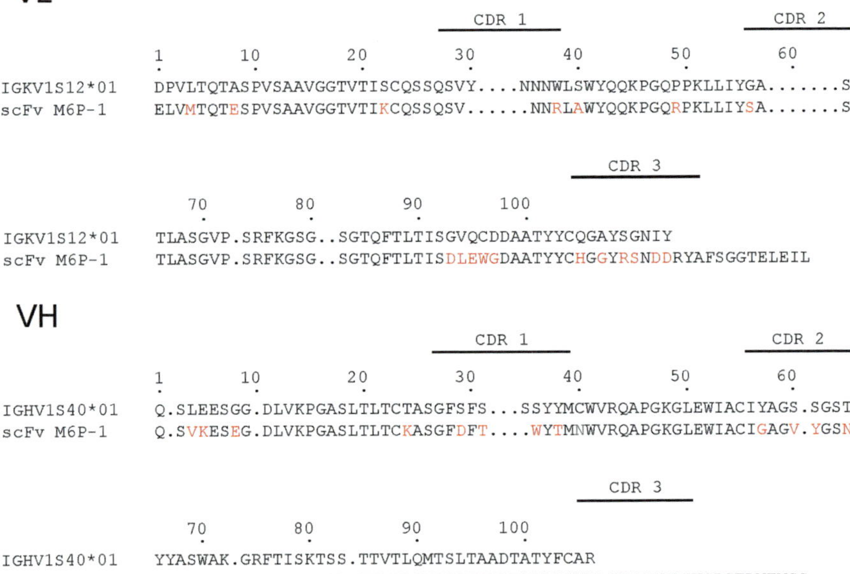

Fig. 13.4 Primary structure of the scFv M6P-1 deduced from its cDNA sequence. The CDR of heavy and light chains are indicated and alignment to its germline precursor assigned according to Giudicelli (2006)

monovalent nature of scFv and the often low affinities of anti-carbohydrate antibodies, the ELISA is even more affected by these factors. Thus, when using neoglycoconjugates made with isolated oligosaccharides a high ligand to protein

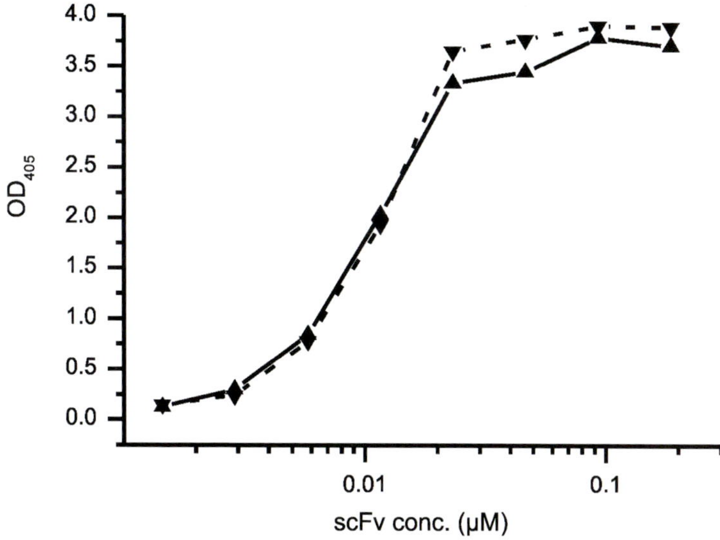

Fig. 13.5 ELISA binding assay of recombinant scFv M6P-1 (*broken line*, *triangle down*) and scFv M6P-1S (*solid line*, *triangle up*) against immobilized PMP-BSA (45 pmol/cup). The scFv starting concentration was 0.18 μM (5 μg/ml)

ratio would be desirable. However, neoglycoconjugates with a high ligand to protein ratio not always give the best results in ELISA binding assays when native BSA is used (own observation). It may thus be advantageous to use denatured and reduced BSA for the generation of neoglycoconjugates (Houen and Jensen 1995) for this purpose.

In any case, to determine the ligand concentration suitable for ELISA the binding reactivity should be tested in an ELISA checkerboard titration in which binding at different scFv starting concentrations is measured against varying concentrations of immobilized ligand. For ELISA using scFv M6P-1 (Fig. 13.5) we have used PMP-BSA (molar ratio of PMP:BSA of 20:1) containing 3–100 pmol of ligand with 45 pmol giving the best result when purified scFv was added at a starting concentration of 5 μg/ml. Bound scFv was detected by incubation with the anti-c-myc mAb 9E10 (gift from Dr. C. R. MacKenzie, NRC, Ottawa, Canada), a HRP-conjugated goat-anti-mouse IgG H + L (Dianova, Hamburg, Germany) and diammonium 2,2′-azino-bis(3-ethylbenzothiazoline-6-sulfonate (AzBTS-$(NH_4)_2$, Sigma-Aldrich) as substrate.

13.2.3.2 ELISA Inhibition

Inhibition of binding in ELISA is performed conveniently by first titrating the inhibitor in buffer in a separate non-treated polystyrene plate (e.g., Nunc V96 MicroWell) starting in the first row at double concentration of the highest inhibitory concentration to be tested in a volume of, e.g., 30 μl. The same volume of antibody is then added at a constant concentration which yields an OD within the linear range of the colour reaction and which is sufficiently strong to allow sampling of the inhibition (OD 1.0–2.0). For best results quadruplicate measurements at each inhibitor concentration should be performed and titrations starting at a concentration sufficiently high to achieve complete inhibition over a few titrations and ending with several dilute concentrations of inhibitor at which no inhibition is seen. After preincubation (1 h, 37°C) 50 μl are then transferred to a plate coated with ligand and developed like a regular ELISA. The ELISA inhibition data should then be analyzed by plotting the OD versus the inhibitor concentration and applying an error-weighted non-linear logistic fitting function as implemented in statistical analysis software.

For ELISA inhibition with scFv M6P-1 (Fig. 13.6) we have used 0.6 μg/ml final concentration of scFv and inhibitor concentrations ranging from 0.01 to 100 mM. Binding was measured against 45 pmol PMP-BSA/well. The amount of bound antibody was then determined as for normal ELISA. Using one plate per inhibitor, data points can be measured in quadruplicates over 22 concentrations spanning six orders of magnitude which is sufficient to sample the whole inhibition curve and determine the concentration yielding 50% inhibition (IC_{50}) by fitting to a logistic function. Such an analysis for scFv M6P-1 is shown in Fig. 13.6 showing the strong

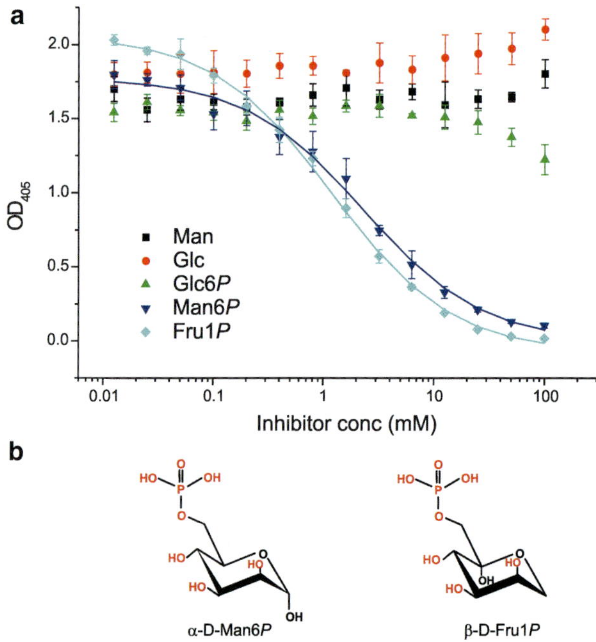

Fig. 13.6 ELISA inhibition data using scFv M6P-1 as primary antibody, PMP-BSA as immobilized antigen and Man6*P*, Glc6*P*, Fru1*P*, Man, and Glc as inhibitors (**a**) at the indicated concentrations. Experimental details are described in Müller-Loennies et al. (2010). Structural comparison of Man6*P* and Fru1*P* (**b**). Fig. (**a**) from Müller-Loennies et al. (2010), with permission

inhibition by Man6*P* and fructose 1-phosphate (Fru1*P*) and no inhibition by Man, Glc and Glc6*P*.

The observed cross-reaction of Man6*P* and Fru1*P* can be explained by the structural similarity due to the same relative orientation of hydroxyl groups at C2-C3-C4, and C3-C4-C5, respectively, with a similar position of the phosphate. Thus, the discrimination between Glc6*P* and Man6*P* is likely due to an unfavourable equatorial position of the C2 OH for binding.

13.2.4 Analysis of Binding by ITC-Microcalorimetry

The comparison of ELISA IC_{50} values allows the ranking of different ligands according to their relative affinities; however, the absolute affinities in terms of K_d cannot be obtained. Therefore we have performed isothermal titration microcalorimetry (ITC) measurements. Using 10 mM of Man6*P* or Fru1*P* as ligands and purified dimeric scFv M6P-1 (11 mg/ml in 100 mM PBS, pH 7.2 containing 150 mM NaCl) we have performed ITC experiments using an ITC200 calorimeter (Microcal Inc., Northampton, MA, USA). As an example, the measurement of scFv M6P-1S against Fru1*P* is shown in Fig. 13.7. For this experiment the measurement cell of the calorimeter was filled with the antibody solution and the ligand loaded into the injection syringe from where it was injected into the cell in 2 μl portions. Twenty injections were performed with 3 min equilibration times between injections and the evolved heat measured with the first injection not considered for data analysis. The heat of dilution was measured for the same number of buffer injections which was subtracted from the sample data. The K_d values of Man6*P* and Fru1*P* were 30 μM for the germline derived scFv sequence (Müller-Loennies et al. 2010) and for the VH Cys/Ser mutant (Fig. 13.7).

13.2.5 Western Blot and Immunoprecipitation

Western blot analysis against the purified lysosomal enzyme arylsulfatase B (kindly provided by M. Vellard, Biomarin, Navato, USA) immobilized on a nitrocellulose membrane at concentrations ranging from 1 to 10 ng revealed that scFv M6P-1 can be used for the detection of lysosomal enzymes with a detection limit of a few ng, depending on the degree of phosphorylation (Fig. 13.8). For comparison the PMP-BSA glycoconjugate used for the immunization and in ELISA binding assays is shown. This is of particular importance for the commercial production of recombinant proteins for enzyme replacement therapy (ERT) of lysosomal storage diseases. By Western blot analysis the expression levels of bioactive enzyme which contains the essential Man6*P* modification can be assessed easily, allowing the selection of clones producing high levels of recombinant protein and therefore leading to a considerable reduction of production costs. A comparison of methods for the quantitative analysis of Man6*P* in glycoproteins revealed that the degree of phosphorylation maybe underestimated in Western blots (Schröder et al. 2010), possibly due to steric hindrance.

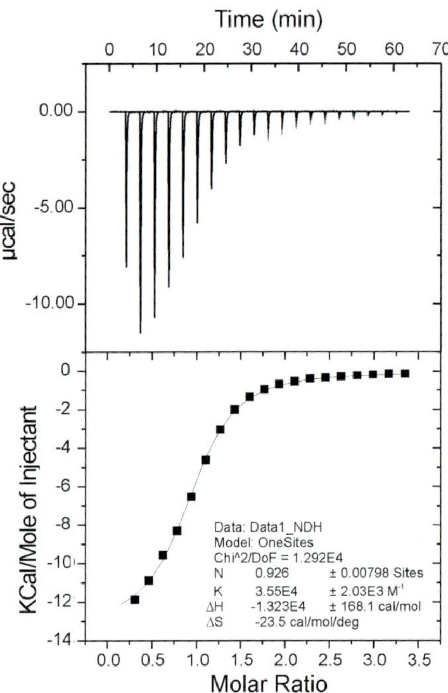

Fig. 13.7 Isothermal titration microcalorimetry (ITC) measurement using scFv M6P-1 in the cell and Fru1*P* as ligand in the injection syringe. The measurement was performed in 100 mM phosphate buffered saline (150 mM NaCl) at pH 7.2. The cell was filled with the antibody solution (11 mg/ml = 0.4 mM) and the ligand (6 mM) loaded into the injection syringe from where it was injected into the cell in 2 μl portions. Twenty injections were performed with 3 min equilibration times between injections and the evolved heat measured with the first injection not considered for data analysis. The data were then subjected to non-linear least squares curve fitting (1 set of binding sites) using MicroCal Origin v. 7.0 analysis software

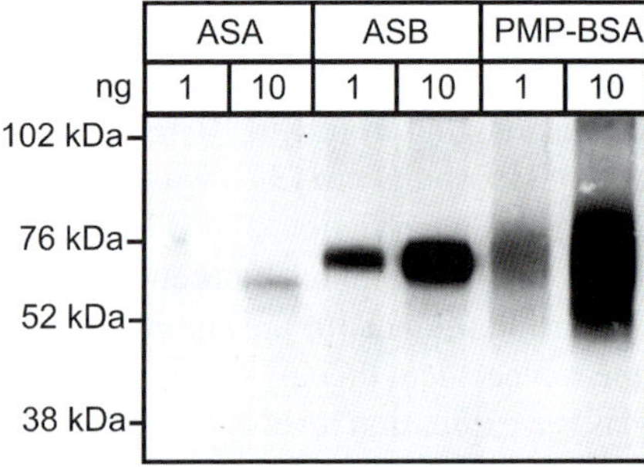

Fig. 13.8 Sensitive detection of Man6*P*-modified lysosomal enzymes. Recombinant lysosomal enzymes arylsulfatase A (ASA), arylsulfatase A (ASB) and a glycoconjugate of pentamannose-6-phosphate and BSA (PMP-BSA) (1 and 10 ng) were separated by SDS-PAGE, blotted onto nitrocellulose and analysed by scFv M6P-1 Western blotting. The positions of the molecular mass marker proteins in kDa are indicated. ASB was kindly provided by M. Vellard, Biomarin, Nevato, CA

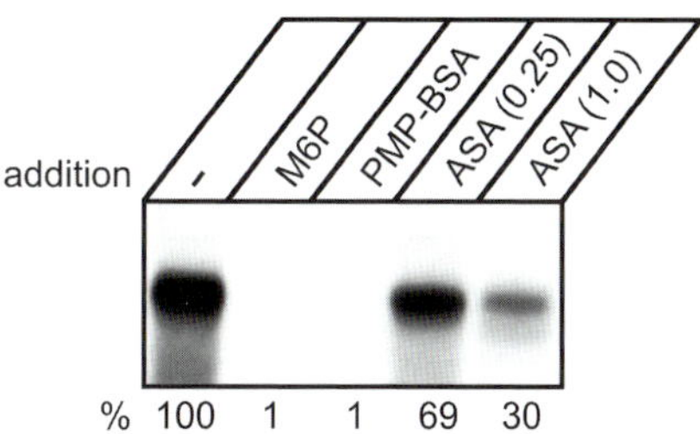

Fig. 13.9 Man6*P*-dependent precipitation of $[^{125}I]$-labelled ASA after incubation with scFv M6P-1-coupled beads in the absence (100%) or presence of the inhibitors Man6*P*, PMP-BSA and arylsulfatase A (ASA). Bound material was eluted, separated by SDS-P AGE, and visualized by autoradiography

As a first step towards the generation of an affinity support for large scale chromatography we have first tested whether it would be possible, in principle, to couple the scFv M6P-1 to beads without its inactivation. ScFv M6P-1 coupled beads allowed the subsequent immunoprecipitation of Man6*P*-containing glycoproteins from conditioned cell culture media. When a solution (0.5 ml) of iodinated arylsulfatase A (ASA) was incubated for 10 h at 4°C with 50 μl of scFv M6P-1S-conjugated Affi-gel 10 beads (BioRad), the ASA could be precipitated with the beads shown by SDS-PAGE and subsequent visualization by autoradiography (Fig. 13.9). Addition of 5 mM Man6*P* to the reaction abrogated the binding indicating that the reaction was Man6*P* specific. Evaluation of the intensity of the $[^{125}I]$-labelled polypeptide bands by densitometry or, alternatively, after excision from the dried gel and γ-counting revealed that 18% of the input was precipitated.

Similar results were obtained when conditioned serum-free media from BHK cells which stably overexpressed human ASA (hASA) or transiently expressed mouse cathepsin D (mCtsD) were used (Müller-Loennies et al. 2010). After mixing aliquots of media (0.25 ml, 1:1 ratio) with medium from non-transfected cells or from the other overexpressing cell line, a Man6*P*-dependent precipitation with 50 μl of scFv M6P-1 coupled beads could be shown by Western blotting using anti-hASA and anti-mCtsD polyclonal antibodies (Fig. 13.10).

13.2.6 Immunofluorescence Microscopy and Immunohistochemistry

The scFv M6P-1 antibody can be used as lysosomal marker colocalizing with lysosomal enzymes such as cathepsin D as showed by double immunofluorescence microscopy (Fig. 13.11a). In cerebellar sections of mouse brain cells Man6*P*-containg proteins are detectable by immunohistochemistry (Fig. 13.11b). The stainings were performed in COS7 cells derived from kidney cells of the African green monkey and mouse tissue demonstrating the species-independence of the antibody.

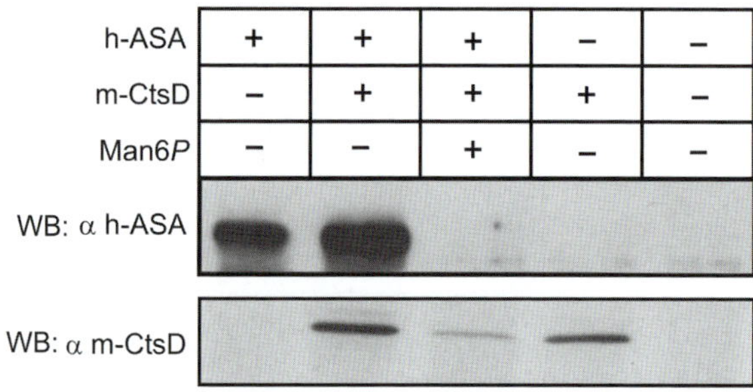

Fig. 13.10 Precipitation of Man6*P*-containing lysosomal enzymes. Purification of Man6*P*-containing lysosomal enzymes from media of overexpressing cells. Serum-free media from BHK cells stably overexpressing human ASA or transiently expressing mouse cathepsin D (mCtsD) were conditioned for 24 h. Aliquots of the media (0.25 ml) were either mixed with 0.25 ml of the other overexpressing cell line or of non-transfected cells and incubated with 50 μl of scFv M6P-1–coupled beads in the presence or absence of Man6*P* (5 mM) for 10 h at 4°C. Then the samples were centrifuged and the supernatant removed. The proteins bound to the scFv M6P-1–coupled beads were solubilized and analyzed by Western blotting using anti-ASA and anti-mCtsD polyclonal antibodies (From Müller-Loennies (2010))

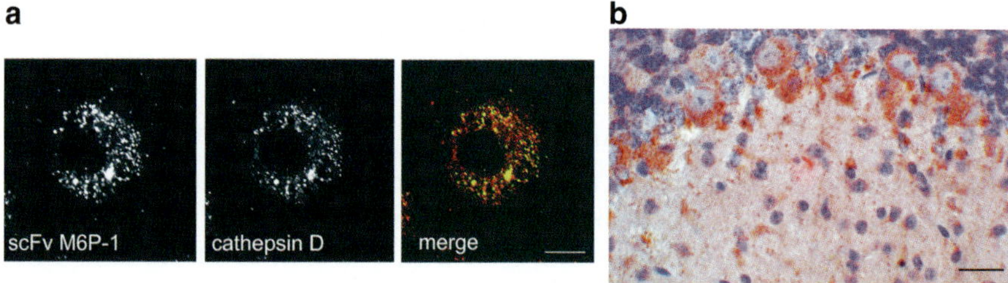

Fig. 13.11 For double immunofluorescence microscopy COS7 cells were fixed, permeabilized and incubated with myc-tagged scFv M6P-1 and the lysosomal marker protein cathepsin D (**a**). The merged picture reveals overlapping distribution (*yellow*). Scale bar, 80 μm. For immunohistochemistry (**b**) paraffin-fixed cerebellar sections of an adult mouse were incubated with myc-tagged scFv M6P-1 and HRP-coupled anti-myc antibodies followed by the peroxidase-diaminobenzidine reaction. The scFv M6P-1 immunostaining is strong in cerebellar Purkinje cells. Scale bar, 80 μm

13.2.7 Diagnostic Application of scFv M6P-1

The high specificity of the scFv M6P-1 antibody for Man6*P* and its ability to recognize these residues on lysosomal enzymes allows its diagnostic application. In MLII and MLIII patients the activity of the GlcNAc-1-phosphotransferase is absent or reduced by mutations in *GNPTAB* or *GNPTG*, respectively. The antibody scFv M6P-1 permits the indirect determination of GlcNAc-1-phosphotransferase activity by western blotting. In detail, cultured fibroblasts obtained from controls and patients clinically diagnosed for MLIII were lysed and cell extracts were separated by SDS-PAGE followed by Western blot analysis. Several Man6*P*-containing

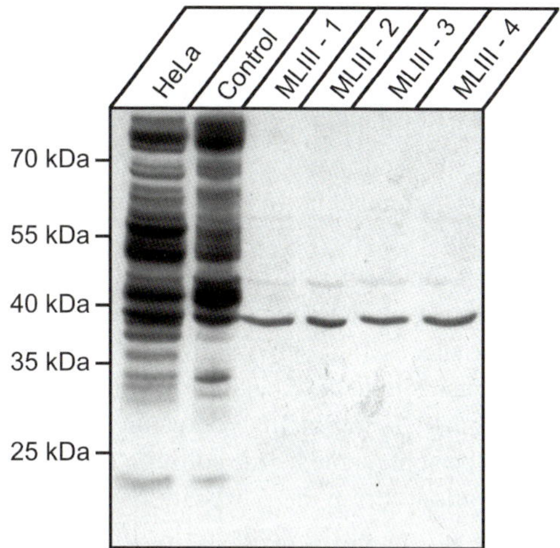

Fig. 13.12 Protein extracts of HeLa cells, and fibroblasts from a healthy control and from four MLIII patients were separated by SDS-PAGE, blotted onto nitrocellulose and analyzed by scFv M6P-1 western blotting. The positions of the molecular mass markers are indicated

proteins in the range between 20 and 100 kDa were detected with different intensities in extracts of human fibroblasts from healthy controls or in HeLa-cells (Fig. 13.12). Man6*P* containing proteins are also detectable in conditioned media of cultured fibroblasts representing secreted lysosomal enzymes (Pohl et al. 2010a). By contrast, extracts of four MLIII gamma patients exhibiting different mutations in the *GNPTG* gene (Persichetti et al. 2009) contained only one prominent Man6*P*-containing protein. The experiment showed that the method is a rapid tool for diagnosis which is less expensive than sequencing of *GNPTAB* and *GNPTG* genes.

13.3 Conclusion and Outlook

The posttranslational modification with Man6*P* is essential for the viability of eukaryotic cells and the generation of functional lysosomes. As such, inherited genetic defects in the biosynthesis of Man6*P* derivatized glycoproteins lead to severe diseases called mucolipidosis. The diagnosis of these diseases has been technically difficult to achieve and could be only carried out in specialized laboratories.

From an immunized rabbit we have isolated by a genetic approach and phage display a novel scFv specifically binding to Man6*P* residues on glycoproteins. Our experiments have shown that the scFv M6P-1 and its derivative M6P-1S can be used for the diagnosis of MLII and MLIII by simple western blotting. Furthermore, the scFv M6P-1S can be used for immunohistological stainings and immunofluorescence microscopy.

Enzyme replacement therapy (ERT) is possible for eight lysosomal storage diseases at present, with recombinant enzymes which have to be expressed in eukaryotic cells and have to be equipped with Man6*P* for cellular uptake with the exception of β-glucocerebrosidase (Keutzer and Yee 2008). The purification of enzymes for ERT requires expensive chromatographic procedures which do not discriminate between therapeutically active and inactive forms, i.e., with or without Man6*P* modification. Since usually only less than 20% of recombinant proteins when expressed in eukaryotic cells are equipped with Man6*P*, and only a fraction contains high level phosphorylation at more than one site, it would also be desirable to enrich such enzymes because it can be anticipated that such preparations yield enzymes binding with higher affinity to the Man6*P*-receptor at the cell surface leading to an efficient uptake and transport to the lysosomes.

The successful use of scFv M6P-1 coupled to beads in immunoprecipitation experiments indicates that they may be of use in a purification procedure of Man6*P*-containing glycoproteins. Conveniently, a very mild elution of bound proteins would be achievable by the addition of Man6*P* or Fru1*P* without the risk of enzyme inactivation during the purification process. Such beads could also prove useful in studies aiming at the characterization of the Man6*P*-proteome of cells and organs as described for a soluble form of the Man6*P*-receptor purified from bovine serum (Sleat et al. 2007; Sleat et al. 2008; Sleat et al. 2009).

References

Barbas CF III, Burton DR, Scott JK, Silverman GJ (2001) Phage display: a laboratory manual. Cold Spring Harbor Laboratory Press, New York

Bird RE, Hardman KD, Jacobson JW, Johnson S, Kaufman BM, Lee SM, Lee T, Pope SH, Riordan GS, Whitlow M (1988) Single-chain antigen-binding proteins. Science 242:423–426

Braulke T, Bonifacino JS (2009) Sorting of lysosomal proteins. Biochim Biophys Acta 1793:605–614

Braulke T, Gartung C, Hasilik A, Von Figura K (1987) Is movement of mannose 6-phosphate-specific receptor triggered by binding of lysosomal enzymes? J Cell Biol 104:1735–1742

Braulke T, Causin C, Waheed A, Junghans U, Hasilik A, Maly P, Humbel RE, Von Figura K (1988) Mannose 6-phosphate/insulin-like growth factor II receptor: distinct binding sites for mannose 6-phosphate and insulin-like growth factor II. Biochem Biophys Res Commun 150:1287–1293

Bretthauer RK, Kaczorowski GJ, Weise MJ (1973) Characterization of a phosphorylated pentasaccharide isolated from *Hansenula holstii* NRRL Y-2448 phosphomannan. Biochemistry 12:1251–1256

Carpenter JF, Prestrelski SJ, Arakawa T (1993) Separation of freezing- and drying-induced denaturation of lyophilized proteins using stress-specific stabilization. I. Enzyme activity and calorimetric studies. Arch Biochem Biophys 303:456–464

Cathey SS, Kudo M, Tiede S, Raas-Rothschild A, Braulke T, Beck M, Taylor HA, Canfield WM, Leroy JG, Neufeld EF, McKusick VA (2008) Molecular order in mucolipidosis II and III nomenclature. Am J Med Genet A 146A:512–513

De Duve C (1963) The lysosome. Sci Am 208:64–72

Dolezal O, Pearce LA, Lawrence LJ, McCoy AJ, Hudson PJ, Kortt AA (2000) ScFv multimers of the anti-neuraminidase antibody NC10: shortening of the linker in single-chain Fv fragment assembled in V(L) to V(H) orientation drives the formation of dimers, trimers, tetramers and higher molecular mass multimers. Protein Eng 13:565–574

Draber P, Draberova E, Novakova M (1995) Stability of monoclonal IgM antibodies freeze-dried in the presence of trehalose. J Immunol Methods 181:37–43

Ferro V, Li C, Fewings K, Palermo MC, Linhardt RJ, Toida T (2002) Determination of the composition of the oligosaccharide phosphate fraction of *Pichia (Hansenula) holstii* NRRL Y-2448 phosphomannan by capillary electrophoresis and HPLC. Carbohydr Res 337:139–146

Fischer HD, Natowicz M, Sly WS, Bretthauer RK (1980) Fibroblast receptor for lysosomal enzymes mediates pinocytosis of multivalent phosphomannan fragment. J Cell Biol 84:77–86

Futerman AH, van Meer G (2004) The cell biology of lysosomal storage disorders. Nat Rev Mol Cell Biol 5:554–565

Giudicelli V, Duroux P, Ginestoux C, Folch G, Jabado-Michaloud J, Chaume D, Lefranc MP (2006) IMGT/LIGM-DB, the IMGT comprehensive database of immunoglobulin and T cell receptor nucleotide sequences. Nucleic Acids Res 34:D781–D784

Glockshuber R, Malia M, Pfitzinger I, Plückthun A (1990) A comparison of strategies to stabilize immunoglobulin Fv-fragments. Biochemistry 29:1362–1367

Goldberg DE, Kornfeld S (1983) Evidence for extensive subcellular organization of asparagine-linked oligosaccharide processing and lysosomal enzyme phosphorylation. J Biol Chem 258:3159–3165

Hasilik A, Neufeld EF (1980) Biosynthesis of lysosomal enzymes in fibroblasts. Synthesis as precursors of higher molecular weight. J Biol Chem 255:4937–4945

Houen G, Jensen OM (1995) Conjugation to preactivated proteins using divinylsulfone and iodoacetic acid. J Immunol Methods 181:187–200

Huston JS, Levinson D, Mudgett-Hunter M, Tai MS, Novotny J, Margolies MN, Ridge RJ, Bruccoleri RE, Haber E, Crea R (1988) Protein engineering of antibody binding sites: recovery of specific activity in an anti-digoxin single-chain Fv analogue produced in *Escherichia coli*. Proc Natl Acad Sci USA 85:5879–5883

Kelly TE, Thomas GH, Taylor HA, McKusick VA, Sly WS, Glaser JH, Robinow M, Luzzatti L, Espiritu C, Feingold M, Bull MJ, Ashenhurst EM, Ives EJ (1975) Mucolipidosis III (pseudo-Hurler polydystrophy): clinical and laboratory studies in a series of 12 patients. Johns Hopkins Med J 137:156–175

Keutzer J, Yee J (2008) Enzyme replacement therapy for lysosomal storage disorders. Hum Gene Ther 19:857

Kollmann K, Pohl S, Marschner K, Encarnacao M, Sakwa I, Tiede S, Poorthuis BJ, Lübke T, Müller-Loennies S, Storch S, Braulke T (2010) Mannose phosphorylation in health and disease. Eur J Cell Biol 89:117–123

Kornfeld R, Kornfeld S (1985) Assembly of asparagine-linked oligosaccharides. Annu Rev Biochem 54:631–664

Kornfeld S, Mellman I (1989) The biogenesis of lysosomes. Annu Rev Cell Biol 5:483–525

Kornfeld S, Sly WS (2001) I-cell disease and pseudo-Hurler polydystrophy: disorders of lysosomal enzyme phosphorylation and localization. In: Scriver CR, Beaudet AL, Sly WS, Valle D, Childs B, Kinzler KW, Vogelstein B (eds) The metabolic and molecular bases of inherited disease. McGraw-Hill, New York, pp 3421–3452

Kudo M, Bao M, D'Souza A, Ying F, Pan H, Roe BA, Canfield WM (2005) The alpha- and beta-subunits of the human UDP-N-acetylglucosamine:lysosomal enzyme *N*-acetylglucosamine-1-phosphotransferase are encoded by a single cDNA. J Biol Chem 280: 36141–36149

Lazzarino DA, Gabel CA (1989) Mannose processing is an important determinant in the assembly of phosphorylated high mannose-type oligosaccharides. J Biol Chem 264:5015–5023

Leroy JG, Demars RI (1967) Mutant enzymatic and cytological phenotypes in cultured human fibroblasts. Science 157:804–806

Luzio JP, Pryor PR, Bright NA (2007) Lysosomes: fusion and function. Nat Rev Mol Cell Biol 8:622–632

MacKenzie CR, To R (1998) The role of valency in the selection of anti-carbohydrate single-chain Fvs from phage display libraries. J Immunol Methods 220:39–49

Müller-Loennies S, Galliciotti G, Kollmann K, Glatzel M, Braulke T (2010) A novel single-chain antibody fragment for detection of mannose 6-phosphate-containing proteins: application in mucolipidosis type II patients and mice. Am J Pathol 177:240–247

Parodi AJ (2000) Role of N-oligosaccharide endoplasmic reticulum processing reactions in glycoprotein folding and degradation. Biochem J 348(Pt 1):1–13

Parolis LA, Duus JO, Parolis H, Meldal M, Bock K (1996) The extracellular polysaccharide of *Pichia* (*Hansenula*) *holstii* NRRL Y-2448: the structure of the phosphomannan backbone. Carbohydr Res 293:101–117

Parolis LA, Parolis H, Kenne L, Meldal M, Bock K (1998) The extracellular polysaccharide of *Pichia* (*Hansenula*) *holstii* NRRL Y-2448: the phosphorylated side chains. Carbohydr Res 309:77–87

Persichetti E, Chuzhanova NA, Dardis A, Tappino B, Pohl S, Thomas NS, Rosano C, Balducci C, Paciotti S, Dominissini S, Montalvo AL, Sibilio M, Parini R, Rigoldi M, Di Rocco M, Parenti G, Orlacchio A, Bembi B, Cooper DN, Filocamo M, Beccari T (2009) Identification and molecular characterization of six novel mutations in the UDP-N-acetylglucosamine-1-phosphotransferase gamma subunit (GNPTG) gene in patients with mucolipidosis III gamma. Hum Mutat 30:978–984

Pohl S, Castrichini M, Müller-Loennies S, Muschol N, Braulke T (2010a) Loss of N-Acetylglucosamine-1-phosphotransferase gamma-subunit due to intronic mutation in GNPTG causes mucolipidosis type III gamma: Implications for molecular and cellular diagnostics. Am J Med Genet A 152A:124–132

Pohl S, Tiede S, Marschner K, Encarnacao M, Castrichini M, Kollmann K, Muschol N, Ullrich K, Müller-Loennies S, Braulke T (2010b) Proteolytic processing of the gamma-subunit is associated with the failure to form GlcNAc-1-phosphotransferase complexes and mannose 6-phosphate residues on lysosomal enzymes in human macrophages. J Biol Chem 285:23936–23944

Raas-Rothschild A, Cormier-Daire V, Bao M, Genin E, Salomon R, Brewer K, Zeigler M, Mandel H, Toth S, Roe B, Munnich A, Canfield WM (2000) Molecular basis of variant pseudo-hurler polydystrophy (mucolipidosis IIIC). J Clin Invest 105:673–681

Reitman ML, Kornfeld S (1981) Lysosomal enzyme targeting. N-Acetylglucosaminylphosphotransferase selectively phosphorylates native lysosomal enzymes. J Biol Chem 256: 11977–11980

Rothman JE, Katz FN, Lodish HF (1978) Glycosylation of a membrane protein is restricted to the growing polypeptide chain but is not necessary for insertion as a transmembrane protein. Cell 15:1447–1454

Ruddock LW, Molinari M (2006) N-glycan processing in ER quality control. J Cell Sci 119:4373–4380

Schröder S, Matthes F, Hyden P, Andersson C, Fogh J, Müller-Loennies S, Braulke T, Gieselmann V, Matzner U (2010) Site-specific analysis of N-linked oligosaccharides of recombinant lysosomal arylsulfatase A produced in different cell lines. Glycobiology 20:248–259

Sleat DE, Zheng H, Lobel P (2007) The human urine mannose 6-phosphate glycoproteome. Biochim Biophys Acta 1774:368–372

Sleat DE, Della Valle MC, Zheng H, Moore DF, Lobel P (2008) The mannose 6-phosphate glycoprotein proteome. J Proteome Res 7:3010–3021

Sleat DE, Ding L, Wang S, Zhao C, Wang Y, Xin W, Zheng H, Moore DF, Sims KB, Lobel P (2009) Mass spectrometry-based protein profiling to determine the cause of lysosomal storage diseases of unknown etiology. Mol Cell Proteomics 8:1708–1718

Spranger JW, Brill PW, Poznanski AK (2002) Bone dysplasias: an atlas of genetic disorders of the skeletal development. Oxford University Press, New York, pp 57–79

Tiede S, Muschol N, Reutter G, Cantz M, Ullrich K, Braulke T (2005a) Missense mutations in N-acetylglucosamine-1-phosphotransferase α/β subunit gene in a patient with mucolipidosis III and a mild clinical phenotype. Am J Med Genet A 137A:235–240

Tiede S, Storch S, Lübke T, Henrissat B, Bargal R, Raas-Rothschild A, Braulke T (2005b) Mucolipidosis II is caused by mutations in GNPTA encoding the α/β GlcNAc-1-phosphotransferase. Nat Med 11:1109–1112

Varki A, Kornfeld S (1983) The spectrum of anionic oligosaccharides released by endo-β-*N*-acetylglucosaminidase H from glycoproteins. Structural studies and interactions with the phosphomannosyl receptor. J Biol Chem 258:2808–2818

Anti-glycolipid Antibodies in Guillain-Barré Syndrome and Related Neuropathies: Therapeutic Strategies for Disease Treatment

14

Robert K. Yu, Seigo Usuki, and Toshio Ariga

14.1 Summary

Guillain-Barré syndrome (GBS) and its variants are autoimmune neuropathies that frequently occur as a result of enteritis resulting from an infectious event caused by bacterial pathogens such as *Campylobacter jejuni*. These neuropathies are classified as several disorders characterized by an immune-mediated attack on the peripheral nervous system, particularly on the myelin sheath and axon of sensory and motor nerves. Increased antibody titers in GBS and its variants are thought to be caused by production of antibodies to *C. jejuni*-containing carbohydrate antigen(s) that also show cross-reactivity with gangliosides of the myelin sheath and the axons of peripheral nerve cells. For this reason, the most common diagnostic test of GBS is to detect circulating anti-glycolipid antibodies in patients thought to have GBS. Pathogenesis of GBS is believed to involve a molecular mimicry mechanism between epitopes on bacterial (e.g., *C. jejuni*) lipo-oligosaccharides (LOSs) and peripheral nerve glycolipids, particularly gangliosides, resulting in demyelination and/or axonal degeneration. It has been reported that sera of 60% of patients with GBS contain one or more anti-ganglioside antibodies. Other glycolipid antigens include sulfatides and sulfated glucuronosyl glycolipids (SGGLs). These antibodies contribute to the pathogenesis of GBS, and their presence represents an important diagnostic marker for GBS. Recently it has been shown that these antibodies are often concealed in certain patients' sera that are "anti-ganglioside antibody negative" but they react with a mixed form of gangliosides (e.g., GD1a and GD1b), and not with individual purified ganglioside alone. This novel class of autoantibodies has been termed anti-ganglioside-complex (GSC) antibodies.

R.K. Yu (✉) • S. Usuki • T. Ariga
Institute of Molecular Medicine and Genetics and Institute of Neuroscience, Medical College of Georgia, Georgia Health Science University, 11 20 15th Street, Augusta, GA 30912, USA
e-mail: ryu@georgiahealth.edu

P. Kosma and S. Müller-Loennies (eds.), *Anticarbohydrate Antibodies*,
DOI 10.1007/978-3-7091-0870-3_14,

These anti-GSC antibodies also are involved in the pathogenesis of GBS and its variants. Antibody- and/or cell-mediated immune responses are believed to induce pathological lesions of the nerve, resulting in loss of conduction velocity or conduction block. Recent studies also revealed that interruption of neurotransmission could occur as a result of interaction of anti-ganglioside antibodies with ion channels at the nodes of Ranvier. Accumulating *ex vivo* electrophysiological evidence suggests that ganglioside molecular mimicry may be responsible for muscle weakness, possibly via the action of anti-ganglioside antibodies on cell-surface ganglioside antigens of the neuromuscular junction. Although plasmapheresis and intravenous immunoglobulin (IVIG) are commonly used for the treatment of patients with GBS, we have recently developed novel and effective therapeutic strategies employing glycomimics such as anti-idiotypic antibodies and phage-displayed peptides to target specific pathogenic antibodies for elimination in an animal model of GBS. These treatment strategies should represent a novel approach for treatment of GBS and related autoimmune disorders.

14.2 Introduction

Glycosphingolipids (GSLs), and their sialic acid-containing derivatives called gangliosides, are a family of diverse, highly complex molecules localized primarily on the plasma membrane and are particularly abundant in the nervous tissues of vertebrates. GSLs are the important constituents of microdomains or lipid rafts of the extracellular leaflet of plasma membranes (Iwabuchi et al. 1998; Hakomori 2000; Simons and Toomre 2000). Research interest in GSLs, including gangliosides, is not limited to their biological functions in the usual condition, such as neurotrophicity, cell-cell recognition and adhesion, cellular differentiation and growth, intercellular signaling, and trafficking and/or sorting (Hakomori 1990, 2003; Yu 1994; Yu et al. 1994a, 2008, 2010) Evidence of research is also focused on the role of GSLs, particularly gangliosides, in the pathogenic mechanisms of several immune-mediated neurological disorders, such as Guillain-Barré syndrome (GBS) (Willison and Yuki 2002; Ariga and Yu 2005; Yu et al. 2006; Kaida et al. 2009) and in those of Alzheimer's disease (Yanagisawa 2007; Ariga et al. 2008). Accumulating evidence for the putative pathogenic roles of GSLs, including gangliosides, in GBS, indicates that: (a) they are localized in peripheral nerve system (PNS) myelin, axolemma, and synapse, and degeneration of myelin and axons accounts for the loss of sensory and motor functions; (b) animal models of peripheral neuropathies can be established using certain pure glycolipids, including gangliosides, as immunogens; (c) sera from patients with GBS include several antibodies that react with human GSLs of PNS, including GM1, GD1a, GD1b, GalNAc-GD1a, GQ1b, cerebroside (GalCer), sulfatide, sulfated glucuronosyl glycolipids (SGGLs); (d) the pathophysiological effects of the antibodies could be due to one or several more of the following mechanisms, including an antibody-mediated, complement-dependent process, a cell-mediated degenerating process, and/or conduction block at the node of Ranvier (Willison and Yuki 2002; Yu et al.

2006). The presynaptic motor nerve terminal at the neuromuscular junction (NMJ) may be a prominent target because it is highly enriched in gangliosides and lies outside the blood-nerve barrier, allowing antibody access (Plomp and Willison 2009).

14.3 Guillain-Barré Syndrome and Related Neuropathies

GBS is the most frequent cause of acute flaccid paralysis in humans, occurring with an annual incidence of 1–2 cases per 100,000 people. GBS is slightly more common in men than in women, occurring at a ratio of 1.3:1. GBS is primarily an immune-mediated disorder of the PNS. The immune system attacks spinal nerve roots, peripheral nerves, and cranial nerves, resulting in focal inflammation, with variable damage to myelin sheaths and axon fibers. In recent years, studies have shed new light on a number of disease aspects that have enhanced understanding of the pathogenic mechanisms of GBS. As an acute inflammatory polyradiculoneuropathy, GBS frequently develops following a gastrointestinal infection. Clinical symptoms often occur 1–3 weeks after a bacterial or viral infection (Willison and Yuki 2002; Yu et al. 2006). The most commonly identified triggering agents are *C. jejuni* (in 13–39% of cases), followed by cytomegalovirus (5–22%), Epstein-Barr virus (1–13%), and *Mycoplasma pneumoniae* (5%) (Hadden et al. 2001; Schwerer 2002; Yu et al. 2006). All of these pathogens have carbohydrate sequences (antigenic epitopes) in common with glycoconjugates of peripheral nerve tissue.

GBS is recognized as several disorders characterized by an immune-mediated attack on the peripheral nerves, particularly in the myelin sheath or Schwann cells of sensory and motor nerves (Yu et al. 2006). Several subtypes of GBS have been characterized based on their clinical manifestations. The most common form is a multifocal demyelinating disorder caused by damage to the myelin sheath of the peripheral nerves and is called acute inflammatory demyelinating polyneuropathy (AIDP). Clinically, AIDP is characterized by progressive areflexic weakness and mild sensory changes. Sensory symptoms often precede motor weakness. About 20% of AIDP patients eventually have respiratory failure. The chronic variant is called chronic inflammatory demyelinating polyneuropathy (CIDP). It is characterized by progressive weakness and impaired sensory function in the legs and arms. Several variants of CIDP are known, including one form that has no sensory involvement, i.e., no numbness or tingling in the hands or feet. This pure motor chronic acquired demyelinating neuropathy variant is also called multifocal motor neuropathy (MMN). Patients with MMN frequently demonstrate signs of conduction block in the peripheral nerves. On the other hand, sensory nerve conduction evaluations are normal in patients with MMN. Other cases of GBS are associated primarily with axonal processes with axonal degeneration and sparing of the myelin; these cases are called acute motor axonal neuropathy (AMAN). However, another form of GBS is found and characterized by an involvement of both sensory and motor axons and is termed acute motor and sensory axonal neuropathy (AMSAN) (Hughes and Cornblath 2005). More than 90% of patients with GBS in Europe and North America have AIDP or CIDP. The most distinct feature that distinguishes MMN from CIDP is the presence in serum of anti-GM1 ganglioside antibodies, which occur in approximately 50% of MMN patients. Some motor neuropathies have been classified as amyotrophic lateral sclerosis (ALS) variants, with predominantly lower motor neuron signs and axonal changes based on electrodiagnostic studies. AMAN occurs in less than 10% of persons with GBS in the Western hemisphere but in more than 40% of those affected in China and Japan (Yu et al. 2006). The incidence of AMSAN is very low, less than 10% of those with AMAN. Miller Fisher syndrome (MFS) is another GBS variant that occurs in about 5% of people affected by GBS. MFS is characterized by ophthalmoplegia, areflexia, ataxia, and, in some cases, facial and bulbar palsy. The incidence of the pharyngeal-cervical-brachial variant, which is characterized by proximal descending weakness, is very low. When IgM M-proteins react with myelin-associated glycoprotein or sulfated glucuronosyl glycolipids (SGGLs), there is a correlation with a specific syndrome called IgM paraproteinemia neuropathy (Freddo et al. 1985; Yu et al. 1990).

14.4 Anti-ganglioside Antibodies in Guillain-Barré Syndrome and Related Neuropathies

Much of the research into GBS over the last decade has focused on the forms that are mediated by anti-ganglioside antibodies (Ariga et al. 2001; Willison and Yuki 2002; Willison 2005a; Kaida et al. 2009). The target antigens for antibodies in GBS have been identified by a solid-phase immunoassay, such as thin-layer chromatography (TLC)-immunostaining and/or enzyme-linked immunosorbent assay, employing purified ganglioside as the test antigens. It has been reported that the sera of 60% of patients with GBS contain one or more anti-ganglioside antibodies. Measurements of these antibody titers are therefore very important for diagnosing GBS and evaluating the effectiveness of clinical intervention (Willison and Yuki 2002; Ariga and Yu 2005; Yu et al. 2006; Yuki 2007). Early studies performed on the basis of elevated anti-ganglioside antibody titers had identified patients with CIDP, ALS, and MMNs (Pestronk et al. 1988). More than 200 publications have reported the presence of serum antibodies against at least 15 individual gangliosides, including GM1, GM1(NeuGc), Fuc-GM1, GM1b, GalNAc-GM1b, GD1a, GalNAc-GD1a, GD1b, 9-*O*-acetyl-GD1b, GD3, GT1a, GT1b, GQ1b, LM1, and GQ1bα. In addition, four other GSLs such as asialo-GM1, galactocerebroside, and SGGLs have also been found to be target antigens (Willison and Yuki 2002; Ariga and Yu 2005).

From the pathological point of view, *C. jejuni* neuritis strains are associated with up to 75% of patients with AMAN accompanied by anti-GM1, anti-GD1a (Ho et al. 1999; Yoshino et al. 2000; Neuwirth et al. 2010), GM1b, and GalNAc-GD1a antibodies (Yuki et al. 1999); 10–15% of patients with CIDP and AIDP develop anti-GM1 (Melendez-Vasquez et al. 1997; Trojaborg 1998). Anti-GD3, GT3, and

9-*O*-acetyl GD3 antibodies were observed in GBS and less in MFS (Koga et al. 1999). In rare cases, anti-GD3 and anti-GT3 antibodies were found in the pathogenesis of CIDP and AIDP (Usuki et al. 2005); 96% of patients with MFS present elevated anti-GQ1b antibody titers (Chiba et al. 1992); patients with the pharyngeal-cervical-brachial variant often develop associated IgG anti-GT1a antibodies (Koga et al. 1998). Salloway et al. (1996) reported that anti-GD3 antibody was observed in a patient with MFS. Pers et al. (2009) reported an overlap syndrome associating MFS and AIDP. The patient presented unusual neurological manifestations including headache, T10 sensory level, urinary urgency, and gadolinium enhancement of the spinal roots. One year follow-up was characterized by clinical recovery and persistent high rates of anti-GQ1b, -GD1b and -GT1b antibodies. In addition, Dewil et al. (2010) reported an unusual presentation of GBS following a cytomegalovirus (CMV) infection associated with IgG monospecific to GD1b. The clinical feature consisted of predominantly asymmetric motor involvement with respiratory insufficiency, limited sensory complaints and the combination of unilateral facial and contralateral abducens palsy. Lardone et al. (2010) recently reported the relationship between anti-GM1 antibodies and clinical severity of GBS. Thirty-four GBS patients with anti-GM1 IgG antibodies were grouped into two categories according to disease severity at nadir: mild (grades 1–3 by Hughes functional scale, n = 13) and severe (grades 4 and 5, n = 21). No differences in antibody titer were found between the two groups. However, the severe group showed a significantly higher frequency (95% vs 46% in the mild group, $p = 0.002$) of specific anti-GM1 antibodies that did not cross-react with anti-GD1b antibodies. Nonetheless, measurements of these GSL antibody titers remain the most effective and reliable way for diagnosing GBS and evaluating the effectiveness of treatment in the clinic (Willison 2005a; Yu et al. 2006; Kaida et al. 2009).

14.5 Antibodies Against Ganglioside Complexes in GBS and Its Variants

Recently, Kaida et al. (2004) reported that 8 of 100 patients with GBS who were tested had little or no antibody reaction based on ELISA against individual ganglioside species, including GD1a and GD1b. However, using the TLC-immuno-overlay technique employing a crude mixture of whole brain gangliosides, they identified a strong immunoreactive band migrating between GD1a and GD1b in these sera. This finding suggests that these patients' sera contain a special antibody reacting to a complex form of GD1a and GD1b, but not reacting to either GD1a or GD1b alone. This novel class of autoantibodies has been termed "anti-ganglioside-complex (GSC) antibodies". The presence of antibody specificity to GD1a/GD1b and/or GD1b/GT1b is significantly associated with severe disability and a requirement for mechanical ventilation (Kaida et al. 2007). Further study revealed that 39 of 234 GBS patients (17%) had IgG anti-GSC antibodies against at least one ganglioside complex such as GD1a/GD1b, GM1/GD1a, GD1b/GT1b, GM1/GT1b, or GM1/

GD1b. Among the 39 patients who were anti-GSC-positive, all had IgG anti-GM1/GD1a antibodies, and 27 had anti-GM1/GT1b antibodies. Sixteen patients had anti-GD1a/GD1b antibodies, 13 had anti-GD1b/GT1b antibodies, and 6 had anti-GM1/GD1b antibodies, 10 patients had both anti-GD1a/GD1b and anti-GD1b/GT1b antibody activities. Anti-GSC-positive GBS had antecedent gastrointestinal infection and lower cranial nerve deficits more frequently than control GBS. These results indicate that the anti-GSC antibodies might have been involved in GBS sera in which anti-ganglioside antibodies were not detected in the past employing a single ganglioside alone. Indeed, GBS sera without anti-ganglioside antibodies contained anti-GSC antibodies against GSC such as GD1a/GD1b, GD1a/GM1, GM1/GT1b, and GD1b/GT1b ((Kaida et al. 2008), see Table 14.1). In this regard, Hamaguchi et al. (2007) reported that a 42-year-old male patient with GBS had anti-GD1a/GD1b antibody, but not antibody to the corresponding individual gangliosides. The clinical features were similar to those patients with anti-GD1a/GD1b antibodies as previously reported by Kaida et al. (2007), including AMAN-type GBS with cranial nerve deficits and severe disability. In addition, Kuijf et al. (2007) reported that 2 of 21 patients with GBS had serum IgG to the GM1/GD1a complex and two other patients had IgG to the GQ1b/GD1a complex. These pairs of patients were clinically distinct. More recently, a CIDP patient accompanied by anti-GD1b IgM presented an additional new reactivity to GT1b/GM1 and GT1b/GM2 GSCs, and in one with peripheral neuropathy who had reactivity to GM2/GD1b IgM but not to individual gangliosides (Nobile-Orazio et al. 2010). The origin of those anti-GSC antibodies remains unknown, and it would be of considerable interest to investigate the epitope they react to and their pathogenic roles in GBS.

MFS is considered a variant of GBS, in which at least three different MFS-associated antibodies are known: anti-GQ1b, anti-GQ1b/GM1, and anti-GQ1b/GD1a. In patients with MFS, not only GQ1b itself but also clustered epitopes of GSCs, including GQ1b, may be considered to be the prime target antigens for serum antibodies. A tendency to escape sensory disturbances is shown by anti-GQ1b/GM1-positive MFS (Kaida et al. 2006; Kanzaki et al. 2008). Further studies indicated that a serum antibody sample from an MFS patient reacted with GA1/GQ1b, but not with GA1, GQ1b, or GT1a, although GA1 had not been considered to be an important antigen in GBS. Thus, anti-GSC antibodies can be used as markers of severe GBS and its variant and may provide a clue to elucidate its pathogenetic role (Kaida et al. 2007) (see Table 14.1). Moreover, in sera without anti-ganglioside antibodies, it may be necessary to examine the antibody activity using appropriate ganglioside complexes and suitable methodologies, such as liposome-incorporated GSLs (Willison 2005b).

Gangliosides, along with other components such as cholesterol, are known to form lipid rafts in which the carbohydrate portions of two different gangliosides may form a novel conformational epitope. Within the rafts, gangliosides are considered to interact with important receptors or signal transducers. The antibodies against ganglioside complexes may therefore directly cause nerve conduction failure and severe disability in GBS (Kusunoki et al. 2008). Structural and functional analyses of epitopes of GSCs in membranes should provide new insights

Table 14.1 Relationship between anti-glycosphingolipid antibodies, putative infectious pathogens, and clinical symptoms

Anti-glycosphingolipid antibodies	Infectious pathogens	Clinical symptoms
GM1	*C. jejuni* (antecedent gastrointestinal infection)	AMAN, injury to motor axons axonal degeneration, occasional persistent motor weakness, distal-dominant weakness of the extremities, rare cranial nerve palsy
		ALS, MN (cross-reactivity with GA1), AIDP/CIDP
GM1 and GD1a	*C. jejuni*	AMAN, injury to motor axons
GA1	*Mycoplasma pneumoniae*	MND, MN, ALS (cross-reactivity with GM1) motor variant of CIDP
GD1b and other b-series gangliosides	*C. jejuni*	MN, ALS (cross-reactivities with GM1 and GA1), chronic sensory ataxia motor and sensory disturbance
		IgM paraproteinemia with chronic Polyneuropathy
GD1a-GalNAc	*C. jejuni* (antecedent gastrointestinal infection)	AMAN, injury to motor axons distal-dominant, weakness, no sensory signs, axonal dysfunction. Pure motor variant of GBS cranial nerve involvement (facial palsy)
GM1b-GalNAc	*C. jejuni* (antecedent gastrointestinal infection)	IgG, axonal degeneration of the motor nerves (cross-reactivity with GD1a-GalNAc)
GM2	CMV (antecedent respiratory infection)	Sensory dysfunction, frequent facial palsy (cross-reactivity with GD1a-GalNAc or GM1b-GalNAc)
GT1a and GM1b	Dysphasia (aspiration pneumonia etc) botulinum toxin	GBS with oropharyngeal involvement pharyngeal-cervical-brachial weakness bulbar palsy, tendon reflexes
GQ1b	*C. jejuni* (antecedent respiratory tract infection)	MFS
		Bickerstaff's brain stem encephalitis, muscle paralysis, ataxia, hyporeflexia, ophthalmoplegia
GM1b, GM1α	*C. jejuni* (gastrointestinal infection)	Acute motor neuropathy, AMAN limb weakness
	Mycoplasma pneumoniae	Flaccid quadriparesis
GQ1bα	*C. jejuni*	GBS with sensory ataxia, IgM
GD3, GT3, OAc-GT3	*C. jejuni*	MFS, cranial nerve and oculomotor nerve involvement
GM3, GD3, GT3	*C. jejuni*	AIDP, CIDP
LM1	*C. jejuni*	IgG, AMSAN/AMAN motor and sensory fiber involvement (cross-reactivities with GM1, GM1b, GD1a, GD1a-GalNAc, GD1b and GQ1b)

(continued)

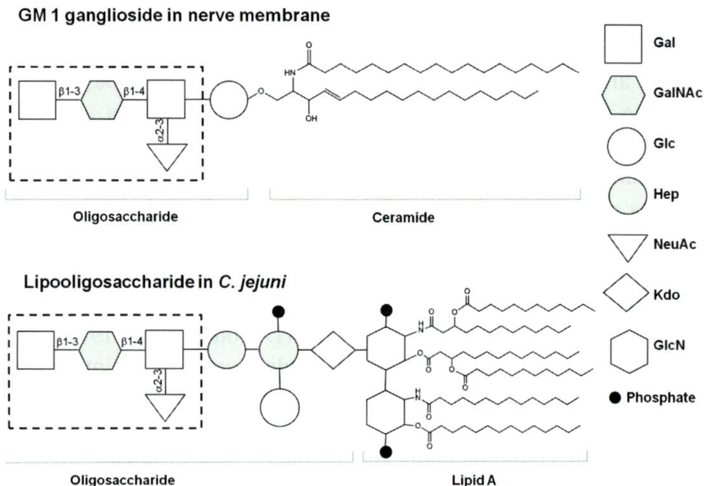

Fig. 14.1 Molecular mimicry of *C. jejuni* LOS and GM1 ganglioside. Gangliosides are highly expressed in nerve cell membranes. They consist of a ceramide portion and a polar head group that contains glucose (Glc), galactose (Gal), *N*-acetyl-galactosamine (GalNAc), and *N*-acetyl-neuraminic acid (NeuAc). Lipo-oligosaccharide-containing ganglioside-like mimics are located in the outer part of the cell wall of Gram-negative bacteria, including *C. jejuni*. The specific structure of gangliosides is crucial in the understanding of the pathogenesis of GBS

suggests that certain infectious agents trigger the disease because clinical symptoms occur frequently after an antecedent infection (for a review, see (Yu et al. 2006)). The most well-studied microbial agent is the Gram-negative bacterium *C. jejuni* which contains a LOS coat that also shares putative antigenic epitopes with those found in human nerve tissues. This resemblance has been termed "molecular mimicry," which is defined as the dual recognition, by a single B- or T-cell receptor, of a microbe's structure and an antigen of the host tissue; this recognition is the mechanism by which infectious agents trigger cross-reactive antibodies or T cells that can lead to autoimmune diseases (Ang et al. 2004) (Fig. 14.1).

The molecular-mimicry hypothesis postulates that a cross-reactive immune response is originally directed to bacterial LOS, and autoantibodies and/or autoreactive T cells induced by infection are initially directed against the microbial antigens (Ang et al. 2004). Subsequently, immune responses against nerve tissue gangliosides are expected as a result of molecular mimicry between gangliosides of the nerve axolemmal membrane and the LOSs of *C. jejuni*. Anti-ganglioside antibodies can arise through molecular mimicry with GBS-associated *C. jejuni* oligosaccharides (Schwerer 2002; Willison and Yuki 2002; Usuki et al. 2006, 2010a, b). This concept has gained strong support from Moran et al. (Moran and Prendergast 2001; Moran et al. 2005), who reported that sera of rabbits immunized with ganglioside-mimicking *C. jejuni* LOSs revealed high titers of anti-LOS antibodies that were cross-reactive with a panel of gangliosides. In addition, sensitization of Lewis rats with a *C. jejuni* LOS bearing the GD3 epitope induced anti-GD3 antibody (Usuki et al. 2006, 2010a, b). These findings strongly support the concept that molecular mimicry between microbial antigens and host tissues represents an attractive mechanism for triggering autoimmune responses in hosts. Initially, Yuki et al. (1993, 1994) reported that the structural mimicry of gangliosides by core oligosaccharides in LOSs from *C. jejuni* has been implicated in inducing cross-reactive anti-ganglioside antibodies. Detailed chemical studies of LOSs from GBS-associated *C. jejuni* isolate, HS:41, using gas chromatography-mass spectrometry and proton nuclear magnetic resonance, identified a tetrasaccharide structure consistent with GM1 mimicry. Several serotypes of *C. jejuni* LOSs and ganglioside mimicry have also been reported, including GM1 and GD2 (serotypes HS:1, HS:2, HS:4; HS:10, HS:19, HS:23, HS:36, and HS:41), asialo-GM1 (serotype HS:41), GD1a (serotypes HS:1, HS:2, HS:4; HS:10, HS:19, HS:23, HS:36, HS41, and HS:19), GD2 (serotypes HS:1, HS:2, HS:4, HS:10, HS:23, HS:36, and HS:41), GD3 (serotypes HS:1, HS:2, HS:4, HS:10, HS:19, HS:19, HS:23, HS:36, and HS:41), GM3 and GD1b (serotypes HS:23, HS:36), GQ1b and GT1a (serotypes HS:2, HS:19, and HS:23) (Yu et al. 2006). Ganglioside-like LOS synthesis is catalyzed by sialyltransferase *Cst-I*, α2,3-sialyltransferase-I; *cgtA*, β1,4-*N*-acetylgalactosaminyltransferase, *Cst-II*, *N*-acetylgalactosaminyltransferase *CgtA*, and galactosyltransferase *CgtB*, all of which have been characterized in *C. jejuni*. In fact, the *cst-II*, *cgtA*, and *cgtB* genes that encode these enzymes have also been cloned (Gilbert et al. 2000), facilitating further studies of the generation of various ganglioside-like epitopes.

In support of the molecular mimicry hypothesis, Yuki et al. (2004) reported that upon sensitization with *C. jejuni* GM1-like LOS (LOS_{GM1}), rabbits developed anti-GM1-like IgG antibody and flaccid limb weakness. Paralyzed rabbits had pathological changes in their peripheral nerves identical with those present in GBS. Immunization with the LOS_{GM1} generated a cross-reacting antibody to GM1 that is located on human peripheral nerves. Thus the carbohydrate mimicry between GM1 and LOS_{GM1} induces the production of pathogenic autoantibodies and the development of GBS (Yuki et al. 2004). The possible pathogenesis of AMAN subsequent to *C. jejuni* enteritis can be envisaged as follows: infection by *C. jejuni* bearing GM1-like epitope induces production of the anti-GM1 IgG antibody, the autoantibody binds to GM1 at the nodes of Ranvier in spinal anterior roots, activated complements are recruited by the anti-GM1 antibodies, which then form a membrane-attack complex. Anti-GM1 antibodies are likely to play a major role in producing nodal membrane damage by complement activation and causing the disruption of sodium channel clusters, followed by disruption of the paranodal structure (Susuki et al. 2007a, b), resulting in muscle weakness in the early phase of illness; in severe cases, Wallerian-like degeneration ensues. To express gangliosides-like LOS epitope, *C. jejuni* requires specific gene combinations that function in sialic acid biosynthesis or transfer. Interestingly, the knockout mutants of these landmark genes of GBS show reduced reactivity with GBS patients' sera and fail to induce an anti-ganglioside antibody response in mice. These genes are crucial for the induction of neuropathogenic cross-reactive antibodies (Komagamine and Yuki 2006). In this regard, Moran et al. (2005) reported that rabbits immunized with *C. jejuni* ganglioside-like LOSs presented high titers of anti-LOS antibodies in sera that were cross-reactive with a panel of gangliosides. Non-ganglioside-mimicking *C. jejuni* LOSs, however, induced a strong anti-LOS response but no anti-ganglioside antibodies. This result suggests that immunization with ganglioside-mimicking *C. jejuni* LOSs may trigger the production of cross-reactive anti-ganglioside antibodies that recognize epitopes at the nodes of Ranvier. Similarly, we have also induced in rats GBS-like experimental neuritis by sensitizing the animals with a highly purified LOS fraction (LOS_{GD3}) that bears structural similarity to GD3 (Usuki et al. 2010a, b). The availability of animal models using defined pure antigens should facilitate a better understanding of the etiology, pathogenic mechanisms, and pathophysiological basis of GBS and the development of effective treatment strategies for GBS (see below).

14.8 Anti-ganglioside Antibodies and the Neuromuscular Junction

The presynaptic neuromuscular junction (NMJ) is considered to be a potential target for autoimmune attack in GBS and peripheral neuropathies for the following reasons (O'Hanlon et al. 2001; Willison and Yuki 2002): (a) NMJ is rich in gangliosides, including GQ1b, GM1, GD3, and GD1a; (b) NMJ lacks the blood–nerve barrier, readily allowing access to circulating autoantibodies; and (c) the NMJ is a vulnerable site for antibody-mediated paralytic diseases, including myasthenia gravis and Lambert–Eaton myasthenic syndrome. Anti-ganglioside antibodies may facilitate studies on the functional roles of gangliosides by inducing specific structural and functional changes in the NMJ. For example, Santafe et al. (2005) reported a monoclonal IgM antibody from a patient with a pure motor chronic demyelinating polyneuropathy that binds specifically to gangliosides GM2, GalNAc-GD1a, and GalNAc-GM1b, all of which have a common epitope of βGalNAc(1→4)[αNeuAc(2→3)]βGal(1→). Thus, it is possible to localize these gangliosides in specific cellular components of the NMJ, describe the anti-ganglioside antibody-induced structural and functional changes in NMJs to gain insights into the role of gangliosides in the synaptic function, and elucidate how these gangliosides are involved in Schwann cell-nerve terminal interactions, including structural stability and neurotransmission. With respect to the membranous cellular components of the nodes of Ranvier, GM1 is present on the cytoplasmic surface of motor neurons and has been specifically identified on paranodal and internodal axolemma, as well as on distal motor nerve terminals (Thomas et al. 1991; Corbo et al. 1992, 1993; Schluep et al. 1998). In some patients with motor axonal GBS, the nodes of Ranvier in intramuscular motor nerve bundles are targeted by anti-GD1a antibody in a gradient-dependent manner, with the greatest vulnerability at distal nodes. These studies provide a detailed mechanism by which loss of axonal conduction can occur in a distal dominant pattern, as observed in certain clinical cases (McGonigal et al. 2010). Similarly, disialogangliosides have been shown to be expressed on internodal axolemma and/or on adaxonal Schwann cell cytoplasm

(Willison et al. 1996). Antibodies to GD1a and GalNAc-GD1a are associated with pure motor axonal neuropathy and preferentially immunostain ventral root (VR) axons rather than dorsal root (DR) axons (Gong et al. 2001; Yoshino et al. 2005). Interestingly, these disialogangliosides are located only in the presynaptic component of the motor end-plates. Taguchi et al. (2004a) also reported that the epitopes recognized by anti-GalNAc-GD1a antibodies were observed in the soma of large neurons in the anterior horn of the adult rat spinal cord and its motor axons, as well as in VRs and NMJs. Kaida et al. (2003) showed that an anti-GalNAc-GD1a antibody immunostained an inner surface of compact myelin and a periaxonal axolemma-related portion in VRs, small-diameter DR fibers, and intramuscular nerves (IMs). These studies suggest that anti-GalNAc-GD1a antibodies in patients' sera may bind to those regions in the VR and IM nerves where GalNAc-GD1a is localized, and the antibodies may function in the pathogenesis of pure motor type GBS. An immune attack directed against antigenic determinants located at the paranodal Schwann cell surface may lead to paranodal demyelination, whereas antigens targeted on the exposed axolemma may result in axonal degeneration, both of which would result in conduction failure. Ligand-binding studies have suggested that GM1, GD1b, and polysialylated gangliosides are enriched in the paranodal myelin loops of the peripheral nerve (Willison and Yuki 2002). In addition, GQ1b is particularly enriched at the nodes of Ranvier (Chiba et al. 1992). In MFS, the serum antibody specifically binds to the disialyl epitope on gangliosides, such as GQ1b, GT1a, and GD3. Since these gangliosides are enriched in synaptic membranes, anti-ganglioside antibodies may target the NMJ, contributing to the disease symptoms (Halstead et al. 2005; Usuki et al. 2005, 2006; Nakatani et al. 2009). *Ex vivo* studies at mouse NMJs revealed that anti-GQ1b-positive MFS serum and human anti-GQ1b monoclonal antibodies induced a dramatic increase in spontaneous quantal acetylcholine (ACh) release, measured as miniature end-plate potential frequency, and subsequent blockade of neuromuscular synaptic transmission, due to a failure of ACh release upon nerve impulses (Goodyear et al. 1999; Jacobs et al. 2002; Taguchi et al. 2004b). The binding of anti-GSL antibodies to nerve terminals also may result in concomitant immunohistological and ultrastructural damage of the terminals (O'Hanlon et al. 2001; Willison and Yuki 2002; Taguchi et al. 2004a; Usuki et al. 2010b). Taguchi et al. (2004a) also reported that anti-GalNAc-GD1a antibodies blocked neuromuscular transmission in muscle-spinal cord co-cultured cells. The ACh-induced potential was not reduced by the addition of antibodies, suggesting that the blockade is presynaptic, probably affecting the ion channels in presynaptic motor axons. As the anti-GA1 antibodies inhibited the voltage-gated Ca^{2+} channel (VGCC) (Taguchi et al. 2004b), anti-GalNAc-GD1a antibodies may block neurotransmission by suppressing VGCC on the axonal terminals of motor nerves.

Although it is not clearly understood how anti-GM1 antibodies cause nerve dysfunction and injury, impairment of sodium and/or potassium ion channels at the nodes of Ranvier has been implicated (Sheikh et al. 1999). Voltage-gated sodium channels (VGSCs) exist at the nodes of Ranvier (Hartung et al. 1995), in which GM1 is colocalized (Apostolski et al. 1994). Several studies have described the relationship between sodium channel block and the development of GBS. Anti-GM1 antibodies induced reduction of the nerve impulse amplitude at common entrapment sites, resulting in frequent Wallerian degeneration or physiological conduction block at the nodes of Ranvier (Kuwabara et al. 1998). Autopsy studies of AMAN patients have indicated that immunoglobulins and complement deposits are frequently located at the nodes of Ranvier, where sodium channels are clustered (Hafer-Macko et al. 1996). In GBS, blocking factors of sodium channels are present in the cerebrospinal fluid, impairing neuron impulse conduction, thereby causing muscle weakness and sensory disturbances in affected patients (Brinkmeier et al. 1992; Wurz et al. 1995). Patch-clamp studies revealed direct inhibition of the ion-conducting pores of VGSCs by exposure to serum from patients with GBS (Weber et al. 2000), resulting in muscle weakness and sensory disturbances in such patients. These studies suggest that inhibition of voltage-gated ion channels should be one of the contributing factors by which nerve conduction is impaired in these patients (Nakatani et al. 2007). Illa et al. (1995) reported that purified anti-GM1 antibodies from patients who exhibited AMAN after immunization with a ganglioside preparation recognized epitopes at the nodes of Ranvier and at the presynaptic nerve terminals of motor end plates from human nerve biopsies. Accumulation of these antibodies at the nodes of Ranvier can cause disruption of Na^+ and K^+ channels and, thus, interference of nerve conduction. Therefore, a causal link between *C. jejuni* infection, the presence of anti-ganglioside antibodies, and development of GBS is considered likely (Willison 2005a). Buchwald et al. (2007) investigated the effects of IgG anti-GM1 and -GD1a monoclonal antibodies on neuromuscular transmission and calcium influx in hemidiaphragm preparations and in cultured neurons, respectively, to elucidate mechanisms of antibody-mediated muscle weakness. As a result, different anti-ganglioside monoclonal antibodies induce distinct effects on presynaptic transmitter release by reducing calcium influx, suggesting that this is one mechanism of antibody-mediated muscle weakness in AMAN. Anti-GM1 antibodies have been shown to mediate complement-dependent disruption of sodium channel clusters in peripheral motor nerves (Takigawa et al. 1995). Thus, anti-ganglioside antibodies, such as anti-GM1, may cause nerve dysfunction and injury by interfering with ion-channel function at the nodes of Ranvier and may contribute to the pathogenic mechanisms of certain neuropathies (Arasaki et al. 1993; Takigawa et al. 1995). Interestingly, Zitman et al. (2008) reported the effects of altered ganglioside profiles in neuronal membranes on synaptic transmission by correlating NMJ functions in GD3 synthase (GD3S)-knockout (KO) mice (lacking b- and c-series gangliosides), and in *N*-acetylgalactosaminyltransferase (GalNAcT) and GD3S double KO (dKO) mice, (lacking all ganglio-series gangliosides other than GM3). Surprisingly, they found no major synaptic deficits in both null mutants; the only changes were some extra degree of rundown of transmitter release at high intensity use at the NMJ in the dKO mice and a temperature-specific increase in quantal content at 35°C in NMJs of GD3S-KO mice, compared with wild type mice. These results indicate that synaptic transmission at the NMJ is not crucially dependent on any particular ganglioside and remains largely intact in the presence of only GM3. Consequently, gangliosides are probably dispensable players in transmitter release, but may modulate the temperature- and use-dependent fine-tuning. Anti-ganglioside antibodies may also target the distal portions of motor axons, including the terminal at the NMJ, causing a synaptopathy that contributes to muscle weakness in GBS/MFS (Plomp and Willison 2009).

Usuki et al. (2005) reported two cases of AIDP or CIDP showing elevated titers of anti-GD3 antibodies, which occur less frequently in GBS. The antibodies showed an inhibitory effect on the spontaneous muscle action potential of the NMJ. To examine the correlation between the anti-GD3 antibody titers and *C. jejuni* infection, Usuki et al. (2006) sensitized female Lewis rats with the LOS fraction from *C. jejuni* HS:19. After 16 weeks of sensitization, animals revealed transient decreases in nerve conduction velocity and conduction blocks and high titers of anti-GM1-like and anti-GD3-like antibodies. As in anti-GD3 antibodies in AIDP and CIDP, this anti-GD3-like antibody also blocked the spontaneous muscle action potential of NMJs in spinal cord-muscle cell co-cultures. To determine the target epitope for GD3-like antibody in the LOS antigen, the LOS fraction containing the GD3 epitope was purified from the total LOSs using an anti-GD3 affinity column. Chemical analysis of the oligosaccharide portion confirmed the presence of a GD3-like epitope with the tetrasaccharide NeuAc-NeuAc-Gal-Hep. The data thus reinforce the concept of carbohydrate mimicry as a potential pathogenic mechanism in peripheral nerve dysfunction (Fig. 14.2).

GBS can be transmitted from animals to humans. For example, campylobacteriosis in chickens can be a preceding event for GBS. Poultry are frequently highly colonized with *C. jejuni* as a major foodborne vehicle for campylobacteriosis. We recently demonstrated the presence of high-titer anti-GM1 antibodies in the serum of a laboratory worker who developed GBS following contact with chickens with campylobacteriosis (Usuki et al. 2008). The microbiologically confirmed strain VLA2/18 (non-serotyped) was isolated from the worker and subsequently inoculated into chickens, resulting in the development of high-titer anti-ganglioside antibodies. Surprisingly, high titers of anti-lipid A-like antibody were also found to be present in the chicken sera together with anti-GM1 and -GM3. Production of anti-ganglioside antibodies is considered to be due to ganglioside-like LOS

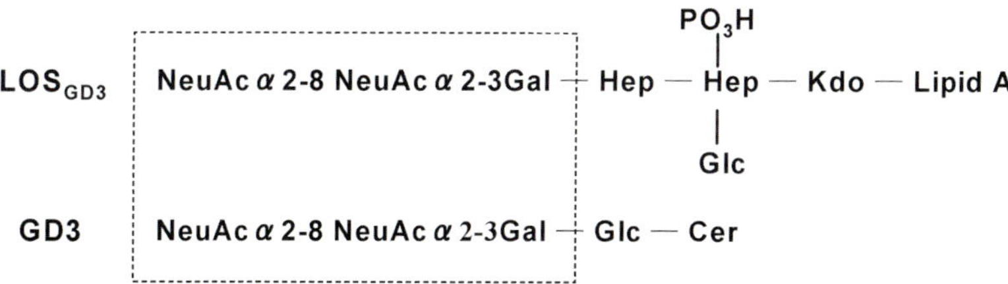

Fig. 14.2 Molecular mimicry of *C. jejuni* LOS (LOS$_{GD3}$) and GD3

antigens. On the other hand, development of anti-lipid A antibody is likely the result of an immune response to the hydrophobic part of LOS antigens. Most interestingly, the anti-lipid A-like antibody revealed an inhibitory effect on VGSCs in whole-cell patch-clamped NSC-34 cells, a motor neuron-like cell line, in culture. Inhibition of *N*-glycan synthesis on the sodium channel protein revealed that the binding site of anti-lipid A antibody is likely located on the protein portion of the sodium channel and, in particular, to Nav1.4 in NSC-34 cells. Thus, the lipid A part of LOSs may also contribute to the immune responses in campylobacteriosis. It would be of considerable interest to survey GBS patients for elevated titers of anti-lipid A antibodies.

14.9 Current Therapeutic Strategies of Anti-glycolipid-mediated GBS and Related Diseases

Currently, plasma exchange, intravenous injection of immunoglobulins (IVIGs), and double-filtration plasmapheresis are the most common treatment paradigms for GBS and its variants (Takigawa et al. 1995; van Doorn et al. 2008; Unal-Cevik et al. 2009). These approaches can bring about a temporary improvement of the clinical symptoms of GBS (Yuki 1998). In clinical trials for reducing anti-ganglioside antibody titers, the mechanism of plasmapheresis is easy to understand, but that of IVIG is unclear, probably involving actions on a number of targets, such as T and B cells, immune cell trafficking, complement factors, and Fc-receptors (Hartung 2008). In addition, IVIG is thought to interfere with and prevent the passage of autoimmune T cells into the blood-nerve barrier (Hartung 2008). Lopez et al. (2000) reported that normal human plasma contains antibodies that specifically block neuropathy-related anti-GM1 IgG antibodies, suggesting that IVIG may be useful in the treatment of a variety of autoimmune diseases. IVIG is slightly safer and much easier to administer than plasma exchange (Hughes et al. 2010). NMJ studies in experimental mouse models showed that IVIG protects the animal from complement-independent inhibition of ACh release by GBS patients' IgG, presumably through neutralization of the antibodies (Buchwald et al. 2002). Plasma exchange after IVIG treatment is sometimes beneficial to patients with severe GBS (Buzzigoli et al. 2010). However, injection of a standard dose of IVIG is not always effective enough to alleviate the symptoms in many GBS patients and sometimes a second IVIG dose is necessary (van Doorn et al. 2010). Recent advances suggest that the use of a combination of agents, such as interferon-β1a (Pritchard et al. 2003) and cyclosporine (Odaka et al. 2005), may be beneficial. Complement-mediated disruption of VGSC clusters has been reported in GBS; therefore, complement-inhibitory agents may have therapeutic potentials for MFS/GBS (van Doorn et al. 2010). Beneficial effects have also been observed with new complement inhibitors in GBS/MFS (Hillmen et al. 2006); it has been shown that these inhibitors can effectively prevent damage caused by anti-GQ1b antibodies at the NMJs (Halstead et al. 2005, 2008a, b). Calpain inhibitors are another class of agents that could play a role in the treatment of anti-GQ1b antibody-dependent complement-mediated peripheral axonal injury, in either proximal or distal sites (O'Hanlon et al. 2003). The complement C5-inhibiting recombinant proteins rRV576 and eculizumab were able to prevent neural injury in a mouse model of MFS and GBS (Halstead et al. 2008a, b; Turatti et al. 2010). Halstead et al. (2008a) assessed the efficacy of the humanized monoclonal antibody eculizumab, which blocks the formation of human C5a and C5b-9, in preventing the immune-mediated motor neuropathy exemplified in an MFS model. Eculizumab completely prevented electrophysiological and structural lesions in anti-GQ1b antibody-pre-incubated NMJs in vitro when normal human serum was used as a source of the complement. Filtration of cerebrospinal fluid may be effective in removing from the fluid inflammatory mediators, autoantibodies, or other factors in GBS (Wollinsky et al. 2001; Manfredi 2002). Circulation immune effectors such as human autoantibodies (anti-GM1 antibodies), which are exogenous to the nervous system, can modulate axon regeneration/nerve repair in GBS. Lopez et al. (2010) reported that passive transfer using cholera toxin B-subunit, which binds to GM1, can effect axonal regeneration/repair after PNS injury in mice. The mechanisms of the beneficial effects of these ligands are not understood, but may be related to blockage of the antibody binding site on the nerve, thus preventing the attachment of antibody-complement attacking complexes. Regardless of the mechanisms, anti-GSL antibodies should be considered as an alternative avenue of treatment for immunosuppressive disorders.

14.10 New Therapeutic Strategies of Anti-ganglioside-mediated GBS Based on Molecular Mimicry Mechanism

With a better understanding of the pathogenic mechanisms of GBS, it is possible to develop more effective therapeutic strategies for this disorder. Willison et al. (2004) synthesized bovine serum albumin (BSA) conjugated with the trisaccharide, αNeuAc(2$\rightarrow$8)αNeuAc(2$\rightarrow$3)Gal common to GQ1b and GD3, named disialylgalactose glycoconjugate (DSG-BSA). It binds anti-GQ1b antibodies in 32/58 (55%) human sera containing IgG or IgM anti-GQ1b antibodies as well as a wide range of mouse monoclonal anti-GQ1b and -GD3 antibodies. When conjugated to Sepharose in mock therapeutic immmunoaffinity columns, the immobilized trisaccharide (DSG-Sepharose) can eliminate anti-GQ1b antibodies from sera immunoreactive to GQ1b. Oligosaccharide-specific immunoadsorption therapy thus provides a new therapeutic approach to anti-GQ1b antibody-associated syndromes that could be applied to clinical practice. Andersen et al. (2004) synthesized truncated ganglioside analogues with GD3, GQ1b and GM2 epitopes that are structural mimics of these gangliosides. Those truncated gangliosides have the ability to neutralize or remove auto-antibodies. Both approaches should be applicable for the therapy in GBS although the synthesis of a large amount of those agents for clinical use is likely to be technically difficult.

In addition to the above, we have demonstrated GD3 ganglioside molecular mimicry in a model of GBS in Lewis rats by sensitization with LOS_{GD3} from

C. jejuni ((Usuki et al. 2006); see Fig. 14.2) and hypothesized that molecular mimicry between the LOS component of *C. jejuni* and gangliosides of PNS may play an important role in the pathogenesis of GBS. Since the neuropathophysiological consequences were largely due to the anti-GD3-like antibodies, we subsequently focused our effort on eliminating the pathogenic antibodies using several novel reagents to mimic GD3 in this model. Two such reagents have been tested in the rat model: the use of anti-idiotypic antibodies against pathogenic antibodies (Usuki et al. 2010b) and peptide glycomimics (Usuki et al. 2010a). Both agents represent excellent "mimics" for GD3 and are expected to provide a means to selectively remove circulating antibodies in animal models of neuropathies.

In general, the first strategy utilizes an anti-idiotypic antibody that mimics a specific GSL. Jerne (1974) proposed that the immune system can be regulated through a network of antibody/anti-idiotype interactions (Fig. 14.3).

One of the implications of the antibody/anti-idiotype model is the existence of anti-idiotype antibodies that carry internal images of every recognizable determinant. Viale et al. (1989) have reported that an anti-idiotype mAb (BEC2) carries the internal image of a carbohydrate-antigenic determinant for GD3 expressed on melanoma-associated GSLs. Recently, Chapman et al. (Chapman and Houghton 1991; Chapman et al. 2004) carried out a phase II clinical trial of BEC2 for patients with melanoma and confirmed the development of anti-GD3 antibodies and an improved survival rate. Similarly, phase III clinical trials are being conducted using BEC2 with adjuvant for the treatment of small cell lung cancer (Giaccone et al. 2005). In our initial proof-of-principle study, we first sensitized Lewis rats with LOS_{GD3} from *C. jejuni* that possesses the same epitope as the trisaccharide NeuAc-NeuAc-Gal of GD3, and injected BEC2 without adjuvant into the sensitized rats that have been induced to produce high titers of anti-GD3 antibodies. In contrast to the clinical trials cited above, our goal was to use BEC2 as a "GD3-mimic." We

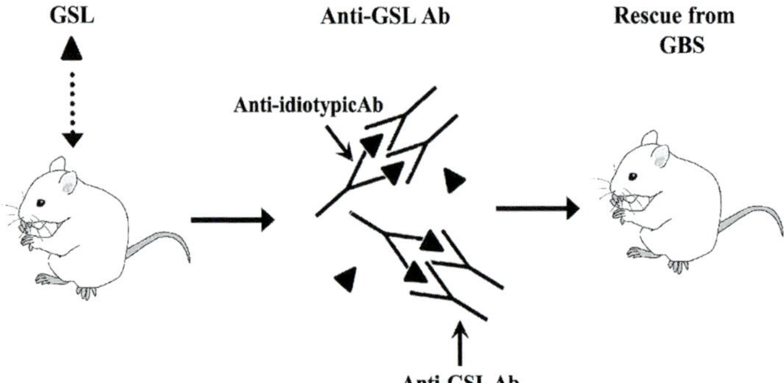

Fig. 14.3 Strategy using anti-idiotypic GD3 antibody (BEC2): The antibody/anti-idiotypic antibody model is based on the existence of an anti-idiotypic GD3 antibody (or other anti-idiotypic antibodies) that carry an internal image of a recognizable determinant, in this case GD3, that specifically "neutralizes" the pathogenic anti-GD3 antibody by competitive inhibition

have previously reported that anti-GD3 antibody elevation is consistent with the clinical severity of the peripheral nerve dysfunction occurring in LOS-sensitized rats (Usuki et al. 2006). Contrary to the cases of patients with melanoma, which showed that BEC2 induces anti-GD3 antibody production, it is expected that BEC2 in the absence of adjuvant will interfere with the binding of anti-GD3 antibodies to endogenous GD3 epitopes in the peripheral nerve. Our study indicated that intraperitoneally injected BEC2 in experimental rats effectively reduced anti-GD3 antibody titers (Fig. 14.4).

Moreover, the injected BEC2 was well tolerated and without adverse effects, consistent with the observation in patients receiving IVIG treatment. Moreover, the effectiveness of BEC2 treatment in the rat has been confirmed by electromyography (Fig. 14.5) and rotarod performance (Fig. 14.6) (Usuki et al. 2010b). Consistent with this model, anti-idiotype mAbs can be identified that carry the internal image of non-protein determinants (Rubinstein et al. 1983; McNamara et al. 1984; Stein and Soderstrom 1984; Viale et al. 1989; Kato et al. 1990; Schreiber et al. 1990).

We propose that in hyper-immune diseases such as GBS or MFS that are accompanied by high titers of anti-ganglioside antibodies, anti-idiotypic mAbs should represent a useful reagent to neutralize anti-ganglioside antibodies by competitive inhibition. The potential mechanisms include a direct binding and inactivation of pathogenic antibodies, induction of anti-idiotypic antibodies, and inhibition of antibody production by inactivating specific B cells primed by GSLs.

The second strategy exploits "mimics" for GSL antigens to selectively remove antibodies. This strategy involves the use of a phage peptide library (Qiu et al. 1999) and requires polypeptides with structures that mimic carbohydrate determinants to provide a surrogate immunogenic. It takes advantage of the method of Scott et al. (Scott and Smith 1990) for efficiently selecting from the peptide library peptide sequences that can bind to target molecules (Fig. 14.7).

This library was first developed for selecting peptides recognized by a mAb or receptor, and was applied by Takigawa and co-workers (2000) to the preparation of peptides that mimic gangliosides. Presumably the peptides may mimic conformations which are adopted by carbohydrate epitopes in the recognition by ganglioside specific antibodies or toxins. Current technology is available to produce peptides mimicking the carbohydrate moiety that are useful to serve as competitive inhibitors for a specific carbohydrate antibody. Mimetic peptides of the L2/HNK-1 carbohydrate epitope (sulfated glucuronosyl paragloboside) have already been identified by phage-display and sequenced by Simon-Haldi et al. (2002). More recently, glycomimetic peptides of GD3 have also been reported (Popa et al. 2006). We treated rats with LOS_{GD3}-induced experimental neuritis by intraperitoneal administration of phage-displayed GD3-like peptides. One of the GD3-like peptides called P_{GD3}-4 of the amino acid sequence RHAYRSMAEWGFLYS was particularly effective in lowering the titer of anti-GD3/anti-LOS_{GD3} antibodies (Fig. 14.4) and ameliorated peripheral nerve dysfunction in the sera of LOS_{GD3}-sensitized rats, as evidenced by improved rotarod performance (Fig. 14.6) and a restoration of motor nerve functions, including an improved histopathology and

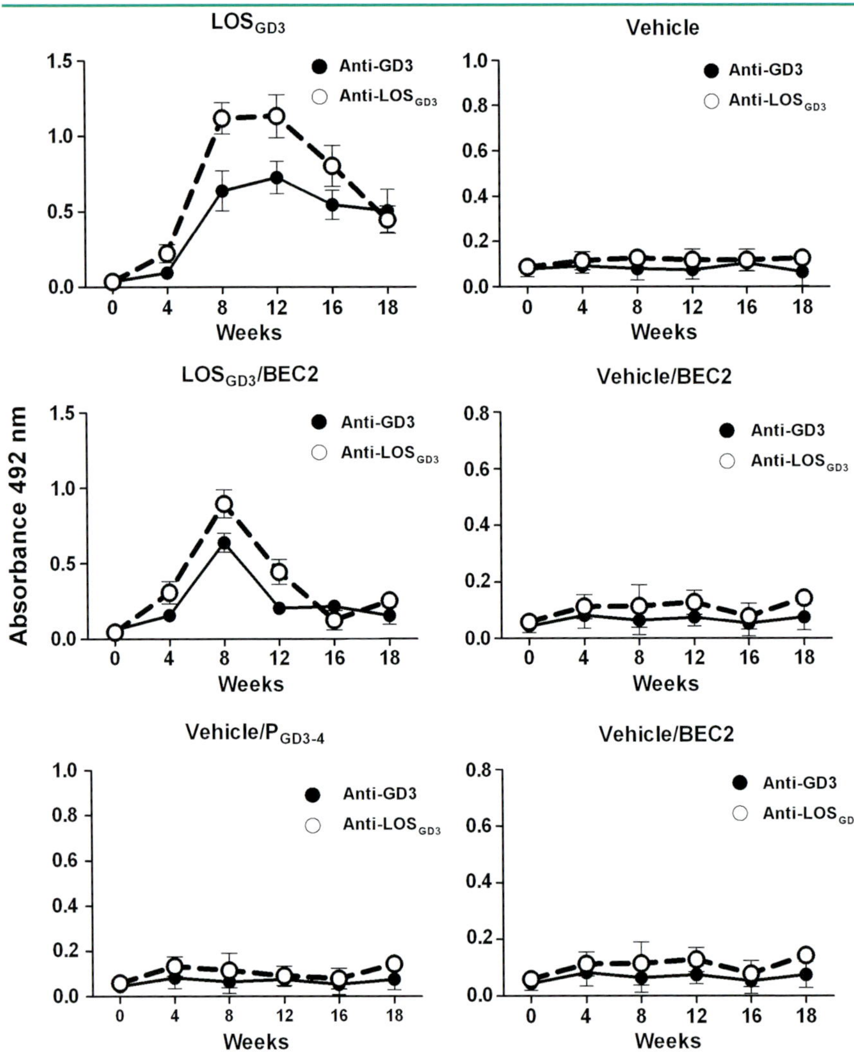

Fig. 14.4 Time course of anti-GD3 and anti-LOS_{GD3} antibody production: Sensitization of Lewis rats was performed according to our established procedure (Usuki et al. 2006) using an emulsion of complete Freund's adjuvant mixed with an immunogen (LOS_{GD3} and keyhole limpet hemocyanin). Subsequently, animals were treated by booster injection at 2-week intervals with incomplete Freund's adjuvant and the immunogen. Anti-GD3 and anti-LOS_{GD3} antibody responses following induction of experimental neuritis using LOS_{GD3} were examined periodically during 18 weeks of experimentation by serum ELISA (sample diluted 1:200). Both antibody titers were elevated after 8 weeks of the primary sensitization. BEC2 and P_{GD3}-4 treatments suppressed the antibody titers. Animal serum samples were obtained at the specified times to test activities of anti-GD3 antibody (*solid circles*) and anti-LOS_{GD3} antibody (*open circles*). Values are means ± SD for four animals (Modified with permission from Usuki et al. 2010a, b)

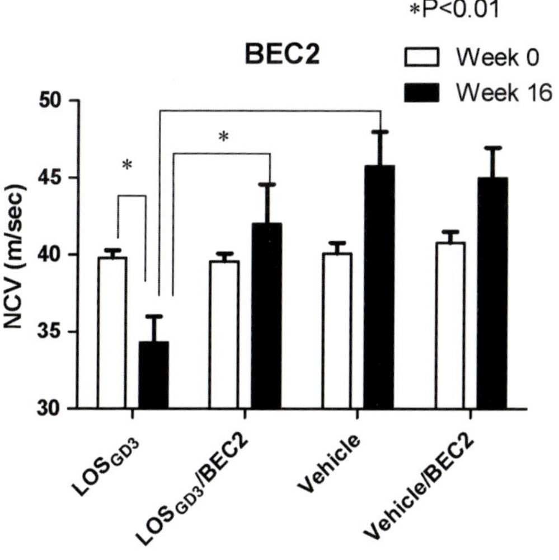

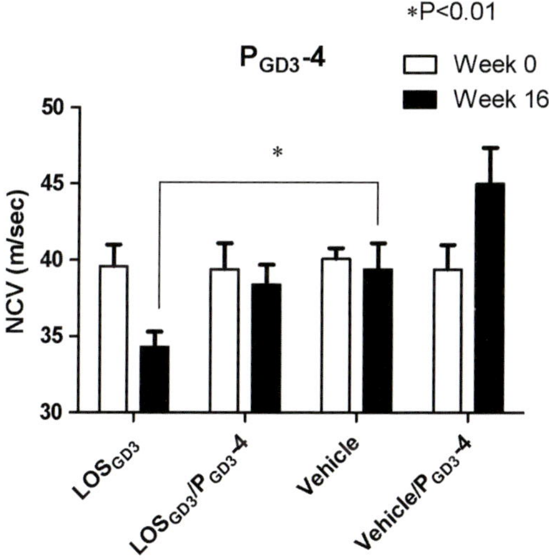

Fig. 14.5 Effect of BEC2 and P_{GD3}-4 on nerve conduction velocity (NCV): Animals underwent electrophysiological measurement by recording NCV (m/sec) in the tail nerve at the beginning and the endpoint according to the experimental schedule. At 16 weeks, the NCV of the LOS_{GD3} group decreased, while BEC2 and LOS_{GD3}/P_{GD3}-4 group improved the NCV (Modified with permission from Usuki et al. 2010a, b)

motor nerve conduction velocity (Fig. 14.5). The data suggest that glycomimetic peptides of GSLs should be potential powerful reagents for therapeutic intervention in GBS. Furthermore, the small peptides have flexible structures and therefore

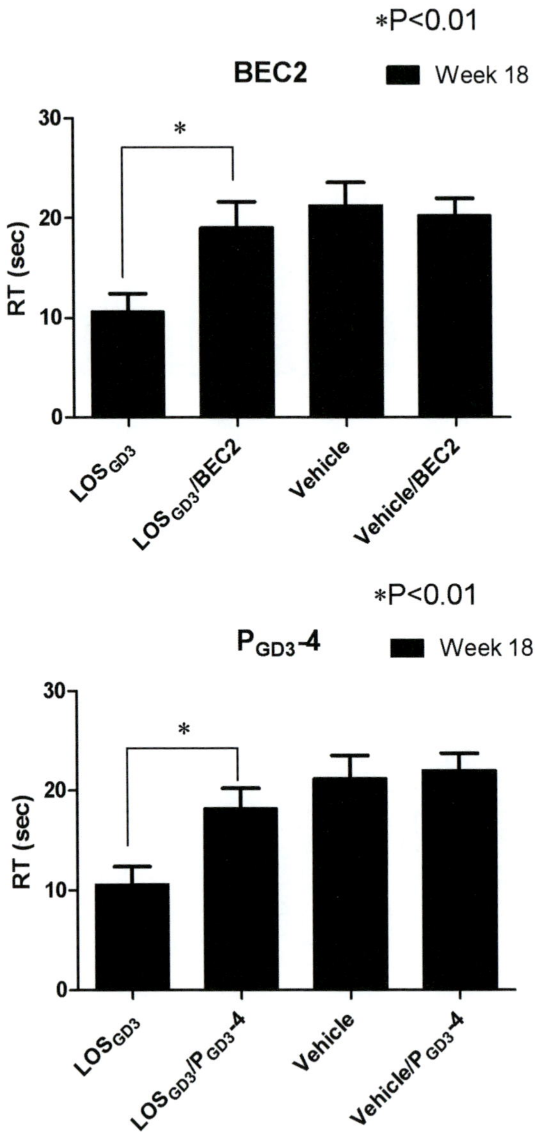

Fig. 14.6 Performance of the rotarod retention time: The rotarod motor test was performed at the endpoint of experiment according to the conventional procedure. A rat was placed on a rotating roller, and the time during which the rat remained on the roller was measured. There is a statistical difference by one-way ANOVA in improved rotarod performance of BEC2 and P_{GD3}-4, respectively, as compared with LOS_{GD3} treatment. Values are means ± SD for four animals (Modified with permission from Usuki et al. 2010a, b)

Fig. 14.7 Strategy using peptide glycomimics of GD3: Peptide mimics for the carbohydrate determinants of GSLs, in this case GD3, provide surrogate antigens to bind specifically the pathogenic anti-GD3 antibody and to neutralize it

no defined conformation and, importantly, are not very immunogenic and elicit minimal known side effects (Usuki et al. 2010a). The small peptides can also be produced cheaply using existing peptide synthesis techniques.

Conclusion

Plasmapheresis and IVIG have been the widely accepted strategies for the treatment of GBS because of their ability to dilute immune effectors such as anti-GSL antibodies in the patient's serum. Those approaches can give rise to a temporary improvement of the clinical symptoms of GBS. The increased antibody titers in GBS are thought to be caused by production of antibodies to bacterial LOSs, particularly that from *C. jejuni*, that exhibit cross-reactivity with gangliosides of the PNS. The epitopes recognized by anti-ganglioside antibodies have been shown to be localized in the nodes of Ranvier of myelinated fibers and in NMJs. Based on the ganglioside mimicry hypothesis, a number of newer therapeutic strategies for treating GBS have been attempted, including immmunoaffinity columns using DSG-BSA-conjugated Sepharose and synthesized truncated gangliosides representative of GD3, GQ1b and GM2 epitopes as methyl glycosides. All those agents have the ability to neutralize or remove auto-antibodies, suggesting that those synthetic compounds can be used for treatment. More recently, we have established, based on a rational design, the use of glycomimetics that have been shown in proof-of-principle studies in a LOS_{GD3}-induced rat model of experimental neuritis that resembles GBS. Those mimics include anti-idiotype antibodies against pathogenic antibodies and glycomimetic peptides (replica peptides). Both reagents "mimic" the carbohydrate epitopes of the respective glycolipid antigens and are expected to provide a means to selectively remove circulating antibodies in animal models of GBS. Rats receiving BEC2 tolerated it well without adverse effects that are consistently observed in patients receiving IVIG treatment. Similarly, animals receiving glycomimetic peptides of GD3 ganglioside showed remarkable recovery from the disease symptoms, indicating their potential efficacy for therapeutic intervention for GBS. Both approaches represent the next generation of strategies for the treatment of GBS and related immune-mediated disorders.

Acknowledgment This study was supported by NIH grants (NS26994, NS11853) to RKY. We thank many former colleagues who contributed to the experimental work that has been carried out in the laboratory of RKY. The editorial assistance of Dr. Rhea Markowitz is also gratefully acknowledged.

Abbreviation

Ach	Acetylcholine
AIDP or CIDP	Acute or chronic inflammatory demyelinating polyneuropathy
ALS	Amyotrophic lateral sclerosis
AMAN	Acute motor axonal neuropathy
AMSAN	Acute motor and sensory axonal neuropathy
BEC2	Anti-idiotype monoclonal antibody against GD3
BSA	Bovine serum albumin
mAb	Monoclonal antibody
MFS	Miller Fisher syndrome
MMN	Multifocal motor neuropathy
PNS	Peripheral nerve system
C. jejuni	*Campylobacter jejuni*
C. coli	*Campylobacter coli*
DSG	Disialylgalactose glycoconjugate
GBS	Guillain-Barré syndrome
GSC	Ganglioside-complex
GSL	Glycosphingolipids
IM	Intramuscular nerve
IVIG	Intravenous immunoglobulin
LPS	Lipopolysaccharide
LOS	Lipo-oligosaccharide
NMJ	Neuromuscular junction
SGGL	Sulfated glucuronosyl glycolipid
SGPG	Sulfated glucuronosyl paragloboside
SGLPG	Sulfated glucuronosyl lactosaminyl paragloboside
VGSC	Voltage-gated sodium channel
VGCC	Voltage-gated Ca^{2+} channel
VR	Ventral root axon

References

Andersen SM, Ling CC, Zhang P, Townson K, Willison HJ, Bundle DR (2004) Synthesis of ganglioside epitopes for oligosaccharide specific immunoadsorption therapy of Guillian-Barre syndrome. Org Biomol Chem 2:1199–1212

Ang CW, Jacobs BC, Laman JD (2004) The Guillain-Barre syndrome: a true case of molecular mimicry. Trends Immunol 25:61–66

Apostolski S, Sadiq SA, Hays A, Corbo M, Suturkova-Milosevic L, Chaliff P, Stefansson K, LeBaron RG, Ruoslahti E, Hays AP et al (1994) Identification of Gal(β 1-3)GalNAc bearing glycoproteins at the nodes of Ranvier in peripheral nerve. J Neurosci Res 38:134–141

Arasaki K, Kusunoki S, Kudo N, Kanazawa I (1993) Acute conduction block in vitro following exposure to antiganglioside sera. Muscle Nerve 16:587–593

Ariga T, Yu RK (2005) Antiglycolipid antibodies in Guillain-Barre syndrome and related diseases: review of clinical features and antibody specificities. J Neurosci Res 80:1–17

Ariga T, Kohriyama T, Freddo L, Latov N, Saito M, Kon K, Ando S, Suzuki M, Hemling ME, Rinehart KL Jr et al (1987) Characterization of sulfated glucuronic acid containing glycolipids reacting with IgM M-proteins in patients with neuropathy. J Biol Chem 262:848–853

Ariga T, Miyatake T, Yu RK (2001) Recent studies on the roles of antiglycosphingolipids in the pathogenesis of neurological disorders. J Neurosci Res 65:363–370

Ariga T, McDonald MP, Yu RK (2008) Role of ganglioside metabolism in the pathogenesis of Alzheimer's disease – a review. J Lipid Res 49:1157–1175

Brinkmeier H, Wollinsky KH, Hulser PJ, Seewald MJ, Mehrkens HH, Kornhuber HH, Rudel R (1992) The acute paralysis in Guillain-Barre syndrome is related to a Na + channel blocking factor in the cerebrospinal fluid. Pflugers Arch 421:552–557

Buchwald B, Ahangari R, Weishaupt A, Toyka KV (2002) Intravenous immunoglobulins neutralize blocking antibodies in Guillain-Barre syndrome. Ann Neurol 51:673–680

Buchwald B, Zhang G, Vogt-Eisele AK, Zhang W, Ahangari R, Griffin JW, Hatt H, Toyka KV, Sheikh KA (2007) Anti-ganglioside antibodies alter presynaptic release and calcium influx. Neurobiol Dis 28:113–121

Buzzigoli SB, Genovesi M, Lambelet P, Logi C, Raffaelli S, Cattano D (2010) Plasmapheresis treatment in Guillain-Barre syndrome: potential benefit over intravenous immunoglobulin. Anaesth Intensive Care 38:387–389

Capasso M, Notturno F, Manzoli C, Yuki N, Uncini A (2010) Reversible conduction failure in pharyngeal-cervical-brachial variant of Guillain-Barre syndrome. Muscle Nerve 42:608–612

Chapman PB, Houghton AN (1991) Induction of IgG antibodies against GD3 ganglioside in rabbits by an anti-idiotypic monoclonal antibody. J Clin Invest 88:186–192

Chapman PB, Williams L, Salibi N, Hwu WJ, Krown SE, Livingston PO (2004) A phase II trial comparing five dose levels of BEC2 anti-idiotypic monoclonal antibody vaccine that mimics GD3 ganglioside. Vaccine 22:2904–2909

Chiba A, Kusunoki S, Shimizu T, Kanazawa I (1992) Serum IgG antibody to ganglioside GQ1b is a possible marker of Miller Fisher syndrome. Ann Neurol 31:677–679

Chou DK, Ilyas AA, Evans JE, Costello C, Quarles RH, Jungalwala FB (1986) Structure of sulfated glucuronyl glycolipids in the nervous system reacting with HNK-1 antibody and some IgM paraproteins in neuropathy. J Biol Chem 261:11717–11725

Chou DK, Schwarting GA, Evans JE, Jungalwala FB (1987) Sulfoglucuronyl-neolacto series of glycolipids in peripheral nerves reacting with HNK-1 antibody. J Neurochem 49:865–873

Corbo M, Quattrini A, Lugaresi A, Santoro M, Latov N, Hays AP (1992) Patterns of reactivity of human anti-GM1 antibodies with spinal cord and motor neurons. Ann Neurol 32:487–493

Corbo M, Quattrini A, Latov N, Hays AP (1993) Localization of GM1 and Gal(β 1-3)GalNAc antigenic determinants in peripheral nerve. Neurology 43:809–814

Dabby R, Weimer LH, Hays AP, Olarte M, Latov N (2000) Antisulfatide antibodies in neuropathy: clinical and electrophysiologic correlates. Neurology 54:1448–1452

Dewil M, Robberecht W, Van Damme P (2010) An unusual presentation of Guillain-Barre syndrome associated with monospecific anti-GD1b antibodies. J Neurol Neurosurg Psychiatry 81:587–588

Dupouey P, Zalc B, Lefroit-Joly M, Gomes D (1979) Localization of galactosylceramide and sulfatide at the surface of the myelin sheath: an immunofluorescence study in liquid medium. Cell Mol Biol Incl Cyto Enzymol 25:269–272

Ferrari S, Morbin M, Nobile-Orazio E, Musso A, Tomelleri G, Bertolasi L, Rizzuto N, Monaco S (1998) Antisulfatide polyneuropathy: antibody-mediated complement attack on peripheral myelin. Acta Neuropathol 96:569–574

Freddo L, Ariga T, Saito M, Macala LC, Yu RK, Latov N (1985) The neuropathy of plasma cell dyscrasia: binding of IgM M-proteins to peripheral nerve glycolipids. Neurology 35:1420–1424

Fredman P, Vedeler CA, Nyland H, Aarli JA, Svennerholm L (1991) Antibodies in sera from patients with inflammatory demyelinating polyradiculoneuropathy react with ganglioside LM1 and sulphatide of peripheral nerve myelin. J Neurol 238:75–79

Fredman P, Lycke J, Andersen O, Vrethem M, Ernerudh J, Svennerholm L (1993) Peripheral neuropathy associated with monoclonal IgM antibody to glycolipids with a terminal glucuronyl-3-sulfate epitope. J Neurol 240:381–387

Giaccone G, Debruyne C, Felip E, Chapman PB, Grant SC, Millward M, Thiberville L, D'Addario G, Coens C, Rome LS, Zatloukal P, Masso O, Legrand C (2005) Phase III study of adjuvant vaccination with Bec2/bacille Calmette-Guerin in responding patients with limited-disease small-cell lung cancer (European organisation for research and treatment of cancer 08971-08971B; Silva study). J Clin Oncol 23:6854–6864

Gilbert M, Brisson JR, Karwaski MF, Michniewicz J, Cunningham AM, Wu Y, Young NM, Wakarchuk WW (2000) Biosynthesis of ganglioside mimics in Campylobacter jejuni OH4384. Identification of the glycosyltransferase genes, enzymatic synthesis of model compounds, and characterization of nanomole amounts by 600-MHz ^{1}H and ^{13}C NMR analysis. J Biol Chem 275:3896–3906

Gong Y, Lunn MP, Heffer-Lauc M, Li CY, Griffin JW, Schnaar RL (2001) Localization of major gangliosides in the PNS: implications for immune neuropathies. J Peripher Nerv Syst 6:142

Goodyear CS, O'Hanlon GM, Plomp JJ, Wagner ER, Morrison I, Veitch J, Cochrane L, Bullens RW, Molenaar PC, Conner J, Willison HJ (1999) Monoclonal antibodies raised against Guillain-Barre syndrome-associated *Campylobacter jejuni* lipopolysaccharides react with neuronal gangliosides and paralyze muscle-nerve preparations. J Clin Invest 104:697–708

Hadden RD, Karch H, Hartung HP, Zielasek J, Weissbrich B, Schubert J, Weishaupt A, Cornblath DR, Swan AV, Hughes RA, Toyka KV (2001) Preceding infections, immune factors, and outcome in Guillain-Barre syndrome. Neurology 56:758–765

Hafer-Macko C, Hsieh ST, Li CY, Ho TW, Sheikh K, Cornblath DR, McKhann GM, Asbury AK, Griffin JW (1996) Acute motor axonal neuropathy: an antibody-mediated attack on axolemma. Ann Neurol 40:635–644

Hahn AF (1998) Guillain-Barre syndrome. Lancet 352:635–641

Hakomori S (1990) Bifunctional role of glycosphingolipids. Modulators for transmembrane signaling and mediators for cellular interactions. J Biol Chem 265:18713–18716

Hakomori SI (2000) Cell adhesion/recognition and signal transduction through glycosphingolipid microdomain. Glycoconj J 17:143–151

Hakomori S (2003) Structure, organization, and function of glycosphingolipids in membrane. Curr Opin Hematol 10:16–24

Halstead SK, Morrison I, O'Hanlon GM, Humphreys PD, Goodfellow JA, Plomp JJ, Willison HJ (2005) Anti-disialosyl antibodies mediate selective neuronal or Schwann cell injury at mouse neuromuscular junctions. Glia 52:177–189

Halstead SK, Humphreys PD, Zitman FM, Hamer J, Plomp JJ, Willison HJ (2008a) C5 inhibitor rEV576 protects against neural injury in an in vitro mouse model of Miller Fisher syndrome. J Peripher Nerv Syst 13:228–235

Halstead SK, Zitman FM, Humphreys PD, Greenshields K, Verschuuren JJ, Jacobs BC, Rother RP, Plomp JJ, Willison HJ (2008b) Eculizumab prevents anti-ganglioside antibody-mediated neuropathy in a murine model. Brain 131:1197–1208

Hamaguchi T, Sakajiri K, Sakai K, Okino S, Sada M, Kusunoki S (2007) Guillain-Barre syndrome with antibodies to GD1a/GD1b complex. J Neurol Neurosurg Psychiatry 78:548–549

Hartung HP (2008) Advances in the understanding of the mechanism of action of IVIg. J Neurol 255(Suppl 3):3–6

Hartung HP, Pollard JD, Harvey GK, Toyka KV (1995) Immunopathogenesis and treatment of the Guillain-Barre syndrome–Part II. Muscle Nerve 18:154–164

Hillmen P, Young NS, Schubert J, Brodsky RA, Socié G, Muus P, Röth A, Szer J, Elebute MO, Nakamura R, Browne P, Risitano AM, Hill A, Schrezenmeier H, Fu CL, Maciejewski J, Rollins SA, Mojcik CF, Rother RP, Luzzatto L (2006) The complement inhibitor eculizumab in paroxysmal nocturnal hemoglobinuria. N Engl J Med 355:1233–1243

Ho TW, Willison HJ, Nachamkin I, Li CY, Veitch J, Ung H, Wang GR, Liu RC, Cornblath DR, Asbury AK, Griffin JW, McKhann GM (1999) Anti-GD1a antibody is associated with axonal but not demyelinating forms of Guillain-Barre syndrome. Ann Neurol 45:168–173

Hughes RA, Cornblath DR (2005) Guillain-Barre syndrome. Lancet 366:1653–1666

Hughes RA, Swan AV, van Doorn PA (2010) Intravenous immunoglobulin for Guillain-Barre syndrome. Cochrane Database Syst Rev CD002063: 6

Illa I, Leon-Monzon M, Agboatwalla M, Ilyas A, Latov N, Dalakas MC (1995) Antiganglioside antibodies in patients with acute polio and post-polio syndrome. Ann N Y Acad Sci 753:374–377

Ilyas AA, Quarles RH, MacIntosh TD, Dobersen MJ, Trapp BD, Dalakas MC, Brady RO (1984) IgM in a human neuropathy related to paraproteinemia binds to a carbohydrate determinant in the myelin-associated glycoprotein and to a ganglioside. Proc Natl Acad Sci USA 81:1225–1229

Ilyas AA, Mithen FA, Dalakas MC, Wargo M, Chen ZW, Bielory L, Cook SD (1991) Antibodies to sulfated glycolipids in Guillain-Barre syndrome. J Neurol Sci 105:108–117

Ilyas AA, Cook SD, Dalakas MC, Mithen FA (1992) Anti-MAG IgM paraproteins from some patients with polyneuropathy associated with IgM paraproteinemia also react with sulfatide. J Neuroimmunol 37:85–92

Iwabuchi K, Handa K, Hakomori S (1998) Separation of "glycosphingolipid signaling domain" from caveolin-containing membrane fraction in mouse melanoma B16 cells and its role in cell adhesion coupled with signaling. J Biol Chem 273:33766–33773

Jacobs BC, Bullens RW, O'Hanlon GM, Ang CW, Willison HJ, Plomp JJ (2002) Detection and prevalence of alpha-latrotoxin-like effects of serum from patients with Guillain-Barre syndrome. Muscle Nerve 25:549–558

Jerne NK (1974) Towards a network theory of the immune system. Ann Immunol (Paris) 125C:373–389

Kaida K, Kusunoki S (2010) Antibodies to gangliosides and ganglioside complexes in Guillain-Barre syndrome and Fisher syndrome: mini-review. J Neuroimmunol 223:5–12

Kaida K, Kusunoki S, Kamakura K, Motoyoshi K, Kanazawa I (2003) GalNAc-GD1a in human peripheral nerve: target sites of anti-ganglioside antibody. Neurology 61:465–470

Kaida K, Morita D, Kanzaki M, Kamakura K, Motoyoshi K, Hirakawa M, Kusunoki S (2004) Ganglioside complexes as new target antigens in Guillain-Barre syndrome. Ann Neurol 56:567–571

Kaida K, Kanzaki M, Morita D, Kamakura K, Motoyoshi K, Hirakawa M, Kusunoki S (2006) Anti-ganglioside complex antibodies in Miller Fisher syndrome. J Neurol Neurosurg Psychiatry 77:1043–1046

Kaida K, Morita D, Kanzaki M, Kamakura K, Motoyoshi K, Hirakawa M, Kusunoki S (2007) Anti-ganglioside complex antibodies associated with severe disability in GBS. J Neuroimmunol 182:212–218

Kaida K, Sonoo M, Ogawa G, Kamakura K, Ueda-Sada M, Arita M, Motoyoshi K, Kusunoki S (2008) GM1/GalNAc-GD1a complex: a target for pure motor Guillain-Barre syndrome. Neurology 71:1683–1690

Kaida K, Ariga T, Yu RK (2009) Antiganglioside antibodies and their pathophysiological effects on Guillain-Barre syndrome and related disorders – a review. Glycobiology 19:676–692

Kanzaki M, Kaida K, Ueda M, Morita D, Hirakawa M, Motoyoshi K, Kamakura K, Kusunoki S (2008) Ganglioside complexes containing GQ1b as targets in Miller Fisher and Guillain-Barre syndromes. J Neurol Neurosurg Psychiatry 79:1148–1152

Kato T, Takazoe I, Okuda K (1990) Protection of mice against the lethal toxicity of a lipopolysaccharide (LPS) by immunization with anti-idiotype antibody to a monoclonal antibody to lipid A from *Eikenella corrodens* LPS. Infect Immun 58:416–420

Koga M, Yuki N, Ariga T, Morimatsu M, Hirata K (1998) Is IgG anti-GT1a antibody associated with pharyngeal-cervical-brachial weakness or oropharyngeal palsy in Guillain-Barre syndrome? J Neuroimmunol 86:74–79

Koga M, Yuki N, Ariga T, Hirata K (1999) Antibodies to GD3, GT3, and O-acetylated species in Guillain-Barre and Fisher's syndromes: their association with cranial nerve dysfunction. J Neurol Sci 164:50–55

Kohriyama T, Kusunoki S, Ariga T, Yoshino JE, DeVries GH, Latov N, Yu RK (1987) Subcellular localization of sulfated glucuronic acid-containing glycolipids reacting with anti-myelin-associated glycoprotein antibody. J Neurochem 48:1516–1522

Komagamine T, Yuki N (2006) Ganglioside mimicry as a cause of Guillain-Barre syndrome. CNS Neurol Disord Drug Targets 5:391–400

Kuijf ML, Godschalk PC, Gilbert M, Endtz HP, Tio-Gillen AP, Ang CW, van Doorn PA, Jacobs BC (2007) Origin of ganglioside complex antibodies in Guillain-Barre syndrome. J Neuroimmunol 188:69–73

Kusunoki S, Kohriyama T, Pachner AR, Latov N, Yu RK (1987) Neuropathy and IgM paraproteinemia: differential binding of IgM M-proteins to peripheral nerve glycolipids. Neurology 37:1795–1797

Kusunoki S, Kaida K, Ueda M (2008) Antibodies against gangliosides and ganglioside complexes in Guillain-Barre syndrome: new aspects of research. Biochim Biophys Acta 1780:441–444

Kuwabara S, Yuki N, Koga M, Hattori T, Matsuura D, Miyake M, Noda M (1998) IgG anti-GM1 antibody is associated with reversible conduction failure and axonal degeneration in Guillain-Barre syndrome. Ann Neurol 44:202–208

Lardone RD, Yuki N, Odaka M, Daniotti JL, Irazoqui FJ, Nores GA (2010) Anti-GM1 IgG antibodies in Guillain-Barre syndrome: fine specificity is associated with disease severity. J Neurol Neurosurg Psychiatry 81:629–633

Lopez PH, Irazoqui FJ, Nores GA (2000) Normal human plasma contains antibodies that specifically block neuropathy-associated human anti-GM1 IgG-antibodies. J Neuroimmunol 105:179–183

Lopez PH, Zhang G, Zhang J, Lehmann HC, Griffin JW, Schnaar RL, Sheikh KA (2010) Passive transfer of IgG anti-GM1 antibodies impairs peripheral nerve repair. J Neurosci 30:9533–9541

Maeda Y, Bigbee JW, Maeda R, Miyatani N, Kalb RG, Yu RK (1991a) Induction of demyelination by intraneural injection of antibodies against sulfoglucuronyl paragloboside. Exp Neurol 113:221–225

Maeda Y, Brosnan CF, Miyatani N, Yu RK (1991b) Preliminary studies on sensitization of Lewis rats with sulfated glucuronyl paragloboside. Brain Res 541:257–264

Manfredi PL (2002) CSF filtration is an effective treatment of Guillain-Barre syndrome: a randomized clinical trial. Neurology 58:988; author reply 988–989

McGonigal R, Rowan EG, Greenshields KN, Halstead SK, Humphreys PD, Rother RP, Furukawa K, Willison HJ (2010) Anti-GD1a antibodies activate complement and calpain to injure distal motor nodes of Ranvier in mice. Brain 133:1944–1960

McNamara MK, Ward RE, Kohler H (1984) Monoclonal idiotope vaccine against *Streptococcus pneumoniae* infection. Science 226:1325–1326

Melendez-Vasquez C, Redford J, Choudhary PP, Gray IA, Maitland P, Gregson NA, Smith KJ, Hughes RA (1997) Immunological investigation of chronic inflammatory demyelinating polyradiculoneuropathy. J Neuroimmunol 73:124–134

Moran AP, Prendergast MM (2001) Molecular mimicry in *Campylobacter jejuni* and *Helicobacter pylori* lipopolysaccharides: contribution of gastrointestinal infections to autoimmunity. J Autoimmun 16:241–256

Moran AP, Annuk H, Prendergast MM (2005) Antibodies induced by ganglioside-mimicking *Campylobacter jejuni* lipooligosaccharides recognise epitopes at the nodes of Ranvier. J Neuroimmunol 165:179–185

Nakatani Y, Kawakami K, Nagaoka T, Utsunomiya I, Tanaka K, Yoshino H, Miyatake T, Hoshi K, Taguchi K (2007) Ca channel currents inhibited by serum from select patients with Guillain-Barre syndrome. Eur Neurol 57:11–18

Nakatani Y, Murata M, Shibata K, Nagaoka T, Utsunomiya I, Usuki S, Miyatake T, Hoshi K, Taguchi K (2009) IgM anti-GQ1b monoclonal antibody inhibits voltage-dependent calcium current in cerebellar granule cells. Exp Neurol 219:74–80

Nemni R, Fazio R, Quattrini A, Lorenzetti I, Mamoli D, Canal N (1993) Antibodies to sulfatide and to chondroitin sulfate C in patients with chronic sensory neuropathy. J Neuroimmunol 43:79–85

Neuwirth C, Mojon D, Weber M (2010) GD1a-associated pure motor Guillain-Barre syndrome with hyperreflexia and bilateral papillitis. J Clin Neuromuscul Dis 11:114–119

Nobile-Orazio E, Hays AP, Latov N, Perman G, Golier J, Shy ME, Freddo L (1984) Specificity of mouse and human monoclonal antibodies to myelin-associated glycoprotein. Neurology 34:1336–1342

Nobile-Orazio E, Manfredini E, Carpo M, Meucci N, Monaco S, Ferrari S, Bonetti B, Cavaletti G, Gemignani F, Durelli L et al (1994) Frequency and clinical correlates of anti-neural IgM antibodies in neuropathy associated with IgM monoclonal gammopathy. Ann Neurol 36:416–424

Nobile-Orazio E, Giannotta C, Briani C (2010) Anti-ganglioside complex IgM antibodies in multifocal motor neuropathy and chronic immune-mediated neuropathies. J Neuroimmunol 219:119–122

O'Hanlon GM, Plomp JJ, Chakrabarti M, Morrison I, Wagner ER, Goodyear CS, Yin X, Trapp BD, Conner J, Molenaar PC, Stewart S, Rowan EG, Willison HJ (2001) Anti-GQ1b ganglioside antibodies mediate complement-dependent destruction of the motor nerve terminal. Brain 124:893–906

O'Hanlon GM, Humphreys PD, Goldman RS, Halstead SK, Bullens RW, Plomp JJ, Ushkaryov Y, Willison HJ (2003) Calpain inhibitors protect against axonal degeneration in a model of anti-ganglioside antibody-mediated motor nerve terminal injury. Brain 126:2497–2509

Odaka M, Tatsumoto M, Susuki K, Hirata K, Yuki N (2005) Intractable chronic inflammatory demyelinating polyneuropathy treated successfully with ciclosporin. J Neurol Neurosurg Psychiatry 76:1115–1120

Pers YM, Taieb G, Ayrignac X, Castelnovo G, Hubert AM, Boucraut J, Labauge P (2009) GQ1b ganglioside antibody-related disorders: a case with a complex phenotype. Acta Neurol Belg 109:330–332

Pestronk A, Adams RN, Clawson L, Cornblath D, Kuncl RW, Griffin D, Drachman DB (1988) Serum antibodies to GM1 ganglioside in amyotrophic lateral sclerosis. Neurology 38:1457–1461

Pestronk A, Li F, Griffin J, Feldman EL, Cornblath D, Trotter J, Zhu S, Yee WC, Phillips D, Peeples DM et al (1991) Polyneuropathy syndromes associated with serum antibodies to sulfatide and myelin-associated glycoprotein. Neurology 41:357–362

Petratos S, Turnbull VJ, Papadopoulos R, Ayers M, Gonzales MF (2000) High-titre IgM anti-sulfatide antibodies in individuals with IgM paraproteinaemia and associated peripheral neuropathy. Immunol Cell Biol 78:124–132

Plomp JJ, Willison HJ (2009) Pathophysiological actions of neuropathy-related anti-ganglioside antibodies at the neuromuscular junction. J Physiol 587:3979–3999

Popa I, Ishikawa D, Tanaka M, Ogino K, Portoukalian J, Taki T (2006) GD3-replica peptides selected from a phage peptide library induce a GD3 ganglioside antibody response. FEBS Lett 580:1398–1404

Pritchard J, Gray IA, Idrissova ZR, Lecky BR, Sutton IJ, Swan AV, Willison HJ, Winer JB, Hughes RA (2003) A randomized controlled trial of recombinant interferon-beta 1a in Guillain-Barre syndrome. Neurology 61:1282–1284

Qiu J, Luo P, Wasmund K, Steplewski Z, Kieber-Emmons T (1999) Towards the development of peptide mimotopes of carbohydrate antigens as cancer vaccines. Hybridoma 18:103–112

Rubinstein LJ, Goldberg B, Hiernaux J, Stein KE, Bona CA (1983) Idiotype-antiidiotype regulation. V. The requirement for immunization with antigen or monoclonal antiidiotypic antibodies for the activation of beta 2 leads to 6 and beta 2 leads to 1 polyfructosan-reactive clones in BALB/c mice treated at birth with minute amounts of anti-A48 idiotype antibodies. J Exp Med 158:1129–1144

Salloway S, Mermel LA, Seamans M, Aspinall GO, Nam Shin JE, Kurjanczyk LA, Penner JL (1996) Miller-Fisher syndrome associated with *Campylobacter jejuni* bearing lipopolysaccharide molecules that mimic human ganglioside GD3. Infect Immun 64:2945–2949

Santafe MM, Sabate MM, Garcia N, Ortiz N, Lanuza MA, Tomas J (2005) Changes in the neuromuscular synapse induced by an antibody against gangliosides. Ann Neurol 57:396–407

Schluep M, van Melle G, Henry H, Stadler C, Roth-Wicky B, Magistretti PJ (1998) In vitro cytokine profiles as indicators of relapse activity and clinical course in multiple sclerosis. Mult Scler 4:198–202

Schreiber JR, Patawaran M, Tosi M, Lennon J, Pier GB (1990) Anti-idiotype-induced, lipopolysaccharide-specific antibody response to *Pseudomonas aeruginosa*. J Immunol 144:1023–1029

Schwerer B (2002) Antibodies against gangliosides: a link between preceding infection and immunopathogenesis of Guillain-Barre syndrome. Microbes Infect 4:373–384

Scott JK, Smith GP (1990) Searching for peptide ligands with an epitope library. Science 249:386–390

Sheikh KA, Deerinck TJ, Ellisman MH, Griffin JW (1999) The distribution of ganglioside-like moieties in peripheral nerves. Brain 122(Pt 3):449–460

Shigeta H, Yamaguchi M, Nakano K, Obayashi H, Takemura R, Fukui M, Fujii M, Yoshimori K, Hasegawa G, Nakamura N, Kitagawa Y, Kondo M (1997) Serum autoantibodies against sulfatide and phospholipid in NIDDM patients with diabetic neuropathy. Diabetes Care 20:1896–1899

Shy ME, Vietorisz T, Nobile-Orazio E, Latov N (1984) Specificity of human IgM M-proteins that bind to myelin-associated glycoprotein: peptide mapping, deglycosylation, and competitive binding studies. J Immunol 133:2509–2512

Simon-Haldi M, Mantei N, Franke J, Voshol H, Schachner M (2002) Identification of a peptide mimic of the L2/HNK-1 carbohydrate epitope. J Neurochem 83:1380–1388

Simons K, Toomre D (2000) Lipid rafts and signal transduction. Nat Rev Mol Cell Biol 1:31–39

Stein KE, Soderstrom T (1984) Neonatal administration of idiotype or antiidiotype primes for protection against *Escherichia coli* K13 infection in mice. J Exp Med 160:1001–1011

Susuki K, Baba H, Tohyama K, Kanai K, Kuwabara S, Hirata K, Furukawa K, Rasband MN, Yuki N (2007a) Gangliosides contribute to stability of paranodal junctions and ion channel clusters in myelinated nerve fibers. Glia 55:746–757

Susuki K, Rasband MN, Tohyama K, Koibuchi K, Okamoto S, Funakoshi K, Hirata K, Baba H, Yuki N (2007b) Anti-GM1 antibodies cause complement-mediated disruption of sodium channel clusters in peripheral motor nerve fibers. J Neurosci 27:3956–3967

Tagawa Y, Yuki N, Hirata K (2000) Anti-SGPG antibody in CIDP: nosological position of IgM anti-MAG/SGPG antibody-associated neuropathy. Muscle Nerve 23:895–899

Taguchi K, Ren J, Utsunomiya I, Aoyagi H, Fujita N, Ariga T, Miyatake T, Yoshino H (2004a) Neurophysiological and immunohistochemical studies on Guillain-Barre syndrome with IgG anti-GalNAc-GD1a antibodies-effects on neuromuscular transmission. J Neurol Sci 225:91–98

Taguchi K, Utsunomiya I, Ren J, Yoshida N, Aoyagi H, Nakatani Y, Ariga T, Usuki S, Yu RK, Miyatake T (2004b) Effect of rabbit anti-asialo-GM1 (GA1) polyclonal antibodies on neuromuscular transmission and acetylcholine-induced action potentials: neurophysiological and immunohistochemical studies. Neurochem Res 29:953–960

Takigawa T, Yasuda H, Kikkawa R, Shigeta Y, Saida T, Kitasato H (1995) Antibodies against GM1 ganglioside affect K^+ and Na^+ currents in isolated rat myelinated nerve fibers. Ann Neurol 37:436–442

Takikawa M, Kikkawa H, Asai T, Yamaguchi N, Ishikawa D, Tanaka M, Ogino K, Taki T, Oku N (2000) Suppression of GD1alpha ganglioside-mediated tumor metastasis by liposomalized WHW-peptide. FEBS Lett 466:381–384

Thomas FP, Trojaborg W, Nagy C, Santoro M, Sadiq SA, Latov N, Hays AP (1991) Experimental autoimmune neuropathy with anti-GM1 antibodies and immunoglobulin deposits at the nodes of Ranvier. Acta Neuropathol 82:378–383

Trojaborg W (1998) Acute and chronic neuropathies: new aspects of Guillain-Barre syndrome and chronic inflammatory demyelinating polyneuropathy, an overview and an update. Electroencephalogr Clin Neurophysiol 107:303–316

Turatti M, Tamburin S, Idone D, Praitano ML, Zanette G (2010) Guillain-Barre syndrome after short-course efalizumab treatment. J Neurol 257:1404–1405

Unal-Cevik I, Onal MZ, Odabasi Z, Tan E (2009) IVIG- responsive multiple cranial neuropathy: a pharyngo-facial variant of Guillain-Barre syndrome. Acta Neurol Belg 109:317–321

Usuki S, Sanchez J, Ariga T, Utsunomiya I, Taguchi K, Rivner MH, Yu RK (2005) AIDP and CIDP having specific antibodies to the carbohydrate epitope (-NeuAcα2-8NeuAcα2-3Galβ1-4Glc-) of gangliosides. J Neurol Sci 232:37–44

Usuki S, Thompson SA, Rivner MH, Taguchi K, Shibata K, Ariga T, Yu RK (2006) Molecular mimicry: sensitization of Lewis rats with *Campylobacter jejuni* lipopolysaccharides induces formation of antibody toward GD3 ganglioside. J Neurosci Res 83:274–284

Usuki S, Nakatani Y, Taguchi K, Fujita T, Tanabe S, Ustunomiya I, Gu Y, Cawthraw SA, Newell DG, Pajaniappan M, Thompson SA, Ariga T, Yu RK (2008) Topology and patch-clamp analysis of the sodium channel in relationship to the anti-lipid A antibody in campylobacteriosis. J Neurosci Res 86:3359–3374

Usuki S, Taguchi K, Gu YH, Thompson SA, Yu RK (2010a) Development of a novel therapy for Lipo-oligosaccharide-induced experimental neuritis: use of peptide glycomimics. J Neurochem 113:351–362

Usuki S, Taguchi K, Thompson SA, Chapman PB, Yu RK (2010b) Novel anti-idiotype antibody therapy for lipooligosaccharide-induced experimental autoimmune neuritis: use relevant to Guillain-Barre syndrome. J Neurosci Res 88:1651–1663

van den Berg LH, Lankamp CL, de Jager AE, Notermans NC, Sodaar P, Marrink J, de Jong HJ, Bar PR, Wokke JH (1993) Anti-sulphatide antibodies in peripheral neuropathy. J Neurol Neurosurg Psychiatry 56:1164–1168

van Doorn PA, Ruts L, Jacobs BC (2008) Clinical features, pathogenesis, and treatment of Guillain-Barre syndrome. Lancet Neurol 7:939–950

van Doorn PA, Kuitwaard K, Walgaard C, van Koningsveld R, Ruts L, Jacobs BC (2010) IVIG treatment and prognosis in Guillain-Barre syndrome. J Clin Immunol 30(Suppl 1):S74–S78

Viale G, Flamini G, Grassi F, Buffa R, Natali PG, Pelagi M, Leoni F, Menard S, Siccardi AG (1989) Idiotypic replica of an anti-human tumor-associated antigen monoclonal antibody. Analysis of monoclonal Ab1 and Ab3 fine specificity. J Immunol 143:4338–4344

Weber F, Rudel R, Aulkemeyer P, Brinkmeier H (2000) Anti-GM1 antibodies can block neuronal voltage-gated sodium channels. Muscle Nerve 23:1414–1420

Willison HJ (2005a) Ganglioside complexes: new autoantibody targets in Guillain-Barre syndromes. Nat Clin Pract Neurol 1:2–3

Willison HJ (2005b) The immunobiology of Guillain-Barre syndromes. J Peripher Nerv Syst 10:94–112

Willison HJ, Yuki N (2002) Peripheral neuropathies and anti-glycolipid antibodies. Brain 125:2591–2625

Willison HJ, O'Hanlon GM, Paterson G, Veitch J, Wilson G, Roberts M, Tang T, Vincent A (1996) A somatically mutated human antiganglioside IgM antibody that induces experimental neuropathy in mice is encoded by the variable region heavy chain gene, V1-18. J Clin Invest 97:1155–1164

Willison HJ, Townson K, Veitch J, Boffey J, Isaacs N, Andersen SM, Zhang P, Ling CC, Bundle DR (2004) Synthetic disialylgalactose immunoadsorbents deplete anti-GQ1b antibodies from autoimmune neuropathy sera. Brain 127:680–691

Wollinsky KH, Hulser PJ, Brinkmeier H, Aulkemeyer P, Bossenecker W, Huber-Hartmann KH, Rohrbach P, Schreiber H, Weber F, Kron M, Buchele G, Mehrkens HH, Ludolph AC, Rudel R (2001) CSF filtration is an effective treatment of Guillain-Barre syndrome: a randomized clinical trial. Neurology 57:774–780

Wurz A, Brinkmeier H, Wollinsky KH, Mehrkens HH, Kornhuber HH, Rudel R (1995) Cerebrospinal fluid and serum from patients with inflammatory polyradiculoneuropathy have opposite effects on sodium channels. Muscle Nerve 18:772–781

Yamawaki M, Vasquez A, Ben Younes A, Yoshino H, Kanda T, Ariga T, Baumann N, Yu RK (1996) Sensitization of Lewis rats with sulfoglucuronosyl paragloboside: electrophysiological and immunological studies of an animal model of peripheral neuropathy. J Neurosci Res 44:58–65

Yamawaki M, Ariga T, Gao Y, Tokuda A, Yu JS, Sismanis A, Yu RK (1998) Sulfoglucuronosyl glycolipids as putative antigens for autoimmune inner ear disease. J Neuroimmunol 84:111–116

Yanagisawa K (2007) Role of gangliosides in Alzheimer's disease. Biochim Biophys Acta 1768:1943–1951

Yoshino H, Miyatani N, Saito M, Ariga T, Lugaresi A, Latov N, Kushi Y, Kasama T, Yu RK (1992) Isolated bovine spinal motoneurons have specific ganglioside antigens recognized by sera from patients with motor neuron disease and motor neuropathy. J Neurochem 59:1684–1691

Yoshino H, Harukawa H, Asano A (2000) IgG antiganglioside antibodies in Guillain-Barre syndrome with bulbar palsy. J Neuroimmunol 105:195–201

Yoshino H, Utsunomiya I, Taguchi K, Ariga T, Nagaoka T, Aoyagi H, Asano A, Yamada M, Miyatake T (2005) GalNAc-GD1a is localized specifically in ventral spinal roots, but not in dorsal spinal roots. Brain Res 1057:177–180

Yu RK (1994) Development regulation of ganglioside metabolism. Prog Brain Res 101:31–44

Yu RK, Ariga T (1998) The role of glycosphingolipids in neurological disorders. Mechanisms of immune action. Ann N Y Acad Sci 845:285–306

Yu RK, Ariga T, Kohriyama T, Kusunoki S, Maeda Y, Miyatani N (1990) Autoimmune mechanisms in peripheral neuropathies. Ann Neurol 27(Suppl):S30–S35

Yu RK, Ariga T, Yoshino H, Katoh-Semba R, Ren S (1994a) Differential effects of glycosphingolipids n protein kinase C activity in PC12D pheochromocytoma cells. J Biomed Sci 1:229–236

Yu RK, Yoshino H, Yamawaki M, Yoshino JE, Ariga T (1994b) Subcellular distribution of sulfated glucuronyl glycolipids in human peripheral motor and sensory nerves. J Biomed Sci 1:167–171

Yu RK, Usuki S, Ariga T (2006) Ganglioside molecular mimicry and its pathological roles in Guillain-Barre syndrome and related diseases. Infect Immun 74:6517–6527

Yu RK, Ariga T, Yanagisawa M, Zeng G (2008) Biosynthesis and degradation of gangliosides in the nervous system. In: Fraser-Reid B, Tasuka K, Thiem J (eds) Glycoscience. Springer, Berlin/Heidelberg, pp 1671–1695

Yu RK, Suzuki Y, Yanagisawa M (2010) Membrane glycolipids in stem cells. FEBS Lett 584:1694–1699

Yuki N (1998) Anti-ganglioside antibody and neuropathy: review of our research. J Peripher Nerv Syst 3:3–18

Yuki N (2007) Ganglioside mimicry and peripheral nerve disease. Muscle Nerve 35:691–711

Yuki N, Taki T, Inagaki F, Kasama T, Takahashi M, Saito K, Handa S, Miyatake T (1993) A bacterium lipopolysaccharide that elicits Guillain-Barre syndrome has a GM1 ganglioside-like structure. J Exp Med 178:1771–1775

Yuki N, Taki T, Takahashi M, Saito K, Tai T, Miyatake T, Handa S (1994) Penner's serotype 4 of *Campylobacter jejuni* has a lipopolysaccharide that bears a GM1 ganglioside epitope as well as one that bears a GD1 a epitope. Infect Immun 62:2101–2103

Yuki N, Tagawa Y, Handa S (1996) Autoantibodies to peripheral nerve glycosphingolipids SPG, SLPG, and SGPG in Guillain-Barre syndrome and chronic inflammatory demyelinating polyneuropathy. J Neuroimmunol 70:1–6

Yuki N, Ho TW, Tagawa Y, Koga M, Li CY, Hirata K, Griffin JW (1999) Autoantibodies to GM1b and GalNAc-GD1a: relationship to *Campylobacter jejuni* infection and acute motor axonal neuropathy in China. J Neurol Sci 164:134–138

Yuki N, Susuki K, Koga M, Nishimoto Y, Odaka M, Hirata K, Taguchi K, Miyatake T, Furukawa K, Kobata T, Yamada M (2004) Carbohydrate mimicry between human ganglioside GM1 and *Campylobacter jejuni* lipooligosaccharide causes Guillain-Barre syndrome. Proc Natl Acad Sci USA 101:11404–11409

Zitman FM, Todorov B, Jacobs BC, Verschuuren JJ, Furukawa K, Willison HJ, Plomp JJ (2008) Neuromuscular synaptic function in mice lacking major subsets of gangliosides. Neuroscience 156:885–897

Computational Techniques Applied to Defining Carbohydrate Antigenicity

15

Robert J. Woods and Austin B. Yongye

15.1 Introduction

The complex shape and dynamic properties of oligo- and polysaccharides, combined with their potential to exhibit functional group modifications, allow these molecules to function pervasively in biology as encoders and recognition molecules (Sharon and Lis 1993; Varki 1993; Dwek 1996). Yet it is this very diversity and flexibility that makes their structural analysis difficult. Carbohydrate recognition may be used in an immunological context to allow a host organism to identify a foreign pathogen, on the basis of the carbohydrates presented on the surface of the pathogen. As such, there is increasing use of polysaccharides isolated from the surface of bacteria, such as *Haemophilus influenzae* (*Hi*), *Streptococcus agalactiae* (*Sa*), also known as group B *Streptococcus*, and *Neisseria meningitidis* (*Nm*), in antibacterial vaccines (Jennings 1992). The increasing use of carbohydrate-based conjugate vaccines is founded on the observation that antibodies against the type-specific bacterial capsular polysaccharides (CPSs) are often protective (Egan et al. 1983; Jennings 1992) and is driven by the increasing prevalence of antibiotic resistant strains. However, the relationships between the carbohydrate sequence

R.J. Woods (✉)
Complex Carbohydrate Research Center, University of Georgia, 315 Riverbend Road, Athens, GA 30602, USA

School of Chemistry, National University of Ireland at Galway, Galway, Ireland
e-mail: rwoods@ccrc.uga.edu1

A.B. Yongye
Complex Carbohydrate Research Center, University of Georgia, 315 Riverbend Road, Athens, GA 30602, USA

Torrey Pines Institute for Molecular Studies, 11350 SW Village Parkway, Port St. Lucie, FL 34987, USA

P. Kosma and S. Müller-Loennies (eds.), *Anticarbohydrate Antibodies*,
DOI 10.1007/978-3-7091-0870-3_15, © Springer-Verlag/Wien 2012

and antigenicity (affinity and specificity for antibody) or immunogenicity (ability to induce an antibody response) are poorly understood.

Computational methods can provide unique insight into the structural features of antigenic oligosaccharides that are responsible for mediating the *affinity* and *specificity* of their interactions with type-specific monoclonal antibodies (mAbs). This is an area of research that presents severe challenges for traditional 3D structural methods; however, simulational methods are well suited to addressing some of these challenges. In particular, they offer the opportunity to generate experimentally inaccessible data, to provide an atomic level interpretation for macroscopic or indirect experimental data, to interpolate between sparse experimental data points, to identify putative antigen – antibody interactions that may be experimentally probed, and to quantify the roles of enthalpy and entropy in driving oligosaccharide antigenicity. Such insight could form a basis for the rational development of more effective antibacterial vaccines and conversely higher affinity engineered carbohydrate-binding antibodies.

Established structural methods, such as X-ray diffraction or NMR spectroscopy face enormous challenges when applied to the study of biologically relevant glycans and glycoproteins. Difficulties in obtaining sufficient material of acceptable purity are compounded by the presence of micro-heterogeneity in the glycans present in all glycoproteins. Further, in the case of co-crystallization experiments between a carbohydrate-binding protein and its ligand, the requirement for a homogeneous carbohydrate sample frequently necessitates the chemical synthesis of the oligosaccharide. This is a far from routine undertaking for any but the smallest glycans. Lastly, even with a supply of protein and ligand, the flexibility of most oligosaccharides detracts from their ability to co-crystallize. While NMR is well suited to work with less homogeneous samples, molecular weight limitations have greatly attenuated its application to large glycoproteins or protein – polysaccharide complexes. In addition, NMR data alone are generally insufficient to completely characterize carbohydrate conformation and are frequently augmented by insight from computational methods, such as molecular dynamics (MD) simulation (Weimar and Woods 2002).

While no method alone is adequate to characterize either the conformation of an oligosaccharide or its complex with a protein, by combining experimental biophysical techniques with current computational methods, an opportunity is provided to deduce structure-function relationships in many areas of glycobiology. Computational methods can contribute unique insight into the relationship between oligosaccharide structure and biological function (Fig. 15.1). Biomolecular simulations offer the potential to make a significant contribution, serving either to assist in the interpretation of otherwise sparse experimental data, or to provide *a priori* models for the structure of oligosaccharides, or insight into the mechanisms of carbohydrate recognition. The models from these simulations are generally able to reproduce experimental NMR data (Vliegenhart and Woods 2006), and may be employed in a predictive capacity.

Predictive accuracy enables MD simulations to be used to probe the relationships between oligosaccharide sequence and structure. The potential benefit

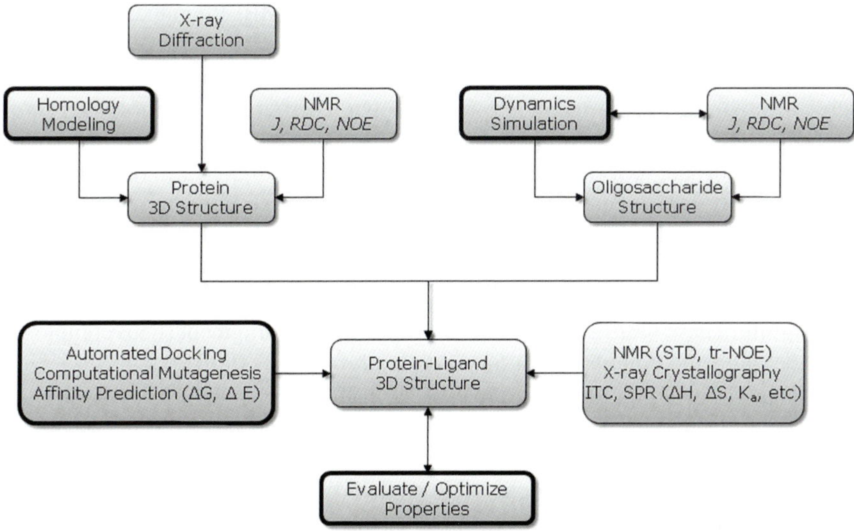

Fig. 15.1 Interplay between traditional biophysical and biochemical techniques and computational methods (*bold outlines*). By appropriately combining techniques, it is possible to establish structure-function relationships in glycans and carbohydrate – protein (e.g., antibody) complexes

of this ability is clearly significant to glycobiology. A more challenging question that immediately arises, once it is possible to predict structure, is whether or not binding affinities may be accurately predicted. This latter question remains a highly active research area of computational chemistry for all classes of interactions. At present there are several methods to calculate binding energies. The most accurate is known as free energy perturbation or thermodynamic integration (TI). TI is limited to examining relative binding energies for very similar ligands; however, it is capable of quantifying the contributions from key structural moieties (Pathiaseril and Woods 2000). An alternative is to compute the ΔG of binding by direct decomposition of the interaction energies between the reactants (Ford et al. 2003). Direct ΔG methods employ implicit solvent models in the calculation of solvation free energy and so are less rigorous than TI calculations, but are more broadly applicable (Gouda et al. 2003). The application of both TI and direct ΔG calculations to carbohydrate-protein complexes have been reviewed recently (Woods and Tessier 2010).

In this chapter we will illustrate the use of computational methods in defining the origin of the structural features that confer specificity and affinity (antigenicity) to carbohydrate antigen – antibody interactions. Not only are such properties of fundamental importance to many host-pathogen interactions, but also, the increasing use of anti-carbohydrate antibodies as diagnostic reagents necessitates well-defined antigenicities, which are not however trivial to confirm. Several popular carbohydrate force fields for molecular simulations have been recently reviewed (Fadda and Woods 2010). Here we will highlight examples employing the

GLYCAM force field (Kirschner et al. 2007) with the AMBER simulation package (Case et al. 2005).

The conformational properties of two bacterial polysaccharides will be described, namely for *S. agalactiae* (also known as group B *Streptococcus*) serotype III (*Sa*III), and *N. meningitidis* serotype B (*Nm*B). Molecular dynamics simulations of the polysaccharides provide unique insight into their solution properties, serving to confirm and characterize the proposed bactericidal epitope in *Sa*III, and to generate models for the highly plastic *Nm*B antigen.

The second two examples will examine the most common types of anti-carbohydrate antibody topologies, namely those that exhibit a cavity or groove type of binding site. These will be illustrated for antigen binding fragment (Fab) complexes with the antigenic epitopes from *Salmonella paratyphi* B (*Sp*B) (cavity-like Fab) and *Shigella flexneri* Y (*Sf*Y) (groove-like). In the *Sp*B system, MD simulations provide an explanation for the conformational differences observed in complexes with this antigen and related Fab and variable fragments (Fv). For the *Sf*Y system, free energy calculations are employed to explain the thermodynamic origin of the affinity data reported for chemical analogs of the native antigen.

It is important to be clear regarding the meanings of the terms antigenicity, epitope, and immunogenicity. Antigenicity (also known as antigenic reactivity) refers to both the *affinity* and *specificity* of an antibody for an antigen (Regenmortel 1989). The term is frequently used to characterize the results of epitope mapping studies. Relative to a given antibody, one epitope might be said to be more antigenic or have higher antigenicity than another. An epitope is that region of an antigen that is in direct contact with the antibody and is therefore responsible for the immunological uniqueness of the antigen. Antigenicity is not synonymous with immunogenicity, which is the ability of an antigen to elicit a humoral or cell-mediated immune response. All substances that are immunogenic are also antigenic; but the reverse is not true. However, since carbohydrates cannot elicit a T-cell response directly, the initial stimulation of the B-cell receptor (BCR) by the carbohydrate antigen is crucial in developing an immune response. Since the BCR shares many features of an antibody, an understanding of the basis of carbohydrate antigenicity may ultimately lead to insight into carbohydrate immunogenicity.

15.2 Example 1. Defining the Conformational Epitope of a Bacterial Polysaccharide (*Sa*III)

Remarkably subtle variations in the carbohydrate sequences among the branched polysaccharides that make up the *Sa* bacterial capsules result in several immunologically distinct serotypes of *Sa*. Due to the large apparent size of the *Sa* epitopes, the differences in the antigenicities of the serotypes are presumed to be due to conformational variations (Kabat et al. 1988; Zou et al. 1999). Notably, the serotypes of *Sa* are compositionally similar, and yet immunologically distinct (see Fig. 15.2). Our research has focused on the capsular polysaccharide associated with *Sa*III. While not the most frequently isolated serotype, *Sa*III exhibits disproportionately high

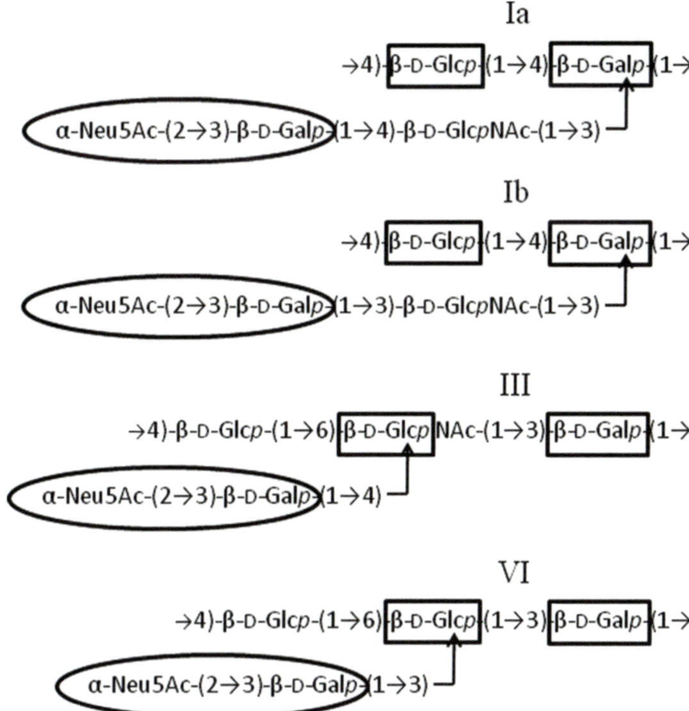

Fig. 15.2 Examples of serotypes of *S. agalactiae* indicating the similarities in the backbone sequence and side chains. The fact that each of these polysaccharides is immunologically distinct highlights the fact that the concept of homology modeling has no role in carbohydrate 3D structure prediction

virulence in infants. A measure of the size of the carbohydrate epitope has been provided by assaying the binding affinities of oligosaccharide repeat units of *Sa*III, for anti-*Sa*III antibodies (Wessels et al. 1987). It was found that oligosaccharide binding increased with the number of repeat units and a conformational epitope was proposed (Wessels et al. 1987).

A complete computational analysis of *Sa*III, with respect to its interaction with mAb 1B1 has been reported, including characterization of the solution conformation of the antigenic fragments (Gonzalez-Outeriño et al. 2005), and of the putative immune complex (Kadirvelraj et al. 2006). Notably, that work provided the first structural and energetic explanation for the observed lack of cross-reactivity between *Sa*III and its close relative *Pneumococcus* type 14. Additionally these studies confirmed that the bactericidal epitope (bound to mAb 1B1) was equivalent to the solution conformational epitope (Kadirvelraj et al. 2006) (Fig. 15.3). The results for *Sa*III illustrate the unique insight that computational methods can bring to the interpretation of carbohydrate antigenicity.

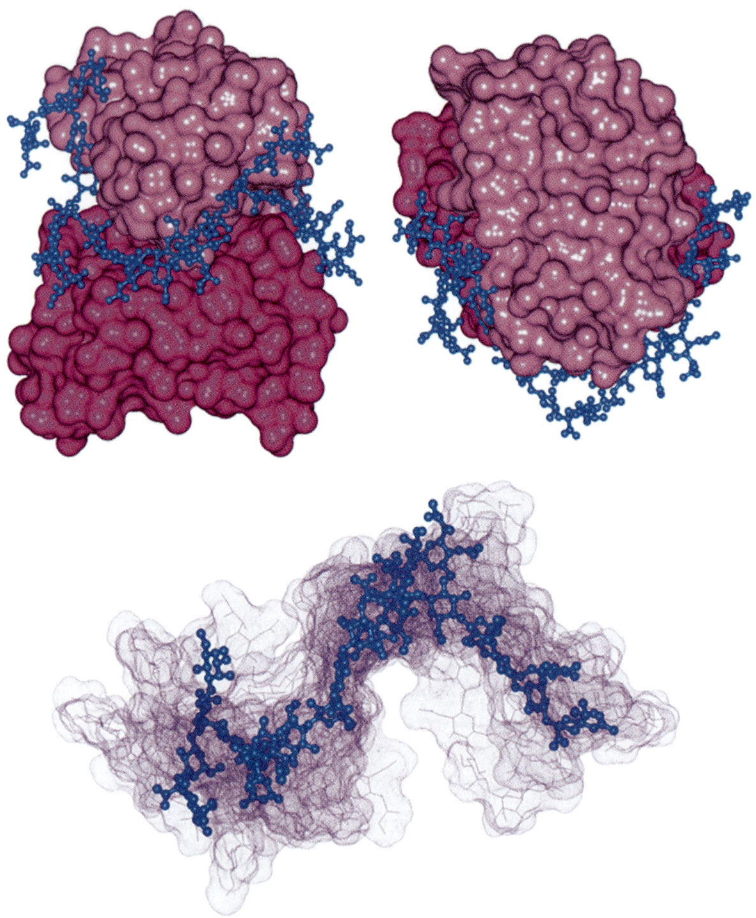

Fig. 15.3 *Upper*: the predicted structures of the immune complex for a 25-mer fragment of *Sa*III (*blue*) bound to a neutralizing mAb (1B1) showing the light chain variable domain V_L (*pink*) and heavy chain variable domain V_H (*purple*) (Kadirvelraj et al. 2006). *Lower*: a comparison of the *Sa*III fragment in its bound conformation (*blue*) with 10 snapshots of the solution conformations of *Sa*III taken from a 25 ns MD simulation (Gonzalez-Outeriño et al. 2005)

Although not a rigid helix, the polymer maintains an overall helical conformation by virtue of the fact that internal rotations associated with the β-D-Glc-(1→6)-β-D-GlcNAc linkage are hampered by stabilizing interactions (arrows) between the side chain terminal Neu5Ac sialic acid residue and the polymer backbone (Fig. 15.4) (Gonzalez-Outeriño et al. 2005). When these interactions are removed, by desialylation, the conformational epitope is destroyed and the recognition motif is reduced to a shorter segment, as seen in *Pneumococcus* type 14 (Gonzalez-Outeriño et al. 2005).

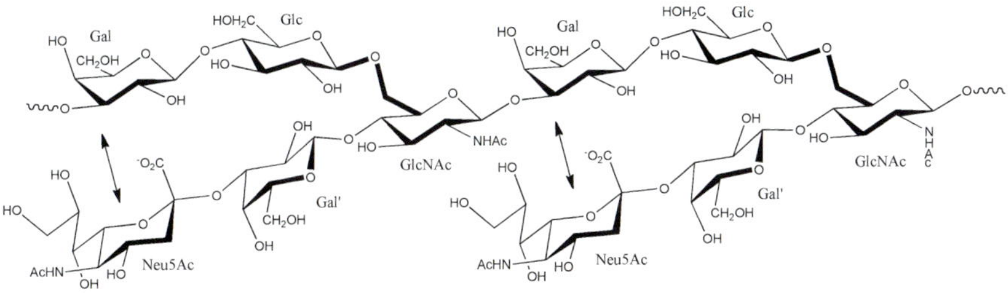

Fig. 15.4 The sequence of a dimeric repeating unit of *Sa*III indicating the side chain – back bone interactions that stabilize the backbone β(1→6)linkage

The conformational analysis of *Sa*III provided unique insight into the 3D structure of the bactericidal epitope, and led to the conclusion that the antibody had evolved to recognize the most frequently populated shape of the polysaccharide. This is entirely consistent with earlier evidence that this polysaccharide exhibited a conformational epitope. The data also suggest that, conversely, an antibody is less likely to evolve to recognize a lengthy segment of a highly disordered polysaccharide, but instead would evolve to recognize shorter segments that display less overall plasticity.

15.3 Example 2. Modeling the Conformational Properties of a Highly Flexible Bacterial Polysaccharide (*Nm*B)

The bacterial serotypes of *Nm* are defined on the basis of their capsular polysaccharides (CPSs), which are invariably polyanionic (see Table 15.1). The CPSs form a shell around the bacterium, but are not toxic themselves. During infection they inhibit phagocytosis by neutrophils, protect the bacterium from antibody recognition, and interfere with adherence of complement. The CPSs are key virulence determinants, due to their location on the outer surface of the bacteria, and constitute the principal antigens in most of the pathogenic bacteria. Virtually nothing is known about the relationship between capsule structure and infectivity. Similarly, there is only a poor understanding of the variation in immunogenicity associated with the various serotypes.

There are two currently available CPS-vaccines for meningococcal disease, one being a mixture of CPSs from groups A and C, and the other a mixture of groups A, C, Y, and W135. A reliable vaccine for group B is still not available. The poor immunogenicity of *Nm*B has been attributed to the structural similarity between the CPS from *Nm*B and human tissue antigens in gangliosides and neural cell adhesion glycoproteins (NCAM) (Finne et al. 1983; Finne and Mäkelä 1985). A protective immune response was elicited from a synthetic derivative of the B-conjugate vaccine, made by replacing the *N*-acetyl groups in the CPS with *N*-propionyl groups (Jennings et al. 1986, see Chap. 3). At first glance these results suggest that the *N*-acetyl and *N*-propionyl groups have little influence on the structure of

Table 15.1 CPS structures for the five most virulent *N. meningitidis* serotypes

Serotype	Oligosaccharide repeat units (anionic residues in bold)
A	→6)α-D-ManNAc(**1→OPO$_3$**→
B	→8)**αNeu5Ac**(2→
C	→9)**αNeu5Ac**(2→
E. coli K92	→8)α**Neu5Ac**(2→9)α**Neu5Ac**(2→
W135	→6)α-D-Gal(1→4)**αNeu5Ac**(2→
Y	→6)α-D-Glc(1→4)**αNeu5Ac**(2→

the epitope. However, when analyzed in terms of antibody class (Krug et al. 2004), it was demonstrated that only IgM class antibodies generated by immunization with the synthetic analogs of *Nm*B maintained the ability to recognize the native antigen. IgG class antibodies produced by the synthetic analog were unable to bind to the native antigen (Liu et al. 2000; Krug et al. 2004). Clearly, there is a trade-off between stimulating the immune system and compromising the 3D structure of the antigen.

Lastly, despite the fact that the CPS from types *Nm*B and *Nm*C (-9-α-D-Neu5Ac-2-) are copolymers of the same carbohydrate, their linkage differences apparently lead to profound 3D structural variations, evidenced by the fact that while mAb 735 recognizes type B, it does not react with type C, yet both polysaccharides cross-react with antisera against *E. coli* K92, which has a CPS composed of an alternating sequence of α(2→8)-, and α(2→9)-linked Neu5Ac residues (Devi et al. 1991).

In order to assess the performance of unrestrained MD simulations on type B antigens, we examined the sialobioside and sialotrioside fragments of *Nm*B by MD and NMR analysis (Yongye et al. 2008b). These structures contain the conformationally-critical α(2→8)-linkages that are present in the *Nm*B homopolymer. Simulations of these fragments serve the important function of establishing the accuracy limits of the computational and experimental protocols.

Data from MD simulations of the antigenic fragments (Fig. 15.5) are presented for comparison with NMR homonuclear *J*-couplings (Table 15.2), experimentally-derived rotamer distributions (Table 15.3), and NOE intensities (Table 15.4).

The level of agreement between the experimental and theoretical values is reasonable, given the sources of errors, although not ideal. The overall conformation of *Nm*B is influenced by the ω_7 and ω_8 torsion angles in the exocyclic glyceryl side chains in the Neu5Ac residues, but not directly by ω_9, which is effectively a free rotor. Scalar couplings were recorded for ω_9 in the trisaccharide and were similar to those from the disaccharide. Additionally, it is important to observe that ω_7 displays markedly different conformational properties depending on whether O8 is free, or whether it participates in a glycosidic linkage. These differences are most apparent in the H6-H7 homonuclear ^3J-couplings (Table 15.2), and it is notable that the unrestrained MD simulations were able to correctly reproduce this difference in rotamer preferences.

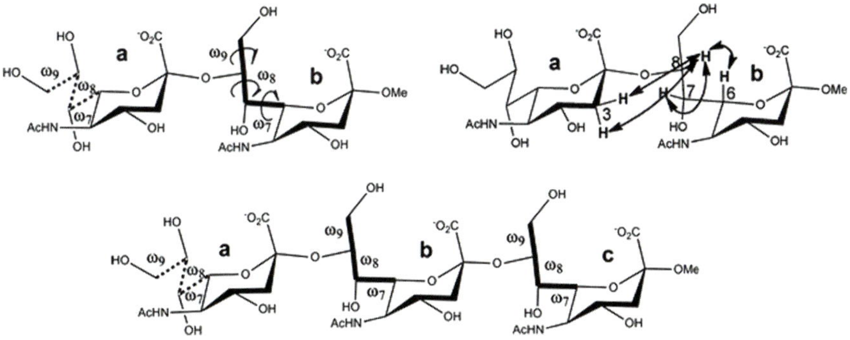

Fig. 15.5 *Upper Left*: Definition of inter-residue ω-torsion angles (terminal sequences shown in with *dashed lines*, internal with bold). *Upper Right*: An indication of the key inter-residue NOEs (*arrows*) pertinent the data in Tables 15.2–15.4. *Lower*: sialotrioside showing internal and terminal ω-angles

Table 15.2 NMR and computed $^3J_{HH}$ coupling constants (Hz) for inter-residue torsion angles in fragments of *Nm*B. Conformation-defining intra-residue *J*-couplings are highlighted in grey

Angle	Linkage	Spins	NMR	MD (100 ns)[a]	REMD (20 ns)[a]
Sialobioside αNeu5Ac(2→8)αNeu5Ac→OMe					
ω_7	Terminal	aH6-aH7	1.4 ± 0.1	1.0 ± 0.8	1.0 ± 0.8
	Internal	bH6-bH7	<1.0	1.2 ± 0.9	1.2 ± 0.9
ω_8	Terminal	aH7-aH8	9.5 ± 0.9	7.9 ± 0.6	8.1 ± 0.6
	Internal	bH7-bH8	1.5 ± 0.2	2.0 ± 0.7	2.0 ± 0.7
ω_9	Terminal (free rotor)	aH8-aH9$_R$	6.1 ± 0.6	6.7 ± 1.5	5.9 ± 1.5
		aH8-aH9$_S$	2.4 ± 0.2	3.7 ± 0.9	3.6 ± 0.9
	Internal (free rotor)	bH8-bH9$_R$	6.1 ± 0.6	7.3 ± 1.6	7.4 ± 1.7
		bH8-bH9$_S$	4.1 ± 0.4	2.9 ± 1.3	2.9 ± 1.3
Sialotrioside (a-b-c) αNeu5Ac(2→8)αNeu5Ac(2→8)αNeu5Ac→OMe					
ω_7	Terminal	aH6-aH7	1.5 ± 0.2	1.0 ± 0.8	1.0 ± 0.8
	Internal	bH6-bH7	<1.0	0.9 ± 0.8	0.9 ± 0.7
	Internal	cH6-cH7	<1.0	1.1 ± 0.9	1.3 ± 1.0
ω_8	Terminal	aH7-aH8	9.6 ± 1.0	7.7 ± 0.6	8.1 ± 0.5
	Internal	bH7-bH8	<4.0	3.6 ± 0.9	1.9 ± 0.9
	Internal	cH7-cH8	<4.0	2.1 ± 0.7	2.1 ± 0.8

[a]REMD simulations were performed at eight temperatures for a total of 160 ns

Conversion of the experimental *J*-values into populations was performed as described earlier (Yongye et al. 2008) and indicated that the ω_7 angle is effectively rigid (Table 15.3). This is a characteristic feature in the NMR of Neu5Ac residues and has been identified (Poppe and van Halbeek 1991) as being due to a strong hydrogen bond between HO7 and the NAc moiety. A hydrogen bond between HO8 and the carboxylate group at C2 has also been identified as stabilizing the ω_8 angle in a predominantly *trans*-orientation (Poppe and van Halbeek 1991). These

Table 15.3 NMR-based and computed populations (%) for inter-residue torsion angles in fragments of *Nm*B

Angle	Linkage	NMR[a, b] *gauche/trans/-gauche*	MD (100 ns) $g/t/-g$	REMD (20 ns) $g/t/-g$
Sialobioside (a-b) α-Neu5Ac-(2→8)-α-Neu5Ac→OMe				
ω_7	Terminal a	100/0/0	100/0/0	100/0/0
ω_7	Internal b	100/0/0	100/0/0	100/0/0
ω_8	Terminal a	0/100[c]/0	13/80/7	13/83/4
ω_8	Internal b	96 ± 3/3 ± 3/0	90/10/0	90/10/0
ω_9	Terminal a	54 ± 8 /0/50 ± 12	61/18/21	52/16/32
ω_9	Internal b	55 ± 8/24 ± 9/20 ± 15	73/2/25	75/4/21
Sialotrioside (a-b-c) α-Neu5Ac-(2→8)-α-Neu5Ac-(2→8)-α-Neu5Ac→OMe				
ω_7	Terminal a	100/0/0	100/0/0	100/0/0
ω_7	Internal b	100/0/0	100/0/0	100/0/0
ω_7	Internal c	100/0/0	100/0/0	100/0/0
ω_8	Terminal a	0/100[c]/0	15/74/7	14/82/4
ω_8	Internal b	60 ± 9 / 25 ± 3 / 0	70/30/0	92/8/0
ω_8	Internal c	66 ± 5 / 31 ± 9 / 0	89/11/0	82/10/8

[a]Range is consistent with the estimated error in the experimental *J*-values, only one symmetric solution is presented

[b]NMR populations derived by employing limiting *J*-values from rotational isomeric states computed from traditional MD (the REMD simulations did not give significantly different limiting *J*-values)

[c]Estimated based on the magnitude of the *J*-value

properties are well reproduced by the MD simulations. It is very significant that when HO8 is involved in a glycosidic linkage, it can no longer participate in the internal hydrogen bond and the orientation of the ω_8 angle changes from *trans-* to mostly *gauche*. The ω_8 angle is not constrained by strong internal hydrogen bonds in solution (Poppe and van Halbeek 1991) and is able to populate all three staggered rotamers with a preference for the *gauche*. That these features are correctly reproduced here indicates that the force field is able to reproduce the delicate energetic balance between intramolecular and solvent-mediated hydrogen bonds (Kirschner and Woods 2001).

The agreement between the theoretical and experimental NOE data for the sialobioside (Table 15.4) suggests that the discrepancies between the computed and theoretical *J*-values do not arise from inaccurate conformational data (since both MD and REMD data sets give very similar results), but from approximation associated with converting the MD data to *J*-values.

In the sialotrioside, there are additional rotatable bonds, and we begin to see a dependence of the computed NOEs on sampling. While quantitative agreement with rotamer populations has not yet been achieved, the simulations have been able to identify the preponderant rotamer in each state and were generally able to correctly rank the populations.

Table 15.4 Experimental NOE distances (Å)[a] and average inter-proton distances from MD and REMD simulations for fragments of *Nm*B. Conformation-defining intra-residue NOEs are highlighted in grey[b]

Spins	NMR	MD 100 ns	REMD 20 ns	Spins	NMR	MD 100 ns	REMD 20 ns
Sialobioside (a–b) α-Neu5Ac-(2→8)-α-Neu5Ac→OMe							
bH8 – bH6	2.6	2.5 ± 0.2	2.5 ± 0.2	bH8 – bH7	2.3	2.6 ± 0.2	2.6 ± 0.2
aH3$_{ax}$ – bH8	2.7	2.9 ± 0.7	3.0 ± 0.8	aH3$_{eq}$ – bH8	4.0	3.9 ± 0.4	3.4 ± 0.4
aH3$_{ax}$ – aH3$_{eq}$	1.7	1.7 ± 0.1	1.7 ± 0.1	aH3$_{ax}$ – aH5	2.6	2.7 ± 0.2	2.7 ± 0.2
aH3$_{ax}$ – aH4	2.9	3.0 ± 0.1	3.0 ± 0.1	aH3$_{eq}$ – aH4	2.5	2.5 ± 0.1	2.5 ± 0.1
bH3$_{ax}$ – bH4	3.1	3.0 ± 0.1	3.0 ± 0.1	bH5 – bNMe	4.3	4.5 ± 0.1	4.5 ± 0.1
bH3$_{ax}$ – bH5	2.6	2.7 ± 0.2	2.7 ± 0.2	bH9R – bH8	2.3	2.5 ± 0.2	2.9 ± 0.3
Sialotrioside (a–b–c) α-Neu5Ac-(2→8)-α-Neu5Ac-(2→8)-α-Neu5Ac→OMe							
cH8 – bH3$_{ax}$	2.6	3.3 ± 0.8	2.6 ± 0.7	bH6 – bH8	2.3	2.6 ± 0.3	2.5 ± 0.1
bH3$_{eq}$ – cH8	3.5	4.1 ± 0.5	3.8 ± 0.5	aH3$_{ax}$ – bH8	3.0	3.4 ± 0.8	2.8 ± 0.7
bH6 – bH7	2.2	2.4 ± 0.1	2.4 ± 0.1	aH3$_{eq}$ – bH8	3.4	4.2 ± 0.4	3.8 ± 0.4

[a]Derived using the isolated spin-pair approximation (ISPA)

[b]Conformationally insensitive NOEs for the sialotrioside were similar to the sialobioside values, and are omitted

15.3.1 MD Simulations of a 12-mer Fragment of *Nm*B

In order to extrapolate the modeling to a fragment that mode accurately captured the properties of a polysaccharide, 12-mer fragment of *Nm*B was subjected to 25 ns MD simulation. By comparing the NMR data for the sialotrioside (Table 15.5), it appears that the ω-angles in the polysaccharide, and in the 12-mer, populate approximately the same states as the internal ω-angles in the trisaccharide. The initial MD data are qualitatively in agreement with the experimental data; however, further MD data are required before the simulations may be considered converged. Precise characterization of the rotational isomeric states in the polysaccharide is impossible with the available NMR data.

The *Nm*B case illustrates a very important point, namely that for a flexible antigen, characterizing only the solution states is unlikely to lead to the identification of the bactericidal epitope. To make that identification likely requires an examination of the antigen in the presence of at least one protective mAb.

Previously, various perfectly helical structures were suggested for *Nm*B, which were in qualitative agreement with the available NMR data (Evans et al. 1995). More recently (Henderson et al. 2003), both helical and random models were

Table 15.5 Inter-glycosidic homonuclear ^3J-couplings in methyl α(2→8)-dodecasialoside from a 25 ns MD simulation compared to experimental data for the intact polysaccharide.

Angle	Linkage	Spins	MD[a] (average)	NMR[b] intact polysaccharide (colominic acid)	Sialotrioside NMR internal linkages	Sialotrioside NMR terminal linkages
ω_7	Internal	H6-H7	**2.2 ± 0.8**	<3	<**1.0**	**1.5 ± 0.2**
ω_8	Internal	H7-H8	**3.4 ± 1.2**	<3	<**4.0**	**9.6 ± 1.0**
ω_9	Free rotor	H8-H9S	**3.8 ± 1.8**	**5**	2.8 – 4.5	<**4.0**
		H8-H9R	**6.1 ± 1.4**	**6**	6.0 – 6.3	6.2 ± 0.6

[a]Theoretical values computed for the central six internal linkages only
[b]Michon et al. (1987)

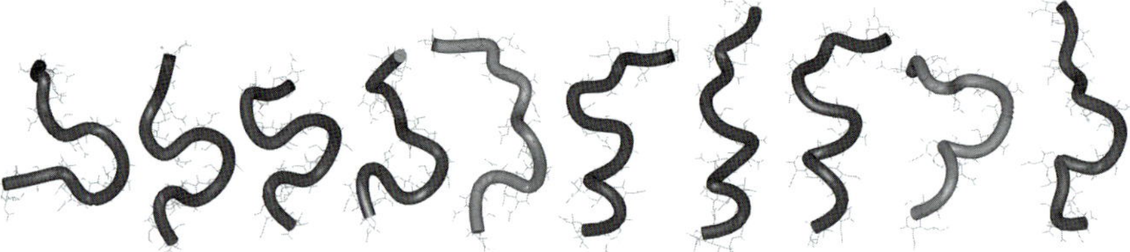

Fig. 15.6 Snapshots from a 25 ns MD simulation of a 12-mer of *Nm*B selected at 2.5 ns intervals illustrate the plasticity of this polysaccharide. Multiple conformational states are present with regions of helical structure transitioning (*grey*) between more convoluted conformations

compared to NMR relaxation data and it was concluded that a random coil model was in best agreement. The present MD studies indicate that the CPS is very unlikely to be a rigid helix, but rather, as seen in the smaller fragments, likely interconverts between multiple well-defined rotameric states (Fig. 15.6). This dynamic model is consistent with, albeit limited, experimental scalar *J*-coupling data for the polysaccharide, and is consistent with the well characterized di- and trisaccharide fragments.

15.4 Example 3. Docking and MD Simulations of Carbohydrate-Antibody Structures (the *Sp*B – Se155 Antibody System)

The 3D structures of antibody-carbohydrate complexes can be used to identify the conformation of the bactericidal epitope. However, because oligosaccharides are generally refractory to crystallization, such complexes are difficult to generate for analysis by x-ray diffraction. For this reason, there is interest in using computational docking methods to predict the orientation of the antigen in the binding site (Paula et al. 2005; Kadirvelraj et al. 2006), given only the 3D structure of the protein (Fig. 15.1). However, computational docking is prone to false positives (Woods and Tessier 2010), and the current algorithms do not include potential functions that correctly predict the conformational properties of oligosaccharides, such as arise from the exo-anomeric effect (Wolfe et al. 1979). In this section we will examine the case of the compact carbohydrate antigen from the O-chain polysaccharide of *Salmonella* serotype B in complex with mAb Se155-4 (Fig. 15.7). This antibody appears to have matured to recognize this immunodominant antigen by forming a remarkably hydrophobic cavity, which is nevertheless able to satisfy all of the hydrogen bond requirements of the immune-dominant abequose (Abe) residue. This is a particularly interesting system because, in the crystal structure with the Fv fragment (Zdanov et al. 1994), a water molecule

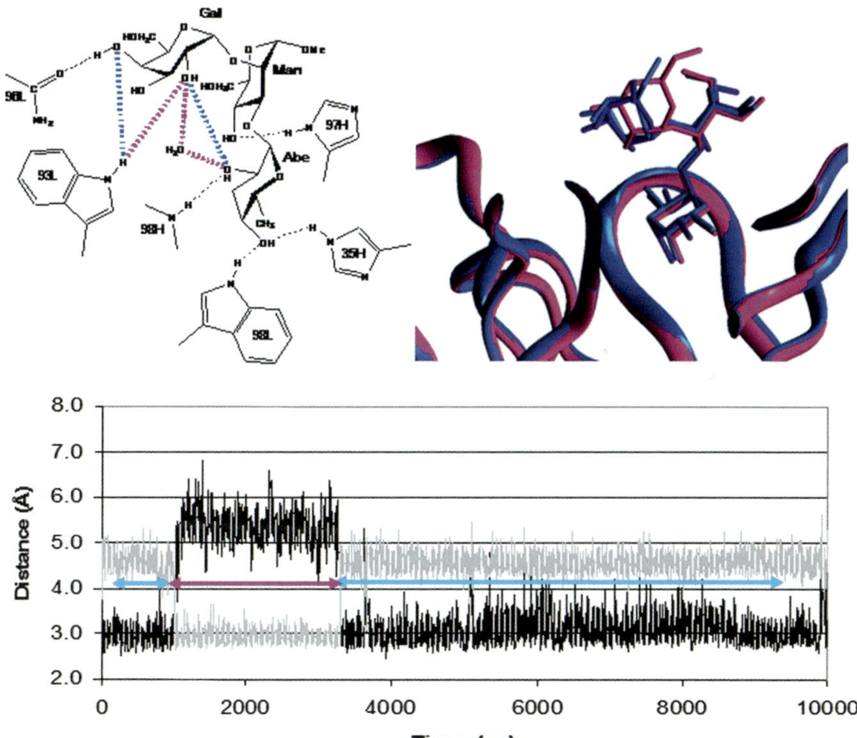

Fig. 15.7 *Upper Left*: The hydrogen bonding network in the Fv (*pink*) and Fab (*light blue*) complexes of Se155-4. Interactions unique to the Fv are shown in pink; those unique to the Fab in light blue. *Upper Right:* A view of the trisaccharide antigen in the binding site of the Fv and Fab structures. The lowest energy pose from the docking is illustrated in *dark blue*. *Lower*. Time dependence of the Gal O2 – Abe O2 interatomic separation (*black*) and the Gal O2 – Trp93L Nε interaction indicating the interconversions between the Fab-like (*light blue*) and Fv-like (*pink*) conformations

mediates the interaction between two monosaccharide residues in the antigen, while in the Fab structure this water is absent (Bundle et al. 1994). In the absence of this water, two new hydrogen bonds are formed and one is broken.

15.4.1 Molecular Docking

Since docking experiments are normally performed without prior knowledge of bound water molecules, we chose to dock to the Fv structure, but with all waters removed. The docking should either predict a ligand orientation as in the Fab complex (as might be expected, since the Fab complex lacks a water-mediated interaction), or as in the Fv, or a hybrid of the two.

The trisaccharide was docked to the Fv fragment using Autodock, following reported protocols (Kadirvelraj et al. 2006), allowing all inter-glycosidic and hydroxyl torsion angles full rotational freedom. The docking predicted a hybrid orientation between that of the Fv and Fab complexes (Table 15.6 and Fig. 15.7). Superimposition of the coordinates of the Fab, Fv, and docked complexes, indicated that the immunodominant Abe residue was positioned equivalently in each complex, as was the central Man residue. However, the orientation of the terminal Gal residue varied in each complex. It is noteworthy that the docked conformation of the ligand (dark blue in Fig. 15.7) is more similar to that in the Fab complex (light blue). Thus, the docking behaved as might be expected, given that, in the Fab structure, the bridging water between Gal O2 and Abe O2 is absent.

15.4.2 MD Refinement

The lowest energy pose from the docking (dark blue in Fig. 15.7) was then solvated and subjected to a 10 ns MD simulation. The interatomic interactions were monitored over the course of the trajectory and indicated a conformational interconversion (Fig. 15.7). Although the automated docking led to a hybrid conformation, between that of the Fv and Fab structures (Table 15.6), the MD simulation demonstrated that both conformations were populated at room temperature in an aqueous environment.

Analysis of the intermolecular interactions indicated that a Fab-like conformation was present for ~78% of the 10 ns timeframe; a Fv like conformation for 22%. In each case, as seen experimentally, the immunodominant Abe residue remained unaffected by these motions (Table 15.6). MD-refinement removed three false positive hydrogen bonds, predicted by the docking and allowed one to form that docking had missed. The overall data from the MD suggest an antigen whose immunodominant region is well defined, but that can populate at least two distinct conformations, which are both consistent with the two structures observed experimentally.

This system serves to illustrate the fact that automated docking can provide a medium resolution structure for carbohydrate – antibody interactions, but that subsequent MD simulations are able to significantly improve the accuracy of the

Table 15.6 Experimental and computed interatomic distances (Å) between the *Sp*B antigen and mAb Se155-4 with the water-mediated interactions highlighted in grey

Hydrogen bond	X-ray Fv[a]	X-ray Fab[b]	Docking[c] to Fv	MD of docked complex (10 ns)
Abe O2 – G98H N	2.8	2.7	2.9	2.9 ± 0.1, 100%
Abe O4 – W98L Nε	3.0	2.9	2.7	3.1 ± 0.2, 100%
Abe O4 – H35H Nε	3.3	3.5	2.8	3.5 ± 0.2 100%
Gal O2 – Abe O2	4.4	2.9	3.4	5.4 ± 0.3/3.1 ± 0.3
Gal O2 – W93L Nε	2.8	4.4	3.8	2.9 ± 0.1/4.6 ± 0.3
Gal O4 – W93L Nε	5.5	3.3	2.8	6.7 ± 0.5/3.1 ± 0.4
Gal O3 – H34L Nε	5.6	3.6	3.4	6.4 ± 0.4/3.6 ± 0.5
Man O4 – H97H Nδ	2.7	2.9	3.9 (fals negative)	3.2 ± 0.7, 100%
Man O4 – Abe O2	4.0	3.6	3.2 (false positive)	4.2 ± 0.3[d]
Gal O3 – W93L Nε	4.2	4.3	3.0 (false positive)	4.8 ± 0.4[d]
Gal O4 – N96L Oδ	3.6	3.8	2.7 (false positive)	5.2 ± 1.2[d]
False Negatives			**1**	**0**
False Positives			**3**	**0**

[a]1MFA (Zdanov et al. 1994)
[b]1MFD (Bundle et al. 1994). Exists in a water-mediated interaction
[c]In a typical docking run, a grid box with dimensions 30 × 30 × 30 Å and a grid point spacing of 0.375 Å was centered on the complementarity determining region with the ligand positioned initially at the center of the grid. Docking was performed with AutoDock 3.0.5 (Morris et al. 1998) employing the Solis and Wets local search method with a Lamarckian genetic selection algorithm (Solis and Wets 1981). The total number of docking runs was set to 150, while Autodock default values were utilized for all other parameters. The results for the lowest energy poses were selected for analysis
[d]No distances less than 3.2 Å were observed during the simulation

structures. We believe this approach offers much potential for application to this challenging area.

15.5 Example 4: Docking, MD, and Free Energy Simulations of Carbohydrate: Antibody Structures (the *SfY* – SYAJ6 Antibody System)

The *SfY* antigen was selected for analysis by docking, MD, and thermodynamic integration (TI) calculations because it is extremely well-characterized experimentally and represents an example of a co-crystal of a linear oligosaccharide antigen in a groove-like antibody combining site. Experimental crystal structures have been reported for the free Fab (Fab SYAJ6) (Vyas et al. 2002), as well as for complexes of the Fab with synthetic tri- and pentasaccharide analogs of the polysaccharide (Vyas et al. 2002). Additionally, accurate thermodynamic binding data have been reported for several deoxy derivatives of the pentasaccharide (Vyas et al. 2002), which may be employed in the validation of binding energy prediction methods.

15.5.1 Molecular Docking

Presented in Fig. 15.8 are the lowest energy structures from three docking analyses. As a positive control, we began by docking of the pentasaccharide to the Fab structure extracted from the Fab – pentasaccharide crystal structure (α-L-Rha-(1→2)-α-L-Rha-(1→3)-α-L-Rha-(1→3)-β-D-GlcNAc-(1→2)-α-L-Rha) (panel A). Since the protein surface is ideally disposed to receive the oligosaccharide in that structure, the performance of the docking depends only on the sampling of the oligosaccharide conformational states and the energy function. Autodock was selected because it has been shown to perform well on carbohydrate – protein complexes (Laederach and Reilly 2002).

The results of docking the *Sf*Y pentasaccharide to the crystal structure of the free Fab are shown in Fig. 15.8, panel B. The influence of variations in protein side chain orientations on the overall structure is evident, although not profound. In the final experiment (panel C), a model for the Fab was employed that was generated by homology modeling. This is the worst-case, or most optimistic scenario, since the protein structure may include not only non-optimal side chain orientations, but also inaccurate back bone conformations. While the docked oligosaccharide still made contacts with each of the CDR loops, it was displaced and disordered internally, relative to the experimental structure.

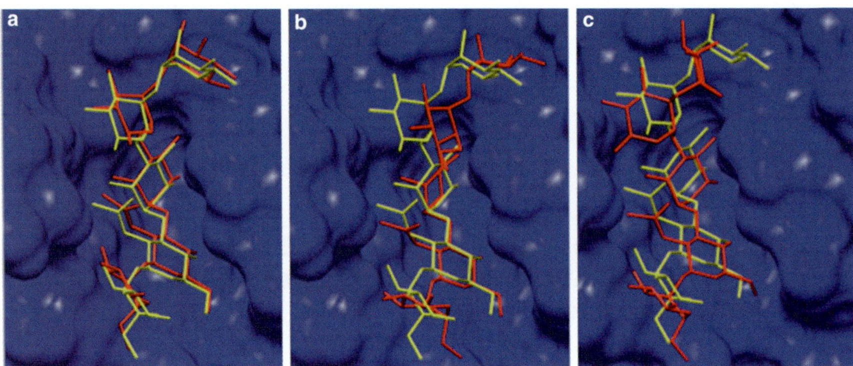

Fig. 15.8 Results from three docking scenarios: (**a**) employing Fab from Fab – oligosaccharide crystal structure (PDB id 1M7I (Vyas, Vyas et al. 2002)); (**b**) Fab from crystal structure of free Fab (PDB id 1 M71 (Vyas, Vyas et al. 2002)); (**c**) homology modeled Fab, generated as described in (Dyekjaer and Woods 2006) using PDB id 1MNU (van den Elsen et al. 1999) for CDR L1 and L2, 1KEG (Yokoyama et al. 2000) for CDR L3; all CDRs in the VH domain were taken from PDB id 1AXT (Barbas et al. 1997). The experimental alignment of the oligosaccharide is presented in *yellow*, the theoretical in *red*

15.5.2 MD Refinement

Each of the docked structures presented in Fig. 15.8 was then subjected to a 10 ns explicitly solvated MD simulation to determine whether the MD refinement would improve the docked orientations. No restraints were applied to either the protein side chains or the ligand during the MD. In all cases, the structures improved, with the most significant improvement seen for the homology modeled Fab complex. When docked to the crystal structure of the free Fab, docking correctly formed only two of the eight intermolecular hydrogen bonds and predicted two incorrect hydrogen bonds (false positives) (see Table 15.7).

A relatively short MD refinement removed the false positives and led to the correct prediction of 6/8 interactions. Notably, with the exception of one hydrogen

Table 15.7 Hydrogen bond distances (Å) in complexes resulting from docking of the pentasaccharide to the crystal structure of the free Fab or to the homology model, followed by MD refinement

Hydrogen bonds	X-ray (Co-complex)	Docking to free fab (after 10 ns MD)	Docking to homology model of fab (after 10 ns MD)
H27 Nε – Rha5 O3	3.21	–[a]	–
		2.9 ± 0.1 (99%)	3.1 ± 0.2 (96%)
Y32 Oγ – Rha2 O4	2.52	–	2.5
		3.2 ± 0.2 (55%)	–
W33 Nε – Rha1 O4	2.70	–	–
		3.2 ± 0.1 (53%)	–
E50 Oε – GlcNAc4 O4	2.81	–	3.3
		3.2 ± 0.2 (8%)	2.7 ± 0.1 (99%)
T91 O – GlcNAc4 N	2.68	3.0	–
		3.0 ± 0.1 (100%)	2.9 ± 0.2 (99%)
T91 Oγ – Rha3 O2	2.92	–	–
		–	–
A97 O – Rha2 O3	3.02	–	2.6
		2.7 ± 0.1 (100%)	3.0 ± 0.2 (34%)
G99 O – Rha3 O2	3.15	2.8	–
		2.9 ± 0.2 (100%)	3.2 ± 0.1 (56%)
Correctly predicted		**2/8 after Docking**	**3/8 after Docking**
		6/8 after MD	**5/8 after MD**
N31 O – Rha2 O4	–	3.0	–
		3.2 ± 0.2 (18%)	–
T92 O – Rha5 O3	–	2.4	–
		–	–
V98 O – Rha3 O2	–	–	2.9
		–	–
False positives		**2 after Docking**	**1 after Docking**
		0 after MD	**0 after MD**

[a]Dashes indicate the H-bond was not observed, based on a 3.2 Å cutoff

bond, the MD simulations initiated with the crystal structure of the complex effectively converged to that initiated from the complex docked to the free Fab.

It is significant that in the case of the relatively low-resolution structure resulting from docking to the homology modeled Fab, even a short MD refinement significantly improved the prediction of intermolecular hydrogen bonds, removing all false positives. It is notable that two hydrogen bonds are absent in the MD structure, but this did not cause the ligand to alter its position significantly (the average RMSD of the oligosaccharide was only 0.7 Å). The loss of some crystallographic hydrogen bonds in MD simulations of carbohydrate – protein complexes is common (Bryce et al. 2001). Several hydrogen bonds appear to lengthen, but nevertheless remain stable over the course of the simulations. For example, while the Tyr32 Oγ – Rha2 O4 hydrogen bond is only present 55% of the time, the average heavy atom separation is stable at 3.5 ± 0.4 Å. While this is obviously a weakened interaction, such long hydrogen bonds are the reason some studies employ hydrogen bond cutoff values of as much as 3.5 Å (Bryce et al. 2001).

15.5.3 Free Energy Calculations

The relative binding energies for two synthetic deoxy oligosaccharides closely related to the native antigen were computed (Table 15.8 and Fig. 15.9). These oligosaccharides were selected because they represent two possible situations; that is, one binds better than the wild-type oligosaccharide (Rha2 2-OH→2-H), and one binds much worse (Rha3 4-OH→4-H). All TI calculations were performed sequentially over 12 values of λ (each step initiated with velocities and coordinates of preceding). They were performed in two steps: (1→2) Charge mutation followed by (2→3) van der Waals and valence property mutation (see Table 15.8 for methodological details).

Table 15.8 Application of TI calculations[a] to the prediction of relative binding free energies of antigenic oligosaccharides from *Sf*Y to mAb SYAJ6

Mutation	ΔG in water	ΔG in protein	**Net affinity (ΔΔG)**
Rha2 2-OH→2-H (Introduction of hydrophobic interactions)			
Coulomb	−46.78 ± 0.4	−48.66 ± 0.3	−1.88 ± 0.5
van der Waals	3.74 ± 0.2	4.48 ± 0.2	0.74 ± 0.3
ΔG Computed	−43.04 ± 0.4	−44.18 ± 0.4	**−1.1 ± 0.6**
Experiment[b]			**−1.6**
Rha3 4-OH→4-H (Loss of a direct H-bond)			
Coulomb	−18.30 ± 0.3	−16.40 ± 0.4	1.90 ± 0.5
van der Waals	2.00 ± 0.3	2.94 ± 0.3	0.94 ± 0.4
ΔG Computed	−16.30 ± 0.4	−13.46 ± 0.5	**2.8 ± 0.6**
Experiment[b]			**Inactive, ΔΔG >> 0**

[a]The perturbations involving the ligand, both free and bound, were performed with electrostatics decoupled from van der Waals and internal properties as described in (Kadirvelraj et al. 2006) with integration using 12 point quadrature, for a total of 5.76 ns for each mutation cycle.
[b]Vyas et al. (2002)

Fig. 15.9 Amino acid color scheme: Positive charge (*blue*), negative (*red*), polar neutral (*white*), aliphatic (*green*), aromatic (*yellow*). The deoxy position in the ligand is indicated by a *pink* ball

Because we were able to employ the crystal structure of the complex in these calculations they provide an optimal situation for establishing the accuracy of the GLYCAM and AMBER force fields and the TI protocols. Under these conditions, the results presented in Table 15.8 provide encouraging support for the use of TI calculations to probe the effects of chemical modifications on antigenicity. Additionally, as seen from the data in Table 15.6, the MD-refined co-crystal structure employed in these TI calculations is effectively equivalent to the MD-refined structure generated by docking of the antigen to the free Fab. Thus, the TI calculations may prove useful in systems that require the antigen first to be docked to the antibody.

Conclusions

When comparing computational and experimental data sets, both theoreticians and experimentalists should be aware that each other's data inevitably contains errors, whether related to precision or accuracy, and it is critical to have some estimate of the statistical reliability of all reported values. In many comparisons it is preferable to derive the experimental observable from the theoretical data, rather than derive a 3D model from the experimental data. For example, NMR data is often too sparse in flexible molecules to be sufficient to derive a well-defined 3D structure, however the theoretical simulations should be consistent with the experimental data (Yongye et al. 2008). With the continued growth of the performance:cost ratio for computers, there is little justification for reporting theoretical data from simulations that have not reached an appropriate level of convergence for the timescale of the experimentally-observed phenomena.

Increasingly, computational chemists are adopting the strategy of including positive and negative controls in MD simulations and free energy calculations. In the case of antigenicities, these may take the case of comparing ligands known to bind as well as those known not to bind (Ford et al. 2003; Kadirvelraj et al. 2006). Such comparisons can greatly bolster confidence in the results when the computational method is employed predictively, and are highly effective at identifying anecdotal results.

Unlike polypeptides, oligosaccharides frequently exist as non-linear polymers. This feature, combined with the configurational diversity associated with carbohydrate linkages prevents the use of sequence homology when predicting the 3D structures of oligosaccharides. In effect, every oligosaccharide must be treated as a unique case. Fortunately, and again in contrast to polypeptides, it is routinely possible to generate qualitatively likely 3D structures for oligosaccharides by imposing established rules for linkage and ring conformation (Rao et al. 1998). However, such initial models are inadequate because they fail to capture the dynamic properties of these molecules. When multiple rotameric states are likely, such as for (1→6)-linkages, MD simulations provide a method for identifying the preferred states, and are often able to quantitatively reproduce their populations (Kirschner and Woods 2001; Gonzalez-Outeriño et al. 2005; Gonzalez-Outeiriño et al. 2006; Kirschner et al. 2007). The successes of such predictions are a testament to the power of computational simulations, but some challenging cases remain, including highly flexible furanosyl rings (Taha et al. 2010).

With regard to protein carbohydrate complexes, automated docking may be employed to predict the pose of the carbohydrate in the binding site, given a 3D structure for the protein. This is an extremely powerful technique in principle, however, in practice, the results are profoundly sensitive to the methodology as well as to the extent to which the carbohydrate induces conformational changes in the orientation of the protein side chains. Provided a reasonable pose has been generated by docking, MD simulations can significantly improve the accuracy of the predicted complex. Given an accurate protein carbohydrate complex, computational methods such as TI, may be employed to predict the effect of structural alterations on the affinity (Woods and Tessier 2010). The ability to rank ligands in order of affinity is essential in understanding the molecular basis for carbohydrate antigenicity, while the ability to determine the quantitative contributions to binding energy arising from modest chemical alterations in the hapten may ultimately guide the development of synthetic vaccines.

References

Anthony BF, Okada DM (1977) The emergence of Group B streptococci in infections of the newborn infant. Ann Rev Med 28:355–369

Barbas CF, Heine A, Zhong G, Hoffmann T, Gramatikova S, Björnestedt R, List B, Anderson J, Stura EA, Wilson IA, Lerner RA (1997) Immune versus natural selection: antibody aldolases with enzymic rates but broader scope. Science 278:2085–2092

Bryce RA, Hillier IH, Naismith JH (2001) Carbohydrate-protein recognition: molecular dynamics simulations and free energy analysis of oligosaccharide binding to concanavalin A. Biophys J 81:1373–1388

Bundle DR, Baumann H, Brisson JR, Gagne SM, Zdanov A, Cygler M (1994) Solution structure of a trisaccharide-antibody complex: comparison of NMR measurements with a crystal structure. Biochemistry 33:5183–5192

Case DA, Cheatham TE III, Darden T, Gohlke H, Luo R, Merz KM Jr, Onufriev A, Simmerling C, Wang B, Woods R (2005) The AMBER biomolecular simulation programs. J Comput Chem 26:1668–1688

Devi SJN, Robbins JB, Schneerson R (1991) Antibodies to poly[(2→8)-α-N-acetylneuraminic acid] and poly[(2→9)-α-N-acetylneuraminic acid] are elicited by immunization of mice with *Escherichia coli* K92 conjugates: Potential vaccines for groups B and C meningococci and *E. coli* K1. Proc Natl Acad Sci USA 88:7175–7179

Dillon HC, Khare S, Gray BM (1987) Group B streptococcal carriage and disease: a 6 year prospective study. J Pediatr 110:31–36

Dwek RA (1996) Glycobiology: toward understanding the function of sugars. Chem Rev 96:683–720

Dyekjaer JD, Woods RJ (2006) Predicting the 3D structures of anti-carbohydrate antibodies: combining comparative modeling and MD simulations. In: Vliegenthart JFG, Woods RJ (eds) NMR spectroscopy and computer modeling of carbohydrates: recent advances, vol 930. American Chemical Society, Washington, D.C, p 18

Egan ML, Pritchard DG, Dillon HC Jr, Gray MB (1983) Protection of mice from experimental infection with Type III Group B *Streptococcus* using monoclonal antibodies. J Exp Med 158:1006–1011

Evans SV, Sigurskjold BW, Jennings HJ, Brisson JR, To R, Altman E, Frosch M, Weisgerber C, Kratzin H (1995) Evidence for the extended helical nature of polysaccharide epitopes. The 2.8 Å resolution structure and thermodynamics of ligand binding of an antigen binding fragment specific for α-(2–8)-Polysialic acid. Biochemistry 34:6737–6744

Fadda E, Woods RJ (2010) Molecular simulations of carbohydrates and protein–carbohydrate interactions: motivation, issues and prospects. Drug Discov Today 15:596

Finne J, Leinonen M, Mäkelä HP (1983) Antigenic similarities between brain components and bacteria causing meningitis – implications for vaccine development and pathogenesis. Lancet 2:355–357

Finne J, Mäkelä PH (1985) Cleavage of the polysialosyl units of brain glycoproteins by a bacteriophage endosialidase – involvement of a long oligosaccharide segment in molecular-interactions of polysialic acid. J Biol Chem 260:1265–1270

Ford MG, Weimar T, Köhli T, Woods RJ (2003) Molecular dynamics simulations of Galectin-1-oligosaccharide complexes reveal the molecular basis for ligand diversity. PROTEINS: Struct Funct Genet 53:229–240

Gonzalez-Outeriño J, Kadirvelraj R, Woods RJ (2005) Structural elucidation of type III group B *Streptococcus* capsular polysaccharide using molecular dynamics simulations: the role of sialic acid. Carbohydr Res 340:1007–1018

Gonzalez-Outeiriño J, Kirschner KN, Thobhani S, Woods RJ (2006) Reconciling solvent effects on rotamer populations in carbohydrates: a joint MD and NMR analysis. Can J Chem 84:569–579

Gouda H, Kuntz ID, Case DA, Kollmann PA (2003) Free energy calculations for theophylline binding to an RNA aptamer: comparison of MM-PBSA and thermodynamic integration methods. Biopolymers 68:16–34

Henderson TJ, Venable R, Egan W (2003) Conformational flexibility of the group B meningococcal polysaccharide in solution. J Am Chem Soc 125:2930–2939

Jennings HJ, Roy R, Gamian A (1986) Induction of meningococcal group-B polysaccharide-specific IgG antibodies in mice by using an N-propionylated-B polysaccharide-tetanus toxoid conjugate vaccine. J Immunol 137:1708–1713

Jennings H (1992) Further approaches for optimizing polysaccharide-protein conjugate vaccines for prevention of invasive bacterial disease. J Infect Dis 165:156–159

Jones C (1998) Capsular polysaccharides from *Neisseria meningitidis* and *Streptococcus pneumoniae*. Carbohydr Eur 21:10–16

Kabat EA, Liao J, Osserman EF, Gamian A, Michon F, Jennings HJ (1988) The epitope associated with the binding of the capsular polysaccharide of the Group-B meningococcus and of *Escherichia coli* K1 to a human monoclonal macroglobulin, IgM nov. J Exp Med 168:699–711

Kadirvelraj R, Gonzalez-Outeriño J, Foley BL, Beckham ML, Jennings HJ, Foote S, Ford MG, Woods RJ (2006) Understanding the bacterial polysaccharide antigenicity of *Streptococcus agalactiae* versus *Streptococcus pneumoniae*. Proc Natl Acad Sci USA 103:8149–8154

Kadirvelraj R, Foley BL, Dyekjaer JD, Woods RJ (2008) Involvement of water in carbohydrate-protein binding: Concanavalin A revisited. J Am Chem Soc 130:16933–16942

Kirschner KN, Woods RJ (2001) Solvent interactions determine carbohydrate conformation. Proc Natl Acad Sci USA 98:10541–10545

Kirschner KN, Yongye AB, Tschampel SM, González-Outeiriño J, Daniels CR, Foley BL, Woods J (2007) GLYCAM06: a generalizable biomolecular force field. Carbohydrates. J Comput Chem 29:622–655

Krug LM, Ragupathi G, Hood C, Kris MG, Miller AV, Allen JR, Keding SJ, Danishefsky SJ, Gomez J, Tyson L, Pizzo B, Baez V, Livingston PO (2004) Vaccination of small cell lung cancer patients with polysialic acid or N-propionylated polysialic acid conjugated to keyhole limpet hemocyanin. Clin Cancer Res 10:916–923

Laederach A, Reilly PJ (2002) Specific empirical free energy function for automated docking of carbohydrates to proteins. J Comp Chem 24:1748–1757

Liu T, Guo Z, Yang Q, Subash S, Jennings HJ (2000) Biochemical engineering of surface α2–8 polysialic acid for immunotargeting tumor cells. J Biol Chem 275:32832–32836

Michon F, Brisson J-R, Jennings HJ (1987) Conformational differences between linear α(2-8)-linked homosialooligosaccharides and the epitope of the group B meningococcal polysaccharide. Biochemistry 26:8399–8405

Morris GM, Goodsell DS, Halliday RS, Huey R, Hart WE, Belew RK, Olson AJ (1998) Automated docking using a Lamarckian genetic algorithm and empirical binding free energy function. J Comput Chem 19:1639–1662

Pathiaseril A, Woods RJ (2000) Relative energies of binding for antibody-carbohydrate-antigen complexes computed from free-energy simulations. J Am Chem Soc 122:331–338

Paula S, Monson N, Ball WJ Jr (2005) Molecular modeling of cardiac glycoside binding by the human sequence monoclonal antibody 1B3. Proteins 60:382–391

Poppe L, van Halbeek H (1991) Nuclear magnetic resonance of hydroxyl and amido protons of oligosaccharides in aqueous solution: evidence for a strong intramolecular hydrogen bond in sialic acid residues. J Am Chem Soc 113:363–365

Rao VSR, Qasba PK et al (1998) Conformation of carbohydrates. Harwood Academic, Amsterdam

Regenmortel MHV (1989) The concept and operational definition of protein epitopes. Phil Trans R Soc Lond B 323:461–466

Sharon N, Lis H (1993) Carbohydrates in cell recognition. Sci Am 268:82–89

Taha HA, Castillo N, Sears DN, Wasylishen RE, Lowary TL, Roy PN (2010) Conformational analysis of arabinofuranosides: prediction of 3JH, H using MD simulations with DFT-derived spin-spin coupling profiles. J Chem Theory Comput 6:212–222

van den Elsen J, Vandeputte-Rutten L, Kroon J, Gros P (1999) Bactericidal antibody recognition of meningococcal PorA by induced fit. Comparison of liganded and unliganded Fab structures. J Biol Chem 274:1495–1501

Varki A (1993) Biological roles of oligosaccharides: all of the theories are correct. Glycobiology 3:97–130

Vliegenhart JFG, Woods RJ (eds) (2006) NMR spectroscopy and computer modeling of carbohydrates: recent advances, ACS symposium series. American Chemical Society, Washington, DC

Vyas NK, Vyas MN, Chervenak MC, Johnson MA, Pinto BM, Bundle DR, Quiocho FA (2002) Molecular recognition of oligosaccharide epitopes by a monoclonal Fab specific for *Shigella flexneri* Y Lipopolysaccharide: x-ray structures and thermodynamics. Biochemistry 41:13575–13586

Weimar T, Woods RJ (2002) Combining NMR and simulation methods in oligosaccharide conformational analysis. In: Jiménez-Barbero J (ed) NMR of glycoconjugates. Wiley, Weinheim, pp 111–144

Wessels MR, Pozsgay V, Kasper DL, Jennings HJ (1987) Structure and immunochemistry of an oligosaccharide repeating unit of the capsular polysaccharide of type III group B *Streptococcus*. J Biol Chem 262:8262–8267

Wolfe S, Whangbo M-H, Mitchell DJ (1979) On the magnitudes and origins of the "anomeric effects", "exoanomeric effects", "reverse anomeric effects", and C-X and C-Y bond lengths in XCH_2YH molecules. Carbohydr Res 69:1–26

Woods RJ, Tessier MB (2010) Computational glycoscience: characterizing the spatial and temporal properties of glycans and glycan–protein complexes. Curr Opin Struct Biol 20:575–583

Yokoyama H, Mizutani R, Satow Y, Komatsu Y, Ohtsuka E, Nikaido O (2000) Crystal structure of the 64 M-2 antibody Fab fragment in complex with a DNA dT(6–4)T photoproduct formed by ultraviolet radiation. J Mol Biol 299(3):711–723

Yongye AB, Foley BL, Woods RJ (2008a) On achieving experimental accuracy from molecular dynamics simulations of flexible molecules: aqueous glycerol. J Phys Chem A 112(12): 2634–2639

Yongye AB, Gonzales Outeriño J, Glushka J, Schultheis V, Woods RJ (2008b) The conformational properties of methyl α-(2,8)-di/trisialosides and their *N*-acyl analogs: implications for Anti-*Neisseria meningitidis* B vaccine design. Biochemistry 47(47):12493–12514

Zdanov A, Li Y, Bundle DR, Deng S-J, MacKenzie CR, Narang SA, Young NM, Cygler M (1994) Structure of a single-chain antibody variable domain (Fv) fragment complexed with a carbohydrate antigen a 1.7-Å resolution. Proc Natl Acad Sci USA 91:6423–6427

Zou W, MacKenzie R, Therien L, Hirama T, Yang QL, Gidney MA, Jennings HJ (1999) Conformational epitope of the type III group B *Streptococcus* capsular polysaccharide. J Immunol 163(2):820–825

The Interaction of Saccharides with Antibodies. A 3D View by Using NMR

16

Filipa Marcelo, F. Javier Cañada, and Jesús Jiménez-Barbero

16.1 Introduction

The study of molecular recognition phenomena has occupied the minds and the hearts of many scientists during the last decades (Rebek 2009). The understanding of these events is of paramount importance to achieve a better knowledge of the living systems. Nowadays, it is clear that carbohydrates play a key role in a variety of biological processes (Varki et al. 1999). They appear in all cells, in different forms, and they are implicated in many cellular processes, including cell-cell recognition, cellular transport, and adhesion. Carbohydrate-mediated interactions are also concerned in diverse disease mechanisms, especially in the immune system (Avci and Kasper 2010; Engering et al. 2002). Bacteria and viruses contain unique carbohydrates on their surfaces, and these saccharide molecules are often those first recognized by the human immune system. Therefore, carbohydrates would, in theory, be good vaccine candidates educating the immune system to create antibodies (Johnson and Pinto 2008). Additionally to their presence on the surfaces of microbial pathogens, carbohydrates cover the wall of mammalian cells, and altered glycosylation takes place frequently in cancer (Dube and Bertozzi 2005). Certain oligosaccharides are characteristically expressed on cancerous cells and represent excellent targets for anticancer vaccines or drugs (Dube et al. 2006). However, the successful use of carbohydrates as vaccines has been limited for many years due to the weak immunogenic effects usually restricted to IgM antibody response, particularly a T-independent cell response without memory function, and poor response in infants (Lindberg 1999; Alexander et al. 2000). An efficient strategy to overcome these problems has focused on the design of glycoconjugate vaccines, in which an appropriate glycan is covalently attached to a carrier protein or peptide. This approach has proved to be the most effective, since it may induce T-cell responses

F. Marcelo • F.J. Cañada • J. Jiménez-Barbero (✉)
Chemical and Physical Biology, CIB-CSIC, Ramiro de Maeztu 9, 28040 Madrid, Spain
e-mail: jjbarbero@cib.csic.es

P. Kosma and S. Müller-Loennies (eds.), *Anticarbohydrate Antibodies*,
DOI 10.1007/978-3-7091-0870-3_16, © Springer-Verlag/Wien 2012

giving a protective immunity against a wide range of bacterial pathogens, which express a glycocalyx and where antibodies directed against cell surface saccharides are protective (Roy 2008). An alternative strategy consists in the use of peptides as sugar mimetics either to replace the carbohydrate molecule as a vaccine, or to supplement it in order to boost the immune response (Westerink et al. 1995; Pashov et al. 2005; Bolesta et al. 2005; Harris et al. 1997). The study of how complex carbohydrates interact with antibodies represents an important step toward the design of carbohydrate-based vaccines (Serruto and Rappuoli 2006). From the interaction viewpoint, NMR spectroscopy, together with X-ray crystallography, is the technique of choice to disclose, at the molecular level, the interactions between carbohydrates and their protein receptors. Nevertheless, the Ka values of carbohydrate antigens to antibodies are typically weak, in the 10^2–10^6 M^{-1} range, making crystallization of antibody–carbohydrate complexes for use in X-ray crystallography difficult (DeMarco and Woods 2008). This issue can be circumvented with the use of NMR that proved to be extremely useful to obtain new insights into the solution structure and the dynamics of a ligand-antibody complex (Johnson and Pinto 2004). However, due to the intrinsic complexity and flexibility of glycoconjugates, a multidisciplinary strategy combining NMR parameters with molecular modeling protocols should be followed in order to access this information (Poveda and Jiménez-Barbero 1998). In this context the present review focuses on the application of NMR methods to characterize the main structural features that govern the recognition of carbohydrates by antibodies.

16.2 NMR Methods

Different NMR-based approaches may be employed to investigate ligand-receptor interactions, including carbohydrate-antibody recognition events. The method of choice depends on the particular problem and the required structural information. Generally speaking, two global different approaches may be envisaged, ligand-based or receptor-based. In the first one, changes in the NMR parameters of the ligand when passing from the free to the bound state are followed up to disentangle the recognition process form the point of view of the ligand. Alternatively, if the receptor size permits the NMR-based analysis of all or part of their resonance signals can be performed. Thus, the variations in different NMR parameters of the receptor may be employed to deduce key features of the interaction from the perspective of the receptor, including information on the residues directly involved in the interaction. In the latter case, isotopic labeling is required to make specific resonance assignments. From the sugar ligand's perspective, it is well known that NMR measurements are able to detect binding, to elucidate the bound conformation of the ligand, to establish its binding epitope, and to provide dynamic information (Jiménez-Barbero et al. 1999). In fact, in the last decade, NMR spectroscopy has become fundamental in the drug discovery and drug design processes. Logical applications of the established methods have been applied to screen carbohydrate libraries for finding good binders to protein receptors (Kogelberg et al. 2003; Ribeiro et al. 2010). Among the NMR methods currently available to analyze interactions, a combination of transferred NOE (TR-NOESY) (Ni and Zhu 1994) and saturation transfer difference (STD-NMR) (Mayer and Meyer 1999; Mayer and Meyer 2001) experiments have been extensively employed to study the conformations of carbohydrates bound to antibodies and to define their interacting epitopes (Rademacher et al. 2007; Herfurth et al. 2005; Clément et al. 2006; Maaheimo et al. 2000).

From the receptor's viewpoint, antibodies are usually very large macromolecules. Therefore, to gain detailed structural information of a ligand-antibody complex by NMR represents a real challenge. Despite the recent advances in NMR methodology and stable isotope labeling protocols, few examples can be found involving chemical shift perturbation analysis of the resonances of an antibody domain upon oligosaccharide addition (Takahashi et al. 1991). Further detailed information about this methodology has been published in a recent review (Yamaguchi and Kato 2010).

16.2.1 Different NMR Methods to Analyse Sugar-Antibody Interactions: A Brief Description

16.2.1.1 Ligand-Based Methods

TR-NOESY

When a ligand is in a fast chemical exchange between its free and receptor-bound state, its NMR parameters are the weighted average between both states. Therefore, it is possible to detect ligand binding to receptors based on changes in the motion, orientation and diffusion properties of the ligands when passing from being free in solution to being recognized by a macromolecule. NOE is a key parameter to deduce molecular conformations in solution, which depends on the internuclear distances between the nuclei under observation, and on the time scale of motion of the corresponding molecule. It is well known that NOE measurements can be used to estimate distances between protons, and thus, to deduce the conformation of a ligand. If a carbohydrate reversibly binds to a large molecular weight receptor, like an antibody, the observed NOEs for the ligand resonances are averaged between those of the free and bound states. In contrast to the small positive NOE normally found for a small ligand when free in solution, relaxation and NOEs, in the bound state, are governed by the correlation time of the huge receptor, and large negative NOEs are expected (Jiménez-Barbero and Peters 2002). For a ligand exchanging between its free and antibody-bound states, it is possible to find experimental conditions in which the latter dominates the observed NOE, which are dubbed trNOEs for the free-bound chemical exchange system (Fig. 16.1). Then, the interpretation of the NOE information allows to deduce the bound conformation of the ligand. An experimental complication inherent to transferred NOE measurements is related to spin diffusion effects that may arise from indirect interactions between spins. As a result, NOE signals may appear between two protons, which are not actually close in space, but close to one or more counterparts within the ligand or at

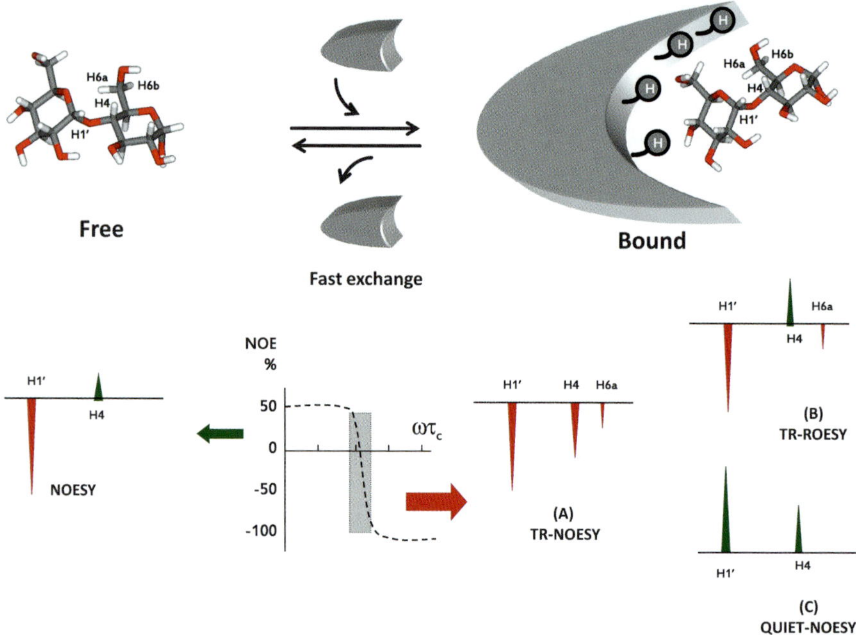

Fig. 16.1 *Left*: 1D NOESY spectrum of the interglycosidic NOE between H1′ (negative sign) and H4 (positive sign) of maltose in the free state. *Center*: representation of NOE curve in function of correlation time (τc) and magnetic field (ω). *Right*: (**A**) 1D TR-NOESY spectrum showing negative trNOE contacts between H1′ and H4 and H6a; (**B**) 1D TR-ROESY spectrum showing a true (positive) trROE cross-peak with H4 and a negative one for H6a; (**C**) 1D QUIET-NOESY showing a cross-peak between H1′ and H4 (both signals are positive), but no cross-peak with H6a

the receptor. These spin-diffusion mediated NOEs may lead to interpretation errors in the analysis of the ligand bound conformation, as exemplified in the analysis of the conformation of a fluorinated disaccharide to its specific antibody (Glaudemans et al. 1990). The first conclusions on the bound conformation had to be corrected later by using an alternative approach, called TR-ROESY (Arepalli et al. 1995). In a TR-ROESY experiment, direct NOE effects have positive sign while indirect NOEs display negative signs (Fig. 16.1). Hence, the application of this experiment allows to discriminate direct and indirect effects.

As key example of this application, Milton and Bundle combined TR-NOESY and TR-ROESY experiments with modeling data to investigate the conformation of a *Salmonella*-type oligosaccharide complexed to the antibody Se155-4 (Milton and Bundle 1998). This antibody recognized the repeating unit of the *Salmonella* serogroup B O antigen [3-α-D-Gal*p*(1→2)[α-D-Abe*p*(1→3)]α-D-Man*p*(1→4)α-L-Rha*p*(1→]. The conformation of a *Salmonella*-type pentasaccharide in the bound state was deduced from TR-NOESY, and the cross-peaks that arise from spin diffusion were distinguished by the acquisition of a TR-ROESY. Interestingly, the authors were able to show that the monoclonal antibody (mAb) selects one high-energy conformation of the α-D-Man*p*(1→4)α-L-Rha*p* glycosidic linkage (see chapter 1).

Nevertheless, sometimes the TR-NOESY/TR-ROESY combination is not sufficient to rule out spin diffusion. An alternative strategy consists in selective elimination of certain spins from relaxation pathways during the mixing time of a TR-NOESY experiment (Macura et al. 1992). For this purpose, NMR experiments have been developed, such as MINSY (Mixing Irradiation during NOESY) and QUIET-NOESY (Quenching of Undesirable External Trouble in NOESY) experiments (Massefski and Redfield 1988; Zwahlen et al. 1994; Vincent et al. 1996). While in MINSY experiments the spins suspected to be involved in spin diffusion pathways are removed by saturation using a low-power pulse, in QUIET-NOESY a double or multiple selective shaped 180° pulses during the NOESY mixing time are applied. In other words, both experiments permit to eliminate all indirect dipolar interactions only leaving those cross-peaks that correspond to the direct NOE effects (Fig. 16.1).

Indeed, Peters and co-workers have illustrated that a careful examination of spin diffusion effects should be considered when bioactive conformations of carbohydrates are analysed (Haselhorst et al. 1999). As leading example, TR-NOESY, TR-ROESY, QUIET-TR-NOESY and MINSY experiments have been used to disclose the bound conformations of a synthetic disaccharide, αKdo(2→4)α Kdo(2→O)-allyl (**1**) (Fig. 16.2), present on the surface of Gram-negative bacteria belonging to the family *Chlamydiaceae*, to the two mAb S25-2 and S23-24.

Two major conformations of the disaccharide (A and B) are present in the free state (Fig. 16.3a, b). Fittingly, the TR-NOESY of disaccharide **1** in the presence of mAb S25-2 (Fig. 16.2b) revealed a completely different NOE pattern than that observed in aqueous solution in the absence of the antibody (Fig. 16.2a). The combination of the TR-NOESY data with those obtained from TR-ROESY spectra permitted to postulate the existence of a conformation close to minimum B. However, the subsequent analysis of the MINSY and QUIET-TR-NOESY experiments demonstrated that disaccharide **1** adopts a different conformation (C) upon binding to the S25-2 antibody (Fig. 16.3c, d). This conformer is not populated, at least in a detectable amount, in the free state in aqueous solution. The bound state conformation of disaccharide **1** was also investigated in the presence of mAb S23-24. Interestingly, in this case, the TR-NOESY data was very similar to those obtained in aqueous solution (Fig. 16.2c). Indeed, the mAb S23-24 bound conformation of **1** is closely related to conformer A, which is the most populated in the free state.

In the end, this work points out the remarkable flexibility of carbohydrate molecules, which are able to bind in different conformations, depending on the architectures of the receptor's binding sites and the occurring interactions.

STD-NMR

A related technique, but now employing inter-instead of intramolecular NOE transfer, is the saturation transfer difference (STD NMR) experiment (Fig. 16.4). In this method, two 1D-NMR spectra are recorded, with and without selective saturation of the receptor (antibody) protons. Selective saturation of the protein

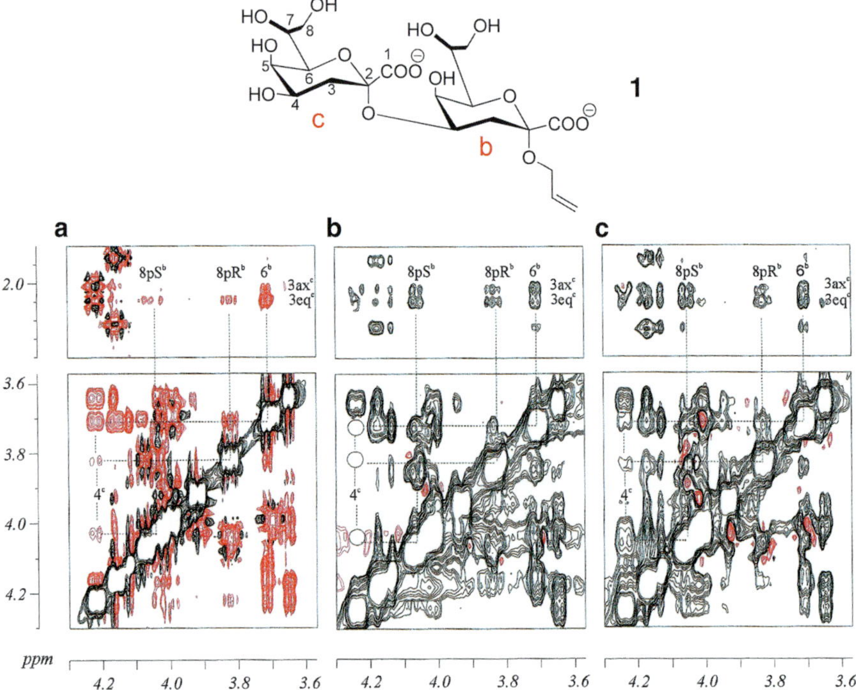

Fig. 16.2 Disaccharide α-Kdo-(2→4)-α-Kdo(2→O)-allyl (**1**); 2D NOESY and 2D TR-NOESY spectra of **1** (310 K, 500 MHz): (**a**) aqueous solution, (**b**) in the presence of mAb S25-2, and (**c**) in the presence of mAb S23-24. Mixing times were (**a**) 900, (**b**) 150, and (**c**) 150 ms. Positive contours are *red*, and negative contours are *black* (Spectra taken from: Peters T. and co-workers; 1999 Copyright © 1999 American Chemical Society, license number: 2624691381502)

results in a spread of magnetization throughout the entire protein by spin diffusion, reaching the binding site and, therefore, also affecting the nuclei of any interacting ligand. Thus, the intermolecular transfer of magnetization from the antibody to protons of the bound ligand lead to decreased ligand resonance intensities. This decrease can be better detected in a difference spectrum that results from subtraction of this spectrum from one recorded without saturation of the protein.

The only condition is that the selective saturation pulse should be set at frequencies at which no small ligand resonances are present. The STD technique may allow to identify a binding compound in a mixture, as well as to define the part of ligands which is in closer contact with the protein, the epitope (Meyer and Peters 2003). Therefore, STD-NMR has proved to be extremely useful to characterize the binding of carbohydrates to lectins, enzymes, and antibodies.

In a recent example, application of STD-NMR revealed the structural features of the interaction between a *Bacillus anthracis* tetrasaccharide and a mAb (Oberli et al. 2010). This tetrasaccharide contains three rhamnose residues and an atypical

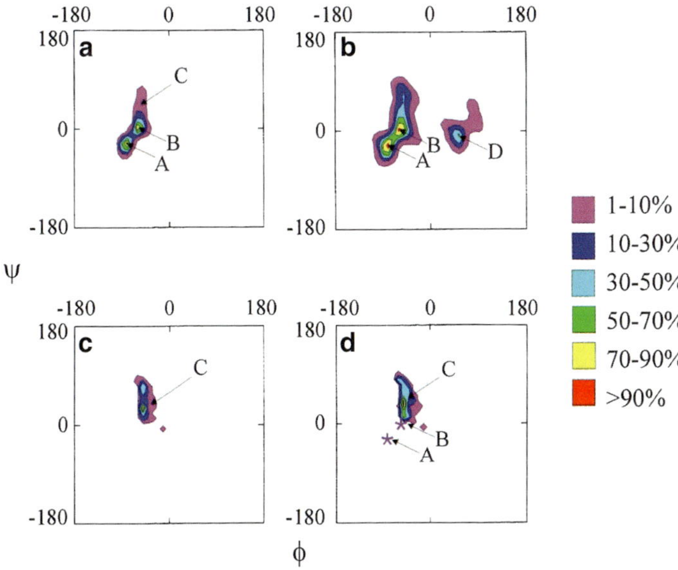

Fig. 16.3 Contour plots showing the relative population of conformational space around the (2→4)-glycosidic linkage in **1**. The versus maps were divided into bins of 10° in the ϕ and ψ directions, and the number of conformations in each bin was counted. Then, contour levels were calculated relative to the highest populated bin (global minimum). The contour levels are color-coded. Magenta represents 1–10%, *dark blue* 10–30%, *light blue* 30–50%, *green* 50–70%, *yellow* 70–90%, and *red* more than 90% of the number of conformations in the most populated bin. (**a**) MMC simulation at 600 K. (**b**) MMC simulation at 2000 K. (**c**) and (**d**) Possible conformations of 1 bound to mAb S25-2 (Plots taken from: Peters T. and co-workers; 1999 Copyright © 1999 American Chemical Society, license number: 2624691381502)

terminal saccharide, named anthrose, which after immunization of mice yielded mAb MTA1-3 (Tamborrini et al. 2006; Werz and Seeberger 2005). A multidisciplinary approach involving microarray screening, surface plasmon resonance (SPR) and STD-NMR led to structural insights into the molecular recognition of carbohydrate-antibody interactions. SPR and microarray analysis of various synthetic *Bacillus anthracis* tetrasaccharide type glycans demonstrated that the anthrose residue is essential for recognition. The STD results supported this conclusion and pointed out that tight-binding sites were found within the β-anthrose (1→3)Rha fragment (see Chap. 2).

Nevertheless, STD, as well as TR-NOESY experiment, presents certain tight kinetic requirements. In fact, they properly work when the off-rate is fast in the relaxation time scale of the ligand. Thus, for slow dissociation kinetics, these methods do not provide information, since the build up of STD or (NOE) effect is not transferred to the free state, due to fast relaxation in the binding site. Since slow dissociation rates are usually linked to the existence of high-affinity constants, STD and TR-NOESY methods are not useful for dissociation constants in the low micromolar or nanomolar ranges. In these cases, the methods of choice from the NMR point of view are those based on observation of the resonances of the receptor.

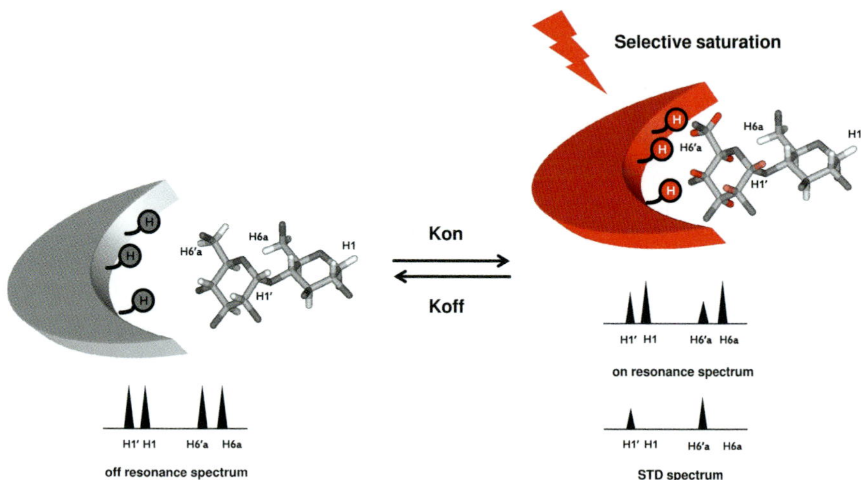

Fig. 16.4 STD-NMR experiment. Resonances of the protein are selectively saturated (represented by *red arrow*) and rapidly transferred by spin diffusion throughout the protein. Intermolecular NOE transfer results in a decrease in the signal intensity of ligand's protons in close contact contact with the protein (protons in red). Graphically in the example it is only shown H1′ and H6′a resonances. These changes are visibly detected after subtraction of the on- to off-resonance spectrum in order to obtain a difference spectrum called STD spectrum that allow an unambiguous epitope determination

In any case, the estimation of binding affinities can be derived by STD analysis. A detailed protocol has been recently reported towards this aim (Angulo et al. 2010).

The NMR spectra of carbohydrates are frequently difficult to analyze in a direct manner, due to overlapping signals. Therefore, combinations of STD with other NMR pulse sequences to provide concatenated techniques, such as STD-TOCSY and STD-HMQC have permitted the investigation of the interacting epitope of oligosaccharide ligands when bound to different antibodies. For instance, STD-1D-TOCSY was applied by Johnson and Pinto to the epitope mapping of oligosaccharides interacting with a mAb directed against the cell-wall polysaccharide of group A *Streptococcus* (GAS) (Johnson and Pinto 2002). A branched trisaccharide and a hexasaccharide were found to share the same epitope, and it was possible to detect that, besides the GlcNAc residue, also Rha moieties established contacts at the antibody binding site. The obtained results were in agreement with immunological studies that pointed out that at least a pentasaccharide is required for effective production of anti-GAS antibodies (Reimer et al. 1992).

Other Experiments

As mentioned above, STD-NMR and TR-NOESY have shown modest success for analyzing the structural features of high affinity ligands. Assuming that the association rate is under molecular diffusion control (k_{on} typically $10^8\ M^{-1}\ s^{-1}$), for the fast exchange condition to be held, systems with dissociation constants beyond 0.1 μM would be intrinsically difficult to be detected by these methods (Lundquist and Toone 2002).

However, other NMR methods might be employed. For ligand-protein systems, displaying an intermediate exchange rate (Kd $\approx$ 1 μM) in the chemical shift scale, the observed resonance frequencies of the signals do not shift when the concentration of the ligand is varied; however, they experience a significant loss in the signal intensity, due to line broadening (Gemmecker 1999). The large size of the ligand-protein complex produces an increase of the transverse relaxation rate, thus originating large line widths for the signal resonances. This methodology has been employed to monitor the interaction of MUC1 glycopeptides with the fragment antigen unity (FAB) of the anti-MUC1 mAb B27.29. ^{1}H NMR-monitored titrations of the glycopeptides, complemented with additional biochemical studies, showed a stronger interaction for the glycosylated versus the non-glycosylated peptide (Grinstead et al. 2002). The protons preferentially bound to the antibody binding pocket suffered a significant decrease of their signal intensities, relative to those far from the antibody recognition site.

In addition, the relative NMR resonance linewidths within a given molecule can be regarded as monitors of relaxation rates, and thus, molecular motions. On this basis, the analysis of the transverse relaxation rates can be very useful to disclose, for example, the dynamics of *N*-glycans of antibodies, as elegantly exemplified by Barb and Prestegard (2011). Earlier X-ray and NMR structural data had suggested that the α(1→6)Man linked branch of the *N*-glycan attached to IgG Fc fragments was firmly bound to the protein surface, whereas the α(1→3)Man linked branch was more dynamic (Deisenhofer 1981; Yamaguchi et al. 1998; Wormald et al. 1997). Nevertheless, the availability of both of these terminated glycans to several glycan-modified enzymes contradicts this hypothesis (Scallon 2007; Barb et al. 2009). Actually, Prestegard's group has recently demonstrated that both glycan branches (α(1→3)- and α(1→6)Man) are in fact accessible and highly dynamic. Selective isotope labeling of the *N*-glycans was required to unequivocally demonstrate the exchange of the α(1→6)Man-linked branch between a protein-bound and unbound state. Relaxation dispersion and temperature-dependent chemical shift perturbation experiments pointed out the existence of two distinct chemical environments for the α(1→6)Man linked branch so that a dynamic model of the glycans on the Fc fragment of IgG is more consistent with the enzymatic observations.

16.3 Case Studies

STD-NMR has also been employed to directly study the interaction between ganglio-oligosaccharides and autoantibodies in patient sera. It has been described that the sugar moieties on the bacterial cell surface often resemble those present on the host cell, and can lead to the production of antibodies that cross-react with epitopes common to pathogen and host leading to autoimmune diseases (Ang et al. 2004; Yuki 2005). In this context, immune-mediated neuropathologies, such as the Guillain–Barré and Fisher syndromes occur as a result of the presence of autoantibodies that target gangliosides, the glycosphingolipids predominantly found in the nervous system. Thus, STD-NMR, in combination with SPR, allowed the definition of the molecular interaction between purified IgG autoantibodies and gangliosides (Houliston et al. 2007). Interestingly, since a large amount of pure antibody can be difficult to get, STD-NMR also offers the possibility of direct detection of ganglioside-antibody interactions using untreated serum (Houliston et al. 2009). In this particular case, sera samples from two patients were collected. It was demonstrated, also employing immunological screening methods that the antibodies of one patient (P1) targeted two distinct gangliosides, GM1 {β-D-Gal*p*(1→3)-β-D-Gal*p*NAc(1→4)[αNeu5Ac (2→3)]-β-D-Gal*p*(1→4)-β-D-Glc*p*(1–1)Cer} and GM2 {β-D-Gal*p*NAc(1→4) [αNeu5Ac(2→3)]-β-D-Gal*p*(1→4)-β-D-Glc*p*(1–1)Cer}. On the other hand, antibodies of P2 were more reactive against GM1. The analysis of the STD-NMR response of GM1 when added to P1 and P2 sera indicated a similar binding mode of the ganglioside towards both antibodies. The data were interpreted in terms of a simultaneous interaction of two sequentially separated regions: the terminal β-D-Gal*p*(1→3)-β-D-Gal*p*NAc and the αNeu5Ac residue (Fig. 16.5).

Noteworthy, the STD-NMR signals from the αNeu5Ac residue of GM1 were much weaker for the interaction with P2- than for P1-antibodies. This fact permitted to interpret the absence of interaction between P2-antibody and GM2, since this ganglioside lacks the terminal Gal residue that presented the major STD response in the complex of GM1 with this P2 antibody. Moreover, the STD-NMR experiments revealed that the majority of the binding contacts between P1-antibodies and GM2 proceeded through the αNeu5Ac moiety. These results pointed out similar protocols that could be eventually relevant for diagnostic purposes.

As a paradigmatic case for the use of STD-NMR, to analyze the interactions of carbohydrates with antibodies has been recently described in the solution NMR study of the interactions of oligomannosides with the anti-HIV 2G12 antibody. It is

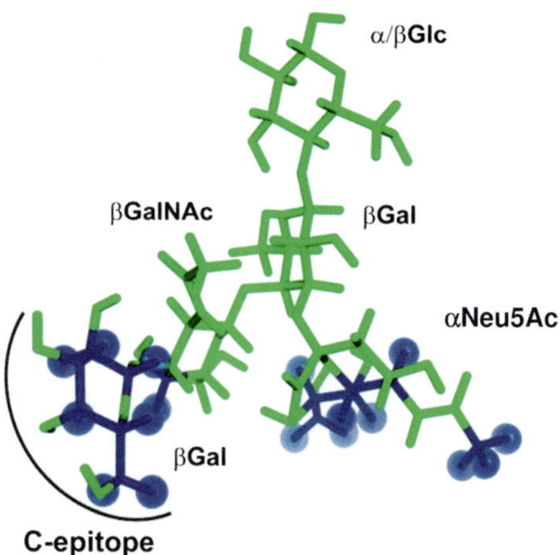

Fig. 16.5 Molecular representation of oligo-GM1. Protons shaded *blue* correspond to those saturated upon binding with P1 mAb. The C-epitope is almost identically targeted by both patient antibodies (Molecular representation taken from Jarrell HC and co-workers; 2009 Copyright © 2008 American Chemical Society, licence number: 2625250015413)

well known that the binding of HIV to its target cells is mediated by the exposed envelope gp120 glycoprotein, which is highly decorated by oligomannosides (Douek et al. 2009; Barin et al. 1985). In addition, it has been demonstrated that the 2G12 antibody, isolated from some infected individuals, recognizes these oligomannose clusters present at the surface of gp120 (Trkola et al. 1996; Sanders et al. 2002). Hence, the study of molecular recognition of these natural mannose glycans and related synthetic derivatives by the 2G12 antibody is extremely important for designing carbohydrate-based vaccines (see Chap. 6). Indeed, X-ray crystallographic structures of the Fab 2G12 bound to different mannosides are available (Calarese et al. 2003, 2005). In this context, the NMR-based work has explored the interactions of five synthetic oligomannose derivatives, structurally related to the natural $Man_9(GlcNAc)_2$ (Scheme 16.1), with the 2G12 antibody by means of STD-NMR and TR-NOESY (Enriquez-Navas et al. 2011) supported by

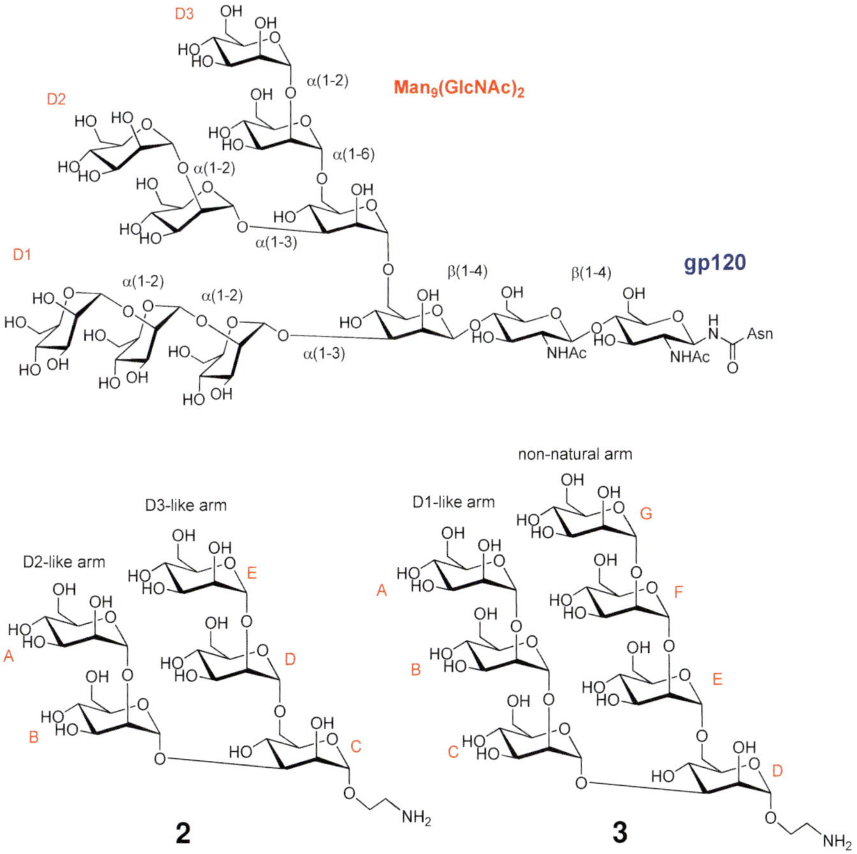

Scheme 16.1 Natural undecasaccharide $Man_9(GlcNAc)_2$ present in the HIV envelope glycoprotein gp120 and its structural relative mannosides, the branched penta- (**2**) and heptamannoside (**3**)

full-matrix relaxation calculations using the CORCEMA-ST program (Jayalakshmi and Krishna 2002, 2004).

The authors demonstrated that the linear oligosaccharides present the same single binding mode, where the non reducing terminal disaccharide [αMan (1 → 2)αMan] makes the closest contacts with the antibody. Theoretical STD-NMR signal intensities from crystal structures of 2G12/dimannoside and 2G12/ tetramannoside (D1-like) obtained using CORCEMA-ST showed a very good agreement between STD-NMR results in solution and the crystallography models. In contrast, for the branched mannoside **2,** the solution NMR data revealed two alternative binding modes, whereas the X-ray study described a single binding mode, in which the D3-arm binds to the antibody and the D2-arm is solvent exposed. The inconsistency between the solution state STD-NMR data and the single binding mode determined by X-ray (D3-bound) was quantitatively confirmed using CORCEMA-ST. In fact, only when the CORCEMA analysis included both bound conformations as a simple sum of STD-NMR signal intensities of the D3-and D2-bound conformations, the experimental data could be explained (Fig. 16.6). Moreover, an unequivocally outcome was provided by TR-NOESY. Intermolecular NOEs, between both anomeric protons of both A and E mannose rings and the aliphatic amino acid side chain region of 2G12 were observed, indicating the interaction of these residues with the antibody (Fig. 16.6). Remarkably, in the case of the branched oligomannoside analogue **3** the antibody preferentially recognized the D1-arm, although the same trisaccharide motif is present in both arms.

Fittingly, STD-based titrations showed that the branched oligosaccharides **2** and **3** presented lower affinity constants than linear ligands (D1-like tri- and tetramannoside). From all the obtained data, it was suggested that the αMan(1→2)αMan(1→2)Man trisaccharide motif seems to be the minimum structural requisite to provide significant binding affinity towards the antibody 2G12. This study complements the previous solid state investigations, furnishing new and important structural and dynamic information.

Finally, NMR methods have also been applied to investigate mucin structure, as well as to study the antibody recognition of tumor-specific glycopeptide antigens. In a normal tissue, MUC-1, an extensively *O*-glycosylated protein that includes a tandem repeating domain of conserved 20 amino acids, is characterized by highly branched oligosaccharides with a GalNAc-unit directly α-*O*-linked to serine (Ser) or threonine (Thr) amino acids (Hanisch and Müller 2000; Gendler 2001). In tumour cells, the expression of MUC-1 is usually increased and its carbohydrate side-chains are truncated, due to incomplete glycosylation. The observation of different exposed epitopes, such as the Tn antigen (αGal*p*NAc(1→*O*-Ser/Thr), allowed the development of a variety of mAb able to specifically interact with malignant cells (Springer 1984; Senapati et al. 2010; Danussi et al. 2009). Therefore, a detailed knowledge of mucin structure has become vital in vaccine strategies that target tumor-associated mucin motifs. Indeed, several NMR investigations supported by molecular modelling have been carried out to disclose mucin architecture, (Live et al. 1999; Coltart et al. 2002) as well as for the access to the conformation and dynamics features of Tn antigen's clusters (Corzana et al. 2009, 2011). The analysis of different NMR parameters for the free and bound

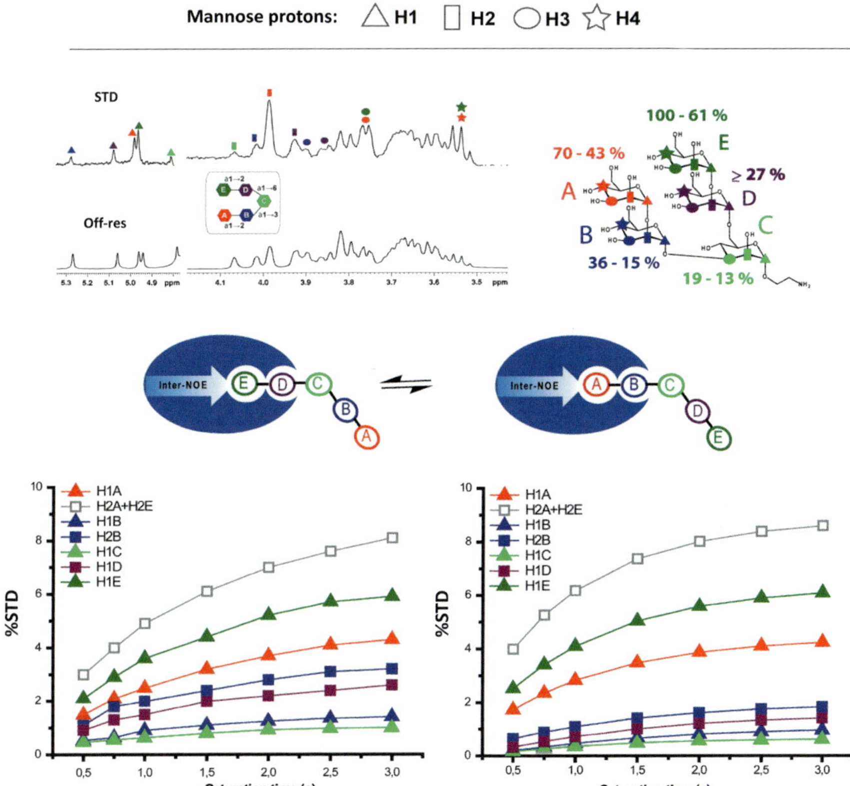

Fig. 16.6 Binding of branched oligomannoside **2** to the human mAb 2G12 in solution. *Top:* ^{1}H STD NMR spectrum and ^{1}H NMR equilibrium signals (*left*); epitope of the ligand, normalized levels of saturation (%) received by each ligand residue upon binding to 2G12 (*right*); *Center:* cartoon showing the bimodal binding model for the molecular recognition of **2** by 2G12; *Bottom*: experimental (*left*) and theoretical (*right*) STD buildup curves of compound **2**. The theoretical calculations were preformed assuming contributions from both binding modes (60% for D3-like arm; 40% for D2-like arm) (Figure kindly prepared by Dr. Jesús Angulo, Department of Bioorganic Chemistry, Instituto de Investigaciones Químicas (CSIC-US))

states for unglycosylated and Tn-glycosylated MUC-1 peptides can be very useful to determine the effect of glycosylation on MUC-1 humoral immune recognition. For instance, Campbell and co-workers have demonstrated that the increase in binding affinity shown by the glycosylated peptides is not merely due to the carbohydrate stabilizing conformation and backbone dynamics of the peptide, but also due to additional contacts of the Tn moieties (Grinstead et al. 2002). Hence, it seems reasonable to think that MUC-1 glycopeptides might be better vaccine candidates than their unglycosylated counterparts. Also, STD-based experiments combined with docking calculations have been used by Meyer's group (Möller et al. 2002) to determine the binding epitope of MUC-1 glycopeptides bound to the breast cancer-selective mAb SM3. The results pointed out the existence of an extended conformation of the peptide, with the carbohydrate interacting via the *N*-acetyl group.

Acknowledgements We thank MICINN (grant CTQ2009-08536) and CESGA for financial support. Filipa Marcelo thanks to Fundação para a Ciência e Tecnologia for the Post-Doc research grant (SFRH/BPD/65462/2009). We also would like to thank to all the colleagues in all parts of the world that have contributed with their work to the elaboration of this review.

References

Alexander J, del Guercio M-F, Maewal A, Qiao L, Fikes J, Chesnut RW, Paulson J, Bundle DR, DeFrees S, Sette A (2000) Linear PADRE T helper epitope and carbohydrate B cell epitope conjugates induce specific high titer IgG antibody responses. J Immunol 164:1625–1633

Ang CW, Jacobs BC, Laman JD (2004) The Guillain-Barré syndrome: a true case of molecular mimicry. Trends Immunol 25:61–66

Angulo J, Enriquez-Navas PM, Nieto PM (2010) Ligand-receptor binding affinities from saturation transfer difference (STD) NMR spectroscopy: the binding isotherm of STD initial growth rates. Chem Eur J 16:7803–7812

Arepalli SR, Glaudemans CPJ, Davis DG, Kovac P, Bax A (1995) Identification of protein-mediated indirect NOE effects in a disaccharide-Fab' complex by transferred ROESY. J Magn Reson B 106:195–198

Avci FY, Kasper DL (2010) How bacterial carbohydrates influence the adaptive immune system. Annu Rev Immunol 28:107–130

Barb AW, Prestegard JH (2011) NMR analysis demonstrates immunoglobulin G N-glycans are accessible and dynamic. Nat Chem Biol 7:147–153

Barb AW, Brady EK, Prestegard JH (2009) Branch-specific sialylation of IgG-Fc glycans by ST6Gal-I. Biochemistry 48:9705–9707

Barin F, McLane MF, Allan JS (1985) Virus envelope protein of HTLV-III represents major target antigen for antibodies in AIDS patients. Science 228:1094–1096

Bolesta E, Kowalczyk A, Wierzbicki A, Rotkiewica P, Bambach B, Tsao CY, Horwacik I, Kolinski A, Rokita H, Brecher M, Wang X, Ferrone S, Kozbor D (2005) DNA vaccine expressing the mimotope of GD2 gangliside induces protective GD2 cross-reactive antibody responses. Cancer Res 65:3410–3418

Calarese DA, Scanlan CN, Zwick MB, Deechongkit S, Mimura Y, Kunert R, Zhu P, Wormald MR, Stanfield RL, Roux KH, Kelly JW, Rudd PM, Dwek RA, Katinger H, Burton DR, Wilson IA (2003) Antibody domain exchange is an immunological solution to carbohydrate cluster recognition. Science 300:2065–2071

Calarese DA, Lee HK, Huang CY, Best MD, Astronomo RD, Stanfield RL, Katinger H, Burton DR, Wong CH, Wilson IA (2005) Dissection of the carbohydrate specificity of the broadly neutralizing anti-HIV-1 antibody 2G12. Proc Natl Acad Sci U S A 102:13372–13377

Clément M-J, Fortune A, Phalipon A, Marcel-Peyre V, Simenel C, Imberty A, Delepierre M, Mulard LA (2006) Towards a better understanding of the basis of molecular mimicry of polysaccharide antigens by peptides: the example of *Shigella flexneri* 5A. J Biol Chem 281:2317–2332

Coltart DM, Royyuru AK, Williams LJ, Glunz PW, Sames D, Kuduk SD, Schwarz JB, Chen X-T, Danishefsky SJ, Live DH (2002) Principles of mucin architecture: structural studies on synthetic glycopeptides bearing clustered Mono-, Di-, Tri-, and Hexasaccharide domains. J Am Chem Soc 124:9833–9844

Corzana F, Busto JH, de Luis MG, Jiménez-Barbero J, Avenoza A, Peregrina JM (2009) The nature and sequence of the amino acid aglycone strongly modulates the conformation and dynamics effects of Tn antigen's clusters. Chem Eur J 15:3863–3874

Corzana F, Busto JH, Marcelo F, de Luis MG, Asensio JL, Martín-Santamaría S, Jiménez-Barbero J, Avenoza A, Peregrina JM (2011) Engineering O-Glycosylation points in non-extended peptides: implications for the molecular recognition of short tumor-associated glycopeptides. Chem Eur J 17:3105–3110

Danussi C, Coslovi A, Campa C, Mucignat MT, Spessotto P, Uggeri F, Paoletti S, Colombatti A (2009) A newly generated functional antibody identifies Tn antigen as a novel determinant in the cancer cell-lymphatic endothelium interaction. Glycobiology 19:1056–1057

Deisenhofer J (1981) Crystallographic refinement and atomic models of a human Fc fragment and its complex with fragment B of protein A from *Staphylococcus aureus* at 2.9- and 2.8-Å resolution. Biochemistry 20:2361–2370

DeMarco ML, Woods RJ (2008) Structural glycobiology: a game of snakes and ladders. Glycobiology 18:426–440

Douek DC, Roederer M, Koup RA (2009) Emerging concepts in the immunopathogenesis of AIDS. Annu Rev Med 60:471–484

Dube DH, Bertozzi CR (2005) Glycans in cancer and inflammation: potential for therapeutics and diagnostics. Nat Rev Drug Discov 4:477–488

Dube DH, Prescher JA, Quang CN, Bertozzi CR (2006) Probing mucin-type *O*-linked glycosylation in living animals. Proc Natl Acad Sci U S A 103:4819–4824

Engering A, Geijtenbeek TB, van Kooyk Y (2002) Immune escape through C-type lectins on dendritic cells. Trends Immunol 23:480–485

Enriquez-Navas PM, Marradi M, Padro D, Angulo J, Penadés S (2011) A solution NMR study of the interactions of Oligomannosides and the Anti-HIV-1 2G12 antibody reveals distinct binding modes for branched ligands. Chem Eur J 17:1547–1560

Gemmecker G (1999) NMR Spectroscopy in Drug Development and Analysis. In: Holzgrabe U, Wawer I, Diehl B (eds) NMR as a tool in drug research. Wiley, New York, pp 140–141

Gendler SJ (2001) MUC1, the renaissance molecule. J Mammary Gland Biol Neoplasia 6: 339–353

Glaudemans CPJ, Lerner L Jr, Dares GD, Kovac P, Venable R, Bax A (1990) Significant conformational changes in an antibody carbohydrate epitope upon binding to a monoclonal antibody. Biochemistry 29:10906–10911

Grinstead JS, Koganty RR, Krantz MJ, Longenecker BM, Campbell AP (2002) Effect of glycosylation on MUC1 humoral immune recognition: NMR studies of MUC1 glycopeptide-antibody interactions. Biochemistry 41:9946–9961

Hanisch F-G, Müller S (2000) MUC1: the polymorphic appearance of a human mucin. Glycobiology 10:439–449

Harris SL, Craig L, Mehroke JS, Rashed M, Zwick MB, Kenar K, Toone EJ, Greenspan N, Auzanneau F-I, Marino-Albernas J-R, Pinto BM, Scott JK (1997) Carbohydrate cross-reactivity: evidence for discrimination by peptides between closely related anti-carbohydrate antibodies. Proc Natl Acad Sci U S A 94:2454–2459

Haselhorst T, Espinosa J-F, Jiménez-Barbero J, Sokolowski T, Kosma P, Brade H, Brade L, Peters T (1999) NMR experiments reveal distinct antibody-bound conformations of a synthetic disaccharide representing a general structural element of bacterial lipopolysaccharide epitopes. Biochemistry 38:6449–6459

Herfurth L, Ernst B, Wagner B, Ricklin D, Strasser DS, Magnani JL, Benie AJ, Peters T (2005) Comparative epitope mapping with saturation transfer difference NMR of sialyl Lewis(a) compounds and derivatives bound to a monoclonal antibody. J Med Chem 48:6879–6886

Houliston RS, Yuki N, Hirama T, Khieu NH, Brisson J-R, Gilbert M, Jarrell HC (2007) Recognition characteristics of monoclonal antibodies that are cross-reactive with gangliosides and lipooligosaccharide from *Campylobacter jejuni* strains associated with Guillain-Barré and Fisher syndromes. Biochemistry 46:36–44

Houliston RS, Jacobs BC, Tio-Gillen AP, Verschuuren JJ, Khieu NH, Gilbert M, Jarrell HC (2009) STD-NMR used to elucidate the fine binding specificity of pathogenic anti-ganglioside antibodies directly in patient serum. Biochemistry 48:220–222

Jayalakshmi V, Krishna NR (2002) Complete relaxation and conformational exchange matrix (CORCEMA) analysis of intermolecular saturation transfer effects in reversibly forming ligand–receptor complexes. J Magn Res 155:106–118

Jayalakshmi V, Krishna NR (2004) CORCEMA refinement of the bound-ligand conformation within the protein binding pocket in reversibly forming weak complexes using STD-NMR intensities. J Magn Res 168:36–45

Jiménez-Barbero J, Peters T (2002) NMR spectroscopy of glycoconjugates. Wiley, Weinheim

Jiménez-Barbero J, Asensio JL, Cañada FJ, Poveda A (1999) Free and protein-bound carbohydrate structures. Curr Opin Struct Biol 9:549–555

Johnson MA, Pinto BM (2002) Saturation transfer difference 1D-TOCSY experiments to map the topography of oligosaccharides recognized by a monoclonal antibody directed against the cell-wall polysaccharide of group A Streptococcus. J Am Chem Soc 124:15368–15374

Johnson MA, Pinto BM (2004) NMR spectroscopic and molecular modeling studies of protein-carbohydrate and protein-peptide interactions. Carbohydr Res 339:907–928

Johnson MA, Pinto BM (2008) Structural and functional studies of peptide–carbohydrate mimicry. Top Curr Chem 273:55–116

Kogelberg H, Solís D, Jiménez-Barbero J (2003) New structural insights into carbohydrate–protein interactions from NMR spectroscopy. Curr Opin Struct Biol 13:646–653

Lindberg AA (1999) Glycoprotein conjugate vaccines. Vaccine 17(suppl 2):S28–S36

Live DH, Williams LJ, Kuduk SD, Schwarz JB, Glunz PW, Chen X-T, Sames D, Kumar RA, Danishefsky SJ (1999) Probing cell-surface architecture through synthesis: an NMR-determined structural motif for tumor-associated mucins. Proc Natl Acad Sci USA 96: 3489–3493

Lundquist JJ, Toone EJ (2002) The cluster glycoside effect. Chem Rev 102:555–578

Maaheimo H, Kosma P, Brade L, Brade H, Peters T (2000) Mapping the binding of synthetic disaccharides representing epitopes of chlamydial lipopolysaccharide to antibodies with NMR. Biochemistry 39:12778–12788

Macura S, Fejzo J, Hoogstraten CG, Westler WM, Markley JL (1992) Topological editing of cross-relaxation networks. Isr J Chem 32:245–256

Massefski W, Redfield AG (1988) Elimination of multiple-step spin diffusion effects in two-dimensional NOE spectroscopy of nucleic acids. J Magn Reson 78:150–155

Mayer M, Meyer B (1999) Characterization of ligand binding by saturation transfer difference NMR spectroscopy. Angew Chem Int Ed 38:1784–1788

Mayer M, Meyer B (2001) Group epitope mapping by saturation transfer difference NMR to identify segments of a ligand in direct contact with a protein receptor. J Am Chem Soc 123:6108–6117

Meyer B, Peters T (2003) NMR spectroscopy techniques for screening and identifying ligand binding to protein receptors. Angew Chem Int Ed 42:864–890

Milton MJ, Bundle DR (1998) Observation of the *anti-* conformation of a glycosidic linkage in an antibody bound oligosaccharide. J Am Chem Soc 120:10547–10548

Möller H, Serttas N, Paulsen H, Burchell JM, Taylor-Papadimitriou J, Meyer B (2002) NMR-based determination of the binding epitope and conformational analysis of MUC-1 glycopeptides and peptides bound to the breast cancer-selective monoclonal antibody SM3. Eur J Biochem 269:1444–1455

Ni F, Zhu Y (1994) Accounting for ligand-protein interactions in the relaxation-matrix analysis of transferred nuclear overhauser effects. J Magn Reson B 103:180–184

Oberli MA, Tamborrini M, Tsai Y-H, Werz DB, Horlacher T, Adibekian A, Gauss D, Möller HM, Pluschke G, Seeberger PH (2010) Molecular analysis of carbohydrate-antibody interactions: case study using a *Bacillus anthracis* tetrasaccharide. J Am Chem Soc 132:10239–10241

Pashov A, Canziani G, MacLeod S, Plaxco J, Monzavi-Karbassi B, Kieber-Emmons T (2005) Targeting carbohydrate antigens in HIV vaccine development. Vaccine 23:2168–2175

Pellecchia M, Sem DS, Wüthrich K (2002) NMR in drug discovery. Nat Rev Drug Discov 1:211–219

Poveda A, Jiménez-Barbero J (1998) NMR studies of carbohydrate-protein interactions in solution. Chem Soc Rev 27:133–144

Rademacher C, Shoemaker GK, Kim H-S, Zheng RB, Taha H, Liu C, Nacario RC, Schriemer DC, Klassen JS, Peters T, Lowary TL (2007) Ligand specificity of CS-35, a monoclonal antibody that recognizes mycobacterial lipoarabinomannan: a model system for oligofuranoside-protein recognition. J Am Chem Soc 129:10489–10502

Rebek J (2009) Introduction to the molecular recognition and self-assembly special feature. Proc Natl Acad Sci U S A 106:10423–10424

Reimer KB, Gidney MAJ, Bundle DR, Pinto BM (1992) Immunochemical characterization of polyclonal and monoclonal *Streptococcus* group A antibodies by chemically defined glycoconjugates and synthetic oligosaccharides. Carbohydr Res 232:131–142

Ribeiro JP, André S, Cañada FJ, Gabius H-J, Butera AP, Alves RJ, Jiménez-Barbero J (2010) Lectin-based drug design: combined strategy to identify lead compounds using STD NMR spectroscopy, solid-phase assays and cell binding for a plant toxin model. ChemMedChem 5:415–419

Roy R (2008) Carbohydrates-based vaccines. ACS symposium series 989. ACS books, Washington DC

Sanders RW, Venturi M, Schiffner L, Kalyanaraman R, Katinger H, Lloyd KO, Kwong PD, Moore JP (2002) The mannose-dependent epitope for neutralizing antibody 2G12 on human immunodeficiency virus type 1 glycoprotein gp120. J Virol 76:7293–7305

Scallon BJ (2007) Higher levels of sialylated Fc glycans in immunoglobulin G molecules can adversely impact functionality. Mol Immunol 44:1524–1534

Senapati S, Das S, Batra SK (2010) Mucin-interacting proteins: from function to therapeutics. Trends Biochem Sci 35:236–245

Serruto D, Rappuoli R (2006) Post-genomic vaccine development. FEBS Lett 580:2985–2992

Springer GF (1984) T and Tn, general carcinoma autoantigens. Science 224:1198–1206

Stockman BJ, Dalvit C (2002) NMR screening techniques in drug discovery and drug design. Prog Nucl Magn Reson 41:187–231

Takahashi H, Igarashi T, Shimada I, Arata Y (1991) Preparation of the Fv fragment from a short-chain mouse IgG2a anti-dansyl monoclonal antibody and use of selectively deuterated Fv analogues for two-dimensional ^{1}H NMR analyses of the antigen-antibody interactions. Biochemistry 30:2840–2847

Tamborrini M, Werz DB, Frey J, Pluschke G, Seeberger PH (2006) Anti-carbohydrate antibodies for the detection of anthrax spores. Angew Chem Int Ed 45:6581–6582

Trkola A, Purtscher M, Muster T, Ballaun C, Buchacher A, Sullivan N, Srinivasan K, Sodroski J, Moore JP, Katinger H (1996) Human monoclonal antibody 2G12 defines a distinctive neutralization epitope on the gp120 glycoprotein of human immunodeficiency virus type 1. J Virol 70:1100–1108

Varki A, Cummings R, Esko J, Freeze H, Hart G, Marth J (1999) Essentials of glycobiology. Cold Spring Harbor Laboratory, New York

Vincent SJF, Zwahlen C, Bodenhausen G (1996) Suppression of spin diffusion in selected frequency bands of nuclear Overhauser spectra. J Biomol NMR 7:169–172

Werz DB, Seeberger PH (2005) First total synthesis of a *Bacillus anthracis* tetrasaccharide antigen – creation of an Anthrax vaccine. Angew Chem Int Ed 44:6315–6318

Westerink MAJ, Giardina PC, Apicella MA, Kieber-Emmons T (1995) Peptide mimicry of the meningococcal group C capsular polysaccharide. Proc Natl Acad Sci USA 92: 4021–4025

Wormald MR, Rudd PM, Harvey DJ, Chang S-C, Scragg IG, Dwek RA (1997) Variations in oligosaccharide-protein interactions in immunoglobulin G determine the sitespecific glycosylation profiles and modulate the dynamic motion of the Fc oligosaccharides. Biochemistry 36:1370–1380

Yamaguchi Y, Kato K (2010) Dynamics and interactions of glycoconjugates probed by stable-isotope-assisted NMR spectroscopy. Methods Enzymol 478:305–322

Yamaguchi Y, Kato K, Shindo M, Aoki S, Furusho K, Koga K, Takahashi N, Arata Y, Shimada I (1998) Dynamics of the carbohydrate chains attached to the Fc portion of immunoglobulin G as studied by NMR spectroscopy assisted by selective ^{13}C labeling of the glycans. J Biomol NMR 12:385–394

Yuki N (2005) Carbohydrate mimicry: a new paradigm of autoimmune diseases. Curr Opin Immunol 17:577–582

Zwahlen C, Vincent SJF, Di Bari L, Levitt MH, Bodenhausen G (1994) Quenching spin diffusion in selective measurements of transient Overhauser effects in nuclear magnetic resonance. Applications to oligonucleotides. J Am Chem Soc 116:362–368

17 Determination of Antibody Affinity by Surface Plasmon Resonance

Roger MacKenzie and Sven Müller-Loennies

17.1 Introduction

Over the past two decades surface plasmon resonance (SPR) has emerged as gold standard technology for the analysis of biomolecular interactions. In the monoclonal antibody (mAb) development area SPR is employed from the early screening stages to detailed characterization of binding kinetics and affinities to epitope mapping to final product testing. This label free technology provides high quality kinetic and affinity data and, in some instances, other unique information not obtained by alternative methods such as ELISA. SPR is well-suited to the study of protein-carbohydrate interactions which are often of low affinity and not easily characterized by other methods.

Monoclonal antibodies rank as the top-selling class of biologics with US sales of almost $17 billion in 2009 and an annual growth rate approaching double digits. Over 30 mAbs have been approved by the FDA and hundreds more are in various stages of clinical development as researchers strive to develop mAbs to address other indications and unmet medical needs (Aggarwal 2010). In humans, most cell surface proteins, which are generally preferential targets for antibody drug development, are glycosylated and quite frequently it is the glycan component of the glycoprotein that is indispensable for biological function. Altered glycosylation is a feature of many cancer types and targeting aberrant glycosylation patterns or overexpression of certain carbohydrate moieties with therapeutic vaccines or antibody

R. MacKenzie (✉)
Institute for Biological Sciences, National Research Council Canada, 100 Sussex Drive, Ottawa, ON K1A OR6, Canada
e-mail: roger.mackenzie@nrc-cnrc.gc.ca

S. Müller-Loennies
Research Center Borstel, Leibniz-Center for Medicine and Biosciences, Parkallee 1-40, 23845 Borstel, Germany

P. Kosma and S. Müller-Loennies (eds.), *Anticarbohydrate Antibodies*,
DOI 10.1007/978-3-7091-0870-3_17,

drugs is an attractive therapeutic option (reviewed in Schietinger et al. 2008 and Astronomo and Burton 2010).

Many pathogenic bacteria present cell surface carbohydrates from which carbohydrate-based vaccines are derived. Anti-carbohydrate antibodies against capsular polysaccharide or lipopolysaccharide (LPS, endotoxin) are generally responsible for protection against bacteria presenting these structures. The demonstrated capacity of conjugate vaccines, comprised of carbohydrate covalently coupled to a protein carrier, to confer long lasting immunity against *Haemophilus influenzae*, *Neisseria meningitidis*, *Salmonella typhi* and *Streptococcus pneumoniae* is the kingpin of carbohydrate vaccine technology. Significant efforts, fuelled by glycomics research, are now underway to develop conjugate vaccines against other infectious diseases as well as certain cancers (reviewed in Astronomo and Burton 2010).

There are specific challenges associated with the characterization of carbohydrate-protein recognition mainly due to their often low affinity with K_D values in the micromolar range, the presence of multiple binding sites on the same molecule leading to avidity effects and the availability of only small amounts of material. SPR is a suitable technique to address some of these challenges and aid in the development of e.g. carbohydrate vaccines and therapeutic anti-carbohydrate mAbs for which precise measurements of affinities and specificities are required. For carbohydrate vaccine design protective carbohydrate epitopes need to be identified. Rather than providing an in depth review of biosensor technology which can be found elsewhere in the literature (Karlsson and Fält 1997; Karlsson 2004; Rich and Myszka 2010) and references therein] in this chapter we discuss experimental design and highlight pitfalls that must be avoided in order to collect high quality SPR data and we describe a few examples how we have successfully applied SPR for the characterization of anti-carbohydrate antibodies related to infectious diseases.

17.2 Protein-Carbohydrate Interactions

The recognition of carbohydrates by proteins is widespread in nature. In these interactions carbohydrates bind to lectins from plants, invertebrates, mammals (mannose receptor of macrophages, surfactant proteins, sperm adhesion, galectins, siglecs), bacteria (outer membrane proteins, toxins, fimbriae) and bacteriophages. Also, the immune system often targets carbohydrate epitopes, producing anti-carbohydrate antibodies, e.g. against capsular polysaccharides and O-antigens of LPS from Gram-negative bacteria.

Structural analyses by X-ray crystallography of carbohydrate binding proteins in complex with ligand have shown that they frequently possess carbohydrate recognition sites which interact with terminal or branch-point monosaccharides and which are buried in a deep or shallow pocket with only a few additional carbohydrate residues directly involved in the interaction (Cygler et al. 1991; Villeneuve et al. 2000; Vyas et al. 2003; Calarese et al. 2003; Ramsland et al. 2004; Van Roon et al. 2004; Vulliez-Le Normand et al. 2008; Brooks et al. 2008b, 2010a, b, c; Farrugia et al. 2009; Gerstenbruch et al. 2010; Evans et al. 2011; Blackler et al. 2011). These structures have shown that the contact surface area of antibodies which interact with carbohydrates is generally smaller in comparison to antibody-protein interactions. Characteristically, stacking interactions between aromatic amino acid side chains and carbohydrates play an important role in carbohydrate recognition (Toone 1994) in addition to electrostatic ionic interactions for charged ligands. There is generally a favourable enthalpy contribution to the free energy of binding (Bundle and Young 1992) but this is largely counteracted by an unfavourable entropy factor attributed to loss of carbohydrate flexibility and unfavourable solvent re-arrangement upon binding (Carver 1993). Rearrangement of water and especially desolvation, i.e. release of surface bound water into the bulk solvent, are key features of complex formation (Toone 1994; Homans 2007). Consequently, protein-carbohydrate interactions typically are of relatively low intrinsic affinity and rely on multivalency for adequate functional affinities.

17.3 Analysis of Biomolecular Interactions

Specificity and affinity are the key factors which describe molecular recognition. In the simplest case of a 1:1 interaction (Langmuir binding), a binding event can be formally described as:

$$\mathrm{A} + \mathrm{L} \underset{k2}{\overset{k1}{\rightleftarrows}} \mathrm{AL}$$

According to the law of mass action an equilibrium constant K can be calculated and thus the strength of binding may be expressed as a binding constant (affinity association constant K_A or dissociation constant K_D, where $K_\mathrm{A} = 1/K_\mathrm{D}$). The constant K is related to the standard free energy of binding, ΔG^0, by the equation $\Delta G^0 = RT - \ln K_\mathrm{A}$ and consists of entropy and enthalpy contributions since $\Delta G^0 = \Delta H^0 - T\Delta S^0$ (a detailed description can be found in Homans 2007). Hence, specificity may be determined by comparison of binding constants at equilibrium and describes the ability of a molecule to preferentially form a complex with one binding partner over another.

The constant K can also be determined from the rate constants of complex formation (k_a) and dissociation (k_d). Apart from providing insight into the mechanism of complex formation, determination of rate constants is of biological relevance since it was shown that the half-life of complexes formed between MHC presented peptides and T-cell receptors ($t_{1/2} = \ln 2/k_\mathrm{d}$) rather than the K_D correlated with biological activity, i.e. activation of T-cells (Kalergis et al. 2001). In this case cell activation was efficient only within a certain half-life-effect curve with a Gaussian distribution. The negative effect of very slow k_d (high affinity) was explained by the occupancy of the receptor binding site longer than necessary for its stimulation. This was presumed to slow down the turnover of receptors which over the duration of the interaction became incapable of further triggering intracellular signalling events (Foote and Eisen 2000; Malissen 2001). In general, it is important to keep in mind that affinity describes an equilibrium state which is seldom reached in biological systems.

It is evident that the successful design of novel therapeutic drugs will require the identification of ligands with a biologically meaningful affinity and binding kinetics. On the other hand for diagnostic applications apart from a high selectivity an affinity as high as possible is required in order to maximize signal intensities and minimize the amounts needed thereby minimizing cost. Apart from a high intrinsic affinity of the individual carbohydrate binding site this may be achieved by an enhanced avidity by oligo- or multimerization of both binding partners.

In addition to SPR, many methods such as isothermal titration microcalorimetry (ITC), nuclear magnetic resonance (NMR) spectroscopy, fluorescence spectroscopy, ELISA, equilibrium dialysis, analytical ultracentrifugation, affinity gel electrophoresis, and even mass spectrometry can be employed to estimate or determine the binding strength of molecular interactions, in principle. Compared to these methods SPR has the advantage of requiring relatively little amount of unlabelled material and providing additional insight into the kinetics of binding. SPR analyses may be performed at varying temperatures and therefore in principle SPR allows the determination of thermodynamic parameters.

17.4 Surface Plasmon Resonance

Surface plasmon resonance offers many advantages in the study of biological recognition events, including protein-carbohydrate interactions. SPR measures complex formation and dissociation events in real time without a requirement for labelling and provides a means of deriving rate constants, affinity constants and the quantitation of complex formation. SPR-based biosensors are a proven technology for the generation of reliable, high quality and informative data on the nature of a wide range of molecular interactions.

17.4.1 General Principles

The phenomenon of SPR was first exploited by Biacore AB for the study of biological interactions and is the detection method used in the widely used Biacore instruments. In these instruments, a wedge of polarized light is reflected from a thin gold layer supported on glass and contained in a removable sensor chip. SPR causes a reduction in the intensity of reflected light at a very specific angle of incident light and the angle at which this reduction occurs is sensitive to refractive index changes on the non-illuminated side of the gold film. A description of the physical background behind SPR and further technical developments has been published (Englebienne et al. 2003). In conventional SPR analysis, molecules (ligand) are captured or coupled at the sensor chip surface and the subsequent binding of interacting partners (analytes) to the ligand can then be monitored in real time. A microfluidics cartridge is interfaced with the sensor chip to permit continuous delivery of buffer, coupling or capture reagents and potential binding partners to the sensor chip surface. In recent years several other SPR-based instruments for biomolecular interaction analysis have been launched in the marketplace by a number of vendors (for a list see Rich and Myszka 2010).

17.4.2 Immobilization Techniques

Ligands can be coupled to the carboxylated dextran matrix on the most commonly used Biacore sensor chips by standard coupling chemistries that utilize carboxylate, amino, aldehyde or thiol groups on the ligand. Carbohydrates can be conveniently immobilized as glycoconjugates. Polysaccharides conjugated to carrier proteins can be coupled via amino groups on the protein to CM5 sensor chips activated with *N*-hydroxysuccinimide (NHS) and *N*-ethyl-*N′*-(dimethylaminopropyl)-carbodiimide (EDC). Another strategy that has been used for immobilization of carbohydrates involves reductive amination through the reducing end followed by coupling through the introduced amino group or coupling after biotinylation on a NeutrAvidin™ chip. Several Biacore sensor chips are available in addition to the standard dextran matrix and SA chips (http://www.biacore.com/lifesciences). These include chips with less dextran, dextran with more or less carboxylation, no matrix, an alkane thiol layer to which liposomes can be fused to form hybrid bilayers and a lipophilic C_{18} for immobilizing liposomes and lipophilic molecules.

17.4.3 Guidelines for High Quality Data Collection

Unfortunately the scientific literature on the analysis of biomolecular interactions by SPR contains a disproportional amount of low quality data (Rich and Myszka 2010). Avoiding a number of well-established pitfalls highlighted in Box 17.1 and mentioned below as appropriate would alleviate this problem. This has been repeatedly emphasized by others (O'Shannessy 1994; Karlsson 2004; Rich and Myszka 2010) but is also highlighted here because of its fundamental importance. For several years now the Journal of Molecular Recognition has published an annual review of the optical biosensor literature in which this issue has been discussed extensively. The latest review covered the 2008 literature (Rich and Myszka 2010).

Appropriate reference surfaces must be chosen and serve several purposes – determination of refractive index differences between the sample and the running buffers, baseline drift, matrix effects and measurement of non-specific binding. In order for the non-specific binding measurement to be accurate the reference and active surfaces should be as similar as possible – for example, similar levels of matrix activation. To avoid overcrowding on the sensor chip surface, immobilized ligand densities should be the minimum required to give sufficiently high responses

Box 17.1 Collection of High Quality SPR Data

- Ensure that the instrument is properly maintained and cleaned on a regular basis
- Use only high quality reagents
- Minimize nonspecific binding and baseline drift
- Avoid avidity effects when deriving intrinsic affinities by immobilizing multivalent molecules and ensuring that analytes are free of aggregates
- Use proper reference surfaces
- Apply double referencing against buffer injections and reference surface
- For collection of kinetic data, use low ligand surface densities and high flow rates
- Replicate and randomize samples

for ligand-analyte complex formation. This also ensures efficient delivery of the analyte to the sensor chip surface and for the same reason flow rates should be as fast as possible.

Analyses can be performed under a range of buffer conditions, temperatures and flow rates. However, the most commonly used buffer is 10 mM HEPES, pH 7.4, containing 150 mM NaCl, 3.3 mM EDTA and 0.005% P-20 detergent. Although most Biacore instruments permit data collection from 4°C to 40°C, which allows for the derivation of thermodynamic parameters, analyses are typically performed at 25°C.

When the objective is to determine the intrinsic affinities and rate constants of protein-carbohydrate interactions, experiments should be designed to generate data that are described by a simple one-to-one interaction model. Therefore, analytes should be in general monovalent due to the multivalency of the sensor chip surface. Multivalent proteins used as analytes should be produced as monovalent fragments when possible, e.g. for antibodies Fab, or single-chain fragments of the variable domains (scFv). The preparations have to be purified by size exclusion chromatography immediately prior to analysis to minimize the presence of aggregates which can introduce multivalent binding and seriously compromise data quality. However, if it is impossible to obtain monovalent carbohydrate binding fragments, as is the case for lectins, the protein macromolecule should be immobilized and the carbohydrate used as the analyte. As analytes carbohydrates have the advantage of little tendency to form aggregates. The binding of carbohydrates as small as disaccharides to proteins can be monitored with the latest Biacore instruments which have improved sensitivity compared to the older instruments.

When the objective is to determine the functional affinities of protein carbohydrate interactions, experimental conditions should be optimized to maximize multivalent binding in order to quantify the avidity effect – i.e. the ratio of multivalent to monovalent binding. The carbohydrate ligand should be immobilized at a sufficiently high surface density and the multivalent carbohydrate binding protein should be injected over the carbohydrate surface at relatively low concentrations to minimize competition for available carbohydrate ligand.

High quality SPR data can be fitted to suitable interaction models for the calculation of rate and affinity constants, typically with BIAevaluation software from GE Healthcare. However, for protein-carbohydrate interactions, the kinetics are often too rapid for determination of rate constants. The BIACORE instruments are capable of measuring k_a rates in the 10^3–10^8 M^{-1} s^{-1} range and k_d rates in the 10^{-5}–1 s^{-1} range.

17.4.4 Protein Binding to Immobilized Carbohydrate

Carbohydrates may be directly immobilized on sensor chips if suitable functional groups are available and the chemical reaction does not destroy the epitope. For the preparation of immunogens for induction of antibodies in animals carbohydrates usually have to be conjugated to carrier protein. These conjugates can be readily immobilized on sensor chips.

One of the first anti-carbohydrate antibodies studied by SPR was mAb Se155-4, an IgG antibody specific for the *Salmonella* serogroup B O-polysaccharide (MacKenzie et al. 1996). As for many of the serotype-specific *Salmonella* LPS antibodies, the immunodominant carbohydrate in this interaction is a branching 3,6-dideoxyhexose residue, which is for the serogroup B LPS an abequose. This study showed that the relatively low affinity of the monovalent interaction between 4 and 8 μM K_D values was due to a rapid dissociation (k_d 0.25 s^{-1}) of the complex. Whereas it might have been anticipated that mainly the k_d is affected by valency this example showed that the on-rate may also be altered. The same observation was made in a recent investigation of lectin-carbohydrate interactions by SPR and ITC (Murthy et al. 2008). A comparison of purified monomeric (monovalent) with dimeric (bivalent) scFv revealed a 20-fold slower k_d in the presence of free ligand during the analysis and a fivefold increased k_a, thus yielding an avidity of approximately two orders of magnitude higher. The k_d determination for the dimeric scFv in the absence of free ligand (MacKenzie et al. 1996) showed that the gain in avidity from the monomer to dimeric scFv is approximately 1,000-fold. Furthermore, it was shown that even when using purified scFv dimers a biphasic dissociation phase may be observed. It became evident that some monovalent binding may occur because the faster k_d was identical to the k_d observed for the purified monomer. One possible explanation for this observation is a steric hindrance between analyte molecules preventing access to bivalent binding of immobilized ligands.

We have studied the epitope recognition of high affinity anti-carbohydrate antibodies against small negatively charged oligosaccharides from *Chlamydia* LPS by SPR and ELISA binding assays to complement crystallographic structural analyses (see Chap. 4, Blackler et al.). Chlamydiae are Gram-negative bacteria which contain a LPS of di- to tetrasaccharides of 3-deoxy-D-*manno*-oct-2-ulopyranosonic acid (Kdo) (Brade 1999). The structures of these oligosaccharides

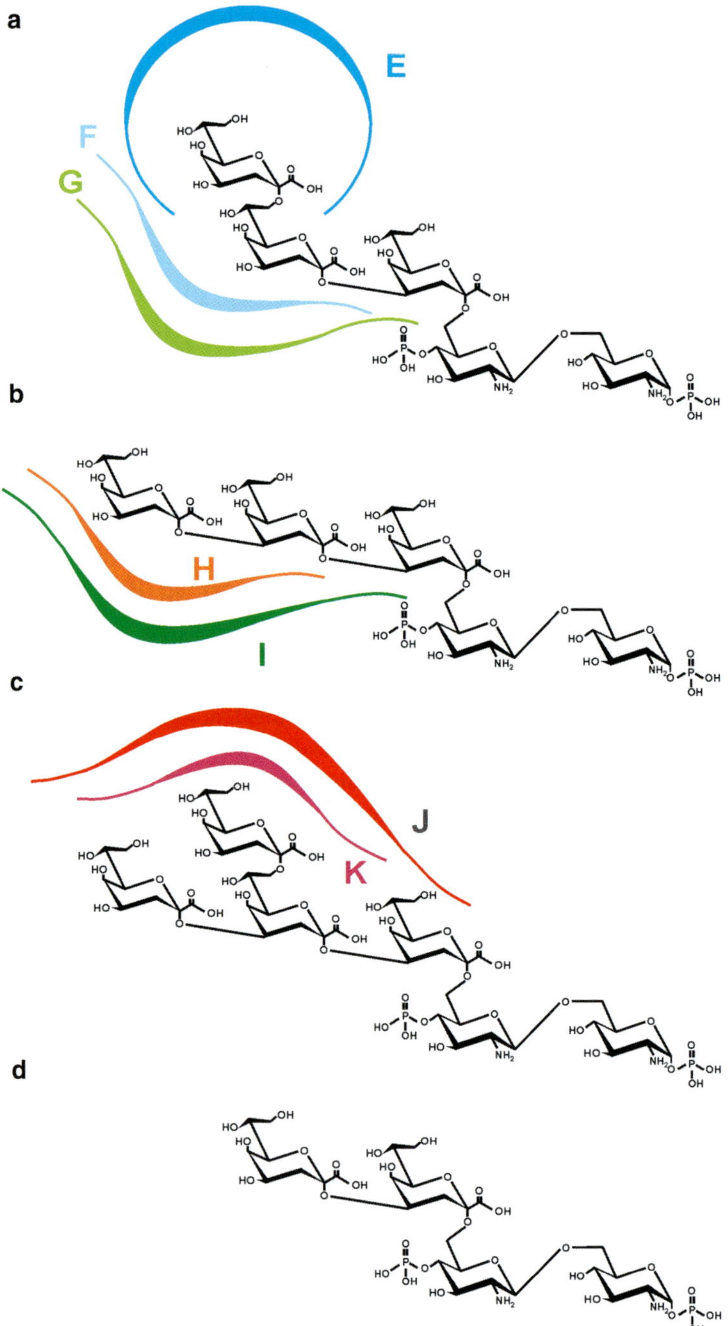

Fig. 17.1 Chemical structures of oligosaccharides obtained after deacylation of chlamydial LPS. All chlamydial species investigated so far contain the pentasaccharide shown in (**a**) and which incorporates the Kdo(2→8)Kdo(2→4)Kdo trisaccharide which is the *Chlamydia* family specific

are depicted in Fig. 17.1 and occur in Chlamydiae as Kdo(2→8)Kdo(2→4)Kdo (a family specific epitope of *Chlamydiaceae*), Kdo(2→4)Kdo(2→4)Kdo or a branched Kdo(2→4)[Kdo(2→8)]Kdo(2→4)Kdo bound to lipid A. All of these oligosaccharides are antigenic and upon natural infection or experimental immunization the formation of antibodies is induced which derive from several distinct germline families (unpublished observation) with different epitope specificities (Brade 1999).

Glycolipids such as LPS are amphiphiles and form micelles above the critical micellar concentrations. They are therefore multivalent in solution at the concentrations used in SPR binding assays. They may be coated directly on hydrophobic HPA sensor chips to obtain a homogeneous surface. However, the generation of a suitable control surface may be difficult to achieve. Alternatively, they may be chemically deacylated and subsequently covalently linked to carrier proteins such as BSA. Such conjugates are suitable for immunization, ELISA and also SPR therefore allowing the use of the same antigen in each instance and a direct comparison of binding assays. This approach is particularly suited for LPS which can be deacylated by strong alkaline treatment without hydrolysis of the carbohydrate linkages. Such treatment generates free amines within the lipid A sugar backbone (phosphorylated GlcN-disaccharide) which has been used for the conjugation to BSA after introduction of a glutaraldehyde spacer (Brade et al. 1993). These neoglycoconjugates were then used for experimental immunization and immobilization on CM5 sensor chips for SPR analysis using monovalent antibody fragments (scFv and Fab) as analytes. These experiments showed that a close-to-germline antibody, mAb S25-2, and a matured mAb specific for the family specific for consistency epitope, S25-23, had, in comparison to other anti-carbohydrate antibodies, an unusual high affinity with K_D values in the nanomolar range [Table 17.1, (Müller-Loennies et al. 2000)].

Despite the collection of monomeric scFv of S25-2 by gel filtration immediately prior to the SPR analysis deviation from the 1:1 interaction model became apparent during the fitting routine. This deviation was enhanced in the analysis of low affinity interactions with smaller oligosaccharide structures presenting only parts of the epitope due to the higher analyte concentrations needed. Therefore, several precautions had to be taken to ensure the reliability of the biosensor data. Importantly, global fitting of sensorgrams at several analyte concentrations ranging up to

Fig. 17.1 (continued) epitope. The structures shown in (**b**) and (**c**) occur only in *Chlamydia psittaci* and represent species-specific epitopes. The structurally related Re-type LPS of enterobacterial deep rough mutants (**d**) contains only a 2→4-linked Kdo disaccharide. The epitopes recognized by mAbs are indicated and comprise Kdo (E), Kdo(2→8)Kdo (F), Kdo(2→8)Kdo (2→4)Kdo (G), Kdo(2→4)Kdo (H), Kdo(2→4)Kdo(2→4)Kdo (I), Kdo(2→8)[Kdo(2→4)]Kdo (2→4)Kdo (J) and Kdo(2→8)Kdo(2→4)Kdo (K) (Modified from (Brooks et al. 2010b), copyright 2010, with permission from the American Chemical Society)

Table 17.1 Kinetics of Kdo(2 → 8)Kdo(2 → 4)Kdo binding by IgG, Fab and scFv forms of S25-2 and S25-23 as determined by SPR (Reprinted from Müller-Loennies et al. (2000), with permission, Copyright © 2000, Oxford University Press)

	S25-2			S25-23		
Antibody form	k_a, M^{-1} s^{-1}	k_d, s^{-1}	K_D, M	k_a, M^{-1} s^{-1}	k_d, s^{-1}	K_D, M
IgG	1.3×10^5 ($\pm 24^a$)	8.8×10^{-4} (± 8.1)	6.7×10^{-9}	4.5×10^4 (± 5.5)	1.9×10^{-4} (± 16)	4.1×10^{-9}
Fab	2.0×10^5 (± 11)	1.2×10^{-1} (± 8.3)	6.0×10^{-7}	5.2×10^4 (± 13)	8.7×10^{-3} (± 2.1)	1.7×10^{-7}
scFv	1.3×10^5 (± 14)	7.5×10^{-2} (± 2.7)	5.9×10^{-7}	5.9×10^4 (± 23)	1.2×10^{-2} (± 4.2)	2.2×10^{-7}

[a]% standard deviation

tenfold over the K_D was applied and satisfied a 1:1 interaction model. Furthermore the consistency of K_D values was confirmed by a comparison of results from kinetic analysis and equilibrium binding. The SPR analyses showed that the high affinity of the antibody was due to fast association rates ($1.0 \times 10^5\ M^{-1}\ s^{-1}$) and relatively slow dissociation rates for monovalent binding, ranging from 0.3 to 0.07 s^{-1}.

Sequence analysis of mAb S45-18, which binds the epitope Kdo(2→4)Kdo (2→4)Kdo with high specificity (Nguyen et al. 2003), showed that it derived from the same set of germline genes as S25-2 but underwent extensive affinity maturation. Most importantly, a phenylalanine residue introduced into the combining site was involved in a hydrophobic stacking interaction with all three Kdo residues (Nguyen et al. 2003). These structural changes of the combining site were shown by SPR analysis of Fab binding to immobilized glycoconjugate to accelerate the k_a to $1.2 \times 10^7\ M^{-1}\ s^{-1}$ with an almost unaltered k_d of 0.05 s^{-1} yielding a K_D of 4 nM (Gerstenbruch et al. 2010). A sequence comparison between mAb S45-18 and mAb S69-4, an antibody which is able to distinguish the branched Kdo tetrasaccharide from the linear Kdo(2→4)Kdo(2→4)Kdo trisaccharide and which therefore could be used for the selective immunostaining of *C. psittaci* (Müller-Loennies et al. 2006), showed that it also contained a phenylalanine residue at an equivalent position in VH CDR3. Despite this, SPR analysis revealed only very weak binding with fast kinetics which did not allow the determination of rate constants. The K_D values determined from steady state binding were 10 μM for the tetrasaccharide and 100 μM for the trisaccharide indicating that the positioning of the phenylalanine was altered by the different loop structure. Thus the use of a different set of diversity and joining genes played a major role in affinity maturation of the mAb S45-18 antibody. Substitution of the four amino acids immediately following PheH97 (scFv S69-4 $H3_{post}$) led to a 1,000-fold affinity increase to a K_D of 10 nM for the monovalent interaction [Table 17.2 and Fig. 17.2 (Gerstenbruch et al. 2010)]. Simultaneously a loss of selectivity for the branched structure was observed. This indicated that due to the high affinity the tolerance of subtle conformational changes in the epitope was lost raising the question of whether high affinity and selectivity against these closely related carbohydrate epitopes preclude each other. We have therefore attempted to isolate by phage display a high affinity antibody that is still able to distinguish these two structures (Gerstenbruch et al. 2010). The isolated scFv NH2240-31 showed very high affinity for the branched Kdo tetrasaccharide (K_D of 6 nM) while binding the linear trisaccharide with a K_D of 15 nM. Immunofluorescence staining of bacteria and ELISA confirmed the selectivity for the branched structure. The sequence and crystal structure analysis (Brooks et al. 2008a; Gerstenbruch et al. 2010) revealed a significantly shortened CDR3 VH and an altered positioning of an aromatic side chain residue, possibly allowing a different stacking interaction with the tetrasaccharide ligand than observed with PheH97. Crucial to the successful SPR analyses performed on these antibody fragments was the reduction of immobilized neoglycoconjugate to a maximum of 10–20 RU for the R_{max} as well as double referencing against an appropriate ligand. When higher amounts were immobilized severe subtraction artefacts at the beginning of the injection and the initial phase of dissociation were observed, preventing kinetic analysis.

Table 17.2 SPR binding data of scFv against immobilized neoglycoconjugates (Reprinted from Gerstenbruch et al. (2010), with permission, Copyright © 2010, Oxford University Press)

Analyte	Ligand[a]	k_a (M^{-1} s^{-1} $\times 10^6$)	SE k_a ($\times 10^4$)	k_d ($s^{-1} \times 10^{-3}$)	SE k_d ($\times 10^{-3}$)	K_D ($M \times 10^{-9}$)	Rmax (RU)	SE (Rmax)	$t_{1/2}$ (s)
NH2240-31	HS4*P*	5.4	16	30	0.9	6	11	0.03	23
	2.4/ 2.4PS4*P*	4.6	7.1	70	1.1	15	19	0.02	10
scFv S69-4 $H3_{post}$[b]	HS4*P*	4.7	2.4	50	0.2	10	11	0.01	14
	2.4/ 2.4PS4*P*	6.2	4.9	60	0.5	10	19	0.03	12
Fab S45-18	HS4*P*	4.1	15	30	0.9	7	19	0.09	23
	2.4/ 2.4PS4*P*	12.0	110	50	5	4	27	0.20	14

[a]Abbreviations HS4P and 2.4/2.4PS4*P* refer to the BSA-conjugated branched Kdo tetrasaccharide and the linear 2.4/2.4-linked trisaccharide linked to the 4′-phosphorylated lipid A backbone (GlcN-disaccharide)

[b]In this scFv the four amino acids following PheH97 of CDR3 VH in the low affinity antibody S69-4 have been changed to the sequence of the high affinity antibody S45-18

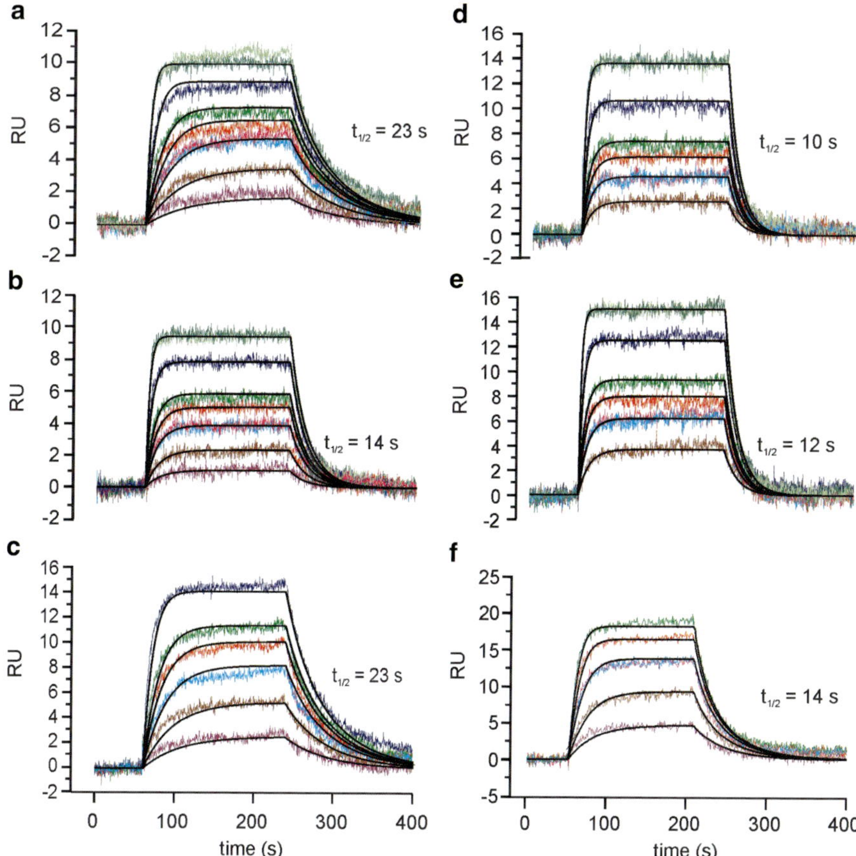

Fig. 17.2 SPR sensorgrams of scFv against immobilized neoglycoconjugates. NH2240-31 (**a** and **d**), scFv S69-4 H3post (**b** and **e**) and Fab S45-18 (**c** and **f**) against the 4′-monophosphorylated hexasaccharide (**a**, **b**, **c**) and the Kdo(2→4)Kdo(2→4)Kdo trisaccharide (**d**, **e**, and **f**) conjugated to BSA by reductive amination after enzymatic dephosphorylation at C1; for oligosaccharide structures see Fig. 17.1b and c. Sensorgrams recorded for protein concentrations of 1, 2.5, 5, 7.5, 10, 20, and 40 nM are shown in **a** and **b**. Identical concentrations are displayed with same colors. Proteins were purified by gel filtration immediately prior to the analysis (Reprinted from Gerstenbruch et al. (2010), Copyright © 2010, with permission from Oxford University Press)

It may not always be possible to generate neoglycoconjugates without destruction of the epitope of interest. An elegant way to immobilize glycolipids on conventional CM5 sensor chips is the capture on surfaces precoated with antibody. This procedure has been successfully applied for the immobilization of the asialo-GM1 glycolipid (Harrison et al. 1998) for the determination of antibody binding kinetics. Liposomes formed using dimyristoylphosphatidylcholine (DMPC) and a small amount of the antigen of interest, e.g. the asialo-GM1 glycolipid, were prepared and a small amount of a second glycolipid, in this case LPS from *Salmonella* serogroup B LPS, was incorporated into the liposomes. After immobilization of the LPS specific antibody on

CM5 sensor chips liposomes could be captured and yielded a stable surface for the SPR measurements. This setup could also be used for inhibition experiments with soluble carbohydrates. The results from such experiments revealed that an increased inhibitor concentration may in some instances promote higher avidity binding, as shown by the addition of a monovalent tetrasaccharide inhibitor which led to lower total amount of bound antibody but simultaneously resulted in a decreased k_d. Thus, low valency inhibition of binding can promote higher avidity antibody-carbohydrate interactions, presumably as there is less competition for available immobilized antigen at lower binding levels.

17.4.5 Carbohydrate Binding to Immobilized Protein

The immobilization of carbohydrates by conjugation to protein yields a multivalent surface which requires the use of monovalent analytes to satisfy the requirements for the application of a 1:1 interaction model. In some instances the preparation of monovalent fragments can be difficult to achieve, such as for IgM antibodies of which Fab fragments cannot be obtained by papain digestion. Also the cloning and soluble expression of monovalent scFv has been shown to be difficult or even impossible for some antibodies. Such problems can be circumvented by the immobilization of the multivalent antibody and then injecting carbohydrates as analytes. The improved sensitivity of modern SPR instruments with a lower mass limit of detection below 500 Da allows the analysis of haptens as small as monosaccharides provided surfaces with theoretical R_{max} of approximately 10 RUs or more can be obtained. This approach led to the accurate determination of affinities of anti-blood group A specific antibodies which could not be obtained as monovalent preparations (Thomas et al. 2002). This study provided first evidence that amino acids not directly contacting antigen can substantially increase the affinities and thus play an important role in affinity maturation against the blood group A determinant. A comparison of monovalent vs. bivalent binding led to the determination of the affinity gain by bivalency, which for this antibody was ~75-fold. An avidity effect of the same order of magnitude was determined by SPR for the mAb Se 155-4 (MacKenzie et al. 1996).

A recent structural analysis of the tumor-specific mAb 237 in complex with a Tn-antigen containing glycopeptide from podoplanin (Brooks et al. 2010c) revealed that the antibody's exquisite specificity stems from the recognition of the terminal GalNAc residue in a small binding pocket. The mAb did not crystallize in complex with the peptide alone or with a glycopeptide carrying a GalNAc substituted with a βGal. These data indicated that only the Tn-glycopeptide is bound. This was confirmed by SPR. Immobilization of the Fab fragment at high ligand density and using an unrelated Fab fragment as control surface allowed the determination of K_D constants by steady state binding and kinetic analysis. Binding was only observed for the natural glycopeptide ($K_D \approx 140$ nM) but not for the unglycosylated peptide or free GalNAc. The lack of observable binding of free GalNAc may have been either due to its small size or the low affinity for the monovalent interaction with the carbohydrate. This could then be excluded by using a multivalent GalNAc carrying

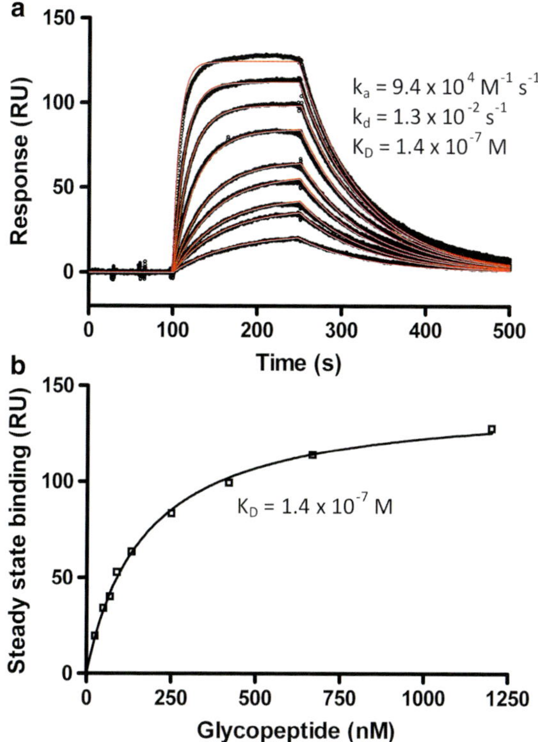

Fig. 17.3 (**a**) Surface plasmon resonance analysis of 25, 50, 70, 90, 130, 250, 420, 670 and 1,200 nM glycopeptide peptide binding to 237 mAb. The *black lines* indicate observed data points and the *red lines* fitting of the data to a 1:1 interaction model. (**b**) Fitting of the binding data to a steady state affinity model (Reprinted from (Brooks et al. 2010c), copyright 2010, with permission from the national Academy of Sciences of the United States of America)

glycoconjugate with unrelated peptide structure as analyte. The multivalency of such an interaction and the greater mass change at the sensor chip surface would have resulted in measurable binding. Since this was not the case the low affinity of the GalNAc binding pocket on the mAb 237 could be proven (Fig. 17.3).

17.4.6 Solution Affinity Analyses

The determination of K_D values from steady state binding or rate constants requires the immobilization of one binding partner. It may however not always be possible to immobilize the ligand in a suitable form or the analyte may be too small to allow for such binding assays. An alternative in such a case is the determination of the free analyte concentration in preincubated mixtures of antibody and ligand. It has been shown that under mass transport limiting conditions, i.e. slow flow-rates and high ligand density, the initial rate of complex formation is directly proportional to the free analyte concentration (Adamczyk et al. 2000). This procedure requires the generation of a standard curve by determining the maximum response at equilibrium and a given ligand density using increasing analyte concentrations. The determination of K_D values for any ligand can then be determined from the free analyte concentration present in a pre-equilibrated mixture of ligand and analyte. This assay should be applied only to monovalent analytes because an accurate correction for the fractional occupancy is not always possible (Adamczyk et al. 2000).

We have applied an adaptation of this procedure to compare affinities of antibodies against Kdo-containing oligosaccharides from *Chlamydia* (Brooks et al. 2008b). When S25-2 Fab was injected over a surface of immobilized Kdo (2→8)Kdo(2→4)Kdo–BSA in the range of 5–150 nM (Fig. 17.4a) binding proportional to the Fab concentration was observed (Fig. 17.4b). From this standard curve of free Fab concentrations (Fig. 17.4c) the solution affinity of a variety of Kdo analogues was then determined. Affinities for the *Chlamydia*-specific trisaccharide antigen Kdo(2→8)Kdo(2→4)Kdo were obtained by Fab binding to glycoconjugate (Table 17.3) and the solution affinity method (Table 17.4) and compared to those determined earlier using immobilized glycoconjugates [Tables 17.1 and 17.3, (Müller-Loennies et al. 2000)]. For this ligand all values were in a similar range showing the validity of the approach.

To characterize the epitopes of small ligands we compared mAb S54-10, a highly specific antibody for Kdo(2→4)Kdo(2→4), and S73-2, a multi-specific antibody capable of recognizing the two trisaccharide structures Kdo(2→4)Kdo(2→4) and Kdo(2→8)Kdo(2→4) with high affinity (Brooks et al. 2010b) in SPR binding assays (Figs. 17.5 and 17.6; Table 17.4). To carry out solution affinity analyses we immobilized BSA-glycoconjugates of Kdo(2→8)Kdo(2→4)Kdo and Kdo(2→4) Kdo(2→4)Kdo on CM5 sensor chips and obtained standard curves of free Fab concentrations binding to the immobilized glycoconjugates. The K_D constants determined for both antibodies by solution affinity analysis using a number of structurally related natural and artificial ligands revealed that S73-2 required the presence of the (2→4)-linkage for high affinity binding. Whereas this mAb was fully cross-reactive with the two trisaccharides, mAb S54-10 was highly specific for the Kdo(2→4)Kdo (2→4) trisaccharide (Table 17.5).

17.4.7 Epitope Mapping

Antibodies often recognize conformational epitopes within polysaccharides which are influenced by the length of the polymer and its chemical structure. Such dependencies can be resolved by SPR which has been successfully employed to map protective conformational epitopes on the type III group B streptococcal polysaccharide and group B meningococcal polysaccharide (Zou et al. 1999; MacKenzie and Jennings 2003). In addition to the identification of the protective epitope the group B streptococcal polysaccharide study further revealed that oligosaccharides with chain lengths shorter than seven oligosaccharide repeating

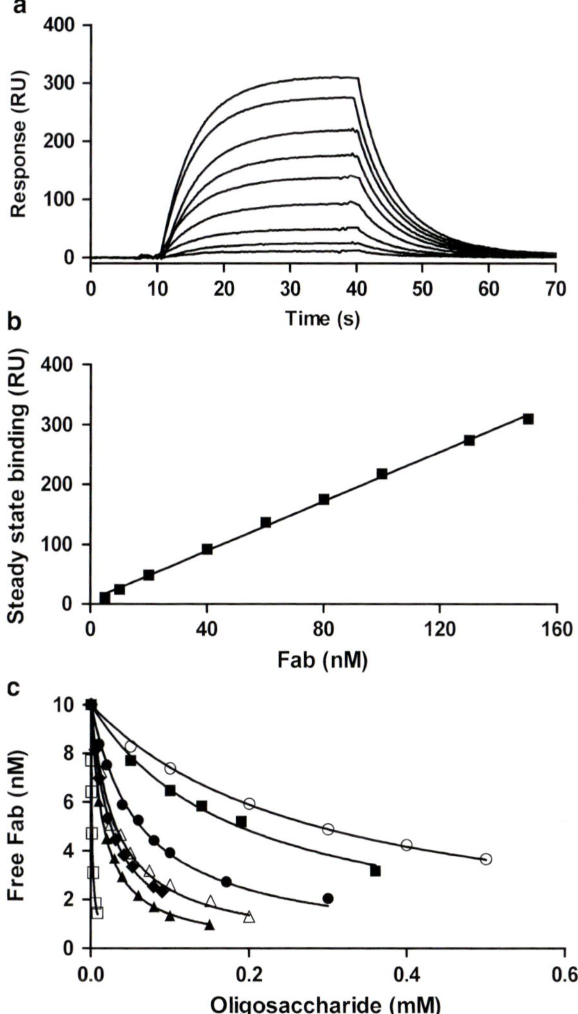

Fig. 17.4 Surface plasmon resonance analysis of S25-2 affinity for Kdo antigens. (**a**) Sensorgrams of 5, 10, 20, 40, 60, 80 and 100 nM S25-2 Fab binding to immobilized Kdo(2→8)Kdo(2→4)Kdo-BSA. (**b**) Standard curve of S25-2 Fab binding to Kdo(2→8)Kdo(2→4)Kdo-BSA used to determine free Fab concentrations for solution affinity of synthetic Kdo analogues. (**c**) Concentration of free Fab vs. concentration of synthetic Kdo analogues for determination of solution affinity. (●) Kdo(2→4)Kdo(2→4)Kdo; (■) Ko(2→4)Kdo; (♦) 3,4-dehydro-3,4,5-trideoxy-Kdo(2→8)Kdo; (▲) 5-deoxy-4-epi-2,3-dehydro-Kdo(4→8)Kdo; (Δ) Kdo(2→4)KdoC1red; (□)Kdo(2→4)Kdo(2→4)Kdo; (○)KdoC1red(2→4)Kdo (Reprinted from (Brooks et al. 2008b), copyright 2008, with permission from Elsevier Ltd.)

units displayed a single epitope while larger oligosaccharides became multivalent. This work is described in more detail in another chapter (Chap. 3, H. Jennings) in this book.

Table 17.3 Binding of S25-2 to synthetic Kdo antigens as determined by SPR (Reprinted from Brooks et al. (2008b), copyright 2008, with permission from Elsevier Ltd)

Antigen[a]	K_D ($\times 10^{-6}$ M)
Kdo	15[b]
Kdo(2→8)Kdo	1.8[b]
Kdo(2→8)Kdo(2→4)Kdo	1.4[c], 0.6[b], 1.6[d]
Kdo(2→4)Kdo	1.1[b]
Kdo(2→4)Kdo(2→4)Kdo	63[c]
Ko(2→4)Kdo	190[c]
Kdo(2→4)KdoC1red[e]	31[c]
KdoC1red(2→4)Kdo	290[c]
3,4-dehydro-3,4,5-trideoxy Kdo(2→8)Kdo	25[c]
5-deoxy-4-epi-2,3-dehydro-Kdo(4→8)Kdo	16[c]

[a]Allyl glycosides were used for solution affinity studies
[b]Determined previously using Fab and immobilized BSA glycoconjugates (Müller-Loennies et al. 2000)
[c]Solution affinity
[d]Determined using Fab and immobilized BSA glycoconjugate
[e]Carboxyl-reduced Kdo

Table 17.4 Kinetic and binding constants of S73-2 and S54-10 for immobilized glycoconjugates determined by SPR (Reprinted from Brooks et al. (2010b), copyright 2010, with permission from the American Chemical Society)

Antibody	Immobilized glycoconjugate[a]	k_a ($\times 10^6$ M^{-1} s^{-1}) $\pm$ SE	k_d (s^{-1}) $\pm$ SE	K_D ($\times 10^{-7}$ M) $\pm$ SE
S54-10	Kdo(2→4)Kdo(2→4)Kdo[b]	2 ± 0.01	0.07 ± 0.0003	0.3 ± 0.01
S73-2	Kdo(2→8)Kdo(2→4)Kdo[c]	1 ± 0.02	0.4 ± 0.03	3 ± 0.3
S73-2	Kdo(2→4)Kdo[d]	N/A[e]	N/A	2 ± 0.2

[a]BSA glycoconjugates
[b]Collected on a conjugate surface density of 280 RUs
[c]Collected on a conjugate surface density of 164 RUs
[d]Collected on a conjugate surface density of 980 RUs
[e]Dissociation rate too fast for kinetic analysis

Since the discovery of structural similarities between LPS structures among pathogenic bacteria attempts have been made to generate cross-reactive and cross-protective antibodies against enterobacterial LPS in the fight against Gram-negative sepsis (reviewed in Müller-Loennies et al. 2007). Based on the chemical characteristics structural regions are distinguished within the LPS molecule, called lipid A, the inner and outer core and the O-polysaccharide (reviewed in Holst and Müller-Loennies 2007). Potentially protective epitopes within the lipid A are cryptic in LPS molecules of pathogenic Gram-negative bacteria (Brade et al. 1997). The isolation of mAb WN1 222-5 which protects against experimental endotoxemia in animals and which is able to neutralize cellular responses also

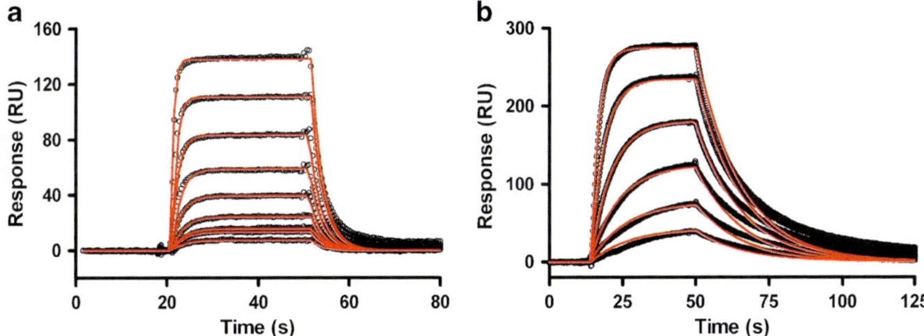

Fig. 17.5 Surface plasmon resonance analysis of S73-2 and S54-10 Fab binding to different Kdo antigens. Sensorgram overlays for the binding of (**a**) 10, 20, 40, 80, 160, 320, 640 and 1,280 nM S73-2 Fab to 160 RUs of immobilized Kdo(2→8)Kdo(2→4)Kdo-BSA and (**b**) 5, 10, 20, 40, 80 and 160 nM S54-10 Fab to 280 RUs of immobilized Kdo(2→4)Kdo(2→4)Kdo-BSA. The *open black circles* are the data points and the *red curves* the fitting of the data to a 1:1 interaction model (Reprinted from (Brooks et al. 2010b), copyright 2010, with permission from the American Chemical Society)

observed during septic shock *in vitro*, such as the release of proinflammatory cytokines, proved the presence of a protective epitope within the core region of enterobacterial LPS common to *Escherichia coli*, *Salmonella* and *Shigella* which is accessible to antibody binding (Di Padova et al. 1993). In support of ELISA binding studies using structurally characterized oligosaccharides, SPR aided in the definition of this epitope within the core region (Müller-Loennies et al. 2003). In order to identify the epitope we obtained structurally related oligosaccharides from *E. coli* J-5 (Fig. 17.7), a mutant strain synthesizing a short chain LPS, and from LPS of four *E. coli* strains synthesizing LPS molecules containing the same inner core structure but with an outer core oligosaccharide (core types R1 to R4) of varying structure without an O-polysaccharide (Fig. 17.8).

The comparison of affinities towards mAb WN1 222-5 by SPR revealed that of the smaller oligosaccharides only an octasaccharide with four phosphates (octasaccharide 4*P*) bound with high affinity (Table 17.6). Larger oligosaccharides with an attached outer core were all bound with significantly higher affinity showing a contribution of the outer core to the binding. Whereas the R1, R3, and R4 core types were bound with a similar 5-fold to 10-fold increase in affinity, the R2 core oligosaccharide was bound 29-fold stronger. This significant increase may be attributed to the substitution with an outer Gal at the first Glc residue in this core type which might be involved in the interaction with the antibody combining site. The similar increase for the structurally diverse R1, R3 and R4 core oligosaccharides have indicated an influence on the conformation of the epitope rather than a direct involvement in hydrogen bond formation with the antibody.

During the WN1 222-5 study we have observed that SPR measurements at an increased salt concentration of 300 mM NaCl yielded substantially higher affinities (0.6–25-fold) than those measured at 150 mM salt. At the lower salt concentration rate constants could not be determined at all for the smaller oligosaccharides. This could

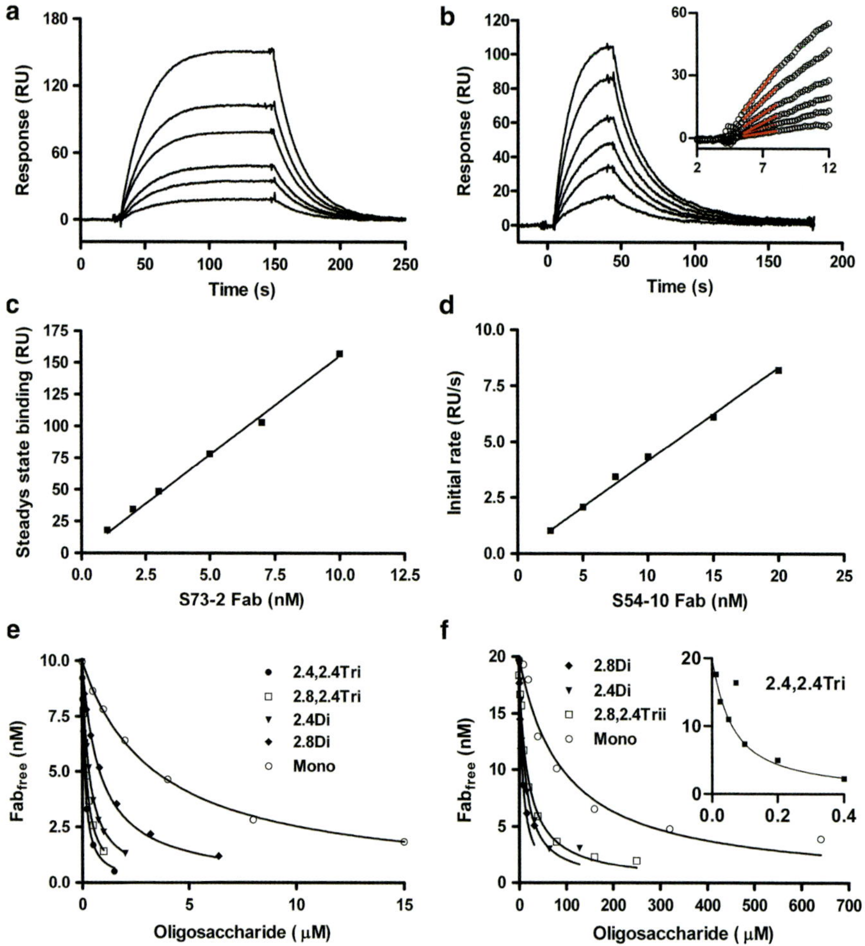

Fig. 17.6 Sensorgram overlays for the binding of (**a**) 1, 2, 3, 5, 7 and 10 nM S73-2 Fab to 2,460 RUs of immobilized Kdo(2→8)Kdo(2→4)Kdo-BSA and (**b**) 2.5, 5, 7.5, 10, 15 and 20 nM S54-10 Fab binding to immobilized Kdo(2→4)Kdo(2→4)Kdo-BSA. Standard curves for (**c**) S73-2 Fab concentration assay based on the steady state binding data from (**a** and **d**) S54-10 Fab concentration assay based on initial mass transport limited rates from the sensorgrams in (**b**) – the inset shows linear fitting (*red lines*) of the initial data points (*open black circles*). Fitting to a solution affinity model of data for the inhibition of (**e**) S73-2 Fab binding to 1,650 or 2,460 RUs of immobilized Kdo(2→8)Kdo(2→4)Kdo-BSA and (**f**) S54-10 Fab binding to 280 RUs of immobilized Kdo(2→4)Kdo(2→4)Kdo-BSA by various saccharides (Reprinted from Brooks et al. (2010b), copyright 2010, with permission from the American Chemical Society)

be explained by the high charge to mass ratio of these molecules possibly leading to an electrostatic repulsion by the sensor chip surface. Indeed, the higher affinities observed at higher salt concentration were attributable to faster on-rates, supporting this assumption. The true affinities thus remained uncertain. To resolve such problematic cases the determination of affinity by other methods is necessary. Among the

Table 17.5 Solution affinities of S73-2 and S54-10 Fab for free Kdo ligands determined by SPR (Reprinted from Brooks et al. (2010b), copyright 2010, with permission from the American Chemical Society)

Antigen	K_D (× 10^{-7} M) ± SE of mAb	
	S54-10[a]	S73-2[b]
Kdo	900 ± 100	30 ± 0.6
Kdo(2→4)Kdo	90 ± 8	3 ± 0.1
Kdo(2→8)Kdo	60 ± 6	8 ± 0.4
Kdo(2→4)Kdo(2→4)Kdo	0.5 ± 0.03	1 ± 0.05
Kdo(2→8)Kdo(2→4)Kdo	200 ± 10	2 ± 0.03

[a]Data collected using Kdo(2→4)Kdo(2→4)Kdo-BSA surface density of 280 RU
[b]Data collected using Kdo(2→8)Kdo(2→4)Kdo-BSA surface density of 1,700 and 2,400 RU

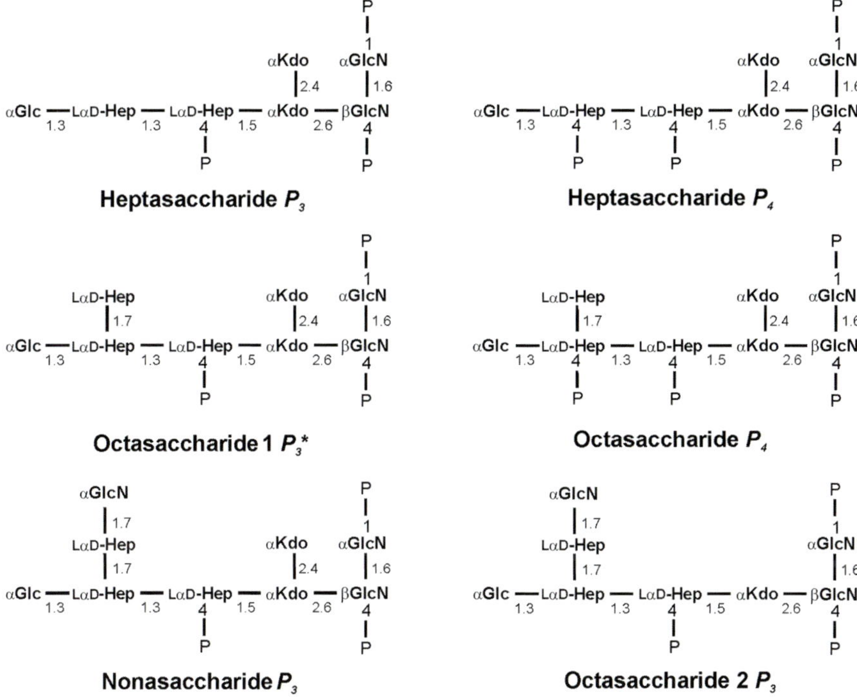

Fig. 17.7 Chemical structures of core oligosaccharides obtained after alkaline deacylation of *E. coli* J-5 LPS. The *E. coli* J-5 mutant is a derivative of *E. coli* O111:B4 which expresses a defective UDP-galactose-4-epimerase and is therefore unable to incorporate galactose into its LPS. The separation of LPS into individual molecular species is so far not possible due to the amphiphilic nature of LPS. After successive de-*O*- and de-*N*-acylation LPS oligosaccharides can be separated by HPAEC and the depicted oligosaccharides were obtained from the J-5 mutant. Octasaccharide 1 P_3, marked with an *asterisk*, was only obtained after chemical deamination of LPS before the deacylation and is not naturally present in LPS from *E. coli* J-5 (Reprinted from (Müller-Loennies et al. 2003), Copyright © 2003, with permission from the American Society for Biochemistry and Molecular Biology)

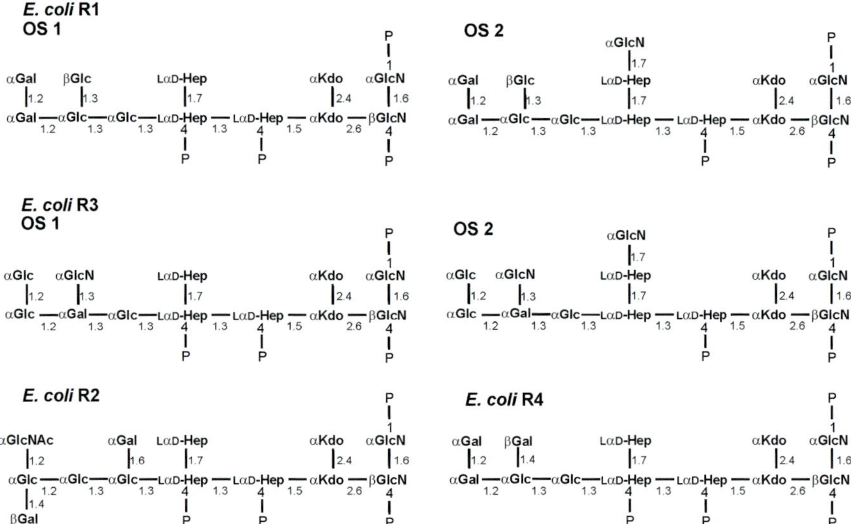

Fig. 17.8 Chemical structures of core-oligosaccharides obtained after alkaline deacylation of *E. coli* LPS. Separation of deacylated LPS from *E. coli* strains F470 (R1), F576 (R2), F653 (R3), and F2513 (R4), by HPAEC identified the depicted oligosaccharides as major components. Whereas LPS from *E. coli* F470 and F653 contain two oligosaccharides (OS 1 and 2) differing in the side chain heptose substitution with GlcN, this modification is absent in LPS of the other strains (Reprinted from (Müller-Loennies et al. 2003), Copyright © 2003, with permission from the American Society for Biochemistry and Molecular Biology)

manifold methods for affinity determination, ITC is particularly suited because label free binding can be studied in solution and it yields additional information about the energetics of the binding event. Using ITC we could confirm the general conclusions drawn from the SPR analyses and showed that the increased salt concentration used during the SPR experiment to prevent electrostatic repulsion at the negatively charged sensor chip surface did not affect complex formation. However, whereas the relative affinities were very similar the absolute affinities determined by ITC were generally higher (Müller-Loennies et al. 2003). Thus, in combination with ELISA binding data SPR analysis using LPS partial structures revealed important structural elements of an epitope at the junction of the inner and outer core in enterobacterial LPS which is accessible to high affinity antibody binding even in the presence of structurally diverse outer core oligosaccharides and O-polysaccharides.

17.5 Summary and Outlook

In this chapter we have attempted to give a brief overview of our work related to the characterization of anti-carbohydrate antibody binding to a variety of diverse ligands. In each case certain technical difficulties have been encountered and we have described appropriate solutions to these problems. We have shown that

Table 17.6 Determination of binding constants of the interaction of enterobacterial LPS oligosaccharides with WN1 222-5 at different salt concentrations and of the relative strengths of binding by SPR and ITC microcalorimetry. Reprinted from Müller-Loennies et al. (2003), Copyright © 2003 with permission from the American Society for Biochemistry and Molecular Biology

		Surface plasmon resonance							Microcalorimetry
Analyte[a]	Salt (mM)	Flow rate (μl min^{-1})	*ka* (M^{-1} s^{-1})	*kd* (s^{-1})	K_D (M)	K_D eq.[b] (M)	K_D rel. to 150 mM salt	Relative to R3[c]	K_D (M)
Heptasaccharide P_3	150				nd	nd			
	300	10	1.5e3	5.1e−2	3.3e−5	4.8e−5		0.01	
Heptasaccharide P_4	150				nd	nd			
	300	10	3.0e3	5.8e−2	2.0e−5	5.8e−5		0.02	
Octasaccharide 1 P_3	150	10	2.2e3	5.9e−2	2.7e−5	nd		0.01	
	300	40	7.7e3	2.2e−2	2.8e−6	1.9e−5	10	0.13	
Octasaccharide P_4	150				nd	nd			
	300	40	9.8e4	9.4e−2	9.5e−7	1.2e−6		0.38	
Nonasaccharide P_3	150				nd	nd			
	300	10	1.1e3	3.9e−2	3.6e−5	nd		0.01	
E. coli R1 (OS 1)	150	5	1.1e4	4.3e−2	3.9e−6	4.5e−6		0.05	
	300	40	1.6e5	2.8e−2	1.7e−7	7.0e−7	25	2.12	
E. coli R2	150	5	1.7e4	4.3e−3	2.6e−7	nd		0.81	5.5e−9
	300	40	1.4e5	4.6e−3	3.2e−8	nd	8	11.25	
E. coli $R3_{GlcN}$ (OS 2)	150	5	2.7e2	6.6e−3	2.5e−5	nd		0.01	
	300	40	6.4e2	8.6e−3	1.4e−5	nd	1.9	0.03	
E. coli R3 (OS 1)	150	5	1.6e5	3.4e−2	2.1e−7	2.4e−7		1.00	5.6e−8
	300	40	8.7e4	3.1e−2	3.6e−7	3.8e−7	0.6	1.00	
E. coli R4	150	5	1.5e4	4.7e−2	3.2e−6	3.1e−6		0.06	4.8e−8
	300	40	1.6e5	4.8e−2	2.9e−7	3.3e−7	11	1.24	7.4e−8

[a]For structures of analytes see Figs. 17.1 and 17.2; *E. coli* $R3_{GlcN}$ refers to the *E. coli* R3 core oligosaccharide (*OS*) 2 containing Glc*p*N on the side-chain heptose

[b]Determined at steady state equilibrium in SPR

[c]SPR data compared at the same salt concentration and in relation to the values obtained for oligosaccharide 1 (Fig. 17.1) from *E. coli* R3. *nd* not determined

when experimental design is carefully performed, SPR is able to contribute substantially to carbohydrate vaccine development for the induction of protective anti-carbohydrate antibodies. The identification and structural description of protective epitopes on carbohydrates represents a first step in the development process. However, as highlighted in a review by van Regenmortel (2002), antigenicity and immunogenicity are not always related and thus active immunization strategies may not be directly deduced from binding data. Nevertheless, the development of passive immunization strategies is straightforward. We have shown how binding data acquired by SPR in combination with structural analyses and molecular biology can contribute to the identification of molecular mechanisms underlying affinity maturation of antibodies, the kinetic effects associated with multivalent binding and the identification of anti-carbohydrate antibodies which can be used as diagnostic tools in the identification of bacterial pathogens such as *Chlamydia*.

The technical difficulties often encountered in obtaining accurate K_D values for carbohydrate-protein interactions due to low affinities and multivalency have been partly overcome by the introduction of SPR as a routine technology requiring relatively little amounts of substance. Prior to the introduction of SPR instruments, isothermal titration microcalorimetry (ITC) had been widely used to study carbohydrate-protein interactions (Christensen and Toone 2003). A major drawback of ITC, preventing its use as a routine technology, has been its low sensitivity in comparison to other methods putting a high demand on the amount of substance needed, usually several milligrams of purified protein per single experiment. The recent marketing of instruments with higher sensitivity has improved the situation considerably and the collection of thermodynamic data may become more routine and in combination with SPR will certainly help to resolve important fundamental questions associated with carbohydrate-protein interactions. However, as has been seen after the introduction of SPR biosensors, neglecting technical and theoretical requirements of proper experimental design, data collection and, last but not least, data analysis may prevent the acquisition of high-quality data. In order to really contribute to a better understanding of carbohydrate-protein binding utmost care must be taken to assure the generation of high quality data instead of purely a large body of data. If this premise will be widely accepted, both methods will surely contribute to a better scientific understanding of carbohydrate recognition by antibodies and hopefully the development of new antibody drugs and improved vaccines against infectious and non-infectious diseases such as cancer.

References

Adamczyk M, Moore JA, Yu Z (2000) Application of surface plasmon resonance toward studies of low-molecular-weight antigen-antibody binding interactions. Methods 20:319–328

Aggarwal S (2010) What's fueling the biotech engine-2009–2010. Nat Biotechnol 28:1165–1171

Astronomo RD, Burton DR (2010) Carbohydrate vaccines: developing sweet solutions to sticky situations? Nat Rev Drug Discov 9:308–324

Blackler RJ, Müller-Loennies S, Brooks CL, Evans DW, Brade L, Kosma P, Brade H, Evans SV (2011) A common NH53K mutation in the combining site of antibodies raised against chlamydial LPS glycoconjugates significantly increases avidity. Biochemistry 50:3357–3368

Brade H (1999) Chlamydial lipopolysaccharide. In: Brade H, Opal SM, Vogel SN, Morrison DC (eds) Endotoxin in health and disease. Marcel Dekker, New York/Basel, pp 229–242

Brade L, Holst O, Brade H (1993) An artificial glycoconjugate containing the bisphosphorylated glucosamine disaccharide backbone of lipid A binds lipid A monoclonal antibodies. Infect Immun 61:4514–4517

Brade L, Engel R, Christ WJ, Rietschel ET (1997) A nonsubstituted primary hydroxyl group in position 6′ of free lipid A is required for binding of lipid A monoclonal antibodies. Infect Immun 65:3961–3965

Brooks CL, Blackler RJ, Gerstenbruch S, Kosma P, Müller-Loennies S, Brade H, Evans SV (2008a) Pseudo-symmetry and twinning in crystals of homologous antibody Fv fragments. Acta Crystallogr D Biol Crystallogr 64:1250–1258

Brooks CL, Müller-Loennies S, Brade L, Kosma P, Hirama T, MacKenzie CR, Brade H, Evans SV (2008b) Exploration of specificity in germline monoclonal antibody recognition of a range of natural and synthetic epitopes. J Mol Biol 377:450–468

Brooks CL, Blackler RJ, Sixta G, Kosma P, Müller-Loennies S, Brade L, Hirama T, MacKenzie CR, Brade H, Evans SV (2010a) The role of CDR H3 in antibody recognition of a synthetic analog of a lipopolysaccharide antigen. Glycobiology 20:138–147

Brooks CL, Müller-Loennies S, Borisova SN, Brade L, Kosma P, Hirama T, MacKenzie CR, Brade H, Evans SV (2010b) Antibodies raised against chlamydial lipopolysaccharide antigens reveal convergence in germline gene usage and differential epitope recognition. Biochemistry 49:570–581

Brooks CL, Schietinger A, Borisova SN, Kufer P, Okon M, Hirama T, MacKenzie CR, Wang LX, Schreiber H, Evans SV (2010c) Antibody recognition of a unique tumor-specific glycopeptide antigen. Proc Natl Acad Sci U S A 107:10056–10061

Bundle DR, Young NM (1992) Carbohydrate-protein interactions in antibodies and lectins. Curr Opin Struct Biol 2:666–673

Calarese DA, Scanlan CN, Zwick MB, Deechongkit S, Mimura Y, Kunert R, Zhu P, Wormald MR, Stanfield RL, Roux KH, Kelly JW, Rudd PM, Dwek RA, Katinger H, Burton DR, Wilson IA (2003) Antibody domain exchange is an immunological solution to carbohydrate cluster recognition. Science 300:2065–2071

Carver JP (1993) Oligosaccharides: how can flexible molecules act as signals? Pure Appl Chem 65:763–770

Christensen T, Toone EJ (2003) Calorimetric evaluation of protein-carbohydrate affinities. Methods Enzymol 362:486–504

Cygler M, Rose DR, Bundle DR (1991) Recognition of a cell-surface oligosaccharide of pathogenic *Salmonella* by an antibody Fab fragment. Science 253:442–445

Di Padova FE, Brade H, Barclay GR, Poxton IR, Liehl E, Schuetze E, Kocher HP, Ramsay G, Schreier MH, McClelland DB, Rietschel ETh (1993) A broadly cross-protective monoclonal antibody binding to *Escherichia coli* and *Salmonella* lipopolysaccharides. Infect Immun 61: 3863–3872

Englebienne P, van Hoonacker A, Verhas M (2003) Surface plasmon resonance: principles, methods and applications in biomedical sciences. Spectroscopy 17:255–273

Evans DW, Müller-Loennies S, Brooks CL, Brade L, Kosma P, Brade H, Evans SV (2011) Structural insights into parallel strategies for germline antibody recognition of LPS from *Chlamydia*. Glycobiology 21:1049–1059

Farrugia W, Scott AM, Ramsland PA (2009) A possible role for metallic ions in the carbohydrate cluster recognition displayed by a Lewis Y specific antibody. PLoS One 4(11):e7777

Foote J, Eisen HN (2000) Breaking the affinity ceiling for antibodies and T cell receptors. Proc Natl Acad Sci U S A 97:10679–10681

Gerstenbruch S, Brooks CL, Kosma P, Brade L, MacKenzie CR, Evans SV, Brade H, Müller-Loennies S (2010) Analysis of cross-reactive and specific anti-carbohydrate antibodies against lipopolysaccharide from *Chlamydophila psittaci*. Glycobiology 20:461–472

Harrison BA, MacKenzie R, Hirama T, Lee KK, Altman E (1998) A kinetics approach to the characterization of an IgM specific for the glycolipid asialo-GM1. J Immunol Methods 212: 29–39

Holst O, Müller-Loennies S (2007) Microbial polysaccharide structures. In: Kamerling JP, Boons GJ, Lee Y, Suzuki A, Taniguchi N, Voragen AG (eds) Comprehensive glycoscience. Elsevier, New York, pp 123–179

Homans SW (2007) Dynamics and thermodynamics of ligand-protein interactions. Top Curr Chem 272:51–82

Kalergis AM, Boucheron N, Doucey MA, Palmieri E, Goyarts EC, Vegh Z, Luescher IF, Nathenson SG (2001) Efficient T cell activation requires an optimal dwell-time of interaction between the TCR and the pMHC complex. Nat Immunol 2:229–234

Karlsson R (2004) SPR for molecular interaction analysis: a review of emerging application areas. J Mol Recognit 17:151–161

Karlsson R, Fält A (1997) Experimental design for kinetic analysis of protein-protein interactions with surface plasmon resonance biosensors. J Immunol Methods 200:121–133

MacKenzie CR, Hirama T, Deng SJ, Bundle DR, Narang SA, Young NM (1996) Analysis by surface plasmon resonance of the influence of valence on the ligand binding affinity and kinetics of an anti-carbohydrate antibody. J Biol Chem 271:1527–1533

MacKenzie CR, Jennings HJ (2003) Characterization of polysaccharide conformational epitopes by surface plasmon resonance. Methods Enzymol 363:340–354

Malissen B (2001) Les liaisons dangereuses. Nat Immunol 2:196–198

Müller-Loennies S, MacKenzie CR, Patenaude SI, Evans SV, Kosma P, Brade H, Brade L, Narang S (2000) Characterization of high affinity monoclonal antibodies specific for chlamydial lipopolysaccharide. Glycobiology 10:121–130

Müller-Loennies S, Brade L, MacKenzie CR, Di Padova FE, Brade H (2003) Identification of a cross-reactive epitope widely present in lipopolysaccharide from enterobacteria and recognized by the cross-protective monoclonal antibody WN1 222-5. J Biol Chem 278: 25618–25627

Müller-Loennies S, Gronow S, Brade L, MacKenzie R, Kosma P, Brade H (2006) A monoclonal antibody against a carbohydrate epitope in lipopolysaccharide differentiates *Chlamydophila psittaci* from *Chlamydophila pecorum*, *Chlamydophila pneumoniae*, and *Chlamydia trachomatis*. Glycobiology 16:184–196

Müller-Loennies S, Brade L, Brade H (2007) Neutralizing and cross-reactive antibodies against enterobacterial lipopolysaccharide. Int J Med Microbiol 297:321–340

Murthy BN, Sinha S, Surolia A, Indi SS, Jayaraman N (2008) SPR and ITC determination of the kinetics and the thermodynamics of bivalent versus monovalent sugar ligand-lectin interactions. Glycoconj J 25:313–321

Nguyen HP, Seto NO, MacKenzie CR, Brade L, Kosma P, Brade H, Evans SV (2003) Germline antibody recognition of distinct carbohydrate epitopes. Nat Struct Biol 10:1019–1025

O'Shannessy DJ (1994) Determination of kinetic rate and equilibrium binding constants for macromolecular interactions: a critique of the surface plasmon resonance literature. Curr Opin Biotechnol 5:65–71

Ramsland PA, Farrugia W, Bradford TM, Mark HP, Scott AM (2004) Structural convergence of antibody binding of carbohydrate determinants in Lewis Y tumor antigens. J Mol Biol 340: 809–818

Rich RL, Myszka DG (2010) Grading the commercial optical biosensor literature-Class of 2008: 'The Mighty Binders'. J Mol Recognit 23:1–64

Schietinger A, Philip M, Schreiber H (2008) Specificity in cancer immunotherapy. Semin Immunol 20:276–285

Thomas R, Patenaude SI, MacKenzie CR, To R, Hirama T, Young NM, Evans SV (2002) Structure of an anti-blood group A Fv and improvement of its binding affinity without loss of specificity. J Biol Chem 277:2059–2064

Toone EJ (1994) Structure and energetics of protein-carbohydrate complexes. Curr Opin Struct Biol 4:719–728

Van Regenmortel MHV (2002) Reductionism and the search for structure-function relationships in antibody molecules. J Mol Recognit 15:240–247

Van Roon AM, Pannu NS, de Vrind JP, van der Marel GA, van Boom JH, Hokke CH, Deelder AM, Abrahams JP (2004) Structure of an anti-Lewis X Fab fragment in complex with its Lewis X antigen. Structure 12:1227–1236

Villeneuve S, Souchon H, Riottot MM, Mazie JC, Lei P, Glaudemans CP, Kovac P, Fournier JM, Alzari PM (2000) Crystal structure of an anti-carbohydrate antibody directed against *Vibrio cholerae* O1 in complex with antigen: molecular basis for serotype specificity. Proc Natl Acad Sci U S A 97:8433–8438

Vulliez-Le Normand B, Saul FA, Phalipon A, Belot F, Guerreiro C, Mulard LA, Bentley GA (2008) Structures of synthetic O-antigen fragments from serotype 2a *Shigella flexneri* in complex with a protective monoclonal antibody. Proc Natl Acad Sci U S A 105:9976–9981

Vyas NK, Vyas MN, Chervenak MC, Bundle DR, Pinto BM, Quiocho FA (2003) Structural basis of peptide-carbohydrate mimicry in an antibody-combining site. Proc Natl Acad Sci USA 100:15023–15028

Zou W, Mackenzie R, Therien L, Hirama T, Yang Q, Gidney MA, Jennings HJ (1999) Conformational epitope of the type III group B *Streptococcus* capsular polysaccharide. J Immunol 163:820–825

Index

P. Kosma and S. Müller-Loennies (eds.), *Anticarbohydrate Antibodies*, DOI 10.1007/978-3-7091-0870-3, © Springer-Verlag/Wien 2012

M

W

X

Printing: Ten Brink, Meppel, The Netherlands
Binding: Stürtz, Würzburg, Germany